MEDICAL PHARMACOLOGY

PRINCIPLES AND CONCEPTS

SEVENTH EDITION

MEDICAL PHARMACOLOGY

PRINCIPLES AND CONCEPTS

ANDRES GOTH, M.D.

Professor of Pharmacology and Chairman of the Department,
The University of Texas Southwestern Medical School,
Dallas, Texas

with 107 illustrations

THE C. V. MOSBY COMPANY

Saint Louis   1974

SEVENTH EDITION

Copyright © 1974 by The C. V. Mosby Company

All rights reserved. No part of this book may be reproduced in any manner without written permission of the publisher.

Previous editions copyrighted 1961, 1964, 1966, 1968, 1970, 1972

Printed in the United States of America

Distributed in Great Britain by Henry Kimpton, London

Library of Congress Cataloging in Publication Data

Goth, Andres.
  Medical pharmacology.

  1. Pharmacology. I. Title.
[DNLM: 1. Pharmacology. QV4 G684m 1974]
RM300.G65 1974   615′.7   73-20083
ISBN 0-8016-1946-7

TS/CB/B 9 8 7 6 5 4 3

PREFACE

THE SEVENTH EDITION of *Medical Pharmacology* attempts to present current information on drugs that is important and useful for rational therapeutics. The emphasis is on principles and concepts rather than on isolated facts. At the same time sufficient factual information is provided for the practical needs of students and health professionals.

The new edition differs from the previous ones in several respects. A new chapter on drug effects on the respiratory tract has been added, the chapters on digitalis and antiarrhythmic drugs have been completely rewritten, and practically all chapters have been thoroughly updated. With the increasing interest in drug-receptor interactions, several discussions in the new edition have been expanded. For example, the effects of histamine on H_1 and H_2 receptors and the opposing effects of specific antagonists are brought up to date. Also more space is devoted to drugs acting on β-adrenergic receptors, both agonists and antagonists. Factual material is presented increasingly in tabular form, particularly in the chemotherapy chapters. A number of problems are interspersed in the text, largely for the purpose of mental stimulation. These problems often give a reference to the current literature, which may stimulate the reader to go more deeply into the subject.

I am grateful for the many constructive criticisms received from experts in many fields. I generally tried to satisfy these experts, although they should recognize that this book is not aimed at those who are at the forefront of their research areas. With the availability of excellent reviews in almost every field, I felt that I could limit myself to making the reader aware of the forefronts of research as long as references to good reviews and original articles were provided.

Members of the Department of Pharmacology and some other departments of The University of Texas Southwestern Medical School have been very helpful in the preparation of this new edition. I am grateful to them and to the secretarial and technical staff as well. I am especially grateful to Dr. Gregory G. Dimijian for updating his chapter on drug abuse. The response of students and practitioners to previous editions has been very gratifying, and it is my hope that the seventh edition will also be useful to the various readers.

Andres Goth

CONTENTS

SECTION SEVEN

DRUG EFFECTS ON THE RESPIRATORY AND GASTROINTESTINAL TRACTS

SECTION EIGHT

DRUGS THAT INFLUENCE METABOLIC AND ENDOCRINE FUNCTIONS

SECTION NINE

CHEMOTHERAPY

Contents

SECTION TEN
PRINCIPLES OF IMMUNOPHARMACOLOGY

SECTION ELEVEN
POISONS AND ANTIDOTES

SECTION TWELVE
DRUG INTERACTIONS

SECTION THIRTEEN
PRESCRIPTION WRITING AND DRUG COMPENDIA

APPENDIX

MEDICAL PHARMACOLOGY

PRINCIPLES AND CONCEPTS

1 Introduction

Chemical agents not only provide the structural basis and energy supply of living organisms but also regulate their functional activities. The interactions between potent chemicals and living systems contribute to the understanding of life processes and in addition provide effective methods for the treatment, prevention, and diagnosis of many diseases. Chemical compounds used for these purposes are *drugs*, and their actions on living systems are referred to as *drug effects*.

Pharmacology deals with the properties and effects of drugs or, in a more general sense, with the interactions of chemical compounds and living systems. It is a discipline of biology and is closely related to other disciplines, particularly to physiology and biochemistry.

Despite the considerable overlap among the various disciplines of biology, pharmacology is unique in dealing primarily with the mechanisms of action of biologically active substances.

Although the specific aim of pharmacology is to define the biologic activity of chemical compounds, it also contributes greatly to knowledge of living systems. This contribution to the understanding of life processes is valuable to biologic sciences in general and to medicine in particular. An understanding of drugs is necessary for the diagnosis, prevention, and treatment of disease. Some aspects of pharmacology are of remote relevance to the study of medicine. To emphasize this distinction, the title *Medical Pharmacology* was chosen for this book.

SUBDIVISIONS OF PHARMACOLOGY AND RELATED DISCIPLINES

There are several fields of study that may be considered subdivisions of pharmacology or disciplines related to it.

Pharmacodynamics is the study of drug effects and the handling of drugs by the body. This aspect of pharmacology is perhaps the nearest to a basic science of medicine.

Emphasis on mode of action of chemical compounds distinguishes pharmacology from some of the other basic sciences of medicine. As used in medicine, the term *pharmacology* is essentially synonymous with pharmacodynamics.

Chemotherapy is that subdivision of pharmacology which, according to the definition first proposed by Paul Ehrlich, deals with drugs that are capable of destroying invading organisms without destroying the host.

Pharmacy is concerned with the preparation and dispensing of drugs. Today the physician seldom has the need to prepare or dispense his own drugs. Even the pharmacist has very little to do with the preparation of drugs, most of them being manufactured by large companies. The pharmacist may provide useful services, however, as a member of the health team having special knowledge about drug preparations.

1

Therapeutics is the art of treatment of disease. *Pharmacotherapeutics* is the application of drugs in the treatment of disease.

Toxicology is the science of poisons and poisonings. Although toxicology may be viewed as a special aspect of pharmacology, it developed into a separate discipline for a variety of reasons. Forensic and environmental medicine requires the services and knowledge of toxicologists with special training in drug identification and poison control.

HISTORICAL DEVELOPMENT OF PHARMACOLOGY

Although no detailed discussion will be attempted, it should be pointed out that the history of pharmacology can be divided into two periods. The early period goes back to antiquity and is characterized by empirical observations in the use of crude drugs. It is interesting that even primitive people could discover relationships between drugs and disease. The use of drugs has been so prevalent throughout history that Sir William Osler stated (1894) with some justification that "man has an inborn craving for medicine."

In contrast to this ancient period, modern pharmacology is based on experimental investigations concerning the site and mode of action of drugs. The application of the scientific method to studies on drugs was initiated in France by François Magendie and was expanded by Claude Bernard (1813–1878). The name of Oswald Schmiedeberg (1838–1921) is commonly associated with the development of experimental pharmacology in Germany, and John Jacob Abel (1857–1938) played a similar role in the United States.

The growth of pharmacology was greatly stimulated by the rise of synthetic organic chemistry, which provided new tools and new therapeutic agents. More recently, pharmacology has benefited from developments of other basic sciences and in turn has contributed to their growth.

Some of the greatest changes in medicine that have occurred during the last few decades are directly attributable to the discovery of new drugs. Progress in this field has not been without its problems, however. Success in the search for new therapeutic agents has not been matched by equal expertise in the evaluation of their clinical safety and efficacy. Furthermore, the practicing physician has not always been prepared for some of the new drugs whose clinical use requires considerable understanding of basic principles. Nevertheless, in the recent history of pharmacology the many successes more than make up for the problems created by drugs.

PLACE OF PHARMACOLOGY IN MEDICINE

There are several reasons for considering pharmacology one of the increasingly important basic sciences of medicine. Some of these are obvious; others are not yet generally recognized.

Large numbers of drugs are used in the practice of medicine. They cannot be applied intelligently or even safely without some understanding of their mode of action, side effects, toxicity, and metabolism. As powerful new drugs are introduced, the necessity of adequate pharmacologic knowledge on the part of the physician becomes increasingly mandatory. Pharmacologic terms and concepts are used so commonly in the clinical journals that a physician without a good grounding in the subject would find it difficult to read and understand the current medical literature.

Pharmacology is taught in medical schools for other reasons. As a basic science it contributes important concepts to the understanding of various functions in health and disease. In research, drugs are used increasingly as chemical tools for elucidating basic mechanisms. Also, drugs are being utilized more frequently for diagnostic purposes.

Pharmacology is also important in medicine because of the commercial influences that are exerted upon the physician in his selection of drugs. A good understanding of the principles of pharmacology should provide the physician with a critical attitude and the ability to evaluate rationally the claims made for various new drug preparations.

Finally, it is increasingly recognized that many functions of the body are controlled by endogenously produced chemical compounds. In addition to the hormonal agents synthesized by endocrine glands, other endogenous compounds exert regulatory effects on body functions. There is now little doubt that acetylcholine and norepinephrine represent such autoregulator drugs. There are probably many others. It is quite likely that such potent agents as histamine, serotonin (5-hydroxytryptamine), heparin, and kinins may act as endogenous regulators of various functions.

Many pharmacologic agents mimic or oppose the actions of these "local hormones" or else affect their binding or metabolism. The recognition that many body functions are normally regulated by drug action has interesting implications. When viewed in this light, pharmacology is not simply the experimental basis of drug therapy but is a basic science of medicine whose tools are highly active chemical compounds by which physiologic and biochemical processes can be influenced.

Problem 1-1. In view of the importance of pharmacology for the practice of medicine, why is not more time given to it by most curriculum committees? The answer seems to lie in the interdisciplinary nature of the subject and in tradition. Because of its interdisciplinary nature, many areas of pharmacology could be taught in other courses. On the other hand, as has been pointed out by the Nobel Laureate Carl Cori,[1] information on drugs can be taught by experts in various disciplines, but an organized course outside a medical school pharmacology department is difficult.

Tradition is an obstacle to the adequate teaching of pharmacology. It is believed by many medical educators that students will learn about drugs "later," perhaps in residency training or as they pick up information when they need it in their practice. Many critical physicians will admit, however, that what they pick up "later" is some practical information essential for therapeutics but not much basic knowledge of pharmacology, which is often badly needed.

CLINICAL PHARMACOLOGY

Although pharmacology is concerned with drug effects in all species of animals, in medicine there is increasing interest in clinical pharmacology, which concerns itself with pharmacologic effects in man.

There are many reasons for this increasing interest. Results of pharmacologic studies on animals sometimes cannot be applied to human beings because of species variations in the response to the drug or in its metabolism. Clinical pharmacology also provides scientific methods for the determination of usefulness, potency, and toxicity of new drugs in man himself. This is of great practical importance these days when the efficacy and safety of drugs are being reassessed.

Pharmacologic knowledge essential for good medical practice includes not only the findings of clinical pharmacology but also those principles and concepts generally derived from animal experiments, which are necessary for thorough understanding of drug effects. Without these principles and concepts, rational therapeutics is impossible.

Reference

1 Cori, C. C.: The call of science, Ann. Rev. Biochem. **38**:1, 1969.

SECTION ONE

GENERAL ASPECTS OF PHARMACOLOGY

2 Basic mechanisms of drug action

Most drugs differ from inert chemicals or foods in their potency, selectivity, and structural specificity. Digitoxin, reserpine, atropine, LSD, and penicillin are a few examples of potent, selective, and structurally specific compounds. A few milligrams of these drugs can alter normal or pathologic physiology or, as in the case of penicillin, can rid the body of invading microorganisms.

Potency immediately suggests an interaction with a biologic control system; selectivity points to a favored localization, or affinity, for some site of action. Finally, structural specificity brings to mind an interaction of the drug with some cellular constituent that is *complementary* to it in three-dimensional space.

Much of experimental pharmacology suggests that these suppositions are correct. Although the point is seemingly academic, an understanding of current views on the basic mechanisms of drug action should promote a way of thinking about drugs that will favor their correct use in therapeutics.

SITES OF DRUG ACTION ON BIOLOGIC SYSTEMS

The specificity of most drug actions suggests a bond formation, generally reversible, between the drug and some cellular constituent. This cellular constituent is generally referred to as the *receptor*.

The *receptor concept* (recently reviewed by Albert) was first proposed by Langley in 1878[6] and was used extensively by Paul Ehrlich in his studies on chemotherapy. Investigating the opposing actions of pilocarpine and atropine on salivary secretion, Langley hypothesized the presence of some substance in the nerve endings or glands, with which the drugs may combine. To Ehrlich, receptors were groups of protoplasmic macromolecules with which drugs could combine *reversibly* or *irreversibly*. Thus, for arsenicals the mercapto group would be a receptor, although covalent bond formation is not a common drug-receptor interaction. Ehrlich recognized that many potent drugs can be removed easily from tissues and must therefore form *reversible* combinations with receptors.

According to current concepts[15] drug-receptor interactions may be of the following types:

1. Drugs may inhibit enzymes.
2. Some steroid hormones may act by de-repressing a length of inactive DNA, leading to the synthesis of new proteins.
3. Drugs may act as coenzymes. Epinephrine acts on adenyl cyclase, catalyzing the formation of cyclic adenylic acid (3',5'-AMP).
4. Drugs may alter the permeability characteristics of cell membranes by interacting with permeases or carrier mechanisms.

Drug effects are often attributed to a primary interaction with enzymes on the basis of insufficient evidence. Inhibition of an enzyme by a drug in the test tube can be misleading. Its effect in the body may depend upon an entirely different action. Nevertheless, in a few cases drug effects undoubtedly are a result of enzymatic action. The anticholinesterases such as physostigmine or the organophosphorus compounds, the carbonic anhydrase inhibitors such as acetazolamide (Diamox), and the monoamine oxidase inhibitors such as iproniazid exert many pharmacologic effects as a consequence of enzyme inhibition. Also, disulfiram (Antabuse) causes severe effects in a person who drinks alcohol because it blocks the enzyme that catalyzes the oxidation of acetaldehyde, a toxic product of alcohol degradation. The antimetabolites, of great interest in chemotherapy of infections and cancer, compete with normal metabolites for an enzyme.

QUANTITATIVE ASPECTS OF DRUG POTENCY AND EFFICACY

A drug is said to be potent when it has great biologic activity per unit weight. When the dose of a drug is plotted on a logarithmic scale against a measured effect, a sigmoid curve is obtained, usually referred to as a log *dose-response* curve. Any point on such a curve could indicate the potency of a drug, but for comparative purposes, the dose that gives 50% of the total or maximal effect is most often selected. This dose is the ED_{50}, or effective dose$_{50}$. In Fig. 2-1, drugs A and B produced parallel dose-response curves. The ED_{50} of drug B may be ten times greater than that of drug A. As a consequence, it may be said that drug A is ten times as potent as drug B. *It is essential to realize that potencies are compared on the basis of doses that produce the same effect and not by comparing the magnitudes of effects elicited by the same dose.*

A clinically important example of a potency relationship very similar to that given in Fig. 2-1, *A*, is given by the diuretic drugs chlorothiazide and hydrochlorothiazide. One hundred milligrams of hydrochlorothiazide given orally to a patient promotes a significant increase in the urinary output of sodium chloride. It takes about 1 Gm. of chlorothiazide to achieve the same effect. As a consequence, one may say that hydrochlorothiazide is ten times as potent as chlorothiazide.

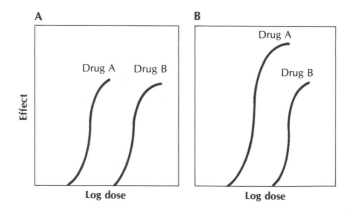

Fig. 2-1. Log dose-response curves illustrating the difference between potency and efficacy. **A,** Drug A is much more potent than drug B, but both have the same maximal effect. **B,** Drug A is not only more potent but has a greater efficacy. It produces a higher peak effect than drug B.

Fig. 2-1, *B*, illustrates another property of a drug that should not be confused with potency. Drug A is not only ten times as potent as drug B but it also has a higher maximum or "ceiling" of activity. The maximum effect is commonly referred to as efficacy, or power, and is illustrated by the following example.

Chlorothiazide as well as hydrochlorothiazide has a definite "ceiling" of activity. Two grams of chlorothiazide will exert its maximal effect on salt excretion, and further increases in dosage will not result in a greater effect. Furosemide, however, has not only greater potency than chlorothiazide but also a higher ceiling. It can cause the excretion of a larger percentage of the total amount of sodium chloride filtered by the glomeruli. Consequently, furosemide not only is more *potent* than chlorothiazide but also has greater *efficacy*, or power.

Potency and efficacy are often confused in medical terminology. Potency alone is an overrated advantage in therapeutics. If drug A is ten times as potent as drug B but has no other virtues, this means only that the patient will take smaller tablets. Pharmaceutical companies often emphasize that a drug is more potent than some other drug. This in itself has very little importance to the physician. On the other hand, if the drug has a greater efficacy, it may accomplish things that are unattainable with a less efficacious compound.

SELECTIVITY

It is a truism in pharmacology that there is no drug with a single action. Nevertheless, it is quite remarkable how selective many of our drugs are. In fact, one of the aims of pharmacology is to provide highly selective therapeutic agents. What is the basis of the selective action of drugs?

When a drug has a much greater effect on some structures than others, one obvious explanation might be that it tends to concentrate in such structures. This simple explanation holds true in only a few cases. For example, the mercurial diuretics tend to concentrate in the renal tubules and exert a diuretic activity at relatively low doses. In the majority of cases, however, selectivity cannot be shown to depend on a special localization of the drug. The affinity for a site of action may be similar to the affinity of dyes for certain materials and not others,[14] the selective permeability of some membranes (this would lead to changes in concentration at subcellular sites), or the existence of specific combining sites in or on the susceptible cells—the *receptors*.

A good example of selectivity due to specific receptors is the effect of acetylcholine on the motor end plate. The direct application of the drug to the end plate results in the production of an action potential. The end plate is so susceptible to the drug that 10^{-15} moles or less will produce a response. At the same time, acetylcholine has no effect when applied to the muscle at a distance from the end plate.[5] It is reasonable to postulate that the end plate must have some combining sites for acetylcholine that the rest of the muscle does not have. This postulate is greatly reinforced by the fact that these sites (receptors) can be blocked by specific antagonists such as *d*-tubocurarine that compete with acetylcholine for the receptor site.

STRUCTURAL SPECIFICITY

The action of most drugs is greatly influenced by slight structural modifications. Furthermore, alterations of structure can cause not only a change in potency but also the formation of compounds that *inhibit* the action of the parent drug. The dependence of drug action on a three-dimensional structure is well illustrated by the greatly differing potencies of stereoisomers. *d*-Amphetamine (Dexedrine) has a greater stimulant effect than *l*-amphetamine (or racemic amphetamine sulfate, Benzedrine). Structural specificity provides evidence that drugs interact with a configurational site, or *receptor*, analogous to the active site of an enzyme.

There is reason to believe, however, that not all drugs act on specific receptors. Some drugs probably distribute themselves in an important phase in or on the surface of the cell and interfere with some function or metabolic process. This nonspecific drug effect differs in many respects from the previously discussed drug actions. The biologic activity of anesthetics, hypnotics, volatile insecticides, and some other drugs depends not on drug-receptor interactions but on the *relative saturation* at some cellular phase (Ferguson's principle).[3] Whenever compounds that are chemically widely different give the same effect when their "thermodynamic activity" is similar, the drugs may be assumed to have a nonspecific or physical type of activity or toxicity. Thermodynamic activity is approximately equal to S_t/S_o, where S_t is the concentration necessary to give a biologic effect and S_o is the solubility of the drug.

In simple terms, if drugs produce the same effect at the same relative saturation, they are not likely to act on specific receptors. It is more probable that by reaching a certain level of saturation at some cellular site (the so-called biophase) they hinder some metabolic function.[3]

DRUG-RECEPTOR INTERACTIONS AS THE MOLECULAR BASIS OF SPECIFIC DRUG ACTION

Receptor theory

As early as 1878 the inhibitory effects of atropine on the actions of pilocarpine were interpreted by Langley[6] as a competition for some "receptive substance." The concept of receptors as a cellular combining site for drugs was effectively used by Ehrlich (see Mautner[21] for details). Mathematical formulations of drug-receptor interactions were postulated by many workers, but especially by Clark,[1] Ariëns,[16] Schild,[12] Stephenson,[13] and Paton.[8]

It has been suggested by Clark[1] that drug-receptor interactions are analogous to adsorption and that drug effect is proportional to drug-receptor combinations. In an extension of this concept and by analogy with enzyme-substrate interactions, it was postulated by Ariëns[16] that

$$[A] + [R] \underset{k_2}{\overset{k_1}{\rightleftharpoons}} AR \xrightarrow{k_3} \text{Response} + [A] + [R]$$

where [A] = agonist, a drug with stimulant properties; [R] = concentration of free receptors; and [AR] = concentration of drug-receptor complex.

As in the formulation by Michaelis and Menten,[7] when the velocity of an enzyme reaction is proportional to the concentration of enzyme-substrate complex, drug effect is proportional to drug-receptor concentration, or [AR].

The varying potencies of members of a homologous series were explained by varying *affinities* of the drugs for the receptor, affinity being the reciprocal of the dissociation constant $(1/K_A)$ of the drug-receptor combination.

Intrinsic activity

Further work has shown, however, that when the potencies of members of a homologous series are compared, in the case of the weaker members not only is the log dose-response curve shifted to the right but the maximum also becomes lower. Because of this finding, it seemed reasonable to postulate that the response was not only dependent on the concentration of drug-receptor complex but also on what is termed *intrinsic activity*,[16] or *efficacy*.[13] Numerically, response $= \alpha RA$, where α is a proportionality constant that determines activity per unit of drug-receptor complex.

Assuming that for a given response a drug occupies only a fraction of the total receptor pool, *efficacy* may be defined as the capacity to stimulate for a given occupancy.[13]

GRAPHIC PRESENTATION OF AFFINITY, INTRINSIC ACTIVITY, AND EFFICACY

Parallel shifts in the log dose-response curve may be attributed to varying affinities, whereas variations in the maximal height of the curves are expressions of varying intrinsic activities, or efficacies. In Fig. 2-1, *B*, drug B is less potent than drug A and has less affinity for the receptor. The relative actions of chlorothiazide, hydrochlorothiazide, and furosemide discussed on p. 9 are examples of the differences between potency and efficacy.

AGONIST, ANTAGONIST, AND PARTIAL AGONIST

An agonist is a drug that has affinity and efficacy. It interacts with receptors and elicits a response. Acetylcholine is a good example of an agonist. However, if a log dose-response curve to acetylcholine is obtained in the presence of atropine (an antagonist), it will be found that atropine has no effects of its own but that it shifts the log dose-response curve of acetylcholine to the right.

Atropine is viewed as competing with acetylcholine for the same receptors, in other

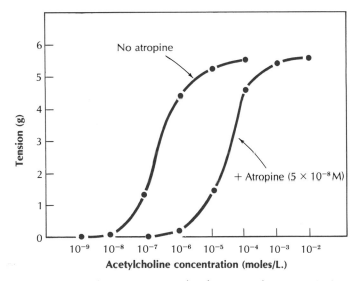

Fig. 2-2. Effect of acetylcholine on tension development of guinea pig ileum. Atropine, a competitive antagonist, caused a parallel shift of the log dose-response curve.

words, the antagonist has affinity but lacks efficacy. This is an example of *competitive* or *surmountable* antagonism. The key feature of this kind of antagonism is *parallel displacement of the log dose-response curve to the right without a shift in the maximum* (Fig. 2-2).

Somewhere between pure agonists and pure antagonists are the drugs termed partial agonists. They have affinity and some efficacy but may antagonize the action of other drugs that have a higher efficacy.

NONCOMPETITIVE ANTAGONISM

In the case of atropine and acetylcholine the antagonist and agonist were competing for the same receptor, as evidenced by the parallel shift in the log dose-response curve without a shift in the maximum. In some instances the antagonist may combine irreversibly with the receptor or a portion of the receptor, in which case increasing the concentration of the agonist will never fully overcome the inhibition. The net effect will be a decrease in the maximum height of the log dose-response curve, which is interpreted to reflect a decrease in the number of drug-receptor complexes.

RATE THEORIES OF DRUG ACTION

In the foregoing discussion it has been assumed that, similar to the Michaelis-Menten kinetics, the response to a drug is proportional to the concentration of the drug-receptor complex. While this theory does not explain how the drug-receptor complex is coupled to the final drug effect, it is quite useful for visualizing the mode of action of competitive antagonists such as atropine, the antihistaminics, and many others.

There are some observations that are difficult to explain by the "receptor occupation" theories. For example, some drugs first stimulate and then act as antagonists. Nicotine does this on ganglionic transmission. Also, many drugs produce their greatest effect at their initial application, with rapid tolerance, or "tachyphylaxis," developing to their action. To explain these effects, which are difficult to visualize according to the receptor occupation theory, several investigators have suggested that drugs contribute a stimulus only during the initial *interaction* with the receptor.[2] As an extension of these concepts, an interesting although not widely accepted theory of drug action has been proposed by Paton.[8] According to the Paton theory, the response to a drug is not dependent on the *concentration* of the drug-receptor complex but on the *rate* of drug-receptor combinations

Paton's rate theory[9] is useful in explaining some facts, such as (1) partial agonists *first* excite *then* block; (2) antagonists are generally slowly washed out from tissues, in contrast to agonists; and (3) at the neuromuscular junction lipid affinity favors a blocking action rather than an excitatory effect. It should be emphasized, however, that it is impossible to be sure of the correctness of either the *receptor occupation theory* or the *rate theory* of drug action.

CURRENT TRENDS IN FUNDAMENTAL PHARMACOLOGY

There is a noticeable trend in modern pharmacology toward studies of basic mechanisms of drug action, sometimes referred to as molecular pharmacology. A few examples may illustrate this trend.

Real advances are being made in the study of pharmacologic receptors. In some instances, such as the cholinergic receptor, efforts are being made at isolating the protein itself. In other instances the existence of a specific receptor is shown by its combination with a labeled antagonist from which it can be displaced by known agonists. The opiate receptor has been studied by this method.[11] Finally, the probable structure of the active site on a receptor macromolecule may be hypothesized from structure-activity relationships of agonists and antagonists that interact with the receptor.

The mode of action of gaseous anesthetics is being studied in relation to the hypothesis that the "structure" of water may be altered by such drugs.[10]

Drug effects on the transport of ions are being studied extensively. Interaction of drugs with endogenous regulators of cellular function is being investigated by many workers. The influence of drugs on the binding and release of catecholamines, serotonin, and histamine is the objective of numerous research efforts. The role of cyclic adenylic acid in the mediation of drug effects is a fertile field of study. The most advanced techniques of protein chemistry are being applied to the study of drug-receptor interactions.[23]

This trend toward molecular pharmacology was envisioned by Claude Bernard in 1865 when he stated that poisons (drugs) are "means of going deeper . . . dealing with the elementary parts of organisms where the elementary properties of vital phenomena have their seat."

References

1 Clark, A. J.: General pharmacology. In Heffter, A., editor: Handbuch der experimentellen Pharmakologie, vol. 4, Berlin, 1937, Springer-Verlag.
2 Croxatto, R., and Huidobro, F.: Fundamental basis of the specificity of pressor and depressor amines in their vascular effects, Arch. Int. Pharmacodyn. 106:207, 1956.
3 Ferguson, J.: Use of chemical potentials as indices of toxicity, Proc. Roy. Soc. [Biol.] 127:387, 1939.
4 Hurwitz, L., and Suria, A.: The link between agonist action and the response in smooth muscle, Ann. Rev. Pharmacol. 11:303, 1971.
5 Katz, B.: Microphysiology of the neuromuscular junction. The chemoreceptor function of the motor end-plate, Bull. Hopkins Hosp. 102:296, 1958.
6 Langley, J. N.: On the mutual antagonism of atropin and pilocarpin, having especial reference to their relations in the sub-maxillary gland of the cat, J. Physiol. 1:339, 1878.
7 Michaelis, L., and Menten, M. L.: Die Kinetik der Invertinwirkung, Biochem. Z. 49:333, 1913.
8 Paton, W. D. M.: A theory of drug action based on the rate of drug-receptor combination, Proc. Roy. Soc. [Biol.] 154:21, 1961.
9 Paton, W. D. M.: Receptors as defined by their pharmacological properties. In Porter, R., and O'Connor, M., editors: Molecular properties of drug receptors, Ciba Foundation Symposium, London, 1970, J. & A. Churchill.
10 Pauling, L.: A molecular theory of general anesthesia, Science 134:15, 1961.
11 Pert, C. B., and Snyder, S. H.: Opiate receptor: demonstration in nervous tissue, Science 179:1011, 1973.
12 Schild, H. O.: Introduction. In de Jonge, H., editor: Quantitative methods in pharmacology, Amsterdam, 1961, North-Holland Publishing Co.
13 Stephenson, R. P.: A modification of receptor theory, Brit. J. Pharmacol. 11:379, 1956.

Recent reviews

14 Albert, A.: Selective toxicity, ed. 3, New York, 1965, John Wiley & Sons, Inc.
15 Albert, A.: Relations between molecular structure and biological activity: stages in the evolution of current concepts, Ann. Rev. Pharmacol. 11:13, 1971.
16 Ariëns, E. J.: Molecular pharmacology, the mode of action of biologically active compounds, vol. 1, New York, 1964, Academic Press, Inc.
17 Burgen, A. S. V.: Receptor mechanisms, Ann. Rev. Pharmacol. 10:7, 1970.
18 Burger, A., and Parulkar, A. P.: Relationship between chemical structure and biological activity, Ann. Rev. Pharmacol. 6:19, 1966.
19 Furchgott, R. F.: Receptor mechanisms, Ann. Rev. Pharmacol. 4:21, 1964.
20 Gourley, D. R. H.: Basic mechanisms of drug action, Fortschr. Arzneimittelforsch. 7:11, 1964.
21 Mautner, H. G.: The molecular basis of drug action, Pharmacol. Rev. 19:107, 1967.
22 Porter, C. C., and Stone, C. A.: Biochemical

mechanisms of drug action, Ann. Rev. Pharmacol. 7:15, 1967.

23 Porter, R., and O'Connor, M., editors: Molecular properties of drug receptors, Ciba Foundation Symposium, London, 1970, J. & A. Churchill.

24 Triggle, D. J.: Chemical aspects of the autonomic nervous system, New York, 1965, Academic Press, Inc.

25 Waud, D. R.: Pharmacological receptors, Pharmacol. Rev. 20:49, 1968.

3

Kinetics of drug distribution

The purpose of drug administration is to ensure an effective level of the therapeutic agent at its site of action. The various factors that will determine such a level will be discussed under the following headings: passage of drugs across body membranes, absorption, distribution of drugs in the body, excretion of drugs, and drug disappearance curves. The quantitative features of drug distribution are sometimes referred to as pharmacokinetics, and much of this chapter deals with that field of knowledge.

PASSAGE OF DRUGS ACROSS BODY MEMBRANES

In order for a drug to reach its site of action it must pass across various body membranes. This can be seen in Fig. 3-1, which depicts the general handling of a drug in the body. Absorption, capillary transfer, penetration into cells, and excretion are all basically examples of the passage of drugs across body membranes.

The great advances that have occurred in our understanding of these processes can only be summarized here. A thorough review of the subject is given in an article by Schanker.[25]

Numerous studies based on such varied techniques as the osmotic behavior of tissues[19] and electron microscopy[24] indicate that the cell membrane consists of a bimolecular lipoid layer attached on both sides to a protein layer. Its thickness is about 100 Ångstroms (Å).

Because of its lipoid nature, the cell membrane is highly permeable to lipid-soluble

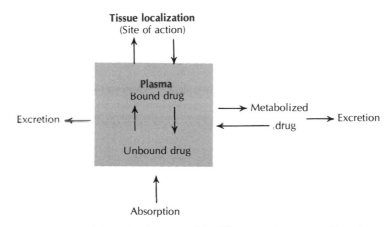

Fig. 3-1. Absorption and fate of a drug. (Modified from Brodie, B. B.: Clin. Pharmacol. Ther. **3**:374, 1962.)

substances. Since the cell is also easily penetrated by water and other small lipid-insoluble substances such as urea, it is postulated that the lipid membrane has pores or channels that allow passage of lipid-insoluble molecules of small dimensions.[26]

In addition to the passive movement of many substances across body membranes, it is necessary to postulate more complex processes for the passage of glucose, amino acids, and some inorganic ions and drug substances. A simplified summary of the various types of passage across body membranes follows:

I. Passive transfer
   1. Simple diffusion
   2. Filtration
II. Specialized transport
   1. Active transport
   2. Facilitated diffusion
   3. Pinocytosis

The essential features of these transfer mechanisms will be described briefly.

PASSIVE TRANSFER

Simple diffusion is characterized by the rate of transfer of a substance across a membrane being directly proportional to the concentration gradient on both sides of the membrane. Both lipid-soluble substances and lipid-insoluble molecules of small size may cross body membranes by simple diffusion. *Filtration* is spoken of when a porous membrane allows the bulk flow of a solvent and the substances dissolved in it, except for those of large size. The glomerular membrane of the kidney is a good example of a filtering membrane.

A special situation exists in the case of partly ionized drugs, since cell membranes are more permeable to the nonionized form of a given drug than to its ionized form because of the greater lipid solubility of the nonionized form. As a consequence, the passage of many drugs into cells and across other membranes becomes a function of the pH of the internal environment and the pK_a of the drug.

The concept of pK_a is derived from the Henderson-Hasselbalch equation. For an acid:

$$pK_a = pH + Log \frac{\text{Molecular concentration of nonionized acid}}{\text{Molecular concentration of ionized acid}}$$

For a base:

$$pK_a = pH + Log \frac{\text{Molecular concentration of ionized base}}{\text{Molecular concentration of nonionized base}}$$

It follows from these equations that, when a substance is half-ionized and half-nonionized at a certain pH, its pK_a is equal to this pH. In other words, a substance is half-ionized at a pH value that is equal to its pK_a.

Although these concepts may seem academic, they have become of great importance in explaining a number of clinically important facts. For example, weak acids such as salicylic acid ($pK_a = 3$) are well absorbed from the stomach, whereas weak bases such as quinine ($pK_a = 8.4$) are not absorbed until they reach the less acidic intestine. The influence of urinary pH on the excretion of salicylic acid and phenobarbital represents another example of the dependence of diffusion on the pK_a of drugs.[28]

Table 3-1. pK$_a$ values for some weak acids and bases (at 25° C.)

Weak acids	pK$_a$	Weak bases	pK$_a$
Salicylic acid	3.00	Reserpine	6.6
Acetylsalicylic acid	3.49	Codeine	7.9
Sulfadiazine	6.48	Quinine	8.4
Barbital	7.91	Procaine	8.8
Boric acid	9.24	Ephedrine	9.36
		Atropine	9.65

Table 3-2. Effect of pH on the ionization of salicylic acid (pK$_a$ 3)

pH	% Nonionized
1	99.0
2	90.9
3	50.0
4	9.09
5	0.99
6	0.10

The pK$_a$ values for a number of acidic and basic drugs are listed in Table 3-1. It should be remembered that for acidic drugs the lower the pK$_a$, the stronger the acid; whereas, for basic drugs the higher the pK$_a$, the stronger the base.

The relationships between pH, pK$_a$, and ionization of an acidic drug are illustrated in Table 3-2, using salicylic acid as an example.

SPECIALIZED TRANSPORT

The passage of many substances into cells and across body membranes cannot be explained simply on the basis of diffusion or filtration. For example, compounds may be taken up against a concentration gradient, great selectivity can be shown for compounds of the same size, competitive inhibition can occur among substances handled by the same mechanism, and in some instances metabolic inhibitors can block the transport processes.

To explain these phenomena the existence of specific *carriers* in membranes has been postulated.[41] *Active transport* is spoken of when, in addition to many other criteria, substances are moving against a concentration or electrochemical gradient. *Facilitated diffusion* is a special form of carrier transport that has many of the characteristics of active transport, but the substrate does not move against a concentration gradient. The uptake of glucose by cells is an example of facilitated diffusion. *Pinocytosis* refers to the ability of cells to engulf small droplets. This process may be of some importance in the uptake of large molecules.

ABSORPTION

The process whereby a drug is made available to the fluids of distribution is referred to as absorption. The rate of this process depends on the method of administration, solubility, and other physical properties of the drug.

ABSORPTION FROM THE GASTROINTESTINAL TRACT

Drugs are administered by the oral route in many different forms—solutions, suspensions, capsules, and tablets with various coatings. When the drug is not in solution, its rate of absorption will be the net result of two processes[16]: the process of solution and the absorption process itself. The solution process can be altered by pharmaceutical manipulations, thus influencing the absorption rate, but the absorption process is a basic characteristic of the membranes of the gastrointestinal tract.

In general, the absorption of drugs from the gastrointestinal tract can be explained by simple diffusion across a membrane having the characteristics of a lipoid structure with water-filled pores. Simple diffusion does not account for the uptake of sugars and other nutrients, in which case absorption can only be explained in terms of active mechanisms. A useful principle, derived from experimental data, is that the limiting membrane is permeable to nonionized lipid-soluble forms of drugs and less permeable to the ionized form. This principle has considerable predictive value.

Weak acids such as salicylates and barbiturates are largely nonionized in the acidic gastric contents and are therefore well absorbed from the stomach. Such weak bases as quinine or ephedrine and the highly ionized quaternary amines such as tetraethylammonium are not significantly absorbed from the stomach. Alkalinization of the gastric contents would be expected to decrease the absorption from the stomach of weak acids and increase that of weak bases.

Absorption from the small intestine is similar in principle to that from the stomach, except that the pH of intestinal contents is usually 6.6. Interestingly, drug distribution studies between plasma and small intestinal fluid would indicate a possible pH value of 5.3 for the area just adjacent to the intestinal absorbing membrane. Weakly acidic and weakly basic drugs are well absorbed from the small intestine, but highly ionized acids and bases are not well absorbed. Special mechanisms exist for the absorption of sugars, amino acids, and compounds related to normal nutrients. Some inorganic ions such as sodium and chloride are well absorbed despite the fact that they are in the ionic form.

In the oral cavity the oral mucosa also appears to behave as a lipid pore membrane, and drugs may be absorbed upon sublingual administration.[29] Nitroglycerin is usually administered in this manner.

Drug effects on gastric emptying may greatly affect absorption. For example, chloroquine has a much higher LD_{50} when given by mouth to rats than after its direct administration into the intestine. This difference is a consequence of inhibition of gastric emptying by chloroquine.[27]

ABSORPTION WITH PARENTERAL ADMINISTRATION

The parenteral injection of drugs has several advantages and also some drawbacks. Drugs that are not absorbed from the gastrointestinal tract must be injected. In addition, the parenteral route prevents destruction of the drug in the alimentary canal and avoids gastric irritation. Also, the rate of absorption can be influenced greatly when injectable drugs are used.

Among the disadvantages of parenteral injection, one should consider local irritation, cost, necessity of sterile technique, and greater likelihood of systemic reaction, particulary when potent drugs are injected by the intravenous route.

When injected intravenously, a drug is rapidly distributed in the body space that is characteristic for it.

The rate of absorption following subcutaneous or intramuscular injection depends largely on two factors: solubility of the preparation and blood flow through the area. Suspensions or colloidal preparations are absorbed more slowly than aqueous solutions. Advantage is taken of this fact in many instances when prolonged absorption is desirable. For example, protamine is added to insulin in order to form a suspension and thereby decrease the rate of absorption from the subcutaneous depot site. The various injectable penicillin suspensions are good examples of prolonging the action of a therapeutic agent by slowing its absorption.

The blood flow through a tissue has much to do with the speed of absorption of a drug from its site of injection. Absorption from a subcutaneous site may be very slow in the presence of peripheral circulatory failure. This has been observed in the subcutaneous administration of morphine to patients in shock. Similarly, the greater blood flow per unit weight of muscle is responsible for the more rapid absorption of drugs from this tissue than from subcutaneous fat.

Certain practical consequences of these facts may be of real clinical importance. Cooling an area of injection will slow absorption, a desirable effect if an excessive dose has been inadvertently injected or if untoward reactions begin to develop in an unusually susceptible patient. On the other hand, massage of the site of injection will speed up absorption.

CLINICAL PHARMACOLOGY OF ABSORPTION: BIOAVAILABILITY

The absorption of a drug from the gastrointestinal tract in man can be estimated fairly accurately, particularly when a reliable method is available for its determination. An approximate idea of the completeness of absorption can be gained by comparing the oral and intravenous doses that produce the same effect. If the two figures are similar, absorption must be fairly complete. On the other hand, if it takes a much larger oral dose to obtain the same end point as by the intravenous route, absorption is probably incomplete.

Drugs used in medicine seem to fall into three categories from the standpoint of absorption. Some are completely absorbed, some are not absorbed significantly, and still others are partially absorbed. Examples of well-absorbed drugs are most sulfonamides, digitoxin, acetylsalicylic acid, and barbiturates. Drugs not absorbed significantly include certain sulfonamides, streptomycin, neomycin, and kanamycin. Examples of partially or variably absorbed drugs are penicillin G, certain digitalis glycosides, and bishydroxycoumarin (Dicumarol).

Drugs that are incompletely and variably absorbed represent a problem to the physician, since he cannot rely on dosage as a guide to adequacy of treatment. In this situation it is very helpful to monitor the concentration of the drug in the blood or to carefully follow a characteristic effect of the drug.

The dosage form of the drug has a great influence on absorption. Solutions are absorbed most rapidly and coated tablets most slowly. Enteric-coated tablets are commonly used in order to provide a sustained level of the drug in the body, but despite the popularity of this dosage form, it cannot be considered a predictable method of administering drugs. There are great individual variations in gastric emptying and rate of dissolution of such preparations. They may even be eliminated unchanged in the feces.

Bioavailability. There is much current interest in observations indicating that various preparations of the same drug administered orally may give different serum concentrations. The term *bioavailability* has been defined[10] as the relative absorption efficiency of a test dosage form relative to a standard oral or intravenous preparation. In one study[10] it was found that digoxin administered in tablet form is only 75% absorbed when compared with an oral solution of digoxin. Considerable variation may exist in tablets of different manufacturers and even in different batches of tablets of the same company. The recognition of the importance of this problem is leading to stricter control of manufacturing processes and the necessity of standardization of products in terms of bioavailability, rather than chemical determination alone.

DISTRIBUTION OF DRUGS IN THE BODY

Once a drug reaches the plasma, its main fluid of distribution, it must pass across various barriers in order to reach its final site of action. The first of these barriers is the capillary wall. Through processes of diffusion and filtration,[14] most drugs rapidly cross the capillary wall, which has the characteristics of a lipid membrane with water-filled pores. Lipid-soluble substances diffuse through the entire capillary endothelium, whereas lipid-insoluble drugs pass through pores, which represent a fraction of the total capillary surface. The capillary transfer of lipid-insoluble substances is inversely related to molecular size. Large molecules such as dextran are transferred so slowly that they can be used as plasma substitutes.

FACTORS CONTRIBUTING TO THE UNEQUAL DISTRIBUTION OF DRUGS

There are several factors that contribute to the unequal distribution of drugs in the body. Some of these are (1) binding to plasma proteins, (2) cellular binding, (3) concentration in body fat, and (4) the blood-brain barrier.

The *binding of drugs to plasma proteins* creates a higher concentration of the drug in the blood than in the extracellular fluid. It also provides a depot, since the bound portion of the drug is in equilibrium with the free form. As the unbound fraction is excreted or metabolized, additional amounts are eluted from the protein. Protein binding prolongs the half-life of a drug in the body, since the bound fraction is not filtered through the renal glomeruli and is not exposed to processes of biotransformation until freed.

The protein-bound fraction of a drug is generally inactive until it becomes free. Thus the protein-bound fractions of sulfonamides and penicillins exert no chemotherapeutic effect. The protein responsible for binding is usually albumin, although globulins may be very important in relation to the binding of some hormonal agents and drugs.

The binding capacity of proteins is not unlimited. Once it becomes saturated, a sudden increase in toxicity may occur with further administration of some drugs. In hypoalbuminemia, toxic manifestations to drugs may appear as a consequence of deficiency in the binding protein.[21]

Drugs may influence the protein binding of other substances or drugs. Thus salicylates decrease the binding of thyroxine to proteins.[30] The binding of bilirubin to albumin may be inhibited by a variety of drugs such as sulfisoxazole or salicylates, the freed bilirubin thereby becoming ultrafiltrable.[17]

Binding to plasma protein influences not only the biologic activity of drugs but also their distribution. A highly protein-bound drug could displace another and increase its pharmacologic activity and toxicity and change its distribution.[1] Fatal kernicterus has occurred in premature infants who were given sulfisoxazole.[17] The sulfonamide displaced bilirubin from plasma protein and thereby promoted the penetration of the bile pigment into the brains of the infants. Recent studies[1] indicate that sulfinpyrazone can increase the concentration of sulfonamides in the fetus by a similar mechanism of displacement on plasma proteins of the mother. Other examples of drug interactions based on displacement in protein binding will be discussed in Chapter 58.

The *cellular binding of drugs is* usually due to an affinity for some cellular constituent. The high concentration of the antimalarial drug quinacrine (Atabrine) in the liver or muscle is probably due to the affinity of this drug for nucleoproteins.

The short duration of action of certain drugs such as the thiobarbiturate intravenous anesthetics has been explained on the basis of the rapid uptake by the brain, followed by a rapid decrease as the concentration of the drug in the blood falls.[6]

The *blood-brain barrier* represents a unique example of unequal distribution of drugs.[4] Even if injected intravenously, many drugs fail to penetrate into the central nervous system, the cerebrospinal fluid, or the aqueous humor as rapidly as into other tissues. Known exceptions to this principle are the neurohypophysis and the area postrema.

The capillaries in the central nervous system are enveloped by glial cells, which represent a barrier to many water-soluble compounds although they are permeable to lipid-soluble substances. Thus quaternary amines penetrate the central nervous system poorly, but the general anesthetics do so with ease.

A fact of great importance in medicine is the change in the permeability of various barriers produced by inflammation. In the early days of penicillin therapy it was known that the administration of large doses to normal persons failed to produce detectable levels of the antibiotic in the cerebrospinal fluid. It was found, however, that penicillin would penetrate into the spinal fluid of patients with meningitis.

Although many drugs do not penetrate the cerebrospinal fluid well, they can move efficiently in the reverse direction when administered by intracisternal injection.[25] Perhaps they are removed from the cerebrospinal fluid by filtration across the arachnoid villi. In addition, the choroid plexus is capable of pumping out certain substances from the cerebrospinal fluid; for example, penicillin.[36]

The passage of drugs into *milk* may be explained by diffusion of the nonionized, nonprotein-bound fraction. Since most drugs are weak electrolytes, they will appear in varying amounts in milk and may exert adverse effects on the breast-fed infant. When taken in larger than average doses by the mother, atropine, bromides, anthraquinones, metronidazole, and ergot alkaloids may cause intoxication in the breast-fed infant. On the other hand, the following drugs appear in milk only in small quantities and are generally of no clinical significance for the infant[34]: morphine, codeine, phenolphthalein, tolbutamide, quinine, and salicylates. Large doses of drugs in general should not be administered to the mother without considering the possible danger to the infant.[34]

EXCRETION OF DRUGS

The most important route of excretion for most drugs is the kidney. Many drugs are also excreted into bile, but are then usually recycled through the intestine, making this route quantitatively unimportant. Excretion of drugs into milk may have some significance for the breast-fed child[34] but is not an important avenue of excretion for the mother. Elimination of drugs through the lungs, salivary and sweat glands, and also in the feces is important only in special cases to be discussed under individual drugs.

Two major mechanisms are involved in the renal handling of drugs: glomerular filtration with variable tubular reabsorption and tubular secretion. The half-life of a drug in the body will be influenced also by such extrarenal factors as plasma protein binding and the existence of tissue depots and, most important, by the rate of drug metabolism.

It has been calculated that without the extrarenal factors the half-life of a drug in the extracellular fluid would be as follows:

70 minutes if excreted solely by glomerular filtration

7 minutes if secreted by the tubules and limited only by renal blood flow

7 days if the drug were reabsorbed by the tubules to the extent that its concentration in the urine is no greater than in plasma

The usual situation is that the drug is filtered through the glomeruli and is partially reabsorbed by the tubules. Since water is reabsorbed to a much greater extent than are most drugs, the concentration of drugs in the urine is most frequently greater than in plasma.

A study of the excretion of weak electrolytes has revealed an interesting connection between the pH of urine and renal handling of these drugs.[9, 14] Generally, drugs that are bases are excreted to a greater extent if the urine is acid, whereas acid compounds are excreted more favorably if the urine is alkaline The magnitude of this pH dependence is influenced also by the dissociation constant of a given drug. To explain these results it has been postulated that the undissociated fraction is reabsorbed more readily than the ionic form of a drug. This thesis is favored by the known lipid solubility of undissociated electrolytes.[25]

A practical application of this knowledge has been proposed in the treatment of phenobarbital poisoning.[28] Since phenobarbital is a weak acid having a pK_a of 7.3, its dissociation is greatly influenced by changes in pH at levels obtainable in mammalian urine. Alkalinization of the urine by the administration of sodium bicarbonate causes a significant increase in the excretion of phenobarbital.

Since urine is normally acid, the excretion of weakly acid drugs by renal handling alone would require a very long time. Fortunately, drug metabolism tends to transform these into stronger acids, thereby increasing the percentage of the ionic forms and hindering their tubular resorption.

In addition to glomerular filtration and passive tubular reabsorption, the renal tubule can actively secrete organic anions and cations. Examples of organic anions are p-aminohippurate, iodopyracet (Diodrast), phenol red, and penicillin, and examples of organic cations are tetraethylammonium, mepiperphenidol (Darstine), and N-methylnicotinamide. These active secretory processes may also handle other anions and cations such as salicylic acid, quinine, and tolazoline (Priscoline).[22] Competition for active tubular secretion exists among the various anions and cations.

Drugs that, in addition to undergoing glomerular filtration, are also secreted by the tubules have a very short half-life in the body. Since this short half-life is a distinct disadvantage in therapy, efforts have been made to inhibit the process of tubular secretion by such drugs as probenecid, which was specifically developed for this purpose. Usually, however, it is simpler to prolong the half-life of drugs by slowing their absorp-

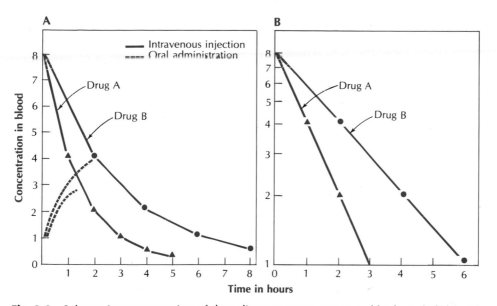

Fig. 3-2. Schematic representation of drug disappearance curves and biologic half-life. The y axis is on the arithmetic scale in **A** and on the logarithmic scale in **B**. Drug A has a biologic half-life of 1 hour. The biologic half-life of drug B is 2 hours.

tion. This is the reason for the development of many penicillin preparations that are absorbed slowly following intramuscular injection.

DRUG DISAPPEARANCE CURVES

The final net effect of absorption, excretion, distribution, and drug metabolism can be described in the form of drug disappearance curves, using blood or tissue concentration data. An understanding of drug disappearance curves and the biologic half-life of various drugs can be of great importance in the design of dosage regimens for therapeutic trials and for evaluation of new drugs. But even in everyday medical practice, the optimal use of many drugs such as the digitalis glycosides or the sulfonamides cannot be achieved without some knowledge of their biologic half-life.

A careful examination of Fig. 3-2 and most other drug disappearance studies indicates that they follow an *exponential decay* curve. Conceptually, this means that the change per unit time is a function of the concentration of the drug. To state it differently, the mean drug concentration in any hour divided by the concentration in the previous hour is constant. It also follows that the period during which the level of the drug falls to one half is also constant. This period is known as the *biologic half-life,* or $t_{1/2}$.

If the disappearance curve is plotted on a semilog scale, a straight line results. The biologic half-life, or $t_{1/2}$, can be easily determined on the straight line given by the semilog plot. For a mathematical treatment of these concepts the reader is referred to Nelson.[15]

It should be emphasized that many drug disappearance curves are not as smooth as the hypothetical ones shown in Fig. 3-2, *A*. Breaks may appear in the curves as a consequence of distributional shifts resulting from the concentration and slow release of drugs by some tissues. It should also be mentioned that the disappearance of some drugs from the blood is not exponential. In the case of alcohol a constant amount is metabolized per hour (p. 255).

IMPLICATIONS OF EXPONENTIAL DRUG DISAPPEARANCE CURVE

The frequency of drug administration to patients is often dependent on the biologic half-life of the drug. This is always the case when a sustained blood level of the drug is desirable. For example, the sulfonamides should be used in such a manner that a sustained blood level is achieved. The frequency with which various members of the sulfonamide group of drugs is administered depends then on the biologic half-life. The $t_{1/2}$ of sulfisoxazole in man is 8 hours, while that of sulfamethoxypyridazine is 34 hours. It is not unexpected, then, that the former is administered orally every 4 hours and the latter every 24 hours. The delay in absorption after oral administration is the main reason why these drugs are administered more frequently than could be predicted from their half-life.

Occasionally the physician wishes to obtain a steadily rising blood or tissue level of a drug until a certain effect is achieved. Quinidine is sometimes given orally every hour for several doses until atrial fibrillation stops. In this case the physician deliberately creates drug cumulation by giving quinidine more frequently than would be justified on the basis of its $t_{1/2}$.

Failure to appreciate the exponential nature of drug disappearance can lead to erroneous ideas in therapeutics. For example, if a drug has a short duration of action, doubling the dose will not double the duration of its effect.

Problem 3-1. A sleeping medication has a half-life of 1 hour. It is administered in a dose of 100 mg., and the patient wakes up when only 12.5 mg. remain in the body. How many hours will the patient sleep? Administering 200 mg. of the same drug, how much longer will the patient sleep? The answer can be found by examining Fig. 3-2. Doubling the dose simply adds one half-life to the duration of sleep.

In general, if a drug has a short duration of action, the following methods are available for prolonging its action:

1. Frequent administration. Most sulfonamides are administered every 4 hours.
2. Slowing absorption. Enteric coating and other pharmaceutical maneuvers can accomplish this.
3. Interfering with renal excretion. Probenecid blocks the excretion of penicillin.
4. Inhibiting drug metabolism. Allopurinol was originally developed for blocking the metabolic degradation of mercaptopurine.

References

1 Anton, A. H., and Rodriguez, R. E.: Drug induced change in the distribution of sulfonamides in the mother and its fetus, Science 180: 976, 1973.
2 Bakay, L.: The blood-brain barrier, Springfield, Ill., 1956, Charles C Thomas, Publisher.
3 Bennett, W. M., Singer, I., and Coggins, C. H.: A practical guide to drug usage in adult patients with impaired renal function, J.A.M.A. 214:1468, 1970.
4 Brodie, B. B., and Hogben, C. A. M.: Some

physicochemical factors in drug action, J. Pharm. Pharmacol. 9:345, 1957.
5 Doluisio, J. T., and Swintosky, J. V.: Drug partitioning. III. Kinetics of drug transfer in an in vitro model for drug absorption, J. Pharm. Sci. 54:1594, 1965.
6 Goldstein, A., and Aronow, L.: The duration of action of thiopental and pentobarbital, J. Pharmacol. Exp. Ther. 128:1, 1960.
7 Gutman, A. B., Yü, T. F., and Sirota, J. H.: A study, by simultaneous clearance techniques, of

salicylate excretion in man. Effect of alkalinization of the urine by bicarbonate administration; effect of probenecid, J. Clin. Invest. **34**:711, 1955.

8 Hogben, C. A. M., Schanker, L. S., Tocco, D. J., and Brodie, B. B.: Absorption of drugs from the stomach. II. The human, J. Pharmacol. Exp. Ther. **120**:540, 1957.

9 Hogben, C. A. M., Tocco, D. J., Brodie, B. B., and Schanker, L. S.: On the mechanism of intestinal absorption of drugs, J. Pharmacol. Exp. Ther. **125**:275, 1959.

10 Huffman, D. H., and Azarnoff, D. L.: Absorption of orally given digoxin preparations, J.A.M.A. **222**:957, 1972.

11 Mark, L. C., Kayden, H. J., Steele, J. M., Cooper, J. R., Berlin, I., Rovenstine, E. A., and Brodie, B. B.: The physiological disposition and cardiac effects of procaine amide, J. Pharmacol. Exp. Ther. **102**:5, 1951.

12 Mayer, S. E., Maickel, R. P., and Brodie, B. B.: Kinetics of penetration of drugs and other foreign compounds into cerebrospinal fluid and brain, J. Pharmacol. Exp. Ther. **127**:205, 1959.

13 Mayer, S. E., Maickel, R. P., and Brodie, B. B.: Disappearance of various drugs from the cerebrospinal fluid, J. Pharmacol. Exp. Ther. **128**:41, 1960.

14 Milne, M. D., Scribner, B. H., and Crawford, M. A.: Non-ionic diffusion and excretion of weak acids and bases, Amer. J. Med. **24**:709, 1958.

15 Nelson, E.: Kinetics of drug absorption, distribution, metabolism and excretion, J. Pharm. Sci. **50**:181, 1961.

16 Nelson, E.: Physicochemical and pharmaceutic properties of drugs that influence the results of clinical trials, Clin. Pharmacol. Ther. **3**:673, 1962.

17 Odell, G. B.: Studies in kernicterus. I. The protein-binding of bilirubin, J. Clin. Invest. **38**:823, 1959.

18 Orloff, J., and Berliner, R. W.: The mechanism of the excretion of ammonia in the dog, J. Clin. Invest. **35**:223, 1957.

19 Overton, E.: Beiträge zur allgemeinen Muskel- und Nervenphysiologie, Pflüg. Arch. Ges. Physiol. **92**:115, 1902.

20 Pappenheimer, J. R., Renkin, E. M., and Borrero, L. M.: Filtration, diffusion and molecular sieving through peripheral capillary membrane: contribution to pore theory of capillary permeability, Amer. J. Physiol. **167**:13, 1951.

21 Petermann, M. L.: Plasma protein abnormalities in cancer, Med. Clin. N. Amer. **45**:537, 1961.

22 Peters, L.: Renal tubular excretion of organic bases, Pharmacol. Rev. **12**:1, 1960.

23 Renkin, E. M., and Pappenheimer, J. R.: Wasserdurchlässigkeit und Permeabilität der Capillarwände, Ergebn. Physiol. **49**:59, 1957.

24 Robertson, J. D.: The ultrastructure of cell membranes and their derivatives, Biochem. Soc. Sympos. **16**:3, 1959.

25 Schanker, L. S.: Passage of drugs across body membranes, Pharmacol. Rev. **14**:501, 1962.

26 Solomon, A. K.: The permeability of red cells to water and ions, Ann. N. Y. Acad. Sci. **75**:175, 1958.

27 Varga, F.: Intestinal absorption of chloroquine in rats, Arch. Int. Pharmacodyn. **163**:38, 1966.

28 Wadell, W. J., and Butler, T. C.: The distribution and excretion of phenobarbital, J. Clin. Invest. **36**:1217, 1957.

29 Walton, R. P.: Sublingual administration of drugs, J. A. M. A. **124**:138, 1944.

30 Wolff, J., Standaert, M. E., and Rall, J. E.: Thyroxine displacement from serum proteins and depressions of serum protein-bound iodine by certain drugs, J. Clin. Invest. **40**:1373, 1961.

Recent reviews

31 Barlow, C. F.: Clinical aspects of the blood-brain barrier, Ann. Rev. Med. **15**:187, 1964.

32 Cserr, H. F.: Blood-brain barrier in vertebrates, Fed. Proc. **26**:1024, 1967.

33 Gosselin, R. E.: Kinetics of pinocytosis, Fed. Proc. **26**:987, 1967.

34 Knowles, J. A.: Excretion of drugs in milk, a review, J. Pediat. **66**:1068, 1965.

35 LaDu, B. N., Mandel, H. G., and Way, E. L.: Fundamentals of drug metabolism and drug disposition, Baltimore, 1971, The Williams & Wilkins Co.

36 Levine, R. R.: Pharmacology: drug actions and reactions, Boston, 1973, Little, Brown & Co.

37 Levy, G.: Dose dependent effects in pharmacokinetics. In Tedeschi, D. H., and Tedeschi, R. E., editors: Importance of fundamental principles in drug evaluation, New York, 1968, Raven Press.

38 Rall, D. P.: Comparative pharmacology and cerebrospinal fluid, Fed. Proc. **26**:1020, 1967.

39 Ther, L., and Winne, D.: Drug absorption, Ann. Rev. Pharmacol. **11**:57, 1971.

40 Weiner, I. M.: Mechanisms of drug absorption and excretion, Ann. Rev. Pharmacol. **7**:39, 1967.

41 Willbrandt, W., and Rosenburg, T.: The concept of carrier transport and its corollary in pharmacology, Pharmacol Rev. **13**:109, 1961.

4 Drug metabolism, enzyme induction, and pharmacogenetics

If the body depended only on its excretory mechanisms for ridding itself of drugs, lipid-soluble compounds would be retained almost indefinitely (p. 22). Fortunately the endoplasmic reticulum of the liver provides enzyme systems for the oxidation of lipid-soluble drugs (Fig. 4-1). The activation of molecular oxygen takes place at a heme protein, cytochrome P_{450}, which is present in large quantities in the endoplasmic reticulum of the liver.

Other drug-metabolizing enzymes are also present in the endoplasmic reticulum, such as esterases, flavin enzymes, and transferases (Table 4-1). Furthermore, acetylations of aromatic amines and the oxidation of alcohol are accomplished by cytoplasmic enzymes. Nevertheless, the cytochrome P_{450}–dependent drug-metabolizing enzymes, being quite nonspecific, play a predominant role in protecting the body against the accumulation of exogenous and some endogenous lipid-soluble compounds by converting them to water-soluble metabolites, which are easily excreted by the kidney.

The drug-metabolizing enzymes, located in the smooth endoplasmic reticulum of the liver, may be induced by numerous drugs such as barbiturates, meprobamate, and griseofulvin. They may be competitively inhibited by drugs and also may become deficient in severe liver disease.

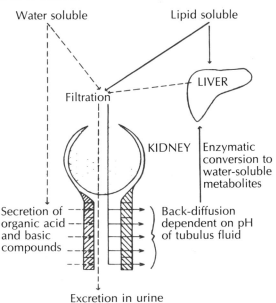

Fig. 4-1. Elimination of drugs. (From Remmer, H.: Amer. J. Med. **49**:617, 1970.)

Table 4-1. Drug metabolism and enzymes of the endoplasmic reticulum*

Drug metabolism	Enzyme
Oxidations of aliphatic and aromatic groups	Cytochrome P_{450}
Barbiturates	
Diazepoxides	
Phenothiazines	
Meprobamate	
Diphenylhydantoin	
Antihistaminics	
Acetophenetidin	
Aminopyrine	
Some synthetic steroids	
Reductions of azo and nitro groups	Flavin enzymes
Hydrolyses of esters and amides	Esterases
Conjugations with glucuronic acid	Transferases
Alcohols	
Phenols	

*Modified from Remmer, H.: Amer. J. Med. **49**:617, 1970.

The application of modern concepts of drug metabolism in medicine is made difficult by the considerable species and individual variations in drug hydroxylations. The human liver contains much less cytochrome P_{450} per unit weight than that of the rat, and the metabolism of many drugs is correspondingly slower in man than in smaller animals. Individual variations in the metabolism of some drugs such as diphenylhydantoin (Dilantin) may be quite large. Although individual variations in drug metabolism make treatment somewhat more difficult, they should not create serious problems if dosage is carefully adjusted to the individual patient's needs and responses.

Some examples illustrate the necessity of studying drug metabolism in man as well as in laboratory animals if the results are to be meaningful to the physician. The effect of a single dose of meperidine in man lasts about 3 or 4 hours, whereas the drug produces only very transitory effects in the dog. This difference is undoubtedly related to the fact that meperidine is metabolized in man at the rate of about 20% per hour, while the corresponding rate in the dog is 90% per hour, as stated by Williams.[67] Other striking differences between drug metabolism in man and certain animals exist. In contrast to man, dogs do not acetylate sulfonamides, and cats have only very slight ability to conjugate drugs with glucuronic acid. Hexobarbital is a short-acting barbiturate in mice or rabbits, whereas it acts for a much longer time in man. Correspondingly, the biologic half-life in minutes for hexobarbital is 19 for mice, 60 for rabbits, and 360 for man.

DRUG METABOLISM

The chemical reactions involved in the metabolism of drugs and foreign compounds may be classified as <u>oxidations, reductions, hydrolyses, and conjugations.</u>[40,54] The various types of drug metabolism will be discussed giving specific examples. In addition, Table 4-1 should be consulted, in which the metabolic reactions limited to the microsomal enzymes are reviewed.

MICROSOMAL ENZYMES

As shown in Table 4-1, the oxidations of a large variety of drugs are linked to the microsomal hydroxylase, cytochrome P_{450}, the properties of which will be discussed in some detail based on the recent review by Remmer.[61]

Microsomal hydroxylase, cytochrome P_{450}. The hydroxylation of numerous drugs by liver microsomes was first demonstrated by Brodie,[2] Cooper,[10] and their co-workers. Subsequently it was shown that a newly discovered cytochrome, named cytochrome P_{450}, was responsible for drug hydroxylations. This enzyme is present in large quantities in the smooth endoplasmic reticulum of the liver and in much smaller quantities in the kidney and other tissues.[61]

The mechanism of drug hydroxylations (Fig. 4-2) may be summarized in the following manner: Cytochrome P_{450} (acting as a mixed-function oxidase) transfers one electron to one atom of oxygen to form water; it also transfers one electron to oxygen which is added to the drug. The formula is as follows:

$$X + 2e^- + 2H^+ + O_2 \xrightarrow{\text{Cytochrome } P_{450}} X{:}O + H_2O$$

where X stands for the drug acted on by the mixed-function oxidase.

The electron donor is reduced NADP. The flavoprotein enzyme, NADPH-dependent cytochrome c reductase is responsible for the flow of electrons from the reduced flavin enzyme to cytochrome P_{450}. The overall reaction for drug X may then be written as follows[61]:

$$X.H + NADPH + H^+ + O_2 \rightarrow X.OH + NADP^+ + H_2O$$

Induction and inhibition of microsomal hydroxylase. The ability of various drugs such as phenobarbital to increase the rate of metabolism of a variety of lipid-soluble

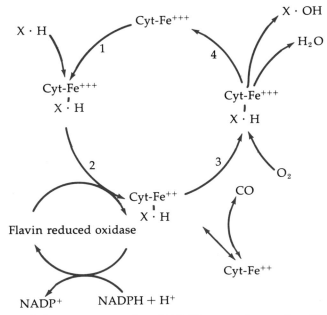

Fig. 4-2. Schema of electron transport from NADPH to cytochrome P_{450}. (From Remmer, H.: Amer. J. Med. **49**:617, 1970.)

drugs is explained at present by the ability of such drugs to cause an hypertrophy of the smooth endoplasmic reticulum and an increase in the amount of microsomal hydroxylase. The low specificity of this enzyme accounts for the ability of one drug to increase the metabolism of even unrelated compounds. The inducing drugs, which include (in addition to phenobarbital) meprobamate, phenylbutazone, diphenyl-hydantoin, griseofulvin, and many others, vary in their power to stimulate enzyme synthesis. Of greatest interest in medicine are the drugs capable of stimulating the formation of microsomal hydroxylase at therapeutic doses. Such is the case for phenobarbital. It is quite likely[61] that most substrates of microsomal hydroxylase can act as inducers if they remain in the liver cells in high enough concentration for long enough periods of time. The short-acting barbiturates may not act as inducers because of their short sojourn in the liver.

Although an increase in microsomal hydroxylase may be induced by a variety of drugs, a deficiency may be encountered in premature infants and sufferers from very severe liver disease and as a consequence of the action of some drugs. A lipid-soluble compound may inhibit the metabolism of another drug competitively. Although there are not many well-studied examples of this type of interaction, it is known that ethyl alcohol, which is not normally metabolized by cytochrome P_{450}, can inhibit drug hydroxylations, undoubtedly because its high concentration in cells makes up for its low affinity for the drug hydroxylase.

OXIDATIVE REACTIONS
Hydroxylation of aromatic rings

Acetanilid is changed to *N*-acetyl-*p*-aminophenol. On the other hand, the naturally occurring compounds L-phenylalanine and tyrosine are hydroxylated by nonmicrosomal enzymes. Phenobarbital is changed to the inactive metabolite *p*-hydroxyphenobarbital.

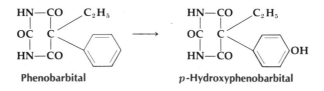

Phenobarbital → *p*-Hydroxyphenobarbital

Aliphatic hydroxylation

Pentobarbital is metabolized to the corresponding carboxylic acid and alcohol, and meprobamate to hydroxymeprobamate.

$$\begin{array}{cc}
\underset{|}{CH_3} & \underset{|}{CH_3} \\
C(CH_2OCONH_2)_2 & \longrightarrow \quad C(CH_2OCONH_2)_2 \\
\underset{|}{} & \underset{|}{} \\
CH_2CH_2CH_3 & CH_2CHOHCH_3 \\
\text{Meprobamate} & \text{Hydroxymeprobamate}
\end{array}$$

N-Dealkylation

Meperidine is metabolized by removal of a methyl group. Mephobarbital is demethylated to phenobarbital.

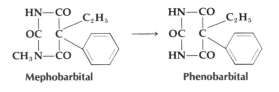

Mephobarbital   Phenobarbital

O-Dealkylation

O-Dealkylation is also known as ether cleavage. Acetophenetidin is transformed into N-acetyl-p-aminophenol, in this case an active metabolite.

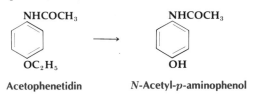

Acetophenetidin   N-Acetyl-p-aminophenol

REDUCTIONS

Chloral hydrate is changed in the body to trichloroethanol, which is an active hypnotic. The azo dye Prontosil is split by reduction, with the formation of sulfanilamide as one of the products.

$$Cl_3CCH(OH)_2 \longrightarrow Cl_3CCH_2OH$$

Chloral hydrate   Trichloroethanol

HYDROLYSES

Esters are commonly hydrolyzed in the body. Thus acetylcholine is metabolized to choline and acetic acid, procaine to p-aminobenzoic acid and diethylaminoethanol, and aspirin to salicylic acid and acetic acid.

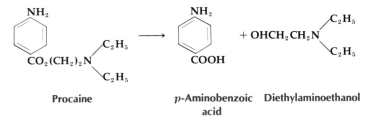

Procaine   p-Aminobenzoic   Diethylaminoethanol
                   acid

CONJUGATION REACTIONS

A number of conjugation reactions have been demonstrated to occur in man. Some of these are important in pharmacology because they inactivate widely used drugs. Conjugation with glucuronic acid, glycine conjugation, methylation, acetylation, and sulfate synthesis belong in this class. Other conjugation reactions that appear to be less important in pharmacology at the present time are glutamine conjugation, mercapturic acid synthesis, and thiocyanate formation.

Glucuronide synthesis

In man, drugs that contain hydroxyl or carboxyl groups may undergo biotransformation to glucuronides. The basic reaction, which takes place in the liver microsomes, may be represented as follows:

$$\text{Uridine diphosphoglucuronate} + \text{ROH} \xrightarrow{\text{Glucuronyl transferase}} \text{RO glucuronide} + \text{Uridine diphosphate}$$

An example of a drug excreted almost entirely as the glucuronide is salicylamide.

Salicylamide   Salicylamide glucuronide

Glycine conjugation

Glycine conjugation is characteristic for certain aromatic acids. It depends on the availability of coenzyme A, glycine, and glycine-*N*-acylase. A typical reaction is as follows:

$$\text{Benzoic acid} \xrightarrow{\text{ATP} + \text{CoA}} \text{Benzoyl-CoA} \xrightarrow{\text{Glycine}} \text{Hippuric acid}$$

Some of the drugs conjugated with glycine in man are salicylic acid, isonicotinic acid, and *p*-aminosalicylic acid. These drugs are metabolized by other pathways also, which may be more important quantitatively than glycine conjugation.

Methylation

Norepinephrine and epinephrine are metabolized in part to normetanephrine and metanephrine by a process of *O*-methylation, whereas nicotinic acid is metabolized to *N*-methylnicotinic acid, an example of *N*-methylation. The source of methyl groups for drug methylations is *S*-adenosylmethionine.

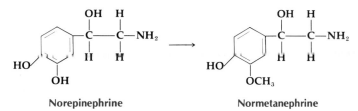

Norepinephrine   Normetanephrine

Acetylation

Derivatives of aniline are acetylated in the body. In addition to sulfanilamide and related compounds, such widely used drugs as *p*-aminosalicylic acid, isonicotinic acid hydrazide, and aminopyrine are transformed by this mechanism. The general reaction involving an amine, acetyl coenzyme A, and a specific acetylating enzyme may be depicted in the following manner:

$$\text{RNH}_2 + \text{CoASCOCH}_3 \xrightarrow{\text{Acetylase}} \text{RNHCOCH}_3 + \text{CoASH}$$

The acetylating ability of different patients may vary considerably. In the case of isonicotinic acid hydrazide a low degree of acetylation shows some correlation with incidence of toxic reactions such as peripheral neuritis.

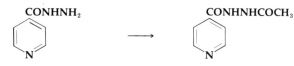

Isonicotinic acid hydrazide   Acetylated isonicotinic acid hydrazide

Ethereal sulfate synthesis

Phenolic compounds may be excreted in part as ethereal sulfates, although the usual metabolic fate of such compounds in man is glucuronide formation. Ethereal sulfate formation is believed to take place in the following manner:

(1) Sulfate + ATP $\longrightarrow$ 3'-Phosphoadenosine-5'-phosphosulfate (PAPS)

(2) Phenol + PAPS $\xrightarrow{\text{Sulfokinase}}$ Phenyl sulfate + 3'-5'-Phosphoadenosine

DRUG METABOLISM AND DETOXICATION

The term *detoxication*, while widely used, fails to give an accurate picture of drug metabolism. The biotransformation of drugs does not always result in a less toxic product. Some drugs such as chlorpromazine, imipramine, and ephedrine are chemically altered but retain their pharmacologic activity. The body may first transform an inactive or moderately active drug into a more active compound and then detoxify it to a harmless form. For example, codeine, a moderately active narcotic, is changed to a small extent to morphine and then to the inactive morphine glucuronide.

Other drugs activated by metabolism in man include acetanilid and acetophenetidin to *p*-acetaminophenol, chloral hydrate to trichloroethanol, Prontosil to sulfanilamide, mephobarbital to phenobarbital, primidone to phenobarbital, and aspirin to salicylic acid.

Finally, the toxicity of some compounds may be caused by a metabolite. The insecticide parathion is changed in the body to the more toxic paraoxon.

An even more remarkable example of the possible deleterious effects of the so-called detoxication process is given by the example of liver damage caused by carbon tetrachloride and probably some other drugs. Carbon tetrachloride is a well-known hepatotoxic agent. The curious finding that newborn rats are more resistant to the toxic effect of carbon tetrachloride[59] along with the observation that phenobarbital increases not only the metabolism of the halogenated hydrocarbon but also its toxicity, suggests that drug metabolism is involved in the hepatotoxicity of the compound. It is believed that free radicals are formed as a result of the interaction of some drugs and the drug-metabolizing enzymes. The free radicals may be directly toxic, perhaps through an interaction with membrane phospholipids. They may also make endogenous proteins antigenic, thus accounting for some forms of drug allergy. There are reasons to believe also that in many drug allergies it is a metabolic product and not the original drug that acts as a haptene.

Details of metabolism must be considered in connection with the individual drugs, but one very interesting generalization has been made concerning the evolutionary importance of certain detoxication mechanisms.

As we have seen in the previous section, the clearance of weakly acid or basic drugs is hindered by the tubular reabsorption of the undissociated molecule. But for terrestrial animals there is no alternate route of excretion. In contrast, aquatic animals have no difficulty with such foreign compounds because the lipid membranes of the gills offer a ready avenue for their excretion. In the course of evolution, terrestrial organisms seem to have solved this problem by utilizing such mechanisms as side chain oxidation and conjugation, which make these foreign compounds more acid and hence more easily rejected by the renal tubules.

The development of detoxication mechanisms appears to have been an evolutionary necessity, since terrestrial animals ingest many foreign compounds with their food. The mechanisms of detoxication, perhaps developed for the handling of such compounds, serve also at the present time for the biotransformation of a large variety of drugs.

FACTORS THAT DELAY THE METABOLISM OF DRUGS

It has been pointed out that drugs are usually metabolized at rates proportional to their plasma levels because at therapeutic levels their concentration is not high enough to saturate the drug-metabolizing enzymes.[54] Any conditions that lower the concentration of drugs at the level of the metabolizing enzymes or decrease the amount or activity of the enzymes would be expected to prolong the biologic half-life of the drug. Several of these factors are of great importance, whereas others may become significant only in particular diseases or in the presence of certain drug combinations. The following are some examples:

1. The reversible protein binding limits drug metabolism. Phenylbutazone, for example, is highly protein bound, up to 98% after therapeutic doses. If the dose is increased so that only 88% of the drug is protein bound, the free portion is metabolized much more rapidly. As a consequence, not much is gained by increasing the dose.

2. Localization of the drug in the adipose tissue (thiopental) or in the liver (quinacrine) protects it against metabolic degradation and prolongs its half-life. Precipitation of the drug in the gastrointestinal tract may similarly prolong its half-life (zoxazolamine).

3. Diseases of the liver and immaturity of drug-metabolizing enzymes during the neonatal period may interfere with the biotransformation of some drugs.

4. A drug may inhibit the metabolism of another drug and thus may prolong and intensify its action. This is why monoamine oxidase inhibitors may cause alarming reactions when tyramine-containing food or beverages are ingested. The very interesting experimental drug SKF-525A (β-diethylaminoethyl diphenylpropylacetate) inhibits the microsomal enzymes that metabolize a large variety of drugs. Iproniazid is another inhibitor of drug-metabolizing enzymes.

ENZYME INDUCTION

When several drugs are used simultaneously in a patient, it is difficult enough to keep in mind their various pharmacologic interactions. An additional difficulty derives from observations indicating that some drugs can induce the formation of microsomal drug metabolizing enzymes. Some cases of tolerance to a drug may be caused by microsomal enzyme induction. There are well-authenticated cases in both the experimental and clinical literature of such drug interactions.

STIMULATION OF DRUG-METABOLIZING ENZYMES BY DRUGS AND FOREIGN COMPOUNDS

It was first shown in 1954[3] that mice fed the carcinogen 3-methylcholanthrene developed an increased capacity for demethylating 3-methyl-4-dimethylaminoazobenzene by liver microsomal enzymes. Several other examples of increased drug metabolism induced by various preparations followed. The long-acting barbiturate phenobarbital was found to stimulate the metabolism of such short-acting barbiturates as hexobarbital.[27] Although the list of compounds that can, under experimental conditions, speed up the metabolism of many other drugs is quite large, species variation is so great that this discussion will be limited to examples of this drug interaction in man. The animal experiments have shown, however, that the inducers cause a marked increase in the smooth endoplasmic reticulum as seen by electron microscopy.[28] They have also established the fact that the inducers do not stimulate the enzymes in the test tube, so there is little doubt that the increased drug metabolism is a consequence of increased formation of the microsomal drug-metabolizing enzymes.

When the endoplasmic reticulum is homogenized, "rough-surfaced" and "smooth-surfaced" microsomes may be separated. The drug-metabolizing enzymes are associated largely with the smooth-surfaced microsomes.

Stimulation of drug metabolism shown in animal experiments cannot always be assumed to occur in man. For example, tolbutamide has a marked stimulatory effect on its own metabolism in the dog, but has only a small stimulatory effect on its own degradation in man.[27]

STIMULATION OF DRUG METABOLISM IN MAN

The following examples of stimulated drug metabolism have been demonstrated in man.

Phenobarbital stimulates the metabolism of diphenylhydantoin (Dilantin),[49] griseofulvin, and bishydroxycoumarin (Dicumarol) (Fig. 4-3). Barbiturates stimulate the glucuronide conjugation of bilirubin in mice; this finding suggested the use of phenobarbital in the treatment of congenital nonhemolytic jaundice in infants.[42] The administration of 15 mg. of phenobarbital two or three times daily lowered the free serum bilirubin concentration in these infants. Additionally, it improved the conjugation of salicylamide in the same infants, another example of glucuronide formation.

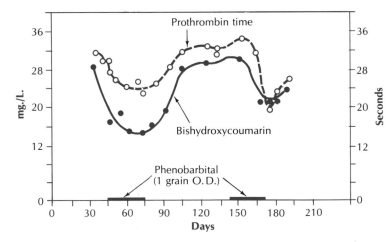

Fig. 4-3. Effect of phenobarbital on plasma levels of bishydroxycoumarin and on prothrombin time in a human subject treated chronically with 75 mg./day of bishydroxycoumarin. (From Cucinell, S. A., Conney, A. H., Sansur, M., and Burns, J. J.: Clin. Pharmacol. Ther. **6**:420, 1965.)

Phenylbutazone speeds the metabolism of aminopyrine.[7] **Meprobamate and glute-thimide** may induce tolerance to their action by enzyme induction.[4]

Diphenylhydantoin interferes with the effect of dexamethasone,[80] probably by promoting microsomal enzyme activity.

The inducers may promote the metabolism of certain hormones as well as that of various drugs and foreign compounds. Oxidative drug-metabolizing enzymes hydroxylate such endogenous compounds as testosterone, estradiol, progesterone, and cortisol.[54] NADPH-requiring microsomal enzymes are involved in the formation or alteration of other endogenous compounds. For example, such enzymes are involved in the synthesis of cholesterol. Clearly, microsomal enzyme induction by drugs may have a much wider significance than the development of tolerance to some therapeutic agents.

Enzyme induction by drugs may not only explain troublesome therapeutic problems of resistance and tolerance to drugs but may also have some useful applications. It is important to point out, however, that there are other mechanisms for the development of drug tolerance that have nothing to do with enzyme induction. The striking examples of tolerance to morphine have no relation to microsomal enzyme induction.

PHARMACOGENETICS

Although several examples of abnormal drug reactions in inherited diseases are well known, the systematic study of pharmacogenetics is of recent origin.[57] Among the well-known examples of adverse drug reaction occurring in certain inherited diseases are the following: Barbiturates may produce severe attacks in congenital porphyria; salicylates are dangerous in individuals in whom glucuronyl transferase is congenitally absent (Crigler-Najjar syndrome); hypersensitivity to atropine occurs in patients suffering from Down's syndrome; and epinephrine or glucagon fail to produce hyperglycemia in individuals who are deficient in the enzyme glucose 6 phosphatase (von Gierke's disease).

A broad classification of pharmacogenetic abnormalities[57] would attribute most genetically conditioned anomalous drug responses to (1) receptor site abnormalities, (2) drug metabolism disorders, (3) tissue metabolism disorders, and (4) anatomic abnormalities.

Although there are not many well-known examples of *receptor site abnormalities,* they must undoubtedly contribute to the variation in drug responses. The resistance of some individuals to the coumarin anticoagulants is probably an example of a receptor site abnormality. The best known examples of pharmacogenetics are provided by *drug metabolism* disorders, in which abnormal blood levels of a drug can be measured after the administration of a normal dose. In *tissue metabolism* disorders an individual may show an adverse reaction to a normal blood level of a drug because of a special vulnerability caused by an abnormality in tissue metabolism. For example, in glucose-6-phosphate dehydrogenase deficiency a usual dose of primaquine may cause hemolytic anemia. Finally, an *anatomic abnormality* may cause adverse drug reactions. For example, in inherited subaortic stenosis digitalis may cause fatal reactions.[57]

The genetic modification of drug metabolism and drug responses is the subject of an increasingly important branch of pharmacology and biochemical genetics. Some of the most striking examples of pharmacogenetics differ from biochemical genetics in that their existence can be revealed *solely* by the use of drugs.

A typical example of how a genetic abnormality is recognized by an unusual response to a drug is that of acatalasia,[31] or lack of catalase in the blood and tissues, cases of which have been reported mostly from Japan. A physician in Japan treating a child for a severe infection of the oral cavity poured some hydrogen peroxide on the wound after excision of the gangrenous tissue. He noted that no bubbles appeared when the hydrogen peroxide came in contact with the blood. The physician suspected immediately that the patient might not have catalase in her blood, a suspicion that was confirmed by laboratory studies. Eventually the genetic basis of this condition was established, and acatalasia is now considered an autosomal recessive trait.[53] Another interesting example of pharmacogenetic abnormality is the failure to taste certain drugs. Phenylthiocarbamide is a bitter unpleasant substance to most individuals of various races. About one third of American Caucasians, however, either cannot taste the substance or do so only at very high concentrations.[55]

CONTINUOUS AND DISCONTINUOUS VARIATION

It is generally recognized that the response to a drug in a population shows *continuous variation*. Drug effects such as the LD_{50} or ED_{50} (p. 42) and rate of destruction of a drug in the body generally show a normal distribution in a population, as shown in Fig. 4-4, *A*. Some of the great discoveries in pharmacogenetics occur when the response to some drug or the metabolism of a drug indicates a *discontinuous variation*, as shown in Fig. 4-4, *B*. Follow-up of such a bimodal distribution often reveals a genetic basis and provides the explanation for unusual responses to drugs, which is more satisfying than simply calling them idiosyncrasies.

EXAMPLES OF PHARMACOGENETIC ABNORMALITIES

Some of the best known genetically determined abnormalities in drug responses are sensitivity to succinylcholine in relation to plasma cholinesterase defects, variations in isoniazid acetylation, hemolytic anemia associated with glucose-6-phosphate dehydrogenase deficiency, and bacterial resistance to drugs. Undoubtedly many other abnormal drug responses will find their explanation in genetic studies.

Succinylcholine and plasma cholinesterases

The muscle relaxant succinylcholine, widely used by anesthesiologists, causes apnea that lasts only a very few minutes. Its short duration of action is a consequence of its enzymatic destruction by plasma cholinesterase. In a few patients, however, the drug produced apnea that lasted for hours.[55] This potentially catastrophic response could have been dismissed as some sort of idiosyncrasy, but an investigation of the plasma cholinesterase activity in some of these patients has revealed that their enzyme level was less than that of normal individuals.

Studies on the cholinesterase activity of the affected individuals, their families, and normal individuals showed considerable overlap until a refinement in technique was introduced.[55] This refinement consists of the determination of the "dibucaine number," or percent inhibition of serum cholinesterase by the drug dibucaine (Nupercaine). The dibucaine numbers of 135 individuals of seven unrelated families gave a trimodal curve with no overlap. It has been postulated that the cholinesterase activity is determined by two alleles, one responsible for the *usual*, the other for the *atypical* form of the enzyme. Most individuals, having a dibucaine number of around 80, are postulated to

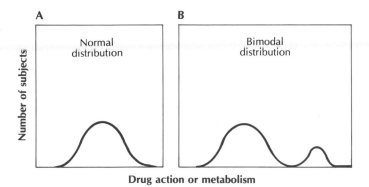

Fig. 4-4. Schematic illustration of *continuous* and *discontinuous* variation. When a standard dose of a drug is given to a large number of persons and a drug effect or metabolism is measured, the usual finding is a normal frequency distribution as in **A.** On the other hand, a discontinuous variation, as exemplified by the bimodal distribution shown in **B,** may indicate a genetically determined abnormality in drug action or metabolism.

have two of the usual alleles, $E_1^u E_1^u$. Individuals of the atypical phenotype, having dibucaine numbers of around 22, have the genotype $E_1^a E_1^a$. Finally, a third or intermediate group, with a dibucaine number of around 62, may have a genotype of $E_1^u E_1^a$.[65]

There are rare individuals who completely lack serum cholinesterase, and their genotype is subject to debate. The existence of some other type of allele is possible.

Practical importance. The practical importance of these studies is the predictive value of laboratory tests for a potentially catastrophic response to succinylcholine. Furthermore, blood transfusion is of value in apnea caused by this muscle relaxant because cholinesterase is stable in stored blood.

Isoniazid acetylation

Isoniazid is very useful in the treatment of tuberculosis. The drug is acetylated in the liver, and both the acetylated and the free form of the drug can be found in the urine. When the percentage of the isoniazid appearing in the urine in the free form was determined in a large group of individuals, it was found that two classes could be distinguished with regard to isoniazid metabolism: slow inactivators and rapid inactivators. Although the two types are fairly evenly distributed among American Caucasians and American Negroes, only 5% of Eskimos and 33% of Latin Americans are slow inactivators.

It is believed that rapid inactivators are normal homozygotes or heterozygotes, whereas slow inactivators are homozygous for a recessive gene that determines a lack of the enzyme which acetylates not only isoniazid but also some sulfonamides.[55]

Practical importance of slow isoniazid inactivation. The slow inactivators are more prone to develop polyneuritis when treated with isoniazid. There is no association between effectiveness of treatment and the genetic abnormality.

Glucose-6-phosphate dehydrogenase deficiency

The antimalarial drug primaquine produces hemolytic anemia, particularly in Negro males. When 30 mg. of the drug is given daily to such an individual, the urine turns dark in 2 or 3 days and the hemoglobin concentration in the blood falls. Extensive investigations of primaquine-induced hemolytic anemia revealed that the susceptible individuals differ from normal individuals in having red cells that are deficient in the enzyme glucose-6-phosphate dehydrogenase. The gene controlling the presence or absence of the enzyme is on the X chromosome and therefore the trait is sex-linked.

Hemolytic anemia caused by the ingestion of the bean *Vicia fava* and reactions to several other drugs have similarly been traced to a deficiency of glucose-6-phosphate dehydrogenase. The following drugs have been suspected: acetophenetidin, acetanilid, probenecid, and others.

Hemoglobin ← Methemoglobin

Reduced glutathione ← Oxidized glutathione

Glycolytic pathway   Glutathione reductase + NADPH   Pentose-phosphate pathway

Glucose   NADP → NADPH

Glucose-6-phosphate dehydrogenase

Glucose-6-phosphate --- 6-Phosphogluconate

Fructose-6-phosphate   Ribose-5-phosphate +

Glyceraldehyde-3-phosphate CO_2

Lactate

As shown in the above schema, the enzyme glucose-6-phosphate dehydrogenase in the red cell is responsible for the formation of NADPH (reduced form of nicotinamide adenine dinucleotide phosphate, or reduced triphosphopyridine nucleotide). NADPH is a cofactor for glutathione reductase, which converts glutathione to the reduced form. When there is a genetically determined deficiency of glucose-6-phosphate in the red cell, severe hemolytic episodes may be caused by the administration of oxidant drugs.

Bacterial resistance to drugs

The study of bacterial genetics and development of resistance to chemotherapeutic agents is of special interest in relation to antibacterial chemotherapy and will be discussed on p. 557.

References

1 Beaser, S. B.: Oral treatment of diabetes mellitus, J.A.M.A. **187**:887, 1964.
2 Brodie, B. B., Gillette, J. R., and La Du, B. N.: Enzymatic metabolism of drugs and other foreign compounds, Ann. Rev. Biochem. **27**:427, 1958.
3 Brown, R. R., Miller, J. A., and Miller, E. C.: The metabolism of methylated aminoazo dyes, J. Biol. Chem. **209**:211, 1954.
4 Burns, J. J.: Implications of enzyme induction for drug therapy, Amer. J. Med. **37**:327, 1964.
5 Burns, J. J., Evans, C., and Trousof, N.: Stimulatory effect of barbital on urinary excretion of L-ascorbic acid and non-conjugated D-glucuronic acid, J. Biol. Chem. **227**:785, 1957.
6 Busfield, D., Child, K. J., Atkinson, R. M., and Tomich, E. G.: An effect of phenobarbitone on blood-levels of griseofulvin in man, Lancet **2**:1042, 1963.
7 Chen, W., Vrindten, P. A., Dayton, P. G., and Burns, J. J.: Accelerated aminopyrine metabolism in human subjects pretreated with phenylbutazone, Life Sci. **2**:35, 1962.
8 Conney, A. H., and Gilman, A. G.: Puromycin inhibition of enzyme induction by 3-methylcholanthrene and phenobarbital, J. Biol. Chem. **238**:3682, 1963.
9 Conney, A. H., Miller, E. C., and Miller, J. A.: Substrate-induced synthesis and other properties of benzpyrene hydroxylase in rat liver, J. Biol. Chem. **228**:753, 1957.
10 Cooper, J. R., Axelrod, J., and Brodie, B. B.:

Inhibitory effects of β-diethylamino-ethyl diphenylpropylacetate on a variety of drug metabolic pathways in vitro, J. Pharmacol. Exp. Ther. 112:55, 1954.

11 Dayton, P. G., Tarcan, Y., Chenkin, T., and Weiner, M.: The influence of barbiturates on coumarin plasma levels and prothrombin response, J. Clin. Invest. 40:1797, 1961.

12 Douglas, J. F., Ludwig, B. J., and Smith, N.: Studies on the metabolism of meprobamate, Proc. Soc. Exp. Biol. Med. 112:436, 1963.

13 Editorial: Hypertensive reactions to monoamine oxidase inhibitors, Brit. Med. J. 1:578, 1964.

14 Fouts, J. R.: Drug-interactions: effects of drugs and chemicals on drug metabolism, Gastroenterology 46:486, 1964.

15 Fouts, J. R., and Brodie, B. B.: On the mechanism of drug potentiation by iproniazid (2-isopropyl-l-isonicotinyl hydrazine), J. Pharmacol. Exp. Ther. 116:480, 1956.

16 Fox, A. L.: The relationship between chemical constitution and taste, Proc. Nat. Acad. Sci. 18: 115, 1932.

17 Fox, S. L.: Potentiation of anticoagulants caused by pyrazole compounds, J.A.M.A. 188:320, 1964.

18 Hertting, G., Axelrod, J., and Whitby, L. G.: Effect of drugs on the uptake and metabolism of H³-norepinephrine, J. Pharmacol. Exp. Ther. 134:146, 1961.

19 Isaac, L., and Goth, A.: The mechanism of the potentiation of norepinephrine by antihistaminics, J. Pharmacol. Exp. Ther. 156:463, 1967.

20 Landsteiner, K.: The specificity of serological reactions, Cambridge, 1945, Harvard University Press.

21 Loeser, E. W., Jr.: Studies on the metabolism of diphenylhydantoin (Dilantin), Neurology 11:424, 1961.

22 Motulsky, A. G.: Drug reactions, enzymes and biochemical genetics, J.A.M.A. 165:835, 1957.

23 Muscholl, E.: Effect of cocaine and related drugs on the uptake of norepinephrine by heart and spleen, Brit. J. Pharmacol. 16:352, 1961.

24 Odell, G. B.: Studies in kernicterus. I. The protein-binding of bilirubin, J. Clin. Invest. 38:823, 1959.

25 Parker, C. W., Shapiro, J., Kern, M., and Eisen, H. N.: Hypersensitivity to penicillenic acid derivatives in human beings with penicillin allergy, J. Exp. Med. 115:821, 1962.

26 Ramboer, C., Thompson, R. P. H., and Williams, R.: Controlled trials of phenobarbitone therapy in neonatal jaundice, Lancet 1:966, 1969.

27 Remmer, H.: Drug tolerance. In Enzymes and drug action, Ciba Foundation Symposium, Boston, 1962, Little, Brown & Co.

28 Remmer, H., and Merker, H. J.: Drug-induced changes in the liver endoplasmic reticulum: association with drug-metabolizing enzymes, Science 142:1657, 1963.

29 Rubin, E., Gang, H., Misra, P. S., and Lieber, C. S.: Inhibition of drug metabolism by acute ethanol intoxication, Amer. J. Med. 49:801, 1970.

30 Sperber, I.: Secretion of organic anions in the formation of urine and bile, Pharmacol. Rev. 11:109, 1959.

31 Takahara, S.: Progressive oral gangrene probably due to lack of catalase in the blood (acatalasemia), Lancet 2:1101, 1952.

32 Vesell, E. S., and Page, J. G.: Genetic control of drug levels in man: phenylbutazone, Science 159:1479, 1968.

33 Vesell, E. S., Passananti, T., and Greene, F. E.: Impairment of drug metabolism by allopurinol and nortryptyline, New Eng. J. Med. 283:1484, 1970.

34 Vogel, F.: Moderne Probleme der Humangenetik, Ergebn. Inn. Med. Kinderheilk. 12:52, 1959.

35 Wadell, W. J., and Butler, T. C.: The distribution and excretion of phenobarbital, J. Clin. Invest. 36:1217, 1957.

36 Walton, R. P.: Sublingual administration of drugs, J.A.M.A. 124:138, 1944.

37 Weiner, I. M., Washington, J. A., II, and Mudge, G. H.: On the mechanism of action of probenecid on renal tubular secretion, Bull. Hopkins Hosp. 106:333, 1960.

38 Werk, E. E., Jr., Choi, Y., Sholiton, L., Olinger, C., and Hague, N.: Interference in the effect of dexamethasone by diphenylhydantoin, New Eng. J. Med. 281:32, 1969.

39 Willbrandt, W., and Rosenberg, T.: The concept of carrier transport and its corollaries in pharmacology, Pharmacol. Rev. 13:109, 1961.

40 Williams, R. T.: Detoxication mechanisms, New York, 1959, John Wiley & Sons, Inc.

41 Wolff, J., Standaert, M. E., and Rall, J. E.: Thyroxine displacement from serum proteins and depression of serum protein bound iodine by certain drugs, J. Clin. Invest. 40:1373, 1961.

42 Yaffe, S. J., Levy, G., Matsuzawa, T., and Baliah, T.: Enhancement of glucuronide-conjugating capacity in a hyperbilirubinemic infant due to apparent enzyme induction by phenobarbital, New Eng. J. Med. 275:1461, 1966.

43 Yu, T. F., Dayton, P. G., and Gutman, A. B.: Mutual suppression of the uricosuric effects of sulfinpyrazine and salicylate. A study in interactions between drugs, J. Clin. Invest. 42:1330, 1963.

Recent reviews

44 Anders, M. W.: Enhancement and inhibition of drug metabolism, Ann. Rev. Pharmacol. **11**:37, 1971.

45 Beutler, E.: The hemolytic effect of primaquine and related compounds: a review, Blood **14**:103, 1959.

46 Brodie, B. B.: Physicochemical and biochemical aspects of pharmacology, J.A.M.A. **202**:600, 1967.

47 Bush, M. T., and Sanders, E.: Metabolic fate of drugs: barbiturates and closely related drugs, Ann. Rev. Pharmacol. **7**:57, 1967.

48 Conney, A. H.: Pharmacological implications of microsomal enzyme induction, Pharmacol. Rev. **19**:317, 1967.

49 Conney, A. H.: Drug metabolism and therapeutics, New Eng. J. Med. **280**:653, 1969.

50 Conney, A. H., and Burns, J. J.: Factors influencing drug metabolism, Advances Pharmacol. **1**:31, 1962.

51 Conney, A. H., and Burns, J. J.: Metabolic interactions among environmental chemicals and drugs, Science **178**:576, 1972.

52 Ebert, R. V.: Oral anticoagulants and drug interactions, Arch. Intern. Med. **121**:373, 1968.

53 Evans, D. A. P.: Pharmacogenetics, Amer. J. Med. **34**:639, 1963.

54 Gillette, J. R.: Biochemistry of drug oxidation and reduction by enzymes in hepatic endoplasmic reticulum, Advances Pharmacol. **4**:219, 1966.

55 Kalow, W.: Pharmacogenetics: heredity and the response to drugs, Philadelphia, 1962, W. B. Saunders Co.

56 Kuntzman, R.: Drugs and enzyme induction, Ann. Rev. Pharmacol. **9**:21, 1969.

57 La Du, B. N.: The genetics of drug reactions, Hospital Practice, p. 97, June, 1971.

58 La Du, B. N., Mandel, H. G., and Way, E. L.: Fundamentals of drug metabolism and drug disposition, Baltimore, 1971, The Williams & Wilkins Co.

59 Recknagel, R. O.: CCl_4 hepatotoxicity, Pharmacol. Rev. **19**:145, 1967.

60 Remmer, H.: The fate of drugs in the organism, Ann. Rev. Pharmacol. **5**:405, 1965.

61 Remmer, H.: The role of the liver in drug metabolism, Amer. J. Med. **49**:617, 1970.

62 Schreiber, E. C.: The metabolic alteration of drugs, Ann. Rev. Pharmacol. **10**:77, 1970.

63 Shuster, L.: Metabolism of drugs and toxic substances, Ann. Rev. Biochem. **33**:571, 1964.

64 Stanbury, J. B., Wyngaarden, J. B., and Fredrickson, D. S.: The metabolic basis of inherited disease, New York, 1960, McGraw-Hill Book Co.

65 Thompson, J. S., and Thompson, M. W.: Genetics in medicine, Philadelphia, 1966, W. B. Saunders Co.

66 Vesell, E. S.: Pharmacogenetics, New Eng. J. Med. **287**:904, 1972.

67 Williams, R. T.: Detoxication mechanisms in man, Clin. Pharmacol. Ther. **4**:234, 1963.

5 Drug safety and effectiveness

The use of any drug carries with it a certain risk. The physician in his therapeutic decisions must weigh this risk against the effectiveness of the drug and the need for its use. The hazards of drug therapy are reduced by regulations that make it difficult to market drugs without considerable critical scrutiny. Valuable as these regulations may be, the ultimate safety and effectiveness of drugs are determined to a great extent by the physician's knowledge of pharmacology.

The physician should be able to evaluate journal articles, claims, and advertisements before he decides to use a drug. That this is not always so is indicated in a recent editorial from the most widely read medical journal.[17] Traditionally the physician relied on such groups of experts as the United States Pharmacopeial Committee, the Council on Drugs of the American Medical Association, and the regulatory bodies for the evaluation of the safety and effectiveness of drugs. Approval by these groups, in addition to the reputation of the manufacturer, gave him a feeling of security in the use of drugs with which he was not familiar.

With the expansion of drug therapy and the introduction of potent agents having complex effects and even more complex interactions with each other, it is increasingly necessary for the physician to have a scientific attitude and considerable knowledge of drug evaluation.

Since the most extensive studies on drug evaluation are carried out in connection with the development of *new* drugs, this subject will be discussed in some detail along with factors that modify drug safety and effectiveness.

DEVELOPMENT OF A NEW DRUG

New drugs originate from many different sources. Accidental observations on natural products, unexpected clinical findings on known compounds, basic physiologic or biochemical investigations, and even test tube experiments have provided leads for great therapeutic discoveries. Most new drugs are discovered today by screening. Large numbers of natural products or synthetic compounds are tested for a variety of possible biologic activities. A highly effective drug that seems safe enough on preliminary testing is then carried through a series of steps:

 I. Animal studies
   1. Acute, subacute, and chronic toxicity
   2. Therapeutic index
   3. Absorption, excretion, distribution, and metabolism
 II. Human studies
   1. Phase 1: preliminary pharmacologic evaluation
   2. Phase 2: basic controlled clinical evaluation
   3. Phase 3: extended clinical evaluation

ANIMAL STUDIES
Acute, subacute, and chronic toxicity

The most common measure of acute toxicity is the median lethal dose (LD_{50}). The LD_{50} is determined by giving various doses of the drug to groups of animals. Ordinarily only a single dose is given to each animal. The percentage of animals dying in each group within a selected period, for example, 24 hours, is plotted against the dose. From this curve the dose that kills 50% of the animals is estimated and is referred to as the LD_{50}. This particular dose-mortality figure is chosen because it can be determined more precisely; the curve approaches a straight line at the LD_{50}. It should be emphasized that the LD_{50} of any drug is of interest only to experimental pharmacologists, not to clinicians.

Customarily at least three different species are used for acute toxicity determinations, and observations are made not only on the LD_{50} but also on the type of toxic symptoms that the animals develop.

In subchronic toxicity studies the mode of administration and dosage depend on the proposed clinical trial. Usually the drug is administered orally. Several doses are used, some within the range of the estimated human dose and others that produce toxic manifestations. Careful observations are carried out on these animals, including a variety of laboratory studies such as hematologic examinations, renal and hepatic function tests, and many others.

The chronic toxicity studies are of long duration. They may last many months and may be carried through several generations to detect the possible teratogenic effect of a drug. Again several species are necessary because even in prolonged studies some species are much more suitable than others for the demonstration of adverse effects. The animals are killed periodically and thorough pathologic studies are performed.

Therapeutic index

The median lethal dose of a drug is not nearly as important as its therapeutic index, or therapeutic ratio. This concept in *animal experiments* refers to the ratio of the median lethal dose to the median effective dose, as illustrated in Fig. 5-1.

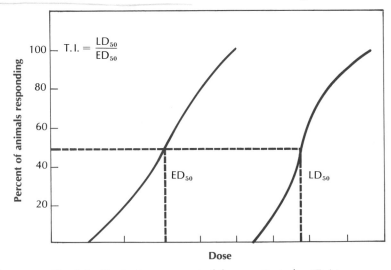

Fig. 5-1. Illustrating concept of therapeutic index (T. I.).

$$\text{Therapeutic index} = \frac{LD_{50}}{ED_{50}}$$

The concept of toxicity in relation to effectiveness, the basis of the therapeutic index, is of interest to clinicians as well as to experimental pharmacologists. A physician may not be greatly interested in the exact number of milligrams of a drug that will produce toxic effects, but he is vitally interested in knowing how far he can exceed the therapeutic dose before he is likely to encounter adverse effects.

There have been attempts at determining therapeutic ratios in human beings. In this instance, toxic dose$_{50}$/effective dose$_{50}$ is ordinarily employed. For example, with increasing doses of digitoxin, nausea develops as a toxic effect. In addition, digitoxin slows the ventricular rate in patients with atrial tachycardia. If the dose-response curves were widely enough separated and did not overlap, such studies would give an indication of a therapeutic ratio and would be suitable for comparing various digitalis preparations. Unfortunately the slopes of these curves are somewhat flat and there is considerable overlap. Furthermore, *biologic variation* is such that an individual could be at the bottom of the toxicity curve and at the top of the effectiveness curve or vice versa. While determination of toxicity in relation to effectiveness has great value in medicine, the therapeutic index as determined by animal experimentation should not be applied uncritically to man.

Absorption, excretion, distribution, and metabolism

The development of analytic methods for determining the absorption, excretion, distribution, and metabolism of a drug in animals adds much to the proper design of animal experiments on the toxicity and efficacy of the drug. In addition, these methods are desirable for the initiation and pursuit of clinical studies.

HUMAN STUDIES—CLINICAL PHARMACOLOGY

Animal studies provide a general profile of the toxicity, pharmacologic activities, and pharmacokinetics of a new drug. Even with all this information available, the initiation of clinical studies is risky. There are numerous examples of drugs that pass all the preclinical criteria for safety but show serious adverse effects in man. The clinical pharmacologist should consider not only the data obtained previously in animals but also the chemical nature of the drug and its possible similarity to hazardous drugs.

The lack of correlation between toxicity data in animals and adverse effects in man is well known. Not only is there great species variation in toxicity, an example of comparative pharmacology, but many adverse effects simply cannot be ascertained in animals. Zbinden[23] claimed that of the 45 most frequent drug-related symptoms observed in 11,000 patients treated with 77 different drugs or drug combinations, at least one half would probably not be recognized in animal experiments. Such symptoms include drowsiness, nausea, dizziness, nervousness, epigastric distress, headache, weakness, insomnia, fatigue, tinnitus, heartburn, skin rash, depression, dermatitis, increased energy, vertigo, lethargy, nocturia, abdominal distention, flatulence, stiffness, and urticaria.

Because of these discrepancies between animal data and human effects, the initial clinical studies on any drug should be undertaken with great care, meticulously planning the methodology and paying special attention to *relevance* (pertinence of data), *representativeness* (selection of material to eliminate bias), and *reliability* (repeatability

43

of results).[11] The new drug application must be filed before any clinical evaluation studies are initiated.

Phase 1: pharmacologic evaluation

Very small doses of the drug are administered to human volunteers in order to obtain a preliminary idea of safety in man. With increasing doses, an attempt is made to extend the previously demonstrated effects in animals to man. The ethical aspects of human experimentation have been the subject of much discussion in recent years and will not be taken up in detail.[22] The important points are, however, that the volunteer must be truly a volunteer (that is, he must be able to give an informed consent) and the investigator must be competent. In some instances it is essential to have methods for the determination of blood levels of the new drug. Without such determinations the investigator could not tell whether lack of effectiveness in man is a consequence of lack of absorption or too rapid excretion and metabolism.

Phase 2: basic controlled clinical evaluation

While the phase 1 studies are usually performed by one or two clinical investigators, in phase 2 a somewhat larger number of clinical investigators attempt to find out in blind or double-blind studies as much information as possible about the safety and efficacy of the new drug. Adverse effects must be reported promptly to the sponsoring company and to the Food and Drug Administration (FDA), and specific studies are sometimes initiated to ascertain the significance of such unexpected findings.

Phase 3: extended clinical evaluation

As many as 50 to 100 physicians participate in the large-scale clinical trial of a new drug. The investigators must not only be competent clinicians but must also have some experience and training in the field of drug evaluation.

Assuming that the phase 3 studies demonstrate to the satisfaction of the FDA that the drug is safe and effective, the investigational drug may be approved to be distributed and used when prescribed by a physician.

It would seem that with all these safeguards a drug approved by the FDA would be free of all hazard. Unfortunately there are many unusual side effects, idiosyncrasies, and drug allergies that show up only after very extensive use in large numbers of patients. Furthermore, it cannot be overemphasized that in addition to the inherent safety of a drug there are many other factors that determine its successful use. Perhaps the most important factor is the competence of the physician and his familiarity with the drug. Other modifying influences are biologic variation, hypersusceptibility, drug idiosyncrasy and drug allergy, age and weight of the patient, disease processes influencing susceptibility and detoxication, and presence of other drugs involving synergism, antagonism, and complex interactions in clinical pharmacology. Also, cumulation, tolerance, tachyphylaxis, and pharmacogenetics can markedly influence the safety and effectiveness of many drugs.

FACTORS INFLUENCING THE SAFETY AND EFFECTIVENESS OF DRUGS
BIOLOGIC VARIATION

Experimental studies in animals show that the dose of a drug which will give an all-or-nothing response (such as the death of the animal) varies considerably. Fig. 5-2 illustrates the gaussian distribution of susceptibility, which can be demonstrated

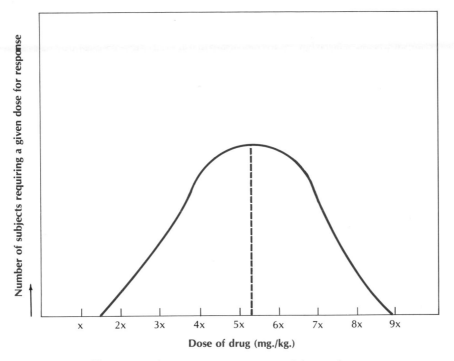

Fig. 5-2. Biologic variation in susceptibility to drugs.

easily in animals. The biologic variation in drug effect is an important reason why dosages must be individualized and treatment adjusted to the requirements of a given patient. The average adult dose recommended by the USP or approved by the FDA is an important guide, but many other factors must be taken into consideration. For this reason a physician well versed in pharmacology often gets better results with the same drug than someone who simply relies on the average doses recommended by the drug compendia.

HYPERSUSCEPTIBILITY

Because of biologic variation, disease, or presence of another medication, some persons may show a much greater than normal response to the ordinary dose of a drug. For example, a thyrotoxic patient may respond with exaggerated cardiovascular response to injected epinephrine. A patient with subclinical asthma may evidence symptoms of bronchial constriction from doses of acetyl-β-methylcholine or histamine that would be innocuous in normal persons. In these cases we are dealing with patients who are at the susceptible end of a normal frequency distribution curve and whose responses are quantitatively different. Hypersusceptibility is sometimes referred to as *drug intolerance*.

DRUG IDIOSYNCRASY AND DRUG ALLERGY

The term *idiosyncrasy* has been used rather vaguely in medicine to cover drug reactions that are *qualitatively* different from the usual effects obtained in the majority of patients and cannot be attributed to drug allergy. Occasionally extreme susceptibility of an individual to the expected pharmacologic effect of a drug has also been included in the drug idiosyncrasies.

With the increasing knowledge of pharmacogenetics, as discussed on p. 35, many drug idiosyncrasies have been found to be genetically conditioned enzymatic deficiencies. Such deficiencies can interfere with the metabolic degradation of a drug, as in prolonged apnea caused by succinylcholine, or they may make certain cells more vulnerable to an adverse effect of a drug, as is the case in hemolytic anemia elicited by primaquine and other drugs in patients whose red cells are deficient in glucose-6-phosphate dehydrogenase.[10]

It is quite likely that all drug idiosyncrasies will turn out to be genetically conditioned abnormalities of enzymes or receptors.

Drug allergy is an altered response to a drug resulting from a previous sensitizing exposure and an immunologic mechanism. It differs from drug toxicity in a number of respects: (1) The altered reaction occurs in only a fraction of the population. (2) Its dose-response is unusual in that a minute amount of an otherwise safe drug elicits a severe reaction. (3) The manifestations of the reaction are different from the usual pharmacologic effects of the drug. Thus aspirin elicits asthma as a presumably allergic reaction in a few individuals. (4) There is a primary sensitizing period before the individual responds with an unusual reaction to a further exposure. (5) When the sensitizing drug is a protein or a compound that forms covalent bonds with proteins, circulating antibodies may be demonstrated in sensitized individuals and skin tests, although hazardous, may show a positive reaction to the offending drug.

The diagnosis of drug allergy is a simple matter when most of the criteria just discussed can be satisfied. This is possible, however, only in the minority of cases. Generally a presumptive diagnosis is made by obtaining a history of a similar reaction on previous exposure to the drug that was characterized by typically "allergic" symptoms such as skin rash, hives, bronchial asthma, or hematologic disturbances. Skin tests with small-molecule drugs (in contrast to tests with proteins) are generally unreliable. An exception to this statement is provided by the anaphylactic hypersensitivity to penicillin. The penicillin *scratch test* is often positive in patients who are highly allergic to the antibiotic. Skin tests utilizing penicilloyl polylysine are discussed in relation to penicillin allergy (p. 531 of the fifth edition).

The differentiation between drug toxicity and allergy is most important, since it should influence the physician's attitude toward subsequent use of the drug. When dealing with drug toxicity, a simple reduction of the dose of a drug may be sufficient to eliminate the adverse effect. In case of drug allergy, reinstitution of treatment with the same drug is always hazardous and may be catastrophic. Some fatal anaphylactic reactions to penicillin could have been prevented if a previous history of reaction to the antibiotic had been recognized as a contraindication to its further use.

The *experimental approach* to drug allergy has produced many interesting findings, but there are many facts that are still unexplained. The most important work on this subject was done by Landsteiner.[6] This investigator showed in animal experiments that small-molecule compounds such as sulfanilic acid are not antigenic by themselves. On the other hand, if such small-molecule compounds are coupled to a protein, they may act as haptenes. Not only do such drug-protein complexes sensitize animals, but complexes of the drug with many different proteins may subsequently elicit antigen-antibody reactions. In other words, the drug has become a determinant group for the antigens. It has also been shown that some cross-reactions occur with drugs of similar structure.

The demonstration[9] that breakdown products of penicillin such as penicillenic acid can be coupled to peptides is a great step forward in the understanding of drug allergy. Although many patients allergic to penicillin have negative reactions to skin tests using the antibiotic, they react positively to the penicillenic acid derivative. It appears then that an individual may be allergic to a drug not because he has antibodies to the drug itself but rather because of a combination of a reactive metabolic breakdown product and some body protein. The problem of penicillin allergy has become more complicated by the demonstration that the antibiotic can form macromolecular complexes, which are antigenic, with or without proteinaceous material.[20]

In most drug allergies it is not known what the complete antigen is or in what form the drug acts as a hapten. A patient may react to the ingestion of a sulfonamide by developing a skin rash and still show no positive reaction to the same drug when injected intracutaneously. This is generally true for drugs of small molecular weight and the *immediate* type of allergies elicited by them. In *contact dermatitis*, on the other hand, positive patch tests are regularly obtained.

Immediate and delayed drug allergies

The terms *immediate* and *delayed reactions* originated from observations of the rapidity with which the positive skin test to allergens becomes manifest. Thus in anaphylactic hypersensitivity, skin test results are immediate, but in delayed states such as tuberculin hypersensitivity, it takes many hours before there is a visible change in the skin where the antigen was injected. In addition, there are profound differences in the immunologic basis of the two types of hypersensitivities. Circulating antibodies are believed to be important in immediate but not in delayed hypersensitivities. The latter can be transferred to normal individuals only by means of sensitized cells.

Among the many types of drug allergies, some are considered immediate, others delayed, and still others are not classifiable at present. *Anaphylaxis, urticaria, angioneurotic edema, drug fever, and asthma* clearly belong in the category of immediate reactions. *Serum sickness* reactions are characterized by a delay in the appearance of manifestations following the initial sensitization to a drug; this same delay is observed after the first administration of a foreign serum. Once an individual is sensitized, however, he often reacts to the same drug rather rapidly. For example, methyldopa (Aldomet) may be taken daily by an individual for a week or two before he develops fever and joint pains. The subsequent administration of a small dose of the drug will produce the same reaction in a matter of hours. *Contact dermatitis* is undoubtedly a delayed allergy. Many other cutaneous reactions and *some* severe hematologic disturbances elicited by drugs probably also belong in the delayed category.

The cross-reactions demonstrated in the experimental studies of Landsteiner are also observed in patients. It is difficult to generalize with respect to these cross-reactions. Occasionally a patient sensitive to one drug will cross-react with many related compounds. In other patients the hypersensitivity is much more specific. Because of these uncertainties, the only safe attitude on the part of the physician is to avoid, whenever possible, not only a drug to which the patient appears to be allergic but also compounds chemically related to it.

AGE AND WEIGHT OF PATIENT

In experimental investigations, drugs are administered on the basis of a certain number of milligrams per kilogram of body weight, since the volume of distribution of a drug is roughly a function of body mass. For the same reason the weight of the patient should be taken into consideration when a dose is calculated. Certain formulas allow adjustment of dosage according to weight. For example, Clark's rule is as follows:

$$\text{Dose for a child} = \text{Adult dose} \times \frac{\text{Weight of child in pounds}}{150}$$

It is assumed in this formula that a child needs a smaller dose because his weight is less, but this is only an approximation. It has been pointed out that the child is not simply a "small adult" and that reactions to drugs in children may result from problems in growth and development rather than size.[19] Catastrophes have resulted from the routine adaptation of adult dosages for children. The gray syndrome caused by chloramphenicol, kernicterus by vitamin K, and blindness by the use of oxygen in premature infants are examples of the peculiar problems of drug use in pediatrics.

The dose of a drug in children is proportional to weight to the 0.7 power.[16] Since body surface is similarly related to body weight, it has been suggested that pediatric dosages should be calculated on the basis of surface area of the body in square meters. Tables relating the weight of a child in pounds to surface area in square meters and approximate percentage of adult dose are available. According to such tables, a 22 lb. child having a surface area of 0.46 sq. m. should receive 27% of the adult dose. A child weighing 121 lb. with a surface area of 1.58 sq. m. would receive 91% of the adult dose.

DISEASE PROCESSES INFLUENCING SUSCEPTIBILITY AND DETOXICATION

Pathologic processes influence susceptibility to drugs. In some instances this can be explained by altered detoxication processes induced by the disease, but in other cases the explanation may be obscure.

It is obvious that in severe renal disease one must use with caution those drugs such as phenobarbital which depend on renal clearance for excretion. In severe liver disease, similar care must be exercised in the use of drugs that are normally detoxified by hepatic processes.

Abnormal susceptibility to drugs in disease states may depend on other mechanisms. The asthmatic patient is said to be hypersusceptible to the bronchoconstrictor action of histamine or methacholine, whereas the thyrotoxic patient is hypersusceptible to epinephrine. Patients with subclinical glaucoma may respond with an acute attack to doses of a mydriatic that would be harmless in a normal person.

In some of these examples the underlying pathologic disturbance offers a reasonable explanation for the hypersusceptible response, but this is not always the case. To put it another way, our knowledge of pathologic physiology is often not sufficiently advanced to explain the varying susceptibility to drugs in disease states. This is still another reason why therapeutics remains an art.

PRESENCE OF OTHER DRUGS—SUMMATION, SYNERGISM, ANTAGONISM, AND COMPLEX DRUG INTERACTIONS IN CLINICAL PHARMACOLOGY

When more than one drug is used in the same patient, their actions may be completely independent of one another. Often, however, the combined effect may be greater than that which could have been obtained with a single drug, or a drug may have even less effect than if it were given alone.

Additive effect, synergism, and potentiation

When the combined effect of two drugs is the algebraic sum of the individual actions, it is referred to as *summation, or additive effect.* Another way of stating the additive effect is in terms of doses rather than effects. If a certain dose of drug A and another dose of drug B produce the same effect quantitatively, the additive effect concept implies that one half the dose of each drug used simultaneously would elicit the same effect. *Synergism* is defined in various ways. To some it means an additive, or greater than additive, effect. Others reserve the term to cases where one drug increases the action of another by interfering with its destruction or disposition, thus greatly increasing its action. *Potentiation* generally means a greater than additive effect. The terms synergism and potentiation are commonly abused in pharmaceutical promotion.

Antagonism

Drug antagonism may be of several types: chemical antagonism, physiologic antagonism, and pharmacologic antagonism.

Chemical antagonism. A drug may actually combine with another in the body. This is the basis of the action of the chemical antidotes. For example, dimercaprol (British anti-lewisite; BAL) can combine with mercury or arsenic in the body. The diuretic effect of a mercurial can be blocked by the injection of BAL.

Physiologic antagonism. Two drugs may influence a physiologic system in opposite directions, one drug cancelling the effect of another. The simultaneous injection of properly adjusted doses of vasodilator and vasoconstrictor drugs may cause no change in blood pressure. Stimulants and depressants of the central nervous system can antagonize each other by a similar mechanism.

Pharmacologic antagonism. Two drugs may compete for the same receptor site, the inactive or weak member of the pair preventing the access of the potent drug. This is the phenomenon of pharmacologic antagonism.

Examples of pharmacologic antagonism are the histamine-antihistaminic drug relationships and also atropine-acetylcholine antagonism. It is quite likely that many examples of competitive antagonism in pharmacology are not competition for enzymes but rather for receptor surfaces.

The key point in pharmacologic antagonism is parallel displacement of the dose-response curve of a drug by a second drug. If the two drugs compete for the same receptor, the curves should remain parallel and the height of the curves should remain the same (p. 12).

Complex drug interactions in clinical pharmacology

A drug may interact with another by many different mechanisms. Some of these are (1) absorption from the gastrointestinal tract, (2) binding to plasma proteins, (3) renal excretion, (4) inhibition of metabolic degradation, (5) promotion of metabolic degradation by enzyme induction, and (6) alteration of electrolyte patterns. These and other drug interactions have acquired such an importance in clinical pharmacology that the problem will be discussed in detail in Chapter 58.

CUMULATION, TOLERANCE, AND TACHYPHYLAXIS

Response to dosage can be greatly influenced by certain special features of drug metabolism such as cumulation, tolerance, and tachyphylaxis.

Cumulation

When a drug is administered at such intervals that the body cannot remove one dose before another is injected, cumulation occurs. This is encountered particularly with drugs having a long half-life in the body. Digitoxin persists in the body for many days, and if given at a daily dose significantly greater than 0.2 mg., it will inevitably accumulate and cause toxic effects because the body eliminates less than this amount every 24 hours.

If we plot in a schematic manner the amount of a cumulative drug in the body against the number of doses, the resulting curve is shown in Fig. 5-3. The plateau in the case of drug *b* (Fig. 5-3) indicates that, in general, the amount of drug metabolized in a day is proportional to the amount in the body.

When we deal with cumulative drugs, the dosage will vary greatly, depending on whether we are administering initial or maintenance doses. The former must be large enough to build up a therapeutically effective level in the body, whereas maintenance doses are adjusted to the daily metabolic and excretory rates.

Tolerance

Tolerance is an interesting phenomenon characterized by the need for increasing amounts of a drug to obtain the same therapeutic effect. Drugs vary greatly in their tendency to induce tolerance; perhaps the best known examples are the opium alkaloids. The adult therapeutic dose of morphine is ordinarily 10 to 15 mg., but if the drug is administered repeatedly to a patient, increasing doses are necessary to obtain the same analgesic effect. Finally, enormous doses are sought by the addict who has gradually

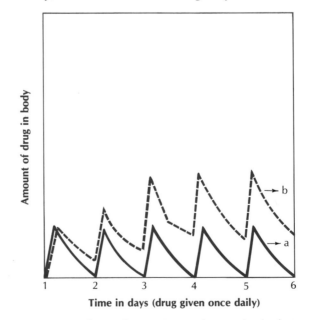

Time in days (drug given once daily)

Fig. 5-3. Illustrating concept of cumulation. Drug a is completely destroyed or excreted in less than 24 hours. Thus it does not accumulate when administered once a day. Drug b requires more than 24 hours for its metabolic degradation or excretion. It is a cumulative drug when it is administered once a day.

developed tolerance. Although it is a well-studied phenomenon, the actual mechanism of tolerance remains mysterious.

Drugs that produce significant tolerance are not numerous. Many are similar to the digitalis glycosides, which can be taken daily for years without tolerance developing.

Tachyphylaxis

Tachyphylaxis is the term reserved for rapidly developing tolerance. This is noted in acute laboratory experiments with certain drugs—for example, vasopressin or certain adrenergic compounds such as amphetamine. In these experiments the first injection of the drug produces a much greater elevation of blood pressure than subsequent injections given after only a brief interval of time.

The mechanism of tachyphylaxis is understood only in some cases. For example, indirectly acting sympathomimetic amines such as amphetamine release norepinephrine from adrenergic nerve endings. Tachyphylaxis probably is a consequence of depletion of available norepinephrine. The same mechanism plays a role in tachyphylaxis to histamine releasers. In other instances the action of a drug may persist at the receptor site, but its overt manifestations are concealed by compensatory reflexes.

PHARMACOGENETICS

Drug effects are greatly influenced by genetically determined variations in susceptibility. Idiosyncrasies in general are most commonly related to pharmacogenetic abnormalities. This subject is discussed in detail on p. 35.

References

1 Abrams, W. B., Bagdon, R. E., and Zbinden, G.: Drug toxicity and its impact on drug evaluation in man, Clin. Pharmacol. Ther. 5:273, 1964.

2 Clark, A. J.: General pharmacology. In Heffter, A., editor: Handbuch der experimentellen Pharmakologie, Berlin, 1937, Springer-Verlag.

3 Dearborn, E. H.: Testing drugs for pharmacologic activity and safety, Biomed. Purview 3:19, 1963.

4 Fouts, J. R., and Brodie, B. B.: On the mechanism of drug potentiation by iproniazid (2-isopropyl-l-isonicotinyl hydrazine), J. Pharmacol. Exp. Ther. 116:480, 1956.

5 Karnofsky, D. A.: Drugs as teratogens in animals and man, Ann. Rev. Pharmacol. 5:447, 1965.

6 Landsteiner, K.: The specificity of serological reactions, Cambridge, 1945, Harvard University Press.

7 Modell, W.: The extraordinary side effects of drugs, Clin. Pharmacol. Ther. 5:265, 1964.

8 Modell, W.: Drug-induced diseases, Ann. Rev. Pharmacol. 5:285, 1965.

9 Parker, C. W., Shapiro, J., Kern, M., and Eisen, H. N.: Hypersensitivity to penicillenic acid derivatives in human beings with penicillin allergy, J. Exp. Med. 115:821, 1962.

10 Prankerd, T. A. J.: Hemolytic effects of drugs and chemical agents, Clin. Pharmacol. Ther. 4:334, 1963.

11 Shaw, D. L.: Clinical evaluation of pharmacologically active compounds, Biomed. Purview 3:30, 1963.

12 Sherlock, S.: Hepatic reactions to therapeutic agents, Ann. Rev. Pharmacol. 5:429, 1965.

13 Zbinden, G.: Experimental and clinical aspects of drug toxicity, Advances Pharmacol. 2:1, 1963.

Recent reviews

14 Barron, B. A., and Bukantz, S. C.: The evaluation of new drugs. Current Food and Drug Administration regulations and statistical aspects of clinical trials, Arch. Intern. Med. 119:547, 1967.

15 Done, A. K.: Perinatal pharmacology, Ann. Rev. Pharmacol. 6:189, 1966.

16 Done, A. K.: Drugs for children. In Modell, W., editor: Drugs of choice 1972-1973, St. Louis, 1972, The C. V. Mosby Co.

17 Editorial: Therapeutic research and the need for a new look, J.A.M.A. 200:547, 1967.

18 Levine, B. B.: Immunochemical mechanisms of drug allergy, Ann. Rev. Med. 17:23, 1966.

19 Shirkey, H. C.: Adverse reactions to drugs—

their relation to growth and development. In Shirkey, H. C., editor: Pediatric therapy, ed. 4, St. Louis, 1972, The C. V. Mosby Co.

20 Stewart, G. T.: Allergy to penicillin and related antibiotics: antigenic and immunochemical mechanisms, Ann. Rev. Pharmacol. 13:309, 1973.

21 Wilson, C. W. M.: The assessment of medical information—a consequence of the drug explosion, J. Irish Med. Ass. 57:147, 1965.

22 Wolfensberger, W.: Ethical issues in research with human subjects, Science 155:47, 1967.

23 Zbinden, G.: Animal toxicity studies: a critical evaluation, Appl. Ther. 8:128, 1966.

24 Zbinden, G.: The significance of pharmacologic screening tests in the preclinical safety evaluation of new drugs, J. New Drugs 6:1, 1966.

SECTION TWO

DRUG EFFECTS ON THE NERVOUS SYSTEM AND NEUROEFFECTORS

6 General aspects of neuropharmacology

It has been estimated that the human nervous system is made up of more than 10 billion neurons.[18] Communication among these neurons is achieved by means of chemical mediators. Since the functions of the nervous system are profoundly dependent on drug effects, it is not surprising that a large variety of compounds act on the nervous system by mimicking the normal chemical mediators or by influencing their actions or metabolism.

The chemical mediators such as acetylcholine and norepinephrine act on postsynaptic or postjunctional membranes by influencing their permeability. Excitatory effects are mediated by permeability changes that lead to depolarization, whereas inhibitory effects are caused by hyperpolarization of the postjunctional membranes. In addition to their postjunctional effects, chemical mediators may exert presynaptic effects that remain to be completely elucidated.

Neuropharmacologic research has provided not only important therapeutic agents, but also valuable tools for the study of the nervous system. We owe much of our knowledge of the autonomic nervous system to studies of neuropharmacologic agents, and the remarkable progress in the understanding of amine metabolism and brain function is largely an outgrowth of investigation on drugs affecting the binding and release of amines in the brain.

In addition to neuropharmacologic agents that influence primarily the action or metabolism of mediators, there are many drugs influencing neural activity by mechanisms that cannot be clearly stated. Nevertheless, they may be classified on the basis of their clinical usage. They will be described under such headings as hypnotics, analgesics, anticonvulsants, general anesthetics, and local anesthetics. Finally, since no drug has a single action, numerous therapeutic agents including hormones may exert effects on the nervous system, although they are not classified as neuropharmacologic drugs.

THE CHEMICAL NEUROTRANSMISSION CONCEPT

The similarity between certain drug effects and those of nerve stimulation was noted prior to this century. Muscarine, from certain mushrooms, was known to slow the heart rate just like vagal stimulation. Adrenal extracts produced effects similar to those following stimulation of sympathetic nerves (Oliver and Shafer, 1895).

Definitive proof of chemical neurotransmission was provided in 1921 by the experiments of Loewi[41] and Cannon.[8] In his classic experiment Otto Loewi demonstrated that when the vagus nerve of a perfused frog heart is stimulated, a substance is released that is capable of slowing a second frog heart with no neural connections to the first. Cannon and Uridil[8] found that sympathetic nerve stimulation of the liver causes the release of a substance similar to epinephrine in many respects. This mediator, at first named "sympathin," is now believed to be norepinephrine. Identification of the neurotransmitter in adrenergic axons as norepinephrine was provided by von Euler.[21]

Acetylcholine was first studied systematically by Dale.[15] The "quantum hypothesis" of acetylcholine release and the role of synaptic vesicles in neuromuscular and synaptic transmission is a contribution of Katz and co-workers.[25,39] The discovery by Brodie and Shore[5] of monoamine release by reserpine led to a great expansion of knowledge regarding the metabolism and function of catecholamines in the nervous system. The uptake of catecholamines by sympathetic nerves is mainly a contribution of Axelrod.[2] The importance of these contributions is attested to by the Nobel Prizes that have been awarded to the great majority of the investigators just cited.

After these discoveries it became apparent that drugs need not necessarily act through nerves to influence an effector organ. In fact, it was then clearly seen that nerves could act by releasing chemical compounds, which in turn influenced the effector structures. Instead of classifying drugs as sympathomimetic and parasympathomimetic, it appeared more reasonable to classify nerves on the basis of the mediator released from them. This led to the concept of cholinergic and adrenergic nerve fibers.[14]

SITES OF ACTION OF CHEMICAL MEDIATORS

The generally accepted sites of action for the neural mediators are as follows:
1. Postganglionic parasympathetic fibers to smooth muscle, cardiac muscle, and exocrine glands: acetylcholine
2. Postganglionic sympathetic fibers to smooth muscle, cardiac muscle, and exocrine glands: norepinephrine (with some exceptions)
3. Synaptic transmission in all autonomic ganglia: acetylcholine (although other amines may modulate transmission)
4. Transmission from motor fibers to skeletal muscle: acetylcholine
5. Central synaptic transmission: acetylcholine is excitatory transmitter at many central synapses; inhibitory transmitters undoubtedly exist; dopamine, norepinephrine, serotonin, and glycine have been postulated as having inhibitory roles at various sites
6. Presynaptic sites: it appears that acetylcholine and the catecholamines may influence mediator release by acting on presynaptic receptors

SYNAPSES AND NEUROMUSCULAR JUNCTIONS

The synapse is the site of transmission of the nerve impulse between two neurons. The axonal terminal is separated from the postsynaptic membrane by a synaptic cleft of about 200 Å in width. Electron micrographs show that the presynaptic element contains numerous vesicles, which are believed to store the transmitter. They also contain some mitochondria.

Transmission of the nerve impulse across the synapse is quite different from axonal conduction. First, transmission is unidirectional. Second, when the axon is stimulated

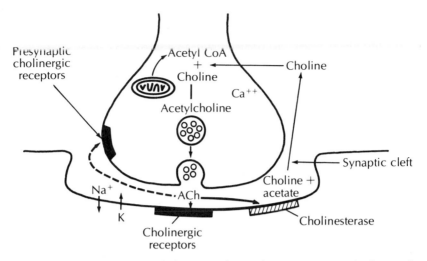

Fig. 6-1. Cholinergic nerve terminal depicting the synthesis, storage, and release of acetylcholine (ACh), its hydrolysis by cholinesterase, and its action on cholinergic receptors on the effector cell and presynaptic receptors.

electrically, there is a delay of about 0.2 second before the postsynaptic element is depolarized.

At somatic motor nerve endings the axon terminal lies within the synaptic gutters. Vesicles containing acetylcholine are present in the axon terminal. Nerve stimulation causes a release of acetylcholine that, diffusing across the gap, causes a change in permeability of the postjunctional membrane to Na^+ and K^+. The release process requires Ca^{++} and is inhibited by Mg^{++}. Botulinus toxin blocks acetylcholine release; hemicholinium, an experimental drug, blocks acetylcholine synthesis, presumably by interfering with the axonal uptake of choline. See Fig. 6-1.

At the terminations of autonomic nerve fibers on smooth muscles, cardiac muscle, or exocrine glands no specialized structures analogous to motor end plates can be seen. The transmitters apparently are discharged at the terminal plexuses into the extracellular space and reach the effector cells by diffusion.

EVIDENCE FOR CHOLINERGIC AND ADRENERGIC NEUROTRANSMISSION

The role of a mediator in neurotransmission is suggested or established by some or all of the following:
1. The presence of the transmitter in the axon along with the enzyme responsible for its production and destruction
2. Similarity of the mediator's effect to that of nerve stimulation
3. Release of the transmitter by nerve stimulation
4. Blockade of the effect of nerve stimulation by drugs that block the transmitter's action

Most of the criteria can be met in studies of neuromuscular transmission and ganglionic transmission. There are formidable difficulties in proving the transmitter role of a substance in the central nervous system by these same criteria.

At *somatic motor nerve endings,* the evidence for the transmitter role of acetylcholine is very convincing. Such nerves contain acetylcholine along with the enzyme choline acetyltransferase. Close intra-arterial injection of acetylcholine elicits a muscle twitch. Release of acetylcholine after motor nerve stimulation can be demonstrated in perfused preparations if the mediator is protected against destruction by the addition of an anticholinesterase. Drugs such as *d*-tubocurarine that block the effect of motor nerve stimulation also block the effect of acetylcholine on skeletal muscle.

At *ganglionic synapses,* the evidence of the transmitter role of acetylcholine is equally as strong as at somatic neuromuscular junctions and is based on observations made on perfused sympathetic ganglia. The adrenal medulla responds to acetylcholine as if it were a modified sympathetic ganglion and secretes epinephrine with smaller quantities of norepinephrine. The secretory process elicited by acetylcholine or stimulation of the splanchnic nerves is blocked by ganglionic blocking agents.

Evidence for the role of acetylcholine at the terminations of *parasympathetic nerves* is substantial, although it is more difficult to obtain because the short postganglionic fibers cannot be directly stimulated. Nevertheless, when the parasympathetic nerve supply to the heart is stimulated, acetylcholine release from the perfused heart can be demonstrated. Similar results have been obtained with some other parasympathetically innervated effector organs. The similarity of the effects of acetylcholine to those of parasympathetic nerve stimulation and the blocking action of atropine further reinforces the concept of cholinergic neurotransmission at parasympathetic endings.

In *sympathetic axon terminals,* the transmitter is undoubtedly norepinephrine. The presence of this catecholamine in such axons and in terminal plexuses can be visualized by fluorescence microscopy (Fig. 8-1). Norepinephrine release by sympathetic stimula-

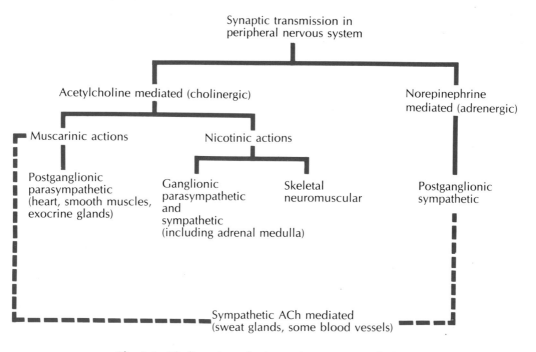

Fig. 6-2. Cholinergic and adrenergic neurotransmission.

tion has been amply demonstrated. Reserpine treatment causes a disappearance of the fluorescent granules from the plexuses and results in decreased sympathetic function. Similarities in the actions of norepinephrine and sympathetic nerve stimulation are well established.

Compared with evidence of actions in the peripheral nervous system, proof of the transmitter role of a compound in the *central nervous system* is extremely difficult to obtain. Acetylcholine is clearly the transmitter to the Renshaw cells from motoneuron collaterals. When applied by iontophoresis, acetylcholine has an effect on the caudate nucleus, supraoptic nucleus, and pyramidal cells of the cortex and other areas.[64] With fluorescence microscopy, adrenergic and serotoninergic pathways have been mapped out by Swedish workers.[12, 70] In addition to the very likely transmitter role for norepinephrine in the central nervous system, there is much evidence for a similar role for dopamine in certain neural pathways. Electrophysiologic effects of various compounds applied by iontophoresis would suggest a bewildering number of potential transmitters in the central nervous system (for details consult reference 64). Glutamate and aspartate have excitatory effects, but glycine, γ-aminobutyric acid, alanine, and serine could conceivably function as inhibitory transmitters. Interestingly, the Chinese restaurant syndrome, characterized by headache and severe discomfort, has been attributed to the high concentration of glutamic acid in Chinese food. The possible role of glycine as a

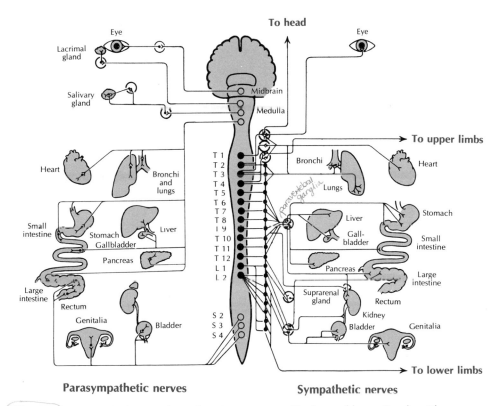

Fig. 6-3. Autonomic innervation of various organs. (Redrawn from a Sandoz Pharmaceuticals publication.)

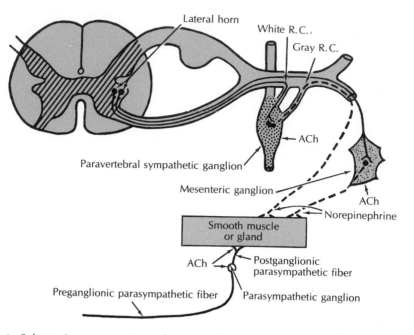

Fig. 6-4. Schematic representation of autonomic innervation of smooth muscle or exocrine gland. *ACh,* Acetylcholine.

spinal inhibitory transmitter is reinforced by observations suggesting that strychnine blocks the effects of glycine on motoneurons of the spinal cord.[16]

Substance P, a polypeptide, is present in brain tissue and in the intestine. It stimulates various smooth muscles, but its role as a transmitter is still unknown.[23]

The autonomic innervation of various organs is indicated in Fig. 6-3, and the likely arrangement of chemical mediators in the peripheral autonomic nervous system is shown in Fig. 6-4.

Additional neural functions for acetylcholine have been postulated but are not generally accepted. A role for acetylcholine in nerve conduction is controversial.[46] There is an interesting suggestion that acetylcholine plays some role even in adrenergic fibers.[7] This suggestion is commonly referred to as the Burn-Rand hypothesis.

MEDIATORS TO SWEAT GLANDS AND ADRENAL MEDULLA

Two apparent exceptions exist to the statement that norepinephrine is the chemical mediator to sympathetically innervated structures. The sweat glands and a few blood vessels, while receiving sympathetic innervation, are known to be activated by cholinergic drugs and inhibited by anticholinergic drugs, atropine being the great inhibitor of sweating. This apparent anomaly has been explained in a satisfactory manner by demonstrating that the particular fibers innervating the sweat glands are cholinergic. In other words, on stimulation they release acetylcholine rather than norepinephrine.

The adrenal medulla is another apparent exception. This structure secretes epinephrine when cholinergic drugs are injected, but its response may be inhibited by ganglionic blocking agents. The explanation of this apparent anomaly is based on embryologic considerations. The adrenal medulla is in reality a modified sympathetic ganglion, and it is therefore not surprising that it should respond to acetylcholine, which is the normal ganglionic mediator for both the sympathetic and parasympathetic nerves.

SEQUENCE OF CHEMICAL EVENTS IN JUNCTIONAL TRANSMISSION

It is well established that the chemical mediators are synthesized by the neurons from precursor substances. The mediators are held in a bound form ready to be mobilized from the nerve endings on the passage of an impulse. Once released, they activate the postsynaptic membrane, probably by altering ionic movements and causing its depolarization. The released mediator is destroyed by specific enzymes, diffuses away from the receptor, or is taken up again by the nerve. In any case, the termination of the action of the mediator allows repolarization of the postsynaptic membrane, making it again responsive to nerve impulses.

The following steps may be distinguished in junctional transmission: (1) synthesis of the mediator, (2) binding of the mediator in a potentially active form, (3) release of the mediator substance, (4) depolarization of postsynaptic membrane, (5) destruction of the mediator, and (6) repolarization of the postsynaptic membrane. Theoretically, at least, drugs could influence junctional transmission by acting at any of the steps, and, indeed, we have examples of many such interactions, as shown in Table 6-1.

It is obvious then that neural transmission is highly vulnerable to drug action, and it is not surprising that we have a large number and variety of neuropharmacologic agents.

PRESYNAPTIC ACTIONS OF DRUGS

Although in the foregoing discussion and in Table 6-1 the postjunctional site of action of drugs is emphasized, there is growing evidence of a presynaptic action of many drugs, particularly in relation to neuromuscular transmission. For example, curare is generally believed to paralyze skeletal muscles by occupying postjunctional cholinergic receptors. On the other hand, several investigators[69] suggest that in addition to the postjunctional effect, curare depresses the release of transmitter from motor nerve terminals by occupying presynaptic receptors. Some even believe that this presynaptic effect is a significant site of action of curare.[72]

Experiments with the venom of the black widow spider also suggest a role for the presynaptic action of acetylcholine.[42, 48] This venom causes a disappearance of the synaptic vesicles and a failure of neuromuscular transmission. Although the postjunctional membrane appears unaffected, its response to exogenous acetylcholine is severely impaired. This experiment suggests that acetylcholine acts on prejunctional receptors to cause further release of acetylcholine, a kind of amplifying mechanism. Although it is impossible to know at present the exact importance of these presynaptic mechanisms of drug action, they are mentioned to indicate that events at junctional transmission are undoubtedly much more complex than has been indicated in the foregoing discussion.

The release of norepinephrine from adrenergic fibers can be inhibited by a presynaptic action exerted on alpha receptors. It appears also that there are presynaptic acetylcholine receptors that can modify the release of mediators from adrenergic fibers.

61

Table 6-1. Sites of drug action in relation to junctional transmission

Site of drug action	Mediator involved	
	Acetylcholine	Norepinephrine
Synthesis of mediator inhibited by:	Hemicholinium*	Methyldopa† α-Methyltyrosine
Binding of mediator in granules inhibited by:		Reserpine Guanethidine
Release of mediator enhanced by:	Carbachol	Tyramine Amphetamine Reserpine Guanethidine
Release of mediator inhibited by:	Botulinus toxin	Bretylium Monoamine oxidase inhibitors (?)

Depolarization of postsynaptic membrane promoted by:	A. Choline esters
	   Pilocarpine
	   Muscarine
	B. Nicotine
	   Dimethylphenyl-
	   piperazinium
	   (DMPP)*
	C. Choline esters
	   Nicotine
	   Phenyltrimethyl-
	   ammonium
	   (PTMA)*
		Catecholamine and related amines

Depolarization of postsynaptic membrane inhibited by:	A. Atropine and related drugs
	
	B. Hexamethonium
	   Nicotine
	C. d-Tubocurarine
	   Succinylcholine
		Alpha-receptor blocking agents: phenoxybenzamine
		Beta-receptor blocking agents: propranolol

*Pharmacologic tool only.
†Major clinical effect due to norepinephrine release rather than inhibition of synthesis.
A. Cholinergic neuroeffector site.
B. Ganglionic site.
C. Skeletal neuromuscular site.

RECEPTOR CONCEPT IN NEUROPHARMACOLOGY

Drugs that inhibit the actions of acetylcholine or norepinephrine at various sites in the body often do so in a selective manner. Thus atropine is very powerful in preventing the actions of acetylcholine on smooth muscles, cardiac muscle, and exocrine glands. At the same time it has very little effect on the actions of acetylcholine on ganglia or skeletal muscle. On the other hand, d-tubocurarine is a potent inhibitor of the skeletal neuromuscular action of acetylcholine, but has very little effect on its smooth muscle actions and blocks ganglionic transmission only in high concentrations. Furthermore, the ganglionic blocking agents such as hexamethonium prevent the effects of acetylcholine on ganglionic transmission without blocking skeletal neuromuscular transmission.

It is reasonable to suppose that there must be at least three receptors for acetylcholine which differ from each other with regard to their interactions with acetylcholine antagonists. Smooth muscles, cardiac muscle, and exocrine glands contain an atropine-sensitive receptor; skeletal muscle, a d-tubocurarine–sensitive receptor; and ganglia, a receptor sensitive to hexamethonium.

Interestingly, there are drugs in nature that appear to have a predilection for one of these receptors. The alkaloid muscarine exerts effects very similar to those of acetylcholine on smooth muscles, cardiac muscle, and exocrine glands without having an effect on ganglionic transmission or skeletal muscle. Nicotine, on the other hand, has a predilection for blocking ganglia following initial stimulation. It also acts on neuromuscular transmission. For these reasons the effects of acetylcholine on smooth muscles, cardiac muscle, and exocrine glands were termed *muscarinic* actions by the pioneer worker Sir Henry Dale, whereas the effects of acetylcholine on ganglia and skeletal muscle were called *nicotinic*. The muscarinic effects are blocked by atropine; the nicotinic effects, by hexamethonium or d-tubocurarine.

The adrenergic receptors are commonly classified as *alpha* and *beta*.[1] When a catecholamine interacts with an alpha receptor, some of the resulting effects are vasoconstriction, pupillary dilatation, and contraction of the nictitating membrane and the splenic capsule. Adrenergic blocking agents that prevent this type of adrenergic drug effect are termed alpha adrenergic blocking agents. Beta receptors for catecholamines mediate such responses as vasodilatation (in skeletal muscle), bronchial relaxation, cardiac acceleration, and positive inotropic effect.

NEWER CONCEPTS ON THE CHOLINERGIC RECEPTOR

A partial isolation of the cholinergic receptor has been achieved[72] as a result of studies on some snake venoms that combine irreversibly with such receptors. It was observed that the alpha toxin of *Bungarus multicinctus,* or bungarotoxin, exerts a postsynaptic blocking action similar to that of d-tubocurarine except that it is irreversible. The toxin can be labeled radioactively and serves admirably for the isolation and study of some cholinergic receptors. It has been estimated from such studies that in an endplate of rat muscle there are about 3×10^7 receptor molecules.

Problem 6-1. What accounts for the muscarinic or nicotinic nature of a cholinergic receptor? Crystallographic analysis of acetylcholine and related agonists provide a tentative answer to this question. Acetylcholine is a flexible molecule and rotation is possible at two different bonds.[72] Muscarinic and nicotinic drugs differ from acetylcholine in the degree of rotation at the sites of torsion. Thus acetylcholine has both muscarinic and nicotinic effects, whereas the purely muscarinic or nicotinic congeners have constraints imposed on them by conformational factors.

FACTORS INFLUENCING RESPONSE OF EFFECTORS TO CHEMICAL MEDIATORS

The response of effector cells may be altered remarkably under certain circumstances. The two conditions that have received attention are sensitization following denervation and sensitization in the presence of other drugs. There are probably many other reasons for the varying susceptibility of different individuals, but the mechanism of this variability is usually quite obscure.

DENERVATION SUPERSENSITIVITY

The supersensitivity of denervated structures is based on several mechanisms. Nonspecific supersensitivity may result from chronically reduced activity in a smooth muscle.[27] For example, chronic treatment of a guinea pig with a ganglionic blocking agent leads in a few days to an increased sensitivity of its isolated ileum to acetylcholine, histamine, potassium, and serotonin.[27] On the other hand, organs deprived of their adrenergic innervation become especially sensitive to catecholamines, probably because of absence of the uptake mechanism for the neurotransmitter (p. 98). Preganglionic denervation, also called deafferentation, is much less effective in increasing the susceptibility of various effectors to catecholamines. In this case the supersensitivity of smooth muscles may be nonspecific, resulting from chronically reduced activity.[27]

A very interesting mechanism appears to be operating in supersensitive skeletal muscle. A week or two following denervation the whole muscle fiber becomes responsive to externally applied acetycholine, whereas only the end plate region was sensitive prior to denervation. It appears as if new acetylcholine receptors had developed as a consequence of denervation.[51]

SENSITIZATION BY DRUGS

In contrast to the supersensitivity induced by denervation and prolonged inactivity, more rapid sensitization to mediators can be produced by certain drugs.

Enzyme inhibitors may be quite effective. The inhibitors of cholinesterase potentiate the actions of acetylcholine. Catechol and pyrogallol may increase the effectiveness of norepinephrine and epinephrine.

Drugs may interfere also with the buffer mechanisms and thereby may allow greater fluctuation in some physiologic parameter such as blood pressure when a neuropharmacologic agent is administered. It has been suggested that protoveratrine can have this action.[33] The ganglionic blocking agents also increase the effectiveness of injected vasoactive drugs, probably by interfering with buffering responses.

The supersensitivity to catecholamines has been studied mostly on the nictitating membrane where two types of supersensitivity may exist.[86] A "presynaptic" supersensitivity develops after surgical denervation and is correlated with the degeneration of adrenergic nerve terminals. It is specific for catecholamines and related amines and develops within 48 hours after denervation. It is undoubtedly related to the absence of the catecholamine uptake mechanism. Another type of supersensitivity, which is nonspecific in that it applies not only to catecholamines but also to acetylcholine and other agonists, develops slowly after surgical denervation or decentralization. It appears to be postsynaptic and requires weeks for its development. This postsynaptic supersensitivity is a consequence of reduced levels of transmitter.

Cocaine,[43,86] antihistaminics,[38] and tricyclic antidepressants cause presynaptic supersensitivity as a consequence of interference with catecholamine re-uptake by the adrenergic terminals. On the other hand, chronic administration of reserpine leads to the postsynaptic type of supersensitivity by chronic depletion of the transmitters. Guanethidine interferes with catecholamine uptake and also produces a long-lasting supersensitivity.[24] It probably exerts both presynaptic and postsynaptic effects.

In general, compounds that have a cocainelike effect on the uptake of catecholamines sensitize effector cells to their pharmacologic effects. The same compounds tend to block the actions of indirectly acting sympathomimetic drugs, such as those of tyramine.

AMINE METABOLISM AND THE NERVOUS SYSTEM

The best known neurotransmitters are nitrogenous bases synthesized by the neuron from precursors and stored in vesicles ready to be released. The active amines do not cross the blood-brain barrier efficiently, whereas the precursor amino acids do.

Only the salient features of biochemical neuropharmacology will be discussed. For greater details specialized texts should be consulted.[64]

ACETYLCHOLINE

The important neurotransmitter acetylcholine is present in certain peripheral nerves and in nerve endings in brain (synaptosomes), where its vesicular localization has been demonstrated.[59]

Acetylcholine is synthesized by the enzyme choline acetyltransferase, previously known as choline acetylase,[47] according to the following schema:

Choline + Acetyl coenzyme A → Acetylcholine + Coenzyme A

Traditionally acetylcholine has been assayed by biologic methods using a skeletal muscle such as the frog rectus abdominis or smooth muscle in the guinea pig ileum as test objects. There are now gas chromatographic techniques available for the same purpose.

During nerve stimulation, *recently* synthesized acetylcholine may be preferentially released. The experimental compound *hemicholinium* blocks the synthesis of the mediator by interfering with the transport of choline across the neuronal membrane.

Acetylcholine released by a nerve impulse must be destroyed rapidly in order to allow the next impulse to act on a repolarized postsynaptic membrane within a few milliseconds. Hydrolysis of acetylcholine reduces the pharmacologic activity of the compound a hundred thousandfold.

Destruction of acetylcholine is accomplished by the *cholinesterases*, which are of two types. *Acetylcholinesterase*, or specific cholinesterase, hydrolyzes acetyl esters of choline more rapidly than butyryl esters. On the other hand, *pseudocholinesterase*, or nonspecific cholinesterase, is sometimes called butyrylcholinesterase because it hydrolyzes butyryl and other esters of choline more rapidly than the acetyl ester. Acetylcholinesterase is localized in neuronal membranes and surprisingly also in membranes of red cells and the placenta, where its function is unknown. Nonspecific cholinesterase is widely distributed in the body. Plasma cholinesterase is of the nonspecific type. Its presence in plasma is not related to neural activity, although its low titer after exposure to anticholinesterase pesticides is a useful method for diagnosing such poisonings. The titer of plasma cholinesterase is depressed also in advanced liver disease, since the enzyme is manufactured in the liver (p. 86).

CATECHOLAMINES

The collective term for norepinephrine (NE), epinephrine, and dopamine is *catecholamine*, since these neurotransmitters are catechols (ortho-dihydroxybenzenes) and contain an amine group in their aliphatic side chain.

Localization

The distribution of catecholamines in the body is well understood, thanks to the availability of suitable methods for their determination, such as the fluorometric assay. In addition, the histochemical fluorescence microscopy techniques developed by Swedish investigators[71] allow an actual visualization of the catecholamine-containing structures (Fig. 8-1), their precise localization, and their susceptibility to drug effects. The fluorescent methods are based on the oxidation of the catecholamines with iodine or, in the case of the histochemical methods, with formaldehyde.

Norepinephrine is present in adrenergic fibers and in certain pathways within the central nervous system. *Epinephrine* constitutes most of the catecholamine present in the human adrenal medulla, although adrenal medullary tumors may contain largely norepinephrine. Small amounts of epinephrine may occur also in various organs and in the central nervous system, but its main function recognized so far has to do with the adrenal medulla. *Dopamine* is present in relatively high concentration in the brain and is particularly concentrated in the caudate nucleus and the putamen.

The distribution of norepinephrine in various organs corresponds well with their adrenergic innervation. Although there is considerable species variation, the heart, arteries, and veins of most mammals contain norepinephrine of the order of 1 μg per gram of tissue.[21] The liver, lungs, and skeletal muscle contain considerably less, whereas the vas deferens has about five to ten times as much.

Table 6-2. Distribution of norepinephrine and dopamine in the human brain (micrograms/gram)*

	Norepinephrine	Dopamine
Frontal lobe	0.00–0.02	0.00
Caudate nucleus	0.04	3.12
Putamen	0.02	5.27
Hypothalamus (anterior part)	0.96	0.18
Substantia nigra	0.04	0.40
Pons	0.04	0.00
Medulla oblongata (dorsal part)	0.13	0.00
Cerebellar cortex	0.02	0.02

*Data from Bertler, A.: Acta Physiol. Scand. **51**:97, 1961.

Biosynthesis

The biosynthesis of catecholamines represents a small but very important portion of the metabolism of tyrosine. Other pathways lead to the formation of thyroxine, p-hydroxyphenylpyruvate, and melanin and to protein synthesis. Tyrosine itself may arise from hydroxylation of phenylalanine or may be taken up directly by the neurons for catecholamine synthesis.

The various steps in the biosynthesis of catecholamines are shown below:

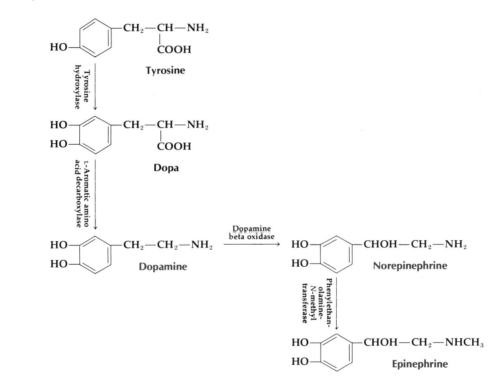

In the order of their functional role in the biosynthesis of catecholamines, the intraneuronal enzymes responsible are tyrosine hydroxylase → L-aromatic amino acid decarboxylase → dopamine-β-oxidase → phenylethanolamine-N-methyl transferase.

Tyrosine hydroxylase[87] appears to be a cytoplasmic enzyme that catalyzes the rate-limiting step in catecholamine biosynthesis. Thus inhibition of this enzyme by amino acid analogues such as α-methyltyrosine leads to a depletion of catecholamines in brain and various sympathetic nerves, with important functional consequences.

L-*Aromatic amino acid decarboxylase* is a cytoplasmic enzyme that decarboxylates a number of substrates in addition to dopa, thereby converting 5-hydroxytryptophan to serotonin and tyrosine to tyramine. As a nonspecific histidine decarboxylase, it also forms histamine in some tissues. Its function in adrenergic neurons is related to the formation of dopamine.

Dopamine-β-oxidase, a copper-containing enzyme bound to the membranes of the exoplasmic granules, catalyzes the conversion of dopamine to norepinephrine. The enzyme is inhibited by copper reagents such as disulfiram and diethyldithiocarbamate. It is generally impossible, however, to lower norepinephrine levels in tissues by the administration of such inhibitors, since dopamine-β-oxidase is not a rate-limiting enzyme in catecholamine biosynthesis. Because the enzyme is associated with the catecholamine vesicles, sympathetic stimulation could lead to the appearance of dopamine-β-oxidase activity in the circulation.[58]

Phenylethanolamine-N-methyl-transferase is a cytoplasmic enzyme present largely in the adrenal medulla where it catalyzes the transfer of a methyl group from S-adenosylmethionine to norepinephrine for the formation of epinephrine.

Negative feedback of catecholamine biosynthesis. Sympathetic nerve stimulation does not cause catecholamine depletion in the axon, suggesting that increased synthesis can keep up with loss. With the discovery of tyrosine hydroxylase as the rate-limiting enzyme in catecholamine biosynthesis, the relative constancy of catecholamine stores can be explained. Norepinephrine and dopamine inhibit tyrosine hydroxylase. It becomes understandable, then, that increased catecholamine release through sympathetic activity will lead to accelerated synthesis of catecholamines at nerve terminals. On the other hand, monoamine oxidase inhibitors, which elevate catecholamine levels in adrenergic neurons, also lead to a slowdown in catecholamine biosynthesis. Since there are reasons to believe that *recently* synthesized catecholamines are preferentially released by sympathetic nerve stimulation, the hypotensive effect of the monoamine oxidase inhibitors (p. 173) may thus become understandable.

Storage and release

Catecholamines are stored in vesicles in association with ATP and a soluble protein *chromogranin*. The vesicles are formed originally in the nerve cell body and are transported to the endings by axoplasmic flow. Constriction of an adrenergic nerve causes the accumulation of vesicles proximal to the ligature.[13] The number of vesicles does not change between two ligatures, an indication again of the need for axoplasmic flow for the transport of the vesicles and their lack of synthesis in the axon. Although the vesicles are probably formed in the cell body and are transported from there, catecholamine biosynthesis undoubtedly takes place in the axonal terminals also. Otherwise one could not explain the failure of nerve stimulation to cause depletion of catecholamines. Axoplasmic flow is of the order of 1 to 10 mm. per hour, calculated by Dahlström[13] for catecholamine-containing vesicles. Such relatively slow movement of catecholamines could not account for the observed constancy of the norepinephrine content of stimulated sympathetic nerves.

Release of catecholamines is believed to take place by a specialized form of exocytosis. During the release process ATP, chromogranin, and dopamine-β-oxidase appear in the perfusate of adrenal medullary tissue[65] in addition to catecholamines. Although these findings suggest that the vesicles empty their content, other evidence indicates that recently synthesized catecholamine is released preferentially. Perhaps only a small portion of the vesicles containing the recently synthesized catecholamine are released under these circumstances.

In contrast with release by exocytosis, reserpine causes the release of the granular catecholamines into the axoplasm, where they are deaminated by the enzyme mono-amine oxidase (MAO) present in the axonal mitochondria.

Catecholamine release requires calcium[65] and is in this respect similar to acetyl-choline release from cholinergic nerves and to histamine release from mast cells.

Disposition of the released catecholamine

The relative constancy of catecholamine stores in adrenergic neurons is not only a consequence of feedback regulation of its biosynthesis. It is also an expression of a remarkable ability of these neurons to take up the amines after their release. More than half the released catecholamine may be conserved by this mechanism, which will be discussed in greater detail (p. 102). The reuptake by the so-called "amine pump" is sodium dependent and is inhibited by ouabain, a known blocker of the Na^+- and K^+-activated membrane ATPase. It is also inhibited by cocaine, desipramine, and some antihistaminics (p. 103). The amine pump is fairly nonspecific, since it transports not only catecholamines but also serotonin, amphetamine, and unnatural isomers of bio-genic amines. What protects the axon from the accumulation of all sorts of amines is a greater specificity of the granular storage mechanism.[81]

The portion of the released catecholamine that escapes the amine pump reuptake is attacked by two enzymes: *catechol-O-methyl transferase* and *monoamine oxidase.* The latter is widely distributed in the body, not only in adrenergic axonal mitochondria but also in nonneural structures. Catechol-O-methyl transferase is also widely dis-tributed and is particularly concentrated in the liver and kidneys. Although the precise relationship of these enzymes to sympathetic function is not understood, it is clearly not as crucial as the acetylcholine-cholinesterase interdependence. For example, inhi-bition of catechol-O-methyl transferase by catechol or pyrogallol does not cause a significant increase in sympathetic activity or potentiation of the action of injected catecholamines. Similarly, drugs that inhibit monoamine oxidase fail to potentiate the action of catecholamines and do not increase sympathetic functions in the periphery. On the other hand, the antidepressant action of these drugs suggests a role for mono-amine oxidase in the central nervous system.

The detailed metabolic pathways of catecholamines are shown in Fig. 6-5. The role of many of these pathways may be appreciated from data on the urinary excretion of catecholamine metabolites in normal humans; the percentages of endogenous cate-cholamines and metabolites are as follows:

Norepinephrine + epinephrine	1.1%
Normetanephrine + metanephrine	7.6%
Vanylmandelic acid (VMA)	91.0%

The 24-hour VMA excretion in normal individuals is 10 mg. Much larger amounts may be excreted by patients with adrenal medullary tumors (p. 106).

Interaction of drugs with catecholamine storage and release mechanisms

Numerous clinically useful drugs interact with the storage and release of cate-cholamines. They are listed in Table 6-3 and will be discussed in some detail in the appropriate chapters.[*]

---

*For an up-to-date review of drug effects on the presynaptic regulation of catecholamine release, see Langer, S. Z.: Presynaptic regulation of catecholamine release, Biochem. Pharmacol. (In press.)

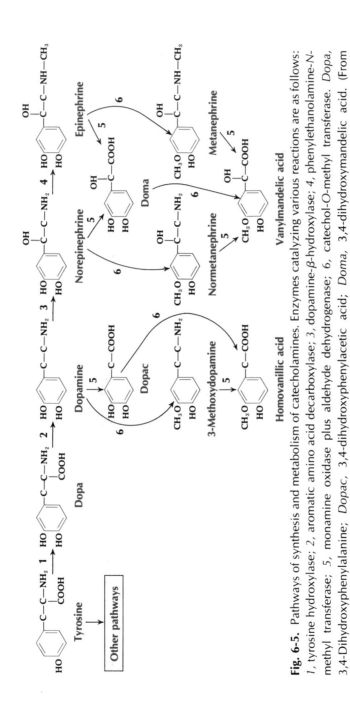

Fig. 6-5. Pathways of synthesis and metabolism of catecholamines. Enzymes catalyzing various reactions are as follows: *1*, tyrosine hydroxylase; *2*, aromatic amino acid decarboxylase; *3*, dopamine-β-hydroxylase; *4*, phenylethanolamine-N-methyl transferase; *5*, monamine oxidase plus aldehyde dehydrogenase; *6*, catechol-O-methyl transferase. *Dopa*, 3,4-Dihydroxyphenylalanine; *Dopac*, 3,4-dihydroxyphenylacetic acid; *Doma*, 3,4-dihydroxymandelic acid. (From Crout, J. R.: Catecholamine metabolism. In Manger, C. W., editor: Hormones and hypertension, Springfield, Ill., 1966, Charles C Thomas, Publisher.)

Table 6-3. Drugs interacting with catecholamine storage and release mechanisms*

Clinical use	Drug	Site of action
Antihypertensive	NE depletors Reserpine Guanethidine	Blockade of intraneuronal storage
Antihypertensive	False transmitters α-Methyldopa	Substitution of NE by false transmitter in storage granules
Antihypertensive	MAO inhibitors Pargyline	Inhibition of NE release by free NE or false transmitter
Antihypertensive	Neuron blockers Bretylium Debrisoquin	Prevention of NE release; also MAO inhibition
Sympathomimetic	Amphetamine Ephedrine	NE release from granules
Antidepressant	Tricyclic drugs Imipramine Amitriptyline	Inhibition of adrenergic neuronal membrane amine carrier system

*Modified from Shore, P. A.: In Jones, R. J., editor: Proceedings of the Second International Symposium, New York, 1970, Springer-Verlag, p. 528.

CHEMICAL SYMPATHECTOMY: 6-HYDROXYDOPAMINE

The administration of 6-hydroxydopamine, an interesting experimental tool, causes an extremely long-lasting depletion of catecholamines in organs innervated by the sympathetic division. Electron microscopic studies indicate that the drug causes a selective destruction of peripheral adrenergic nerve terminals. In newborn animals the whole neuron is destroyed irreversibly, whereas in adults only the terminals are affected so that regeneration of the fibers is possible.[85] To destroy adrenergic terminals in the central nervous system, 6-hydroxydopamine must be injected into the ventricles because it does not cross the blood-brain barrier.

There is every reason to believe that chemical sympathectomy will contribute important information in addition to what has been learned from immunologic and surgical methods already.

SEROTONIN

Serotonin, or 5-hydroxytryptamine, is present in high concentrations in the enterochromaffin cells of the intestinal tract and in the pineal gland. It is also present in the brain, in platelets, and in mast cells of rats and mice. Serotonin occurs also in some fruits such as bananas.

The steps in the biosynthesis of serotonin are as follows:

$$\text{Tryptophan} \xrightarrow[\text{hydroxylase}]{\text{Tryptophan}} \text{5-Hydroxytryptophan} \xrightarrow[\text{decarboxylase}]{\text{L-Aromatic amino acid}} \text{5-Hydroxytryptamine}$$

Serotonin is degraded to 5-hydroxyindolacetic acid by the enzyme monoamine oxidase. The daily excretion of 5-hydroxyindolacetic acid in man is about 3 mg. It may increase greatly in patients with carcinoid tumor or after the administration of reserpine. The ingestion of bananas also results in elevated concentrations of 5-hydroxyindolacetic acid in the urine.

71

In the pineal gland there is not only a high concentration of serotonin but also a biosynthetic product of the amine, 5-methoxy-N-acetyltryptamine, also known as melatonin. This unique product lightens skin color by affecting melanocytes. It also exerts an effect on gonadal functions in female rats. Interestingly melatonin synthesis is greatly influenced by light.[64]

Although the precise function of serotonin in the nervous system is unknown, research on this potential neurotransmitter has had a profound influence on psychopharmacology. For one thing, many hallucinogenic drugs are structurally related to serotonin, such as bufotenine (5-hydroxy-dimethyl-tryptamine) and psilocin (4-hydroxy-dimethyltryptamine). Also, LSD is an indole derivative that antagonizes the effects of serotonin, at least on smooth muscles. In addition, the release of serotonin from the brain by reserpine and the antagonism of many serotonin effects by chlorpromazine added to the general optimism in the late 1950's concerning a role for this biogenic amine in brain function and mental illness.

Unfortunately, a simple connection between serotonin and mental illness is not suggested by studies with a potent inhibitor of serotonin synthesis, para-chlorophenylalanine. This experimental drug blocks the hydroxylation of tryptophan and causes a marked depletion of serotonin in the brain. Despite this fact, its administration to animals or man has failed to produce marked changes in mood and behavior.[20] An apparent aphrodisiac effect has been described in cats,[26] and some changes in mood have been noted in man after the use of p-chlorophenylalanine. These changes, however, were not great enough to explain either the actions of reserpine or those of LSD on the basis of a simple serotonin hypothesis.

For a more detailed discussion of serotonin see Chapter 17.

MISCELLANEOUS POTENTIAL NEUROTRANSMITTERS

In addition to the previously discussed neurotransmitters, several endogenous compounds may play a role in neural function, although the available evidence is hardly sufficient for characterizing them as mediators of neurotransmission.

Histamine is present in the hypothalamus along with serotonin and catecholamines. Its presence in adrenergic nerves is interesting but may be related to the presence of mast cells in close proximity to these nerves. The brain can form histamine from histidine and is rich in the methylating enzyme that inactivates this biogenic amine. Unfortunately no powerful inhibitors of the methylating enzyme are available. Histamine will be discussed in detail in Chapter 15.

Glutamic and *aspartic acid* are remarkably potent in causing depolarization of nerve cells when applied by iontophoresis. Since these amino acids are normally present in the brain, they could conceivably have some neurotransmitter function. Nevertheless, most criteria for proving the neurotransmitter role of a compound cannot be met by these amino acids.

Glycine is recognized increasingly as a probable inhibitory transmitter in the spinal cord. This simple amino acid is present in high concentration in the spinal cord and causes hyperpolarization of motoneurons.[89] Since strychnine is known to antagonize the effects of the naturally occuring inhibitory transmitter released from Renshaw cells to motoneurons, it was of great interest to examine the possible relationship between the alkaloid and glycine.[16] Antagonism of the hyperpolarizing effect of glycine by strychnine applied by microelectrophoresis has been clearly demonstrated. Interestingly, tetanus toxin in the same system does not antagonize the actions of glycine, implying a presynaptic site of action for the toxin.

γ-Aminobutyric acid (GABA) has also received some attention as a naturally occurring amine that may have a role in brain function. This compound is made by brain tissue through decarboxylation of glutamic acid. The structures of glutamic acid and GABA are as follows:

$$NH_2$$
$$HOOC—CH—CH_2—CH_2—COOH \qquad H_2N—CH_2—CH_2—CH_2—COOH$$

Glutamic acid   γ-Aminobutyric acid

Brain tissue contains significant quantities of GABA. Its destruction is accomplished through transamination. The study of the effects of GABA on brain function has been greatly handicapped by the fact that it does not cross the blood-brain barrier effectively when injected. As a consequence, when the drug is injected intravascularly into animals, even in large doses, it is quite inert as far as brain function is concerned. There are indirect reasons for believing that the compound may have some modulating effect on brain function. Since the decarboxylation of glutamic acid requires pyridoxal as a coenzyme, injections of thiosemicarbazide result in a decrease of GABA concentration in the brain. As thiosemicarbazide also causes convulsions, it has been postulated that the convulsions are related to a decreased GABA level in the brain. The convulsions can be antagonized by the injection of pyridoxal.

Crustacean stretch receptors are inhibited by GABA, and studies of Purpura and co-workers[50] suggest that GABA and related omega amino acids may have inhibitory properties on central synaptic transmission when applied directly to the brain surface.

Studies on spinal cord motoneurons do not suggest a role for γ-aminobutyric acid as an inhibitory transmitter. For example, no antagonism between strychnine and γ-aminobutyric acid could be demonstrated,[16] in contrast with strychnine-glycine antagonism. On the other hand, it is conceivable that γ-aminobutyric acid may function as an inhibitory transmitter in areas other than the spinal cord, such as the cerebellum.

Polypeptides such as substance P and kinins have powerful effects on smooth muscles, but little evidence exists at present for their neurotransmitter role. The *prostaglandins*, acidic lipids of great current research interest, also have important actions on smooth muscles. Because they occur in the nervous system, they may play a role in neural function. Nevertheless, all these compounds are more remarkable at present for their pharmacologic actions than for their known physiologic roles. They will be discussed in Chapter 18.

CLASSIFICATION OF NEUROPHARMACOLOGIC AGENTS

Among the hundreds of neuropharmacologic agents, there are many that can be categorized as mimicking or opposing the actions of acetylcholine or norepinephrine.

While the terms *cholinergic* and *adrenergic* are reserved by tradition for nerves rather than drugs, they will also be used in this book as synonyms for cholinomimetic and sympathomimetic, respectively. Thus, in dealing with autonomic nervous system drugs, one may speak of (1) cholinergic (cholinomimetic) drugs, (2) adrenergic (sympathomimetic) drugs, (3) anticholinergic drugs (various types), and (4) adrenergic blocking agents. In addition to these drugs, the adrenergic neuronal blocking agents, histamine, and antihistaminic drugs will also be discussed in this section.

References

1 Ahlquist, R. P.: A Study of the adrenotropic receptors, Amer. J. Physiol. 153:586, 1948.

2 Axelrod, J.: The metabolism of catecholamines in vivo and in vitro, Pharmacol. Rev. 11:402, 1959.

3 Bertler, A.: Occurrence and localization of catechol amines in the human brain, Acta Physiol. Scand. 51:97, 1961.

4 Blaschko, H.: The development of current concepts of catecholamine formation, Pharmacol. Rev. 11:307, 1959.

5 Brodie, B. B., Spector, S., and Shore, P. A.: Interaction of drugs with norepinephrine in the brain, Pharmacol. Rev. 11:548, 1959.

6 Burgen, A., and MacIntosh, F.: The physiological significance of acetylcholine. In Elliott, K. A. C., et al., editors: Neurochemistry, Springfield, Ill., 1955, Charles C Thomas, Publisher.

7 Burn, J. H., and Rand, M. J.: A new interpretation of the adrenergic nerve fiber, Advances Pharmacol. 1:1, 1962.

8 Cannon, W. B., and Uridil, J. E.: Studies on conditions of activity in endocrine glands: some effects on the denervated heart of stimulating nerves of the liver, Amer. J. Physiol. 58:353, 1921.

9 Carlsson, A.: The occurrence, distribution and physiological role of catecholamines in the nervous system, Pharmacol. Rev. 11:490, 1959.

10 Carlsson, A., and Hillarp, N. A.: On the state of catechol amines of the adrenal medullary granules, Acta Physiol. Scand. 44:163, 1958.

11 Curtis, D., Phillips, J., and Watkins, J.: The depression of spinal neurones by γ-amino-n-butyric acid and β-alanine, J. Physiol. 146:185, 1959.

12 Dahlström, A., and Fuxe, K.: Evidence for the existence of monoamine-containing neurons in the central nervous system. I. Demonstration of monoamines in the cell bodies of brain stem neurons, Acta Physiol. Scand (supp. 232) 62:1, 1965.

13 Dahlström, A., and Häggendal, J.: Studies on the transport and life-span of amine storage granules in a peripheral adrenergic neuron system, Acta Physiol. Scand. 67:278, 1966.

14 Dale, H. H.: On some physiological actions of ergot, J. Physiol. 34:163, 1906.

15 Dale, H. H.: The action of certain esters and ethers of choline and their relation to muscarine, J. Pharmacol. Exp. Ther. 6:147, 1914.

16 Davidoff, R. A., Aprison, M. H., and Werman, R.: The effects of strychnine on the inhibition of interneurons by glycine and γ-aminobutyric acid, Int. J. Neuropharmacol. 8:191, 1969.

17 Dengler, H. J., Spiegel, H. E., and Titus, E. O.: Effect of drugs on uptake of isotopic norepinephrine by cat tissues, Nature 191:816, 1961.

18 Eccles, J. C.: The physiology of nerve cells, Baltimore, 1957, The Johns Hopkins Press.

19 Elliott, T. R.: The action of adrenalin, J. Physiol. 32:401, 1905.

20 Engleman, K., Lovenberg, W., and Sjoerdsma, A.: Inhibition of serotonin synthesis by parachlorophenylalanine in patients with the carcinoid syndrome, New Eng. J. Med. 277:1103, 1967.

21 von Euler, U. S.: Noradrenaline: chemistry, physiology, pharmacology and clinical aspects, Springfield, Ill., 1956, Charles C Thomas, Publisher.

22 von Euler, U. S.: Pieces in the puzzle, Ann. Rev. Pharmacol. 11:1, 1971.

23 von Euler, U. S., and Pernow, B.: Neurotropic effects of substance P, Acta Physiol. Scand. 36:265, 1956.

24 Evans, B., Iwayama, T., and Burnstock, G.: Long-lasting supersensitivity of the rat vas deferens to norepinephrine after chronic guanethidine administration, J. Pharmacol. Exp. Ther. 185:60, 1973.

25 Fatt, P., and Katz, B.: Spontaneous subthreshold activity at motor nerve endings, J. Physiol. 117:109, 1952.

26 Ferguson, J., Henriksen, S., Cohen H., Mitchell, G., Barchas J., and Dement, W.: "Hypersexuality" and behavioral changes in cats caused by the administration of p-chlorophenylalanine, Science 168:499, 1970.

27 Fleming, W. W.: Nonspecific supersensitivity of the guinea-pig ileum produced by chronic ganglion blockade, J. Pharmacol. Exp. Ther. 162:277, 1968.

28 Fleming, W. W., and Trendelenburg, U.: Development of supersensitivity to norepinephrine after pretreatment with reserpine, J. Pharmacol. Exp. Ther. 133:41, 1961.

29 Furchgott, R. F.: Receptors for sympathomi-

metic amines. In Adrenergic mechanisms, Ciba Foundation and Committee for Symposium on Drug Action, Boston, 1960, Little, Brown & Co.

30 Galindo, A.: Curare and pancuronium compared: effects on previously undepressed mammalian myoneural junctions, Science 178:753, 1972.

31 Gewirtz, G. P., and Kopin, I. J.: Effect of intermittent nerve stimulation on norepinephrine synthesis and mobilization in the perfused cat spleen, J. Pharmacol. Exp. Ther. 175:514, 1970.

32 Giachetti, A., and Shore, P. A.: Studies in vitro of amine uptake mechanisms in heart, Biochem. Pharmacol. 15:607, 1966.

33 Goth, A., and Harrison, F.: Influence of protoveratrine on effect of vasoactive drugs, Proc. Soc. Exp. Biol. Med. 87:437, 1954.

34 Govier, W. C., Sugrue, M. F., and Shore, P. A.: On the inability to produce supersensitivity to catecholamines in intestinal smooth muscle, J. Pharmacol. Exp. Ther. 165:71, 1969.

35 Harrison, F., and Goth, A.: Effect of reserpine on the hypothalamic pressor response, J. Pharmacol. Exp. Ther. 116:262, 1956.

36 Hertting, G., Axelrod, J., and Whitby, L. G.: Effect of drugs on the uptake and metabolism of H³-norepinephrine, J. Pharmacol. Exp. Ther. 134:146, 1961.

37 Holzbauer, M., and Vogt, M.: Depression by reserpine of the noradrenaline of the hypothalamus of the cat, J. Neurochem. 1:8, 1956.

38 Isaac, L., and Goth, A.: The mechanism of the potentiation of norepinephrine by antihistaminics, J. Pharmacol. Exp. Ther. 156:463, 1967.

39 Katz, B., and Miledi, R.: Propagation of electric activity in motor nerve terminals, Proc. Roy. Soc. [Biol.] 161:483, 1965.

40 Koelle, G. B.: The elimination of enzymatic diffusion artifacts in the histochemical localization of cholinesterases and a survey of their cellular distributions, J. Pharmacol. Exp. Ther. 103:152, 1951.

41 Loewi, O.: Über humorale Übertragbarkeit der Herznervenwirkung, Arch. Ges. Physiol. 189:239, 1921.

42 Longenecker, H. E., Hurlbut, W. P., Mauro, A., and Clark, A. W.: Effect of black widow spider venom on the frog neuromuscular junction, Nature 225:701, 1970.

43 MacMillan, W. H.: A hypothesis concerning the effect of cocaine on the action of sympathomimetic amines, Brit. J. Pharmacol. 14:385, 1969.

44 Maxwell, R. A., Plummer, A. J., Povalski, H., and Schneider, F.: Concerning a possible action of guanethidine (SU-5864) in smooth muscle, J. Pharmacol. Exp. Ther. 129:24, 1960.

45 Miledi, R.: The acetylcholine sensitivity of frog muscle fibers after complete or partial denervation, J. Physiol. 151:1, 1960.

46 Nachmansohn, D.: Studies on permeability in relation to nerve function. I. Axonal conduction and synaptic transmission, Biochim. Biophys. Acta 4:78, 1950.

47 Nachmansohn, D., and Machado, A. L.: The formation of acetylcholine. A new enzyme: "choline acetylase," J. Neurophysiol. 6:397, 1943.

48 Okamoto, M., Longenecker, H. E., and Riker, W. F.: Destruction of mammalian motor nerve terminals by black widow spider venom, Science 172:733, 1971.

49 Palade, G. E., and Palay, S. L.: Electron microscope observations of interneuronal and neuromuscular synapses, Anat. Rec. 118:335, 1954.

50 Purpura, D. P., Girado, M., Smith, T. G., Callan, D. A., and Grundfest, H.: Structure-activity determinants of pharmacological effects of amino acids and related compounds on central synapses, J. Neurochem. 3:238, 1959.

51 Shore, P. A.: Release of serotonin and catecholamines by drugs, Pharmacol. Rev. 14:531, 1962.

52 Shore, P. A., and Olin, J.: Identification and chemical assay of norepinephrine in brain and other tissues, J. Pharmacol. Exp. Ther. 122:295, 1958.

53 Trendelenburg, U.: The supersensitivity caused by cocaine, J. Pharmacol. Exp. Ther. 125:55, 1959.

54 Udenfriend, S.: Amine metabolism and its pharmacological implications. In Neuropharmacology, Transactions of the Fifth Conference, New York, 1960, Josiah Macy, Jr., Foundation.

55 Varma, D. R., and McCullough, H. N.: Dissociation of the supersensitivity to norepinephrine caused by cocaine from inhibition of H³-norepinephrine uptake in cold stored smooth muscle, J. Pharmacol. Exp. Ther. 166:26, 1969.

56 Vogt, M.: Catecholamines in brain, Pharmacol. Rev. 11:483, 1959.

57 Weiner, N., and Trendelenburg, U.: The effect of cocaine and of pretreatment with reserpine on the uptake of tyramine-2-C¹⁴ and DL-epinephrine-2-C¹⁴ into heart and spleen, J. Pharmacol. Exp. Ther. 137:56, 1962.

58 Weinshilboum, R. M., Thoa, N. B., Johnson, D. G., Kopin, I. J., and Axelrod, J.: Proportional release of norepinephrine and dopamine-β-hydroxylase from sympathetic nerves, Science 174:1349, 1971.

59 Whittaker, V.: Identification of acetylcholine and related esters of biological origin. In Heffter, A., and Heubner, W., editors: Handbuch der

experimentellen Pharmakologie, vol. 15, Berlin, 1962, Springer-Verlag.

60 Zeller, E. A.: The role of amine oxidases in the destruction of catecholamines, Pharmacol. Rev. **11**:387, 1959.

Recent reviews

61 Bhagat, B. D.: Recent advances in adrenergic mechanisms, Springfield, Ill., 1971, Charles C Thomas, Publisher.

62 Boura, A. L. A., and Green, A. F.: Adrenergic neuron blocking agents, Ann. Rev. Pharmacol. **5**:183, 1965.

63 Burn, J. H.: Release of noradrenaline from the sympathetic postganglionic fibre, Brit. Med. J. **2**:196, 1967.

64 Cooper, J. R., Bloom, F. E., and Roth, R. H.: The biochemical basis of neuropharmacology, New York, 1970, Oxford University Press, Inc.

65 Douglas, W. W.: Stimulus-secretion coupling: the concept and clues from chromaffin and other cells, Brit. J. Pharmacol. **34**:451, 1968.

66 Eränkö, O.: Histochemistry of nervous tissues: catecholamines and cholinesterases, Ann. Rev. Pharmacol. **7**:203, 1967.

67 Ferry, C. B.: Cholinergic link hypothesis in adrenergic neuroeffector transmission, Physiol. Rev. **46**:420, 1966.

68 Ferry, C. B.: The autonomic nervous system, Ann. Rev. Pharmacol. **7**:185, 1967.

69 Galindo, A.: The role of prejunctional effects in myoneural transmission, Anesthesiology **36**:598, 1972.

70 Ginsborg, B. L.: Ion movements in junctional transmission, Pharmacol. Rev. **19**:289, 1967.

71 Hillarp, N. A., Fuxe, K., and Dahlström, A.: Demonstration and mapping of central neurons containing dopamine, noradrenaline, and 5-hydroxytryptamine and their reactions to psychopharmaca, Pharmacol. Rev. **18**:727, 1966.

72 Hubbard, J. I., and Quastel, D. M. J.: Micropharmacology of vertebrate neuro-muscular transmission, Ann. Rev. Pharmacol. **13**:199, 1973.

73 Izquierdo, I., and Izquierdo, J. A.: Effects of drugs on deep brain centers, Ann. Rev. Pharmacol. **11**:189, 1971.

74 Kirshner, N., and Viveros, O. H.: In Schümann, H. J., and Kroneberg, G., editors: New aspects of storage and release of catecholamines, Berlin, 1970, Springer-Verlag.

75 McLennan, H.: Synaptic transmission, Philadelphia, 1963, W. B. Saunders Co.

76 Pohorecky, L. A., and Wurtman, R. J.: Adrenocortical control of epinephrine synthesis, Pharmacol. Rev. **23**:1, 1971.

77 Riker, W. F.: Pharmacologic considerations in a reevaluation of the neuromuscular synapse, Arch. Neurol. **3**:488, 1960.

78 Rubin, R. P.: The role of calcium in the release of neurotransmitter substances and hormones, Pharmacol. Rev. **22**:389, 1970.

79 Salmoiraghi, G. C., Costa, E., and Bloom, F. E.: Pharmacology of central synapses, Ann. Rev. Pharmacol. **5**:213, 1965.

80 Shore, P. A.: Drugs affecting catecholamine metabolism and storage in the adrenergic neurone. In Jones, R., editor: Atherosclerosis, Proceedings of the Second International Symposium, New York, 1970, Springer-Verlag.

81 Shore, P. A.: Transport and storage of biogenic amines, Ann. Rev. Pharmacol. **12**:209, 1972.

82 Sulser, F., and Sanders-Bush, E.: Effect of drugs on amines in the CNS, Ann. Rev. Pharmacol. **11**:209, 1971.

83 Symposium: Adrenergic mechanisms, Ciba Foundation and Committee for Symposium on Drug Action, Boston, 1960, Little, Brown & Co.

84 Thesleff, S., and Quastel, D. M. J.: Neuromuscular pharmacology, Ann. Rev. Pharmacol. **5**:263, 1965.

85 Thoenen, H., and Tranzer, J. P.: The pharmacology of 6-hydroxydopamine, Ann. Rev. Pharmacol. **13**:169, 1973.

86 Trendelenburg, U.: Mechanisms of supersensitivity and subsensitivity to sympathomimetic amines, Pharmacol. Rev. **18**:629, 1966.

87 Udenfriend, S.: Tyrosine hydroxylase, Pharmacol. Rev. **18**:43, 1966.

88 Volle, R. L.: Pharmacology of the autonomic nervous system, Ann. Rev. Pharmacol. **3**:129, 1963.

89 Willis, W. D.: The case for the Renshaw cell. In Riss, W., editor: Brain, behavior and evolution, vol. 4, Basel, 1971, S. Karger AG.

7 Cholinergic (cholinomimetic) drugs

The various cholinergic drugs can be divided into two major groups: directly acting cholinergic drugs and cholinesterase inhibitors.

DIRECTLY ACTING CHOLINERGIC DRUGS
CHOLINE ESTERS

Although acetylcholine is an essential compound from the standpoint of its role in body physiology, two important considerations render it useless as a drug. First, even when it is injected intravenously, its actions are very brief because of its rapid destruction by the ubiquitous cholinesterases. Second, it has so many diverse effects that no selective therapeutic purpose can be achieved through its use. The various derivatives of acetylcholine, however, differ from the parent compound by being more resistant to the action of the cholinesterases and by having a certain amount of selectivity in their sites of action.

If we depict the acetylcholine-receptor combination in a manner similar to that postulated for acetylcholine-cholinesterase, as shown in Fig. 7-1, it can be seen that slight changes in the structure should alter the union of the drug with the receptor. Some of these changes can prevent an enzymatic attack on the molecule while still allowing an interaction of the drug with some of the receptors.

Drugs in this group that have some importance are the following:

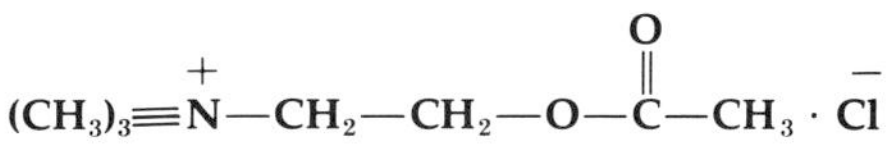

$$(CH_3)_3 \overset{+}{\equiv} N-CH_2-CH_2-O-\overset{\overset{\displaystyle O}{\|}}{C}-CH_3 \cdot \overset{-}{Cl}$$

Acetylcholine chloride

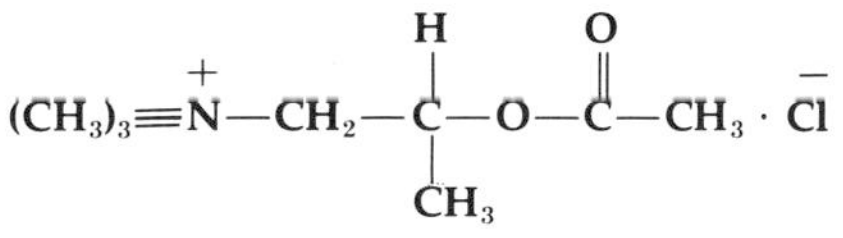

$$(CH_3)_3 \overset{+}{\equiv} N-CH_2-\underset{\underset{\displaystyle CH_3}{|}}{\overset{\overset{\displaystyle H}{|}}{C}}-O-\overset{\overset{\displaystyle O}{\|}}{C}-CH_3 \cdot \overset{-}{Cl}$$

Methacholine chloride

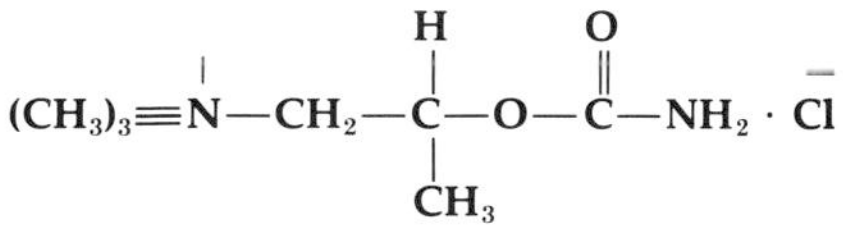

$$(CH_3)_3 \overset{|}{\equiv} N-CH_2-\underset{\underset{\displaystyle CH_3}{|}}{\overset{\overset{\displaystyle H}{|}}{C}}-O-\overset{\overset{\displaystyle O}{\|}}{C}-NH_2 \cdot \overset{-}{Cl}$$

Bethanechol chloride

$$(CH_3)_3 \overset{+}{\equiv} N-CH_2-CH_2-O-\overset{\overset{\displaystyle O}{\|}}{C}-NH_2 \cdot \overset{-}{Cl}$$

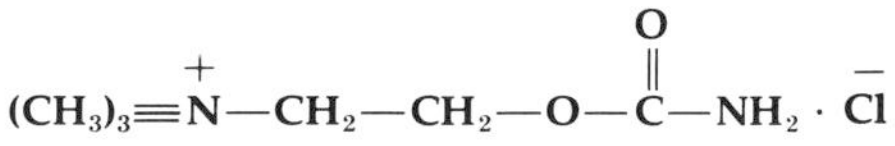

Carbachol chloride

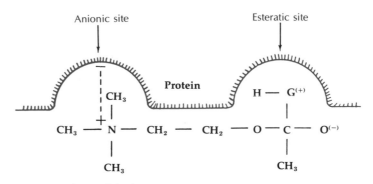

Fig. 7-1. Interaction of acetylcholine and acetylcholinesterase. (From Wilson, I. B.: Neurology [supp. 1] **8**:41, 1958.)

All drugs in this group are quaternary amines. Replacement of the acetyl group by carbamate protects the drug against cholinesterases and thus prolongs its half-life in the body. Substitution in the β-carbon, as in acetyl-β-methylcholine, protects against the action of the nonspecific cholinesterase.

Bethanechol and methacholine have many of the actions of acetylcholine on smooth muscles and glands without significantly affecting ganglia and skeletal neuromuscular transmission.

Bethanechol (Urecholine) has selective effects on the gastrointestinal and urinary tracts and is the parasympathomimetic drug of choice for the treatment of postoperative abdominal distention and postoperative urinary retention. Bethanechol is not destroyed by cholinesterases and thus has prolonged effects. The usual cholinergic side effects are sweating, flushing, salivation, and aggravation of bronchial asthma. Hypotension may be caused by the drug but is not common. Contraindications to its use include bronchial asthma, severe cardiac disease, hyperthyroidism (atrial fibrillation may occur), and mechanical obstruction of the gastrointestinal and urinary tracts. Preparations include tablets of 5, 10, and 25 mg. and solutions for subcutaneous injection, 5 mg./ml. The dosage for adults is 5 to 30 mg. three or four times daily by mouth or 2.5 to 5 mg. three or four times daily by subcutaneous injection.

Methacholine (Mecholyl) has few uses in medicine. It possesses mostly muscarinic activity, especially on the cardiovascular system. Because it is an acetyl ester, it is hydrolyzed by acetylcholinesterase, although more slowly than acetylcholine. Methacholine has been used in the treatment of paroxysmal atrial tachycardia because it abolishes the ectopic focus in the atrium, probably as a consequence of hyperpolarization. It is seldom used for this purpose because it can cause alarming syncopal attacks when injected by the subcutaneous route. Patients with adrenal medullary tumors respond to methacholine with a rise of blood pressure, since it stimulates the output of catecholamines from the tumor. The methacholine test for pheochromocytoma has had some popularity but is seldom used at present. Preparations include tablets containing 200 mg. and powder for injectable solution, 25 mg. For adults the oral dosage is 50 to 600 mg. three or four times daily; the subcutaneous dosage, 10 to 25 mg.

Carbachol is a very potent choline ester having both muscarinic and nicotinic effects. Its only use at present is in the treatment of glaucoma. Solutions of 0.5 to 1%, applied

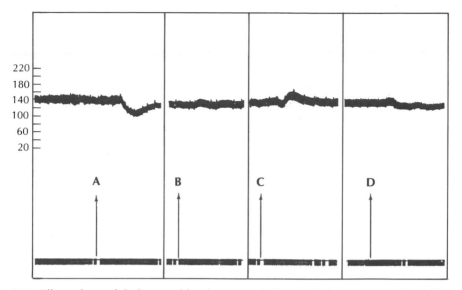

Fig. 7-2. Effect of acetylcholine on blood pressure before and after atropine. The following drugs were administered intravenously to a dog anesthetized with pentobarbital: **A,** acetylcholine, 10 μg/kg.; between **A** and **B,** atropine, 1 mg./kg.; **B,** acetylcholine, 10 μg/kg.; **C,** acetylcholine, 100 μg/kg.; between **C** and **D,** phentolamine, 5 mg./kg.; **D,** acetylcholine, 100 μg/kg. Note that atropine prevented blood pressure lowering induced by small dose of acetylcholine. Large dose of the latter actually caused elevation of blood pressure, the so-called nicotinic effect of acetylcholine. This response is blocked by phentolamine, an adrenergic blocking agent.

to the conjunctiva, cause miosis and reduction of intraocular pressure. The antidote to carbachol is atropine.

The muscarinic and nicotinic actions of the choline esters can be illustrated by a simple experiment. Fig. 7-2 shows the effect of injected choline esters on blood pressure responses of a dog before and after atropine administration.

In summary, the essential actions of the choline esters following subcutaneous injection are cutaneous vasodilatation with flushing, sweating, salivation, and increased tone of the smooth muscle of the gastrointestinal tract and urinary bladder. There are variable effects on heart rate and blood pressure. Some individuals show a precipitous fall of blood pressure, whereas in others the changes in blood pressure and heart rate are slight because compensatory reflexes remain active. It should always be kept in mind that asthmatic patients are particularly susceptible to the bronchoconstrictor action of these compounds. The antidote, atropine, should always be on hand before a choline ester is administered.

PILOCARPINE AND MUSCARINE

The two alkaloids pilocarpine and muscarine have the curious property of acting like acetylcholine on receptors of smooth muscles and glandular cells. Muscarine is present in the mushroom *Amanita muscaria,* along with toxic peptides,[25] whereas pilocarpine is found in the leaves of the plant *Pilocarpus jaborandi.* The structures of these two drugs follow.

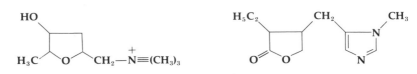

Both alkaloids show the so-called muscarinic effects of acetylcholine without having significant nicotinic action. Atropine blocks these muscarinic effects. Muscarine, being a quaternary ammonium compound, shows some similarity to acetylcholine, but it is puzzling why pilocarpine, which is a tertiary amine, should also mimic the muscarinic effects of acetylcholine. It is well established, however, that this is not the result of cholinesterase inhibition. For molecular aspects of the action of pilocarpine and its quaternary derivative see reference 5.

Although it is generally believed that the pilocarpine effect is exerted directly on cholinergic effectors, some new evidence indicates that ganglia contain atropine-sensitive synapses also, which may be stimulated not only by acetylcholine but also by pilocarpine. Several unexplained effects of pilocarpine become understandable by the existence of a ganglionic action as well as a direct action of the drug on cholinomimetic neuroeffectors.[7]

Of these two drugs, muscarine has only academic interest. Pilocarpine, however, is employed in ophthalmology as a miotic and is occasionally used for stimulating the flow of saliva in patients who complain of dryness of the mouth during therapy with ganglionic blocking agents. For ophthalmologic applications, pilocarpine is employed in a 1% solution. The usual dose for stimulating the secretion of saliva in man is 5 mg., given either orally or by subcutaneous injection. In addition to stimulating the flow of saliva, the drug greatly increases sweating. Its antidote is atropine.

Problem 7-1. The fixed dilated pupil may be an ominous sign caused by an involvement of the third nerve by an intracranial disease. How can this be distinguished from the accidental application to the eye of an anticholinergic (mydriatic) drug? In an interesting recent article,[15] topical application of pilocarpine is used to establish the diagnosis. The pupil responds well to pilocarpine in the case of nerve damage, whereas it is unresponsive if the dilated pupil is caused by the application of a mydriatic drug. Could an anticholinesterase such as physostigmine be substituted for pilocarpine in this diagnostic test?

ANTICHOLINESTERASES

Some drugs inhibit the destruction of acetylcholine and thereby produce a higher concentration of the agent at those sites where it is released. They can also potentiate the action of some of the exogenous choline esters when these are administered.

The cholinesterase inhibitors are of great interest in medicine. They have been found very useful in the treatment of myasthenia gravis and in the management of glaucoma. The group has also yielded some of our most potent insecticides, which are of great toxicologic importance because of their widespread use. Cholinesterase inhibitors are valuable investigative tools. They are also potential chemical warfare agents. Physostigmine is becoming useful also in the treatment of atropine poisoning.

PHYSOSTIGMINE AND NEOSTIGMINE AND RELATED DRUGS

Physostigmine and neostigmine are reversible anticholinesterases. Physostigmine is used almost entirely in the treatment of glaucoma, having been replaced by neostigmine in the management of gastrointestinal and urinary atony.

Physostigmine (eserine), an alkaloid obtained from the seeds of *Physostigma veneno-*

sum, also known as calabar or ordeal bean, has been familiar to pharmacologists since the latter part of the nineteenth century. Early work centered on the ability of this drug to constrict the pupils, and particular attention was paid to the then curious fact that this action requires intact innervation. When the ciliary ganglion is removed, physostigmine does not constrict the pupil. The actions of physostigmine are known to arise from its inhibition of cholinesterase.

Synthesis of compounds related to physostigmine led to the development of neostigmine in 1931.[1] The structures of physostigmine and neostigmine follow:

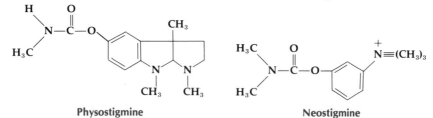

Physostigmine   Neostigmine

Pharmacologic investigations have shown that physostigmine is an antagonist of curare. In 1934 the British physician Mary Walker[16] tried physostigmine in the treatment of myasthenia gravis because of the clinical similarity of this disease to a curarized state. The results were impressive, and when neostigmine became available, it was tried also. The latter drug had many advantages and is used to this day in the treatment of myasthenia, although many new compounds related to neostigmine are available and offer advantages in some cases.

Action and uses of physostigmine

The actions of physostigmine may be attributed entirely to cholinesterase inhibition on the basis of the following considerations. The drug inhibits cholinesterase in vitro. Its affinity for the enzyme may be 10,000 times greater than that of acetylcholine. After combination with the enzyme, it seems to be gradually dissociated and inactivated in the body. Consequently, the drug is a reversible inhibitor of the cholinesterases.

Physostigmine exerts no effect on the denervated pupil or on the denervated skeletal muscle, even when given by close intra-arterial injection.[17] It has potent effects on structures with normal innervation because of its ability to protect the endogenously released acetylcholine.

Neostigmine and related compounds

Neostigmine was developed as a result of synthetic work on physostigmine analogs. Neostigmine is a quaternary ammonium compound, whereas physostigmine is a tertiary amine. This quaternary ammonium structure permits neostigmine to act directly on the neuromuscular junction in addition to inhibiting cholinesterase.

Thus some of the actions of neostigmine are due to cholinesterase inhibition, whereas others are the result of a combination of enzyme inhibition plus a direct acetylcholine-like effect. On the denervated eye, for example, neostigmine acts similarly to physostigmine, producing no pupillary constriction. On the other hand, intra-arterially injected neostigmine will elicit an effect at the neuromuscular junction even when the nerves are degenerated and all cholinesterase has been previously destroyed by diisopropyl fluorophosphate. This evidence suggests that the muscarinic actions of neostigmine are produced by cholinesterase inhibition, whereas the nicotinic actions, at least at the neuromuscular site, are in part due to a direct effect.

The intramuscular injection of 0.5 to 1 mg. of neostigmine methylsulfate (Prostigmin methylsulfate) into a normal human being will produce the usual cholinergic effects: elevation of skin temperature, sweating, salivation, intestinal contractions with a desire to defecate, contraction of smooth muscles of the urinary tract with an urgency to micturate, some slowing of the heart rate with possible hypotension, and muscle fasciculations. Atropine will antagonize the muscarinic effects but not the neuromuscular nicotinic actions of neostigmine. This antidote should be available whenever neostigmine is employed.

Myasthenia gravis is the foremost indication for the use of neostigmine. This will be discussed in connection with the pharmacologic aspects of myasthenia.

The drug has been used also for increasing intestinal tone and in some forms of urinary retention, but bethanechol may be better in these instances. It may be used in paroxysmal auricular tachycardia for the same reasons as methacholine. Neostigmine can also antagonize the action of ganglionic blocking agents.

In addition to the injectable methylsulfate, neostigmine can be given by mouth as the bromide salt. Much larger doses are given orally, 15 to 30 mg., because much of the drug is inactivated in the gastrointestinal tract. Absorption may be variable, and untoward reactions may occur if too much of the drug is suddenly absorbed.

Neostigmine may be used topically in the treatment of glaucoma. Much higher concentrations are necessary than in the case of physostigmine because the drug is less soluble in lipids and does not penetrate biologic membranes as effectively.

Neostigmine has been used in cases of delayed menstruation, in which it may induce bleeding if there is no pregnancy.

Newer drugs related to neostigmine. The anticurare property of neostigmine and its effectiveness in the treatment of myasthenia stimulated interest in the synthesis of many related compounds. Some of these have interesting and useful properties.

The structure of edrophonium (Tensilon) shown below is basically similar to that of neostigmine. This drug has been introduced as an anticurare agent. It also has diagnostic and investigative uses in myasthenia.

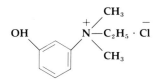

Edrophonium chloride

The essential feature of edrophonium is its very short duration of action. From a practical standpoint if may be considered an extremely short-acting neostigmine. In the myasthenic patient the intravenous injection of 2 to 5 mg. of edrophonium will cause very rapid and transient improvement of muscular strength. This may be used for diagnostic purposes and also for "titrating" the degree of effectiveness of other treatment. The physician may be in doubt whether to increase or decrease the dosage of neostigmine for a myasthenic patient. If intravenous edrophonium causes further improvement in the patient, it is likely that previous therapy has been inadequate. On the other hand, if the reaction to this edrophonium test is unfavorable, indicating overtreatment, increasing the neostigmine dosage would be undesirable. The action of edrophonium in this test lasts only a very few minutes.

The drug is a potent antidote to curare. It acts more rapidly than neostigmine, and its action is more transient. Although the drug has some cholinesterase inhibitory properties, its neuromuscular effect is probably a direct one.

Neostigmine substitutes. A number of substitutes are available for neostigmine in the treatment of myasthenia. At least three of these, pyridostigmine (Mestinon), benzpyrinium (Stigmonene), and ambenonium (Mytelase), have received fairly extensive trials. These compounds act basically the same as neostigmine. Some, for example, ambenonium, may have a longer duration of action and produce fewer muscarinic side effects on the gastrointestinal tract. By having several neostigmine substitutes, the physician is able to select that which is most desirable in a given patient.

Demecarium (Humorsol) is used in glaucoma as a long-acting miotic. It consists chemically of two molecules of neostigmine joined by a decamethylene chain.

Basic differences between physostigmine and neostigmine

Both physostigmine and neostigmine are reversible cholinesterase inhibitors. In addition, neostigmine has a direct effect on acetylcholine receptors at neuromuscular sites. Being a quaternary ammonium compound, neostigmine does not cross biologic membranes as efficiently as physostigmine, which is a tertiary amine. As a consequence, neostigmine is not absorbed as efficiently from the gastrointestinal tract, and large doses are needed for oral administration. Probably for the same reason, higher concentrations of this drug must be used for topical treatment of glaucoma.

ORGANOPHOSPHORUS ANTICHOLINESTERASES

Diisopropyl fluorophosphate (DFP; isofluorophate) and a variety of other alkyl phosphates are highly toxic compounds that produce irreversible inactivation of the cholinesterases. They were developed as potential chemical warfare agents and have had some therapeutic applications, but their principal interest is toxicologic because of their widespread use as insecticides.

The structural formulas of some of the organophosphorus compounds are shown below:

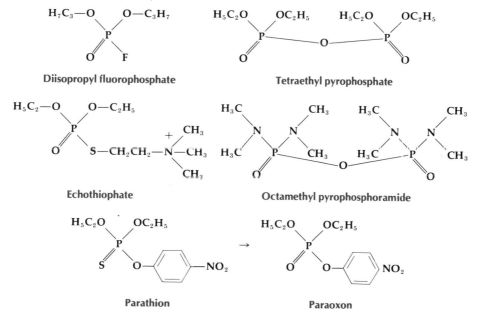

Diisopropyl fluorophosphate

Tetraethyl pyrophosphate

Echothiophate

Octamethyl pyrophosphoramide

Parathion

Paraoxon

Table 7-1. Signs and symptoms of organophosphate poisoning*

Muscarinic manifestations	Nicotinic manifestations	Central nervous system manifestations
Bronchoconstriction	Muscular fasciculation	Restlessness
Increased bronchial secretions	Tachycardia	Insomnia
Sweating	Hypertension	Tremors
Salivation		Confusion
Lacrimation		Ataxia
Bradycardia		Convulsions
Hypotension		Respiratory depression
Miosis		Circulatory collapse
Blurring of vision		
Urinary incontinence		

*Modified from Namba, T., Nolte, C. T., Jackrel, J., and Grob, D.: Amer. J. Med. **50**:475, 1971.

Whereas the reversible anticholinesterases depress enzymatic activity for a few hours following a single administration, the organophosphorus compounds produce an effect that may persist for weeks or months. The difference may be attributed to the fact that the organophosphorus compounds combine with the cholinesterases, which then become phosphorylated. The phosphorylated enzyme is stable, does not hydrolyze, and is inactive against acetylcholine. As a consequence, enzymatic activity will remain reduced until new enzyme material is synthesized, unless some reactivator of cholinesterase is employed as an antidote.

The nonspecific cholinesterase of plasma is affected preferentially and primarily by the alkyl phosphates. With sufficient doses, however, there is increasing destruction of acetylcholinesterase in red cells and in neural tissue. Nonspecific cholinesterase of serum is regenerated by the liver in about 2 weeks. It may take 3 months to regenerate acetylcholinesterase activity at synapses and neuromuscular junctions.

Pharmacologic effects

When DFP or other alkyl phosphate anticholinesterases are injected or inhaled, the clinical picture that develops is a combination of peripheral cholinergic effects and involvement of the central nervous system (Table 7-1). Muscle fasciculations, constricted pupils, salivation, sweating, abdominal cramps, and respiratory distress are consequences of cholinesterase inactivation in the periphery. Anxiety, restlessness, electroencephalographic changes, and perhaps even terminal convulsions may be related to the actions of the inhibitor on the central nervous system. Atropine protects against the peripheral muscarinic effects and the involvement of the central nervous system. It exerts no protective effect against muscle fasciculations and skeletal muscle weakness.[6] The cause of death in organophosphate poisoning is respiratory paralysis.

Antidotal action of pralidoxime

Even though under ordinary circumstances cholinesterase inactivation by the alkyl phosphates is irreversible, compounds have been discovered that are capable of reactivating the enzyme. Pralidoxime (pyridine-2-aldoxime-methiodide; PAM) is a tailor-made molecule developed on the basis of a mechanism postulated by Wilson[18] to explain the action of the alkyl phosphate anticholinesterases.

If we picture the interaction of cholinesterase and acetylcholine as shown in Fig. 7-1, it may be postulated that under normal circumstances the esteratic site is acetylated, but that the acetyl enzyme is quite unstable and is rapidly hydrolyzed. On the other hand, when the esteratic site is phosphorylated as a consequence of interaction with an alkyl phosphate, this combination is highly resistant to hydrolysis and the site becomes unavailable to acetylcholine. Experimental studies have shown that hydroxylamine and oximes are capable of regenerating the enzyme when it is presumably phosphorylated by the alkyl phosphates. With this knowledge, a molecule was designed in which the distance between the quaternary nitrogen and the oxime is the same as that postulated for acetylcholine. It was predicted that such a compound would fit into the cholinesterase enzyme and would act as a more efficient regenerator than would an ordinary oxime. This work led to the synthesis of pralidoxime, the formula of which follows:

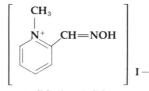

Pralidoxime iodide

The interactions of organophosphates, cholinesterases, and reactivators such as pralidoxime may be visualized in the following manner:

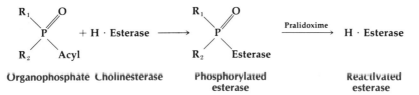

| Organophosphate Cholinesterase | Phosphorylated esterase | Reactivated esterase |

It is of great interest that pralidoxime is capable of protecting experimental animals against otherwise fatal doses of the alkyl phosphates. Atropine is also important because it blocks most of the cholinergic effects, whereas pralidoxime acts to regenerate the enzymes.

Pralidoxime must be administered parenterally. It is usually given by intravenous infusion, 50 mg./kg. of body weight dissolved in 1,000 ml. of saline solution. The drug has some depolarizing effect of its own in addition to reactivation of the phosphorylated cholinesterases.

Other reactivator oximes such as diacetylmonoxime (DAM) and bisquaternary oximes have been studied.

Medical uses of organophosphates

When DFP was developed, it was anticipated by many that it would provide a long-acting preparation for the treatment of myasthenia gravis. Unfortunately, however, this drug and many other related compounds that were investigated have been found to produce many side effects. Among compounds that have been investigated are tetraethyl pyrophosphate (TEPP), hexaethyl tetraphosphate (HETP), and octamethyl pyrophosphoramide (OMPA). None of them is used to any significant extent in the treatment of myasthenia gravis.

DFP, echothiophate, and demecarium are used in the treatment of glaucoma. When applied locally, the action of the drugs remains localized. They may produce a prolonged decrease of intraocular pressure over a period of weeks.

A very high percentage of presently available insecticides contain organophosphorus anticholinesterases. Acute and chronic poisoning due to these pesticides is not uncommon.

The *treatment of organophosphorus poisoning* is as follows: Atropine sulfate, 1 to 2 mg., should be administered as symptoms appear. This antidote may be given every hour up to 25 to 50 mg. in a day. The skin, stomach, and eyes should be decontaminated. Pralidoxime is administered by slow intravenous infusion in a dose of 1 Gm. for adults if the patient fails to respond to atropine. Certain drugs are contraindicated in organophosphorus poisoning. These include morphine, theophylline, or aminophylline. If the patient is cyanotic, artificial respiration should be administered even before atropine.

GENERAL FEATURES OF CHOLINESTERASE INHIBITION

Much has been learned about the importance of the cholinesterases from studies on the action of the anticholinesterases. It appears from these studies that serum cholinesterase is probably of no great physiologic importance but may have a significant effect when exogenous labile choline esters are administered. Serum cholinesterase can be reduced to very low levels with DFP treatment without important consequences. Measurements of serum cholinesterase activity may be altered by disease of the liver or by the previous administration of anticholinesterases. Such measurements are of importance in industrial medicine to evaluate the extent of exposure to anticholinesterases, thus preventing inadvertent poisoning.

The specific acetylcholinesterase appears to exist in excess at the various junctions at which acetylcholine functions as a mediator of neural transmission. Moderate decreases of acetylcholinesterase have little physiologic consequence. On the other hand, a severe reduction of brain cholinesterase, down to 10% of normal, has been observed in animals when death occurs from the administration of an anticholinesterase.

The presence of acetylcholinesterase in the red cell is puzzling since no obvious physiologic reason for it seems to exist. It has been suggested that the acetylcholine-cholinesterase system has a much broader significance than that expected from its neuroeffector function.

Cholinesterase activity of the red cell mass can reflect hematopoietic activity. The regeneration of acetylcholinesterase activity of red blood cells following the administration of irreversible anticholinesterases is directly proportional to the production of new cells.

PHARMACOLOGIC ASPECTS OF MYASTHENIA GRAVIS

Myasthenia gravis has been defined as a chronic disease characterized by weakness and abnormal fatigability of skeletal muscle.[3] The symptoms may be ameliorated by anticholinesterase drugs and "this response serves as the basis for diagnosis and management of the disease."[3]

Although there is increasing evidence that myasthenia gravis may be an autoimmune disease,[13,14] the response of myasthenic patients to a variety of drugs points to a disturbance of neuromuscular transmission as the essential functional manifestation of the underlying pathologic change.

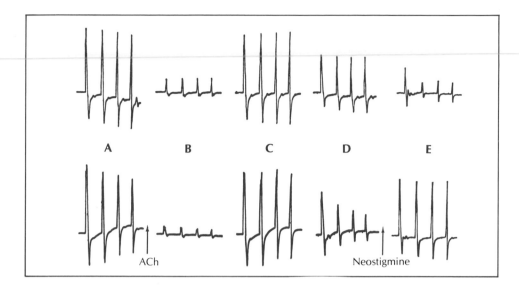

Fig. 7-3. Effect of acetylcholine and neostigmine on the muscle action potential response to nerve stimulation in a normal subject (upper row) and a patient with myasthenia gravis (lower row). **A,** Control response to four supramaximal nerve stimuli at 40-millisecond intervals; **B,** prompt depression 7 seconds after intra-arterial injection of 5 mg. of acetylcholine; **C,** recovery 15 seconds after injection; **D,** late depression 1 hour after injection; **E,** effect of 0.5 mg. neostigmine. (From Grob, D.: J. Chronic Dis. **8**:536, 1958.)

Repetitive stimulation of a motor nerve in a myasthenic patient rapidly leads to fatigue of the muscles innervated by that particular nerve. Intra-arterial injection of acetylcholine, neostigmine, or edrophonium increases the strength of the fatigued muscles. In normal persons the intra-arterial injection of these drugs produces fasciculation and weakness, probably as a result of persistent depolarization of the neuromuscular end plates (Fig. 7-3). Also, myasthenic patients are susceptible to doses of *d*-tubocurarine or quinine that scarcely affect normal persons.

The response of myasthenic patients to various drugs might be explained by postulating a number of different defects in neuromuscular transmission. There may be a defective synthesis or binding of acetylcholine in the synaptic vesicles, acetylcholinesterase may be present in excessive amounts, or some curare-like compound may be present to oppose the actions of acetylcholine on the motor end plate. Interestingly, newborn infants of myasthenic mothers may be similarly affected, but they recover in a matter of days or weeks. This observation has been used to support the postulate that some circulating compound is present that is causally related to the abnormality.

In a study of isolated intercostal muscle from myasthenic patients the significant observation was made that miniature end plate potentials had only one fifth the normal amplitude.[2] This finding suggests that the *amount* of acetylcholine in each synaptic vesicle is abnormally low. The response of these muscles to carbachol and decamethonium was as expected in normal individuals. The conclusion seems to be that myasthenia is a presynaptic disease caused by a deficiency of acetylcholine in the presynaptic vesicles.

Various anticholinesterases are useful for the diagnosis and management of myasthenia. For diagnostic purposes, neostigmine in a dose of 1 to 2 mg. may be injected by the intramuscular route with atropine, 0.6 mg. Smaller doses (0.5 mg.) of neostigmine may be used by the intravenous route. Edrophonium may be given for diagnosis in a dose of 2 to 8 mg. intravenously.

For the management of weakness, neostigmine and related drugs are most useful. Neostigmine bromide is administered orally in doses of 15 to 30 mg., sometimes as often as every 3 hours. (See Table 7-2.) Much smaller doses of neostigmine as the methyl-sulfate suffice when given by the intramuscular route.

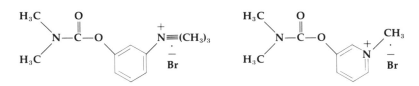

Neostigmine bromide   Pyridostigmine bromide

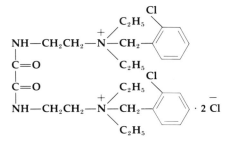

Ambenonium chloride

CHOLINERGIC CRISIS

Excessive doses of anticholinesterases produce what is often called a cholinergic crisis. Its muscarinic signs are miosis, sweating, salivation, lacrimation, and a hyperactive bowel. Its nicotinic signs are revealed by muscle fasciculations and paralysis. The diagnosis of anticholinesterase poisoning can be made on the basis of these symptoms and signs, since there are essentially no other diagnostic possibilities.[4]

An additional difficulty arises during the treatment of myasthenia with the anticholinesterases. It may be difficult to distinguish a cholinergic crisis from severe muscle weakness caused by an exacerbation of the disease. If overdose is suspected, the safest procedure is to withhold medications and maintain adequate airway for artificial respiration. An intravenous injection of 2 mg. of edrophonium may be useful in distinguishing between cholinergic crisis and myasthenic crisis. If the injection is followed by increased strength, it is an indication of undertreatment rather than overtreatment.[10]

Quinine, d-tubocurarine, and decamethonium aggravate the symptoms of the myasthenic. Provocation of these symptoms for diagnostic purposes should be done only under careful supervision with adequate facilities for artificial respiration.

Germine diacetate has been used experimentally in myasthenia (p. 178) but it does not appear promising.

Table 7-2. Anticholinesterase preparations

Drug	Preparations	Usual route of administration
Physostigmine (eserine)	0.1 to 1% solution	Topical (eye)
Neostigmine bromide (Prostigmin bromide)	Tablets, 15 mg.	Oral
Neostigmine methylsulfate (Prostigmin methylsulfate)	Injectable solutions, 0.25, 0.5, and 1 mg./ml.	Subcutaneous or intramuscular
Pyridostigmine (Mestinon)	Tablets, 60 mg.	Oral
Ambenonium (Mytelase)	Tablets, 10 and 25 mg.	Oral
Demecarium (Humorsol)	0.25% solution	Topical (eye)
Edrophonium (Tensilon)	Injectable solution, 10 mg./ml.	Intravenous
Echothiophate (Phospholine)	0.25% solution	Topical (eye)

References

1 Aeschlimann, J. A., and Reinert, M.: Pharmacological action of some analogues of physostigmine, J. Pharmacol. Exp. Ther. **43**:413, 1931.

2 Elmquist, D. M., Hoffmann, W. W., Kugelberg, J., and Quastel, D. M. J.: An electrophysiological investigation of neuromuscular transmission in myasthenia gravis, J. Physiol. **174**:417, 1964.

3 Grob, D.: Myasthenia gravis, J. Chronic Dis. **8**:536, 1958.

4 Hallett, M., and Cullen, R. F.: Intoxication with echothiophate iodide, J.A.M.A. **222**:1414, 1972.

5 Hanin, I., Jenden, D. J., and Cho, A. K.: The influence of pH on the muscarinic action of oxotremorine, arecoline, pilocarpine, and their quaternary ammonium analogs, Molec. Pharmacol. **2**:269, 1966.

6 Kanagaratnam, K., Boon, W. H., and Hoh, T. K.: Parathion poisoning from contaminated barley, Lancet **1**:538, 1960.

7 Levy, B., and Ahlquist, R. P.: A study of sympathetic ganglionic stimulants, J. Pharmacol. Exp. Ther. **137**:219, 1962.

8 Moore, H.: Advantages of pyridostigmine bromide (Mestinon) and edrophonium chloride (Tensilon) in the treatment of transitory myasthenia gravis in the neonatal period, New Eng. J. Med. **253**:1075, 1955.

9 Namba, T., Nolte, C. T., Jackrel, J., and Grob, D.: Poisoning due to organophosphate insecticides, Amer. J. Med. **50**:475, 1971.

10 Osserman, K. E., and Kaplan, L. I.: Studies in myasthenia gravis: use of edrophonium chloride (Tensilon) in differentiating myasthenic from cholinergic weakness, Arch. Neurol. Psychiat. **70**:385, 1953.

11 Quinby, G. E., Loomis, T. A., and Brown, H. W.: Oral occupational parathion poisoning treated with 2-PAM iodide, New Eng. J. Med. **268**:639, 1963.

12 Richter, J. A., and Goldstein, A.: Effects of morphine and levorphanol on brain acetylcholine content in mice, J. Pharmacol. Exp. Ther. **175**:685, 1970.

13 Simpson, J. A.: Myasthenia gravis: a new hypothesis, Scot. Med. J. **5**:419, 1960.

14 Strauss, A. J. L., Seegal, B. C., Hsu, K. S., Burkholder, P. M., Nastuk, W. L., and Osserman, K. E.: Preliminary observations by immu-

nofluorescence technique of a muscle-binding complement-fixing globulin in the serum of patients with myasthenia gravis, Proc. Soc. Exp. Biol. Med. **105**:184, 1960.

15 Thompson, H. S., Newsome, D. A., and Loewenfeld, I. E.: The fixed dilated pupil, Arch. Ophthal. **86**:21, 1971.

16 Walker, M. B.: Case showing effect of prostigmine on myasthenia gravis, Proc. Roy. Soc. Med. **28**:759, 1935.

17 Wescoe, W. C., and Riker, W. F., Jr.: The pharmacology of anti-curare agents, Ann. N. Y. Acad. Sci. **54**:438, 1951.

18 Wilson, I. B.: A specific antidote for nerve gas and insecticide (alkylphosphate) intoxication, Neurology (supp. 1) **8**:41, 1958.

Recent reviews

19 Becker, B., and Ballin, N.: Glaucoma, Ann. Rev. Med. **17**:235, 1966.

20 Glaser, G. H.: Pharmacological considerations in the treatment of myasthenia gravis, Advances Pharmacol. **2**:113, 1963.

21 Koelle, G. B.: Acetylcholine—current status in physiology, pharmacology and medicine, New Eng. J. Med. **286**:1086, 1972.

22 Leopold, I. H., and Keates, E.: Drugs used in the treatment of glaucoma. Part I, Clin. Pharmacol. Ther. **6**:130, 1965.

23 Leopold, I. H., and Keates, E.: Drugs used in the treatment of glaucoma. Part II, Clin. Pharmacol. Ther. **6**:262, 1965.

24 Thesleff, S., and Quastel, D. M. J.: Neuromuscular pharmacology, Ann. Rev. Pharmacol. **5**:263, 1965.

25 Wieland, T.: Poisonous principles of mushrooms of the genus Amanita, Science **159**:946, 1968.

8 Adrenergic (sympathomimetic) drugs

The sympathetic nervous system performs its homeostatic function by releasing norepinephrine at adrenergic nerve endings and epinephrine in the adrenal medulla. Drugs that act directly on adrenergic receptors, or release mediators which then act on the receptors, may be termed sympathomimetic or adrenergic drugs.

CATECHOLAMINES (EPINEPHRINE AND NOREPINEPHRINE)

From a chemical standpoint catecholamines are compounds that contain catechol (*o*-dihydroxybenzene) and an amine. As commonly used in pharmacology, the term refers to norepinephrine, epinephrine, and dopamine, the amines of the sympathetic nervous system.

The information available on epinephrine and norepinephrine will be discussed under the following headings: occurrence and physiologic functions, pharmacologic actions, metabolism, therapeutic applications, and catecholamines and disease states.

Dopamine is discussed on p. 110.

OCCURRENCE AND PHYSIOLOGIC FUNCTIONS

Norepinephrine and epinephrine are catecholamines having the following structural formulas:

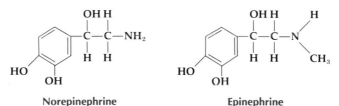

Norepinephrine   Epinephrine

They differ from each other only by the presence of a methyl group on the nitrogen in epinephrine. This small difference, however, results in a considerable change in pharmacologic activity. The prefix *nor* is derived from German chemical terminology. It is the abbreviation of *Nitrogen ohne Radikal*, or "nitrogen without radical," in the case of norepinephrine.

The presence of norepinephrine in adrenergic nerve fibers was demonstrated by von Euler[22] in 1946. It had been suspected that the "sympathin" released following adrenergic nerve stimulation was norepinephrine. The compound has been found in sympathetic ganglia and also in the central nervous system, where its highest concentration is in the hypothalamus.

The relationship between adrenergic nerves and blood vessels and the presence

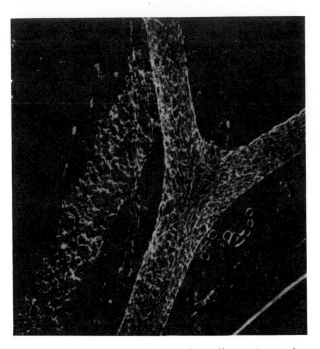

Fig. 8-1. Fluorescent adrenergic terminals around small arteries and a vein in the rat mesentery. (From Falck, B.: Acta Physiol. Scand. [supp. 197] **56:**19, 1962.)

of catecholamines in the nerves is strikingly demonstrated by the fluorescence technique of the Swedish investigators Falck, Hillarp, and Carlsson, as shown in Fig. 8-1.

Epinephrine is highly concentrated in the granules of the adrenal medulla. It is present also in many other organs, probably in chromaffin cells. According to von Euler,[22] sympathetic denervation affects the norepinephrine content of an organ without a significant decrease in epinephrine concentration. From this observation it is suspected that epinephrine is present in chromaffin cells, which have nothing to do with adrenergic innervation. The function of this extraneural epinephrine is not known.

The distribution, storage, and release of catecholamines are discussed on p. 66. The adrenal medullary granules and probably the adrenergic axonal vesicles contain catecholamines along with ATP in the proportion of 4:1. They also contain a special soluble protein, *chromogranin,* and the enzyme dopamine-β-oxidase.

With the development of paper chromatographic methods for the separation of norepinephrine from epinephrine, it was clearly established that the adrenal medulla contains some norepinephrine in addition to epinephrine. In the human adrenal medulla, norepinephrine may represent as much as 20% of the total catecholamine content. It may constitute a much higher percentage in the adrenal medulla of the newborn infant and in tumors of the adrenal medulla.

The main function of norepinephrine appears to be the maintenance of normal sympathetic tone and adjustment of circulatory dynamics. Epinephrine appears to be the great emergency hormone that stimulates metabolism and promotes blood flow to skeletal muscles, preparing the individual for "fight or flight." Among the less well-understood functions are the relationship between norepinephrine of the central nervous system and behavior and the functions of chromaffin cells in various organs.

PHARMACOLOGIC ACTIONS

Since the main physiologic roles of the two catecholamines have to do with circulatory and metabolic adjustments, these same functions will be markedly affected if these compounds are administered. They have, in addition, many miscellaneous effects on the bronchial smooth muscle, on the central nervous system, on eosinophils, and on carbohydrate and fat metabolism.

Adrenergic receptors

There is no drug known that can block all the pharmacologic actions of epinephrine and norepinephrine. Dale[15] demonstrated that certain ergot alkaloids were capable of blocking the excitatory but not the inhibitory actions of epinephrine. He postulated the existence of different receptive mechanisms for epinephrine.

The classification of adrenergic receptors as *alpha* and *beta*, originally proposed by Ahlquist[2] in 1948, is now generally accepted. The concept was based on the order of activity of a series of sympathomimetic drugs at various effector sites and was greatly strengthened when specific blocking agents were developed for each receptor. As

Table 8-1. Receptors mediating various adrenergic drug effects*

Effector organ	Receptor	Response
Heart		
Sinoatrial node	Beta	Tachycardia
Atrioventricular node	Beta	Increase in conduction rate and shortening of functional refractory period
Atria and ventricles	Beta	Increased contractility
Blood vessels		
To skeletal muscle	Alpha and beta	Contraction or relaxation
To skin	Alpha	Contraction
Bronchial muscle	Beta	Relaxation
Gastrointestinal smooth muscle		
To stomach	Beta	Decreased motility
To intestine	Alpha and beta	Decreased motility
Gastrointestinal sphincters		
To stomach	Alpha	Contraction
To intestine	Alpha	Contraction
Urinary bladder		
Detrusor	Beta	Relaxation
Trigone and sphincter	Alpha	Contraction
Eye		
Radial muscle, iris	Alpha	Contraction (mydriasis)
Ciliary muscle	Beta	Relaxation

*Based on data from Epstein, S. E., and Braunwald, E.: New Eng. J. Med. **275**:1106, 1966.

Table 8-2. Cardiovascular effects of small dose of norepinephrine in man

Systolic pressure	Increased
Diastolic pressure	Increased
Mean pressure	Increased
Heart rate	Slightly decreased
Cardiac output	Slightly decreased
Peripheral resistance	Increased

Table 8-3. Cardiovascular effects of small dose of epinephrine in man

Systolic pressure	Increased
Diastolic pressure	Decreased (increased by large dose)
Mean pressure	Unchanged
Cardiac output	Increased
Peripheral resistance	Decreased

shown in Table 8-1, the functions associated with alpha receptors are vasoconstriction, mydriasis, and intestinal relaxation. Beta receptors mediate adrenergic influences for vasodilatation, cardioacceleration, bronchial relaxation, positive inotropic effect, and intestinal relaxation. In addition, alpha receptors are involved in contraction of the nictitating membrane and pilomotor contraction*; glycogenolysis is a beta function.

The effects of the many adrenergic drugs can be explained on the basis of (1) the presence and localization of alpha and beta receptors in various organs, (2) the effect of interaction with each receptor, and (3) the release of endogenous catecholamines by the indirectly acting sympathomimetic amines.

Epinephrine acts on both alpha and beta receptors. In general, norepinephrine acts more on alpha receptors, although its cardiac effects are clearly on beta receptors. Isoproterenol is essentially a pure beta agonist. Tyramine is an indirectly acting amine, causing the release of endogenous catecholamines. Metaraminol is a mixed sympathomimetic drug acting both directly and also by means of release of endogenous catecholamines.

Cardiovascular effects

The actions of norepinephrine and epinephrine on the cardiovascular system may be quite different when both drugs are administered in small doses. They are not very different if large unphysiologic doses are used.

Net effects of small doses in man. When norepinephrine (levarterenol; Levophed) is infused intravenously into a normal person, it is generally given in a solution containing 4 mg. of the drug in 1 L. of isotonic fluid. If this solution containing 4 μg/ml. is infused at such a rate that the patient receives about 10 μg/min., the hemodynamic changes listed in Table 8-2 will be observed. If a similar infusion of epinephrine were to be given to an individual, the changes listed in Table 8-3 would generally be observed. The differences in heart rate elicited by the two drugs are illustrated in Fig. 8-2.

---

*Recent studies indicate that presynaptic alpha receptors mediate inhibition of catecholamine release from peripheral and central adrenergic neurons. For details, consult Starke, K., and Montel, H.: Alpha-receptor mediated modulation of transmitter release from central noradrenergic neurones. Naunyn-Schmiedeberg Arch. Pharmacol. **279**:53, 1973.

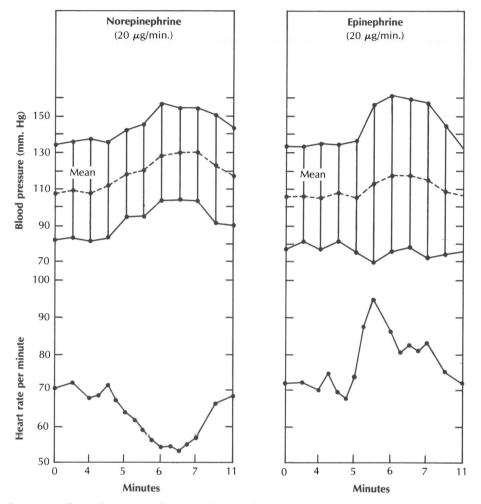

Fig. 8-2. Effect of norepinephrine and epinephrine infusion on blood pressure and heart rate in man. Note increased mean pressure and decreased heart rate following infusion of norepinephrine and also essentially unchanged mean pressure, increase in pulse pressure, and elevated heart rate following infusion of epinephrine. (From Barcroft, H., and Konzett, H.: Lancet **1:**147, 1949.)

The difference between the circulatory effects of epinephrine and norepinephrine reflects their different potency at various sites within the cardiovascular system. Norepinephrine has widespread vasoconstrictor properties, whereas epinephrine constricts some vascular areas and dilates others. The blood pressure elevation produced by norepinephrine brings into play reflexes that will cause bradycardia, which can be eliminated by the administration of atropine.

Epinephrine, on the other hand, stimulates the heart, and since there is no elevation of mean pressure, no reflex mechanisms come into play to slow the heart. The differences observed in man following the infusion of dilute solutions of the two drugs may be attributed to their different peripheral actions, which affect the heart through reflex mechanisms.

Response of heart and various vascular areas. The actions of epinephrine on the heart consist of increased rate,* increased force of contraction, increased irritability, and increased coronary blood flow.

Norepinephrine has cardiac accelerator action also, but this inherent chronotropic effect is opposed by reflex slowing secondary to vasoconstriction and elevated blood pressure. There is some experimental evidence to indicate that the actions of norepinephrine on ventricular automaticity are considerably less than those of epinephrine. It should be mentioned that the cardiac actions of isoproterenol are much more marked than those of epinephrine, whereas other adrenergic drugs such as phenylephrine or methoxamine have even less effect on the heart than does norepinephrine.

The increased coronary blood flow following the injection of epinephrine is largely due to the increased cardiac work and metabolism. It has no usefulness in relieving precordial pain and may even precipitate anginal attacks in patients with coronary atherosclerosis.

The differences between epinephrine and norepinephrine tend to disappear when they are injected in large doses. Under these circumstances both will elevate diastolic pressure, increase peripheral resistance, and reduce blood flow through skeletal muscles.[30]

Despite the fact that epinephrine in small doses can cause decreased total peripheral vascular resistance, its constrictor action in some areas may be greater than that of norepinephrine. The renal arteries and the vessels of the skin and mucous membranes respond with greater constriction to epinephrine than to norepinephrine.

The effects of epinephrine on renal hemodynamics have received considerable attention. It is generally accepted that the drug decreases renal plasma flow but does not influence glomerular filtration, the net effect being an increased filtration fraction.[51] Large doses of epinephrine, however, may decrease the filtration fraction by stopping blood flow through some nephrons. The drug also can induce antidiuresis by stimulating release of the pituitary antidiuretic hormone (ADH).

Cerebral blood flow is affected in a complex manner by norepinephrine and epinephrine. Through their direct action these drugs cause constriction of the cerebral vessels. The elevation of systemic pressure, however, can oppose this direct action to such an extent that no significant change in cerebral blood flow may occur. In normal persons, norepinephrine will reduce cerebral blood flow. If it is given to patients in hypotension following the administration of ganglionic blocking drugs, the reverse may occur as a result of elevation of systemic pressure.[52] It is important to realize that improvement of blood flow in hypotensive states is a consequence of an elevation of systemic pressure. If for any reason systemic pressure is not improved by an infusion of norepinephrine, its direct action on the vessels may further impair the blood supply to vital organs.

Bronchodilator effect

Epinephrine is a dilator of the bronchial smooth muscle; norepinephrine is a much weaker dilator on this particular effector, whereas isoproterenol is a more active bronchodilator than epinephrine. The bronchodilator effect is not important when these

---

*Heart rate may be decreased by epinephrine as a consequence of reflex vagal activity, which can be blocked by atropine.

drugs are administered to a normal individual. It becomes prominent when the bronchi are constricted by some pharmacologic agent such as histamine or methacholine or in disease states such as bronchial asthma. Epinephrine is a time-honored remedy in the latter condition. There is a possibility that, in addition to dilating bronchioles, the drug is beneficial because it constricts bronchial vessels, thereby reducing mucosal edema.

There is a strong clinical impression that repeated administration may produce refractoriness to the useful actions of epinephrine in bronchial asthma. The mechanism of this epinephrine-fastness has not been explained.

Other smooth muscle effects

Under special circumstances epinephrine causes mydriasis by contracting the radial muscle of the iris. This effect does not usually occur upon direct application of the drug, but cocaine sensitizes the radial muscle to topically applied epinephrine. Norepinephrine has less effect on the eye.

The capsule of the spleen is contracted by epinephrine in some animals such as the dog. It is questionable that this effect occurs in human beings.

The catecholamines have some slight inhibitory actions on the gastrointestinal smooth muscle. This action has little physiologic and no therapeutic importance. The same may be said for the complex and variable effects of epinephrine on the uterus.

Effect on glands

Salivary secretion may be stimulated by epinephrine, resulting in a thick saliva. Sweat glands receive cholinergic innervation; consequently, they are not expected to be stimulated by the catecholamines. Nevertheless, intracutaneous injection of catecholamines in man may produce local sweating, which can be blocked by adrenergic blocking drugs. Also, sweating may be a prominent symptom in cases of adrenal medullary tumors. The mechanism of such sweating is not known with certainty. It may be a result of increased metabolism, although the local stimulation of sweat glands suggests a direct effect.

Neural actions

It is believed at present that injected catecholamines do not cross the blood-brain barrier efficiently. Alterations in norepinephrine content in the central nervous system may be associated with altered brain function and behavior, but injected catecholamines do not exert prominent effects. Nevertheless, the injection of epinephrine into normal human beings produces anxiety and weakness. A respiratory stimulant effect has been demonstrated, and its mechanism may be through neural structures. In addition, there is considerable evidence that norepinephrine exerts an inhibitory effect on ganglionic transmission.[45]

It is of interest that certain adrenergic drugs such as amphetamine have a marked stimulant action on the central nervous system.

Effect on eosinophils

It has been shown that the subcutaneous injection of the usual therapeutic dose of epinephrine causes a marked decrease in the number of circulating eosinophils. Since the adrenal glucocorticoids have potent eosinopenic action, it has been postulated that epinephrine causes the release of ACTH, which in turn releases the adrenal glucocorticoids that depress the eosinophil count. This very attractive theory considered epinephrine an important link between stress and adrenocortical activation. However, it has been shown that epinephrine can cause a fall in circulating eosinophils in the adrenalectomized animal. The mechanism of this action and the possible mediation of pituitary-adrenal activation in stress remain mysterious.*

Norepinephrine has considerably less effect than epinephrine on the eosinophil count.

Metabolic actions

It has been mentioned previously that epinephrine is an emergency hormone which produces the kind of metabolic adjustments that are advantageous from a teleologic standpoint for "fight or flight." The most important of these are increased oxygen consumption and elevations of blood sugar, free fatty acids, and plasma potassium.

Oxygen consumption may be increased by 25% following the injection of a therapeutic dose of epinephrine. Norepinephrine has considerably weaker effects on both oxygen consumption and lactic acid production in man.

Epinephrine and isoproterenol, and to a lesser degree norepinephrine, exert complex effects on carbohydrate metabolism. They elevate blood sugar by glycogenolysis and also inhibit glucose utilization.[17,18] By stimulating glycogenolysis, glucose is released from the liver and lactic acid from muscle. The influence on phosphorylase has been studied extensively by Sutherland and Rall.[58-60] It appears that epinephrine in many tissues promotes the formation of a cyclic adenylic acid, adenosine-3',5'-monophosphate, whose structure is as follows:

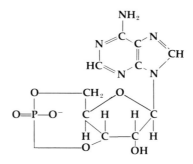

Adenosine-3',5'-monophosphate
(cyclic adenylic acid)

The formation of cyclic adenylate and some of its functions are shown in Figs. 8-3 and 8-4.

Catecholamines promote the release of fatty acids from adipose tissue and elevate the level of unesterified fatty acids in the blood. Thus the sympathetic nervous system, through catecholamine release, provides not only glucose but also free fatty acids as energy sources. The important effect on fatty acid release can be blocked by adrenergic blocking agents.

Marked elevations of plasma potassium may occur following the injection of epinephrine. It is believed that the source of this potassium is the liver.

---

*The effect of epinephrine on eosinophils is blocked by propranolol.[74]

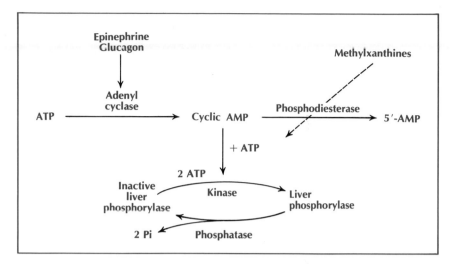

Fig. 8-3. Cyclic AMP and phosphorylase activation. Site of action of epinephrine, glucagon, and methylxanthines. (From Butcher, R. W.: New Eng. J. Med. **279:**1378, 1968.)

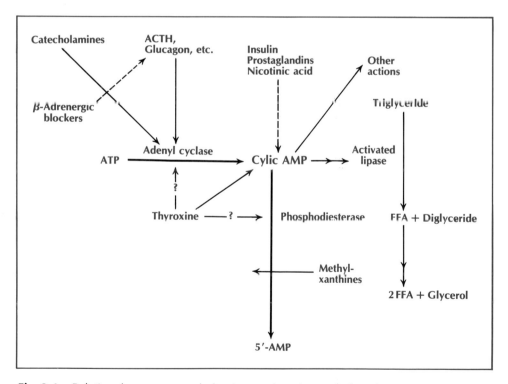

Fig. 8-4. Relation between catecholamines, other drugs, and cyclic AMP, with special reference to lipolytic and antilipolytic agents. (From Butcher, R. W.: New Eng. J. Med. **279:**1378, 1968.)

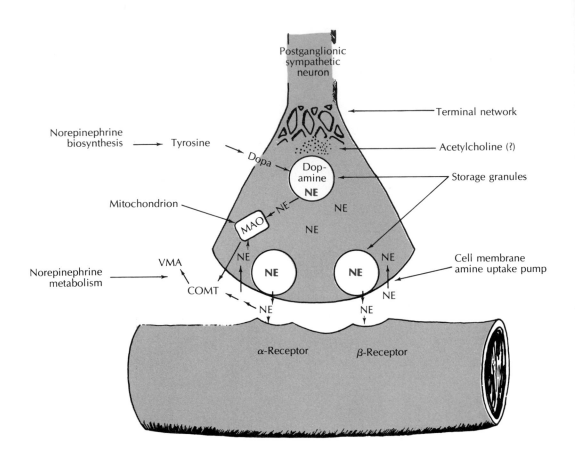

Fig. 8-5. Norepinephrine metabolism in the postganglionic sympathetic neuron. (From Abrams, W. B.: Dis. Chest **55:**148, 1969.)

METABOLISM

Catecholamines are made in the body from tyrosine through a series of steps involving dopa (3,4-dihydroxyphenylalanine), dopamine, norepinephrine, and finally epinephrine (p. 67). It is believed that these catecholamines are synthesized at the sites at which they are stored prior to their release.

The steps in the synthesis of norepinephrine by sympathetic nerves are shown in Fig. 8-5. Norepinephrine synthesis varies directly in relation to nerve stimulation. Catecholamine synthesis is regulated by *tyrosine hydroxylase*, the rate-limiting enzyme. An inhibitor of tyrosine hydroxylase, α-methyltyrosine, blocks the increased catecholamine synthesis that results from nerve stimulation. On the other hand, inhibitors of dopa decarboxylase (aromatic L-amino acid decarboxylase) or dopamine β-hydroxylase have little effect on tissue levels of catecholamines, indicating they are not rate-limiting. Such inhibitors are methyldopa and disulfiram or diethyldithiocarbamate, respectively.

There is much evidence to indicate that norepinephrine inhibits tyrosine hydroxylase.[86] Thus the regulation of norepinephrine synthesis in adrenergic nerves is achieved by end-product inhibition. Norepinephrine synthesis, then, varies directly with nerve activity and inversely with the local concentration of catecholamines.

Table 8-4. Fate of β-^{3}H-epinephrine in man*

Subject	Radioactivity excreted in urine				
	As percent of administered dose	Percent of urinary radioactivity present as			
		Metanephrine			VMA‡
		Free	Conjugated	Total†	
β-^{3}H-epinephrine administered					
R. C.	95	13	46	59	30
D. K.	95	14	38	52	37
R. B.	88	11	36	47	35
D. H.	73	10	49	59	40
β-^{3}H-metanephrine administered					
W. N.	92	16	39	55	24
K. S.	88	11	33	46	25

* From LaBrosse, E. H., Axelrod, J., and Kety, S. S.: Science **128**:593, 1958.

† Metanephrine found after heating in 1N HCl for 30 minutes at 100° C. Conjugated metanephrine represents the difference between free compound and total. A small amount of metanephrine glucosiduronic acid (6%) is included in the conjugated fraction.

‡ 3-Methoxy-4-hydroxymandelic acid. This fraction also contains an unidentified metabolite that represents about 5% of the total radioactivity in the urine.

For years the destruction of the catecholamines in the body was attributed to oxidative deamination through the enzyme amine oxidase. It was even suggested that ephedrine and cocaine sensitize various structures to the action of epinephrine by inhibiting this enzyme.

The amine oxidase theory has become obsolete as a result of discoveries by Armstrong and associates[4] and Axelrod and associates.[5] Armstrong and associates reported that 3-methoxy-4-hydroxymandelic acid, known also as vanylmandelic acid (VMA), was a major metabolite of norepinephrine. Axelrod and associates provided evidence that the principal metabolic pathway of epinephrine is O-methylation to metanephrine. This compound is attacked by monoamine oxidase (MAO), and its oxidative deamination produces VMA.

When 1 mg. of tritium-labeled dl-epinephrine was given by intravenous infusion over a period of 45 minutes to young male subjects, the results listed were noted from urine collected during the following 48 hours:

Total radioactivity	75 to 95% of the administered dose
Metanephrine, or 3-O-methylepinephrine	54% of the radioactivity in the urine
VMA, or 3-methoxy-4-hydroxymandelic acid	36% of the radioactivity of the urine

This experiment indicates that injected epinephrine is excreted in the urine partly as metanephrine and partly as VMA. That metanephrine is a precursor of VMA was demonstrated by a second experiment in which tritium-labeled metanephrine was administered intravenously to normal males. A considerable fraction of the injected metanephrine was excreted as VMA, indicating that metanephrine is further deaminated in the body (Table 8-4).

A most significant observation was that injected metanephrine exerted no demonstrable physiologic or psychologic effects in the volunteers. This shows that even

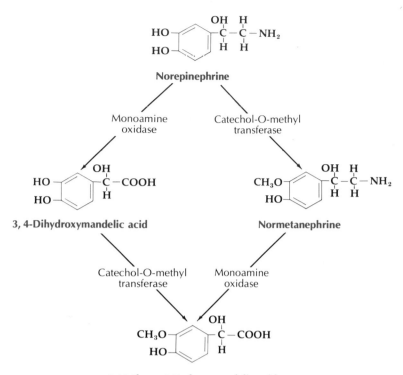

Fig. 8-6. Major pathways of norepinephrine metabolism. MAO actually changes norepinephrine and normetanephrine to the corresponding mandelic aldehydes. These products are then transformed to mandelic acids by aldehyde dehydrogenase. (For other details see text.)

the first step in the metabolism of epinephrine, O-methylation, results in a biologically inactive compound.

Role of MAO in catecholamine metabolism

MAO, localized in mitochondria, is widely distributed in all tissues of the body, one of its functions being the detoxication of monoamines such as tyramine that may be absorbed from the gastrointestinal tract. When this enzyme is inhibited by drugs, the norepinephrine concentration rises in many tissues that have adrenergic innervation.[79] This finding suggests that MAO has an important regulatory function on the norepinephrine stores in adrenergic nerves.

In addition to these important functions, MAO is responsible also for the transformation to VMA of the catecholamines first methylated by the transferase enzyme (Fig. 8-6).

TERMINATION OF ACTION OF CATECHOLAMINES

A number of experimental facts suggest that uptake of catecholamines by nerves is the most important mechanism for the termination of the action of catecholamines. First, the injection of small physiologic doses of tritiated norepinephrine results in its rapid clearance from the blood by the heart and other organs innervated by adrenergic fibers.[32] That this uptake is in adrenergic fibers has been demonstrated by

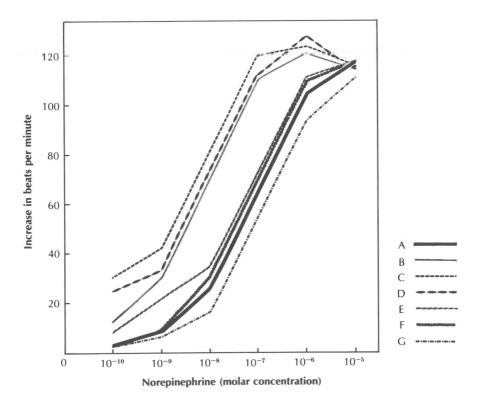

Fig. 8-7. Horizontal displacement of dose-response curves of norepinephrine by cocaine and some antihistaminics, using the isolated rat atrium as the test object. *A,* Saline control; *B,* after cocaine; *C,* after tripelennamine; *D,* after *d*-chlorpheniramine; *E,* after phenindamine; *F,* after pyrilamine; *G,* after promethazine. Cocaine and some antihistaminics potentiate the chronotropic effects of norepinephrine, whereas other antihistaminics have no effect. (From Isaac, L., and Goth, A.: Life Sci. **4:**1899, 1965.)

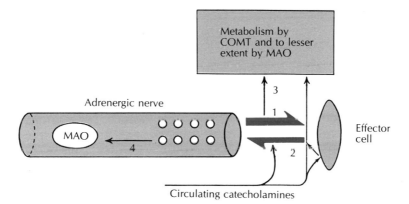

Fig. 8-8. Fate of norepinephrine released from adrenergic nerve. *1,* Release and interaction with receptor on effector cell; *2,* reuptake into the nerve of a portion of released norepinephrine; *3,* metabolism by COMT and to a lesser extent by MAO; *4,* metabolic degradation within the nerve by MAO of norepinephrine released within the axoplasm (such as following ingestion of reserpine).

histochemical techniques in vitro.[3] Furthermore, sympathetic nerve stimulation or reserpine treatment causes release of tritiated catecholamine.

Denervated structures take up only very small quantities of tritiated norepinephrine. Such structures, of course, are supersensitive to the action of catecholamines. Cocaine, imipramine, and certain antihistaminics[36] block the uptake of norepinephrine and potentiate the action of catecholamines (Fig. 8-7). These relationships may become clear by an examination of Fig. 8-8. (See also p. 69.)

THE AMINE PUMP AND FALSE TRANSMITTERS

—The relatively nonspecific amine pump of the adrenergic neuron transports not only catecholamines but also tyramine, metaraminol,[57] α-methyldopa, and even serotonin. Some of these, such as metaraminol, may be held by the axon terminal and released on nerve stimulation, thereby acting as *false transmitters*.[12] The antihypertensive drug α-methyldopa is taken up by the neuron and transformed to α-methyl-norepinephrine, which also acts as a false transmitter when released. A hypotensive action may result from the lower potency of the false transmitters compared with norepinephrine, which they displace.

Despite the low specificity of the amine pump, the adrenergic neuron is protected against the accumulation of all sorts of amines by the much greater specificity of the granular storage mechanism. Thus when tyramine is taken up, it is not only deaminated by monoamine oxidase but the resulting product is also rejected by the granules, since only β-hydroxylated amines are held there. After the use of monoamine oxidase inhibitors, however, tyramine, which is protected against deamination, is transformed by the fairly nonspecific dopamine-β-oxidase into the β-hydroxy derivative *octopamine*, which can be stored in the granules and act as a false transmitter. The hypotensive action of monoamine oxidase inhibitors has been attributed to this mechanism,[76] although the explanation is not entirely satisfying.

Adrenergic nerve terminals can take up compounds that may be injurious to them. The experimental drug *6-hydroxydopamine* causes degenerative changes in adrenergic nerve terminals,[61] leading to *chemical sympathectomy*. Desipramine, a known blocker of the amine pump, prevents these effects.[78]

THERAPEUTIC APPLICATIONS

The therapeutic uses of epinephrine and norepinephrine are based on the vasoconstrictor, cardiac stimulant, and bronchodilator properties of these compounds.

Vasoconstrictor uses

Epinephrine is commonly added to local anesthetic solutions because its vasoconstrictor action delays the absorption of the local anesthetic and thereby restricts its effect to a given area. Because of its vasoconstrictor ability, epinephrine is widely used in the treatment of urticaria and angioneurotic edema.

Norepinephrine has been enthusiastically received as a systemic vasoconstrictor in various hypotensive states. It must be admitted, however, that the intravenous infusion of a vasoconstrictor is not a perfect substitute for normal sympathetic tone because it may actually decrease blood flow to certain vital areas such as the brain unless the rise in systemic pressure is adequate. Norepinephrine is certainly not a substitute for the physiologic management of shocklike states and does not obviate the necessity of correcting such underlying abnormalities as decreased blood volume or fluid balance disturbances.

Cardiac uses

Either epinephrine or the newer drug isoproterenol is indicated in the management of heart block or Adams-Stokes syndrome. These drugs act partly to improve auriculo-ventricular conduction but mostly by stimulating ventricular automaticity, thus producing an increased ventricular rate. Caution should be exercised in the so-called states of prefibrillation, since the drug may precipitate ventricular arrhythmias. It is permissible to inject epinephrine directly into the heart in asystole in an attempt to achieve resuscitation. Cardiac massage is gaining much favor over the simple epinephrine resuscitation.

Bronchodilator action

Epinephrine is a time-honored remedy in the treatment of bronchial asthma. For this purpose it may be given subcutaneously in the amount of 0.2 to 0.5 ml. of a 1:1,000 solution. It may also be given by inhalation. For this purpose a stronger solution (up to 1:100) is employed in a nebulizer. Isoproterenol has been replacing epinephrine in this type of treatment.

Contraindications to the use of epinephrine and norepinephrine exist in hyperthyroidism, in severe hypertension, in various types of heart disease, and if some other drug such as cyclopropane is used that may sensitize the heart to the action of epinephrine.

CATECHOLAMINES AND DISEASE STATES
Hypertension

Since the hemodynamic consequences of norepinephrine infusion are similar to those observed in essential hypertension, it has been suspected that the compound may play a role in hypertensive disease. On the other hand, no increase in catecholamine excretion has been found in the urine of hypertensive patients.

Pheochromocytoma

A rare form of hypertension is caused by tumors of adrenomedullary tissue that secrete norepinephrine with variable amounts of epinephrine. Although pheochromocytoma is a rare tumor, its diagnosis is most important because it represents one of the few forms of completely curable hypertension.

Several tumors have been examined by chemical methods. It appears that most of them contain very high concentrations of norepinephrine and smaller amounts of epinephrine. There may be as much as 10 to 15 mg./gram of tissue, and the total catecholamine content of a large tumor may be more than 1 gram.

Several methods have been introduced during the last few years for the diagnosis of pheochromocytoma. Some of these are based on neuropharmacologic principles and others on the determination of catecholamines in the urine. Although pharmacologic tests are inaccurate and hazardous as compared with chemical tests, they illustrate interesting principles.

Pharmacologic tests. Drug tests for pheochromocytoma are of two types: those that can promote the secretion of catecholamines from the tumor and cause blood pressure elevation and those that inhibit the actions of norepinephrine and thereby cause lowering of the elevated blood pressure.

Among those drugs that elevate blood pressure in patients with pheochromocytoma are histamine, methacholine, and tetraethylammonium. Drugs that lower blood pressure in patients with pheochromocytoma are piperoxan, phenoxybenzamine, and phentolamine.

Histamine, methacholine, and tetraethylammonium lower the blood pressure in normal human beings. They can stimulate adrenomedullary secretion, which causes elevation of blood pressure in patients with pheochromocytoma. This slight effect on the adrenal medulla is overshadowed under normal circumstances by their hypotensive action.

The most widely used drug in diagnosis of pheochromocytoma is phentolamine (Regitine). A dose of 5 mg. is injected intravenously or intramuscularly. If systolic blood pressure falls more than 35 mm. Hg and diastolic pressure more than 25 mm. Hg, the test is considered positive.

Recently tyramine has been added to the list of drugs that cause a marked pressor response in patients with pheochromocytoma.[67]

Chemical tests. Pheochromocytomas secrete norepinephrine and epinephrine. These are metabolized to their respective 3-methoxylated derivatives—normetanephrine and metanephrine. Both of these in turn are converted to VMA. Practically all patients with pheochromocytoma excrete all these compounds in amounts above normal.

The diagnosis of pheochromocytoma may be established by the determination of normetanephrine plus epinephrine or norepinephrine plus epinephrine or VMA in a 24-hour urine specimen. There is a rapid screening procedure for VMA in many labora-

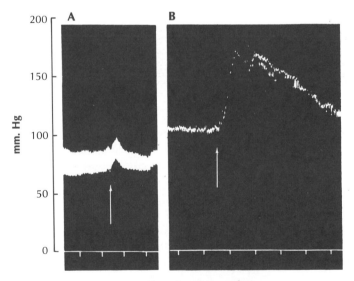

Tyramine (0.5 mg./kg.)

Fig. 8-9. Blood pressure response to tyramine. **A,** Reserpinized cat. **B,** Control cat. Dose of reserpine: 7 mg./kg. subcutaneously. Dose of tyramine: 0.5 mg./kg. intravenously. Arrow indicates time of injection. (From Carlsson, A., Rosengren, E., Bertler, Å., and Nilsson, J.: Psychotropic drugs, Amsterdam, 1957, Elsevier Publishing Co.)

tories, but its diagnostic accuracy is not as great as that of other procedures. Methyldopa, tetracycline, and quinidine may falsely increase norepinephrine plus epinephrine values. MAO inhibitors will increase normetanephrine plus metanephrine. Anxiety and excitement do not elevate the excretion of catecholamines sufficiently to cause diagnostic errors. On the other hand, acute myocardial infarction, surgical trauma, and shock may cause abnormally high urinary output of the catecholamines and their metabolites.[11]

PREPARATIONS OF NOREPINEPHRINE (LEVARTERENOL) AND EPINEPHRINE

Levarterenol bitartrate (Levophed bitartrate) is available for injection in a 0.2% solution equivalent to 1 mg. of base per milliliter in 2 and 4 ml. ampules. For intravenous infusion in adults 4 to 8 ml. of the 0.2% solution is added to 500 ml. of 5% dextrose injection. The infusion rate is regulated to keep the systolic blood pressure somewhat below normal.

Epinephrine hydrochloride (Adrenalin chloride) is a solution containing, for injection, 1 mg./ml. and, for inhalation, 10 mg./ml.

Epinephrine bitartrate is available in special devices (Medihaler-epi) for inhalation, delivering 0.3 mg. per dose.

Epinephrine suspension, aqueous or in oil, for injection contains 2.5 or 2 mg./ml.

Epinephrine bitartrate and epinephrine hydrochloride are also available for opthalmic uses in 1 and 2% solutions.

MISCELLANEOUS ADRENERGIC DRUGS

The various sympathomimetic drugs may act *directly* on alpha and beta receptors or they may act *indirectly* by releasing endogenous catecholamines. Some also have a *mixed* action, both direct and indirect. Some important examples are as follows:

	Alpha agonists	Beta agonists
Direct acting drugs	Methoxamine	Isoproterenol
Mixed acting drugs	Metaraminol	Ephedrine (indirect on alpha receptors)
Indirect acting drugs	Tyramine	
	Amphetamine	

The evidence for this classification is based on various considerations. It has been demonstrated that tyramine, ephedrine, amphetamine, and phenylethylamine, now considered indirectly acting agents, had less effect in animals in whose tissue the norepinephrine content had been depleted by reserpine[7] (Fig. 8-9).

The infusion of norepinephrine restored the capacity of the animals to react to these drugs. In a reserpinized animal the *responses* to some adrenergic drugs are normal or augmented. Other adrenergic drugs are suppressed, and still others are partly antagonized by reserpine.[47] Drugs of the first type include norepinephrine, epinephrine, and phenylephrine. They are direct acting. Among those suppressed by norepinephrine depletion are tyramine, amphetamine, phenylethylamine, and hydroxyamphetamine. Partially suppressed and having presumably a mixed effect are ephedrine and phenylpropanolamine.

Similar results can be obtained with sympathomimetic drugs in animals pretreated with guanethidine.[46]

Another line of evidence that suggests norepinephrine release as the mode of action of many sympathomimetic drugs is the observation that indirectly acting amines are ineffective on chronically denervated structures.

Classification based on clinical usage

A discussion of the sympathomimetic amines may be simplified by placing them into categories based on their clinical usage. There are three such categories: the vasoconstrictors, the bronchodilators, and the central nervous system stimulants. Despite some overlap in these activities, it is possible to select sympathomimetics for therapeutic purposes on the basis of predominant action. Ephedrine, a prototype of the sympathomimetic amines, belongs to a special category. It is used for its cardiovascular, bronchodilator, and stimulant properties.

Adrenergic vasoconstriction is mediated by alpha receptors, and some of the drugs in this group, such as phenylephrine and methoxamine, are largely alpha drugs. Most vasopressors have some effects on beta receptors also. They have cardiac effects, but their vasodilator action is concealed by the more powerful alpha effect.

Bronchodilators in the adrenergic series act on beta receptors. Central nervous system stimulation cannot be explained at present in a satisfactory manner by the receptor theory.

Adrenergic vasoconstrictors are phenylephrine, methoxamine, mephentermine, metaraminol, and the nasal vasoconstrictors phenylephrine hydrochloride, hydroxyamphetamine, phenylpropanolamine, propylhexedrine, cyclopentamine, tuaminoheptane, methylhexaneamine, naphazoline, and tetrahydrozoline. Dopamine is also being advocated in the treatment of hypotension.[44]

Adrenergic bronchodilators are isoproterenol, protokylol, isoetharine, and methoxyphenamine. Related vasodilators are nylidrin and isoxsuprine.

Adrenergic central nervous system stimulants and anorexiants are amphetamine sulfate, dextroamphetamine, methamphetamine, and the related appetite suppressants phenmetrazine and diethylpropion.

Ephedrine

Used in China for centuries and introduced into the United States in 1923, ephedrine is a naturally occurring sympathomimetic drug. It is the most widely used drug in the prevention and treatment of bronchial asthma and acts, at least in part, by releasing catecholamines from their storage vesicles. Its action is similar to that of epinephrine and norepinephrine except for a much longer duration of action, effectiveness after oral administration, central nervous system stimulation, and occurrence of tachyphylaxis on frequent administration. On a weight basis it is about 100 times weaker; thus it is administered in doses of about 25 mg. Its action lasts for hours, and it is well absorbed from the gastrointestinal tract. From the standpoint of intestinal absorption of sympathomimetic drugs, the generalization may be made that the *phenyl* amines are much better absorbed than are the catechol derivatives.

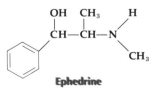

Ephedrine

Ephedrine is an indirectly acting phenylisopropylamine. Its peripheral actions are reduced by intensive pretreatment with reserpine or by sympathetic denervation. Its central nervous system effects, however, are probably direct, since they are not eliminated by reserpine pretreatment. In this respect, ephedrine resembles the amphetamines.

In addition to its vasopressor effects, ephedrine acts on the heart, the heart rate usually increasing. Ephedrine dilates the bronchi and is very useful in the treatment of asthma. It causes mydriasis when applied to the eye, produces central nervous system stimulation with anxiety and wakefulness, and has some slight anticurare action on the skeletal muscles. It is occasionally useful in myasthenia gravis. The compound also has metabolic actions similar to those of epinephrine but is not nearly so potent as the catecholamine in this respect.

Ephedrine is a useful sympathomimetic drug. Its effectiveness following oral administration and its sustained action in the treatment of bronchospasm and some forms of hypotension are distinct advantages over epinephrine. Its central nervous system stimulant effect may be a disadvantage in some patients and may require the simultaneous use of an hypnotic. Ephedrine sulfate USP is available for oral administration in the form of capsules containing 25 and 50 mg. and also as an elixir containing 5 and 10 mg./5 ml. For injection, solutions containing 20, 25, or 50 mg./ml. are available.

ADRENERGIC VASOCONSTRICTORS
Phenylephrine

Phenylephrine (Neo-Synephrine) is closely related chemically to epinephrine. It is a useful vasoconstrictor of sustained action with little effect on the myocardium or the central nervous system. Subcutaneous injection of 5 mg. has been employed extensively to prevent hypotension during spinal anesthesia and for the treatment of orthostatic hypotension. Phenylephrine has a direct action, largely on alpha receptors. Its use as a nasal decongestant is discussed on p. 110.

Methoxamine

Methoxamine (Vasoxyl) differs from many other vasopressors in its remarkable lack of cardiac stimulant properties. When 10 to 20 mg. of methoxamine is injected intramuscularly, the drug produces a sustained pressor effect without cardiac stimulation. It is being employed in various hypotensive states. It does not produce arrhythmias during cyclopropane anesthesia. Methoxamine is available for injection as a solution containing 10 and 20 mg./ml.

Mephentermine

Mephentermine (Wyamine) is a vasopressor drug of prolonged duration of action. It has little effect on the central nervous system but has marked stimulant action on the myocardium, along with its vasopressor action. It has the usual applications in hypotensive states and as a nasal decongestant. Mephentermine sulfate for injection is available in solutions containing 15 and 30 mg./ml.

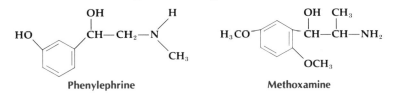

Phenylephrine   Methoxamine

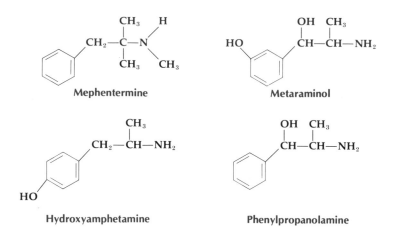

Mephentermine

Metaraminol

Hydroxyamphetamine

Phenylpropanolamine

Metaraminol

Metaraminol (Aramine) resembles phenylephrine in its properties. It is used as a nasal decongestant and a systemic vasopressor and may be administered subcutaneously or intramuscularly in doses of 2 to 10 mg. The uptake of metaraminol by sympathetic fibers is discussed on p. 103. Metaraminol may cause ventricular arrhythmias when used with anesthetics that sensitize the heart to catecholamines. Metaraminol bitartrate is available as an injectable solution containing 10 mg./ml.

Dopamine

Dopamine is a catecholamine of great interest as a chemical mediator in certain parts of the central nervous system (p. 66). It is also the immediate precursor in the biosynthesis of norepinephrine. Its role in Parkinson's disease and the use of L-dopa in this condition are discussed on p. 129.

As an experimental sympathomimetic drug, dopamine activates largely beta receptors. It causes some elevation of blood pressure, mainly in stimulating cardiac output. A unique feature of the action of dopamine is its ability to dilate renal vessels and to produce sodium diuresis.[49]

The dosage required for producing cardiovascular effects varies from 100 to 1,000 μg/min. by constant intravenous infusion.[27] Its use in congestive failure is only experimental.

Nasal vasoconstrictors

Some of the commonly used nasal decongestants are the following.

Phenylephrine hydrochloride (Neo-Synephrine hydrochloride) is available in solutions of 0.125 to 1% for topical application; it may cause rebound swelling of the nasal mucosa. Oral administration of the drug in capsules of 10 and 25 mg. is somewhat unpredictable in its effect.

Phenylpropanolamine hydrochloride (Propadrine hydrochloride) is available in capsules of 25 mg.; it has been used as an anorexiant also, but is ineffective.

Propylhexedrine (Benzedrex) is commonly administered by inhalation. It has many of the properties of amphetamine but with lesser pressor effect and much less central nervous system stimulation.

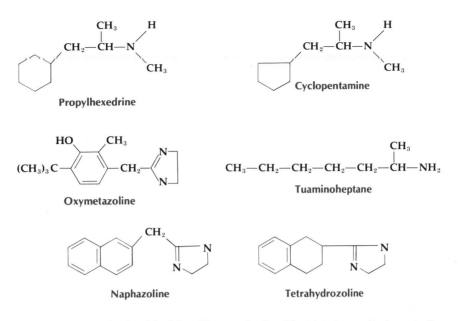

Cyclopentamine hydrochloride (Clopane hydrochloride) is applied topically as a 0.5% solution.

Tuaminoheptane (Tuamine) is available as a 1% solution and also as an inhalant.

Oxymetazoline hydrochloride (Afrin) is available in 0.05% solution as nose drops and spray.

Naphazoline hydrochloride (Privine hydrochloride), an imidazoline derivative, is available in 0.05% solutions as nose drops and a spray. It may cause profound drowsiness and coma in children and also rebound swelling of the mucosa and cardiac irregularities when used excessively.

Tetrahydrozoline hydrochloride (Tyzine) is similar to naphazoline chemically and in its adverse effects.

Current concept of nasal vasoconstrictors

The nasal vasoconstrictors or decongestants are symptomatic medications that have some usefulness but are not harmless. Continued use of these medications may actually induce chronic congestion of the nasal mucosa, probably because ischemia leads to rebound swelling. In excessive doses the nasal decongestants produce the usual adrenergic effects such as increased blood pressure, dizziness, palpitation, and in some cases central nervous system stimulation. In addition, the imidazoline derivatives naphazoline and tetrahydrozoline have produced drowsiness and coma in children.

The nasal decongestants are frequently combined with antihistamines. Thus preparations containing phenylephrine and an antihistamine have become very popular as nasal decongestants that are taken orally. A critical evaluation of these preparations would suggest that there is no advantage in the oral administration of sympathetic amines over their topical application. Furthermore, no definitive evidence of the usefulness or contribution of the antihistamine to the overall effect has been found. Nevertheless, the oral use of nasal vasoconstrictor–antihistamine combinations has become extraordinarily popular, and perhaps further studies may reveal their advantages over topically applied nasal decongestants.

ADRENERGIC BRONCHODILATORS
Isoproterenol

Isoproterenol (isopropylnorepinephrine) is a potent activator of *beta* receptors. It dilates the bronchial smooth muscle and has powerful effects on the heart. It also dilates blood vessels, particularly in skeletal muscle. When used in the treatment of bronchial asthma, it may cause tachycardia, arrhythmias, and hypotension. Some instances of sudden death in asthmatics have been attributed to the excessive use of isoproterenol.

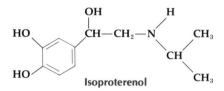

Isoproterenol

The cardiac effects are undesirable when the drug is used in the treatment of bronchial asthma. Palpitations, tachycardia, and anginal pain may occur even after inhalation of the drug. These actions preclude its systemic use by injection. The cardiac actions of the drug may have some usefulness in enhancing deficient auriculoventricular conduction.

In addition to its usefulness as a bronchodilator, isoproterenol is commonly used in the treatment of complete heart block. It should be remembered that isoproterenol, in contrast with most adrenergic drugs, tends to lower peripheral vascular resistance, since it is a *beta* receptor activator.

Isoproterenol hydrochloride (Isuprel hydrochloride) is available in solutions of 1:100 (10 mg./ml.), 1:200 (5 mg./ml.), and 1:400 (2.5 mg./ml.) for oral inhalation; solutions containing 0.2 mg/ml) for injection; and sublingual tablets of 10 and 15 mg. The effects of the tablets are somewhat unpredictable because of erratic absorption.

Other bronchodilators

In addition to isoproterenol, several adrenergic drugs and theophylline derivatives are used as bronchodilators. Epinephrine and ephedrine are widely used and have already been discussed (pp. 105 and 108). Protokylol, isoetharine, and methoxyphenamine are additional adrenergic bronchodilators. Among the theophylline derivatives, aminophylline (theophylline ethylenediamine), oxtriphylline, theophylline in 20% alcohol, and theophylline–sodium glycinate are commonly used in asthmatics. The corticosteroids, although not primarily bronchodilators, are also of great importance in the treatment of severe asthma.

Protokylol (Caytine) resembles isoproterenol in that it may cause cardiac stimulation but no great elevation of blood pressure. It is administered by subcutaneous or intramuscular injection in solution, 0.5 mg./ml.; orally by 2 mg. tablets; or by inhalation of a 1:100 solution (10 mg./ml.).

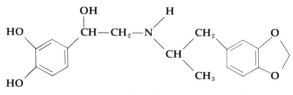

Protokylol

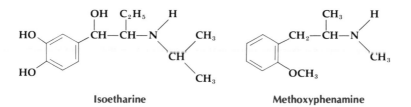

Isoetharine   Methoxyphenamine

Isoetharine (Dilabron) also resembles isoproterenol but is less active. It is used in 1.75% solution for inhalation.

Methoxyphenamine (Orthoxine) has a relatively greater bronchodilator than vasoconstrictor effect when compared with ephedrine. It is used in asthma in doses of 50 mg. Methoxyphenamine hydrochloride (Orthoxine hydrochloride) is available in tablets, 100 mg.; and syrup, 50 mg./5 ml.

Theophylline derivatives. Various naturally occurring xanthines such as caffeine, theophylline, and theobromine exert to a varying extent numerous pharmacologic effects such as central nervous system stimulation, myocardial stimulation, smooth muscle relaxation, and diuresis. Although caffeine has some medical uses as a stimulant, the theophylline derivatives are the most useful drugs in this group as bronchodilators.

The similarities in the actions of adrenergic drugs and theophylline derivatives on the bronchial smooth muscle and on the heart may be related to a basic biochemical effect on cyclic adenylic acid levels in the tissues. As discussed elsewhere (p. 98), catecholamines activate adenyl cyclase, whereas the methylxanthines inhibit phosphodiesterase (p. 99, Fig. 8-3).

Aminophylline (theophylline ethylenediamine) is a highly effective drug for the relief of bronchospasm, particularly when administered by slow intravenous injection. The drug is also given by the oral route and in the form of suppositories. Its absorption from the gastrointestinal tract is somewhat unpredictable.

The most common adverse effects resulting from administration of aminophylline are nausea, vomiting, and epigastric pain. Restlessness and insomnia represent manifestations of central nervous system stimulation. Rapid intravenous injection of aminophylline may cause sudden hypotension and should be avoided.

In addition to its usefulness in the treatment of asthma, aminophylline has other indications. It is a mild diuretic (p. 438). It stimulates the respiratory center and is used occasionally to abolish Cheyne-Stokes respiration. It is found useful also in the treatment of some manifestations of left heart failure, such as paroxysmal nocturnal dyspnea and pulmonary edema.

Preparations of aminophylline include a solution containing 25 mg./ml. for intravenous injection; tablets of 100 and 200 mg. or elixir containing 259 mg./ml. for oral administration; suppositories containing 25, 100, 250, and 500 mg.; and powder for enemas.

Oxytriphylline (Choledyl) is the choline salt of theophylline. It has the same actions as theophylline, but since it is more soluble, its gastrointestinal absorption is better. It is available in tablets of 100 and 200 mg. for oral administration.

Theophylline elixir (Elixophyllin) (theophylline in 20% alcohol) is claimed to be more consistently absorbed from the gastrointestinal tract. It contains 80 mg./15 ml.

Theophylline–sodium glycinate (Glynazan; Theoglycinate) has the same pharmacology as aminophylline. It is claimed to be better absorbed than theophylline and causes less gastric irritation. Preparations include tablets of 324 mg. and elixir containing 324 mg./5 ml. for oral administration.

Adrenal corticosteroids. The adrenal corticosteroids may be remarkably effective in severe asthma that fails to respond to adrenergic drugs or theophylline derivatives. The adrenal corticosteroids will be discussed in Chapter 37.

Clinical pharmacology of bronchodilators

There are significant discrepancies between the potency of the various compounds in experimental preparations and in human bronchial asthma.* The animal investigations show that isoproterenol is ten times as effective as epinephrine and that methoxyphenamine is much more effective than ephedrine. Clinical experience shows, on the other hand, that the differences between these various compounds are not nearly so great. To explain these discrepancies between animal experimentation and clinical experience, some investigators suggest that factors other than bronchial constriction contribute to the obstruction of air flow in the human disease. Some of these factors may be edema of the mucous membrane and the presence of thick secretions, the viscosity of which impedes their removal from the bronchial tree.

Atropine, which has been disappointing in the treatment of asthma, furnished a good illustration of the importance of mucous secretions in the clinical picture of this disease. It is believed by competent clinical investigators that through its drying effect the drug may actually increase the viscosity of mucus, making it more difficult for the patient to cough up the accumulated secretions.

The most effective drugs in human bronchial asthma are isoproterenol, epinephrine, and the theophylline compounds (aminophylline). The adrenal glucocorticoids are remarkably effective also, but their use is reserved for otherwise intractable cases.

The action of these highly effective medications is reinforced by using ephedrine and other bronchodilators, antihistaminics, potassium iodide, and often some sedatives.

ADRENERGIC VASODILATORS

Isoproterenol is a beta adrenergic stimulant that dilates blood vessels while it stimulates the heart. Certain vasodilators have been developed that probably act through a similar mechanism. These are **nylidrin** (Arlidin) and **isoxsuprine** (Vasodilan). Although these drugs can dilate peripheral blood vessels experimentally, their effectiveness in the management of peripheral vascular disease is not universally accepted among clinical investigators. Nylidrin is used orally in doses of 6 mg. and isoxsuprine is also used orally in doses of 10 to 20 mg. Although the action of these drugs resembles that of isoproterenol, they probably act indirectly by releasing catecholamines.

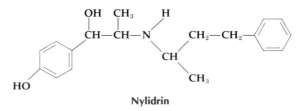

Nylidrin

---

*For a discussion of more selective adrenergic bronchodilators, see p. 448.

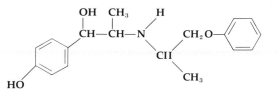

Isoxsuprine

ADRENERGIC CENTRAL NERVOUS SYSTEM STIMULANTS AND ANOREXIANTS
Amphetamines

The amphetamines are powerful stimulants of the central nervous system. *Dextro*-amphetamine has relatively greater central, and less cardiovascular, effects than the *levo* isomer. The drug is used and also abused mainly in relation to its anorexiant effect, and even this use is questioned by many authorities. In addition to being an anorexiant, dextroamphetamine finds some application as an analeptic, in the treatment of narcolepsy, as an antidepressant, in the management of hyperkinetic children, and in postencephalitic reactions.

Numerous anorexiants have been developed and are used by the medical profession, often without the realization that these drugs are essentially weak relatives of dextroamphetamine without significant advantages over the anorexiant prototype. Some of these drugs are methamphetamine (Desoxyn), phenmetrazine (Preludin), diethylpropion (Tenuate; Tepanil), phenylpropanolamine (Propadrine), phentermine (Ionamin; Wilpo), chlorphentermine (Pre-Sate), benzphetamine (Didrex), and phendimetrazine (Plegine). In addition, numerous mixtures of adrenergic stimulants with barbiturates and other depressants have been prepared and are used widely as anorexiants. Despite their popularity, such mixtures are generally not recommended.

The disadvantages in the use of anorexiants are related to the development of psychic dependence and to untoward effects resulting from adrenergic actions. Toxic psychosis may result from large doses of many of these drugs.

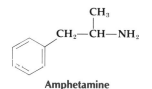

Amphetamine

The racemic form is known as amphetamine and the dextro isomer as dextroamphetamine. The latter is a more potent central nervous system stimulant, whereas the levo isomer has somewhat greater vasopressor activity. The vascular effects of the amphetamines may be attributed to endogenous catecholamine release, since they do not elevate blood pressure in a reserpinized animal. The central nervous system effects are probably not mediated by catecholamine release, since they persist in reserpinized animals. Nevertheless, dextroamphetamine promotes norepinephrine release in the brain.[9] Perhaps it acts on a special norepinephrine pool.

Habituation and tolerance develop to the central nervous system actions of the amphetamines. Withdrawal of the drug leads to marked craving. The amphetamines

115

are well absorbed from the gastrointestinal tract. Amphetamine is metabolized in the liver to p-hydroxyamphetamine. This metabolite may be taken up by adrenergic nerves peripherally and transformed to p-hydroxynorephedrine, which may be stored in the adrenergic vesicles, thus forming a false transmitter.[54] This series of events may explain the tolerance that develops to the pressor actions of amphetamine.

The central nervous system effect of amphetamine is probably related to catecholamine release in the brain and is antagonized — experimentally — by α-methyltyrosine.[20] Although a reserpinized animal still responds to amphetamine with stimulation, this does not prove a direct action of amphetamine. Oral administration of 5 to 10 mg. of dextroamphetamine keeps an individual awake and may elevate his mood, decrease the feeling of fatigue, decrease his appetite, and improve his athletic performance. Large doses produce toxic psychosis.

Methamphetamine (d-desoxyephedrine) is closely related from a structural standpoint to both ephedrine and amphetamine. It is a potent central nervous system stimulant and has a considerable pressor effect on blood vessels. It is used for the same purposes as amphetamine in approximately the same dosage.

Phenmetrazine (Preludin) is used as an appetite suppressant, a questionable approach to the treatment of obesity. It has considerable central nervous system effects.

Diethylpropion (Tenuate; Tepanil) is employed as an anorexigenic agent. It is basically an amphetamine-like drug, although it is claimed that it causes less jitteriness and insomnia and also fewer cardiovascular effects than does amphetamine. The drug is considerably weaker than dextroamphetamine and is used in doses of 25 mg. orally.

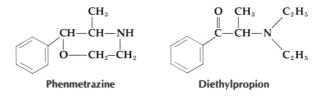

Phenmetrazine   Diethylpropion

STRUCTURE-ACTIVITY RELATIONSHIPS IN ADRENERGIC SERIES

A great deal is known about the relationships between structure and activity in adrenergic drugs. Such knowledge in general is of importance to the pharmaceutical chemist in guiding him in synthetic work on new drugs. Structure-activity relationships are also of fundamental importance in that they should reflect basic characteristics of receptor mechanisms. In the case of adrenergic drugs the problem is complicated by the fact that many sympathomimetic drugs act indirectly through the release of endogenous catecholamines. The differences in action of these drugs may be related to the predominant site of catecholamine release.

A few generalities may serve to illustrate the concept of structure-activity relationships.

The basic adrenergic structure is phenylethylamine.

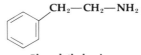

Phenylethylamine

The benzene ring is not essential. Aliphatic chains and ring structures such as naphthalene may be substituted. Hydroxide groups on the benzene ring influence the metabolic rate and also intestinal absorption of the drugs. Sympathomimetic drugs lacking hydroxide groups on the benzene ring are absorbed from the gastrointestinal tract and are not attacked by COMT.

Substitutions on the nitrogen have a great influence on the type of receptor with which the drug will interact. Thus norepinephrine, lacking substitutions, acts on alpha receptors, epinephrine with one methyl group acts on both receptors, and isoproterenol acts almost entirely on beta receptors.

Substitutions on the alpha carbon tend to prolong the action of the drug, probably because of protection against enzymatic destruction. The OH group on the beta carbon is necessary for granular storage in adrenergic neurons.

References

1 Abboud, F. M., Eckstein, J. W., Zimmerman, B. G., and Graham, M. H.: Sensitization of arteries, veins and small vessels to norepinephrine after cocaine, Circ. Res. 15:247, 1964.

2 Ahlquist, R. P.: A study of the adrenotropic receptors, Amer. J. Physiol. 153:586, 1948.

3 Angelakos, E. T.: Histochemical demonstration of uptake of exogenous norepinephrine by adrenergic fibers in vitro, Science 145:503, 1964.

4 Armstrong, M. D., McMillan, A., and Shaw, K. N.: 3-Methoxy-4-hydroxy-D-mandelic acid, a urinary metabolite of norepinephrine, Biochim. Biophys. Acta 25:422, 1957.

5 Axelrod, J., Inscoe, J. K., Senoh, S., and Witkop, B.: O-methylation, the principal pathway for the metabolism of epinephrine and norepinephrine in the rat, Biochim. Biophys. Acta 27:210, 1958.

6 Axelrod, J., and Laroche, M. J.: Inhibitor of O-methylation of epinephrine and norepinephrine in vitro and in vivo, Science 130:800, 1959.

7 Burn, J. H., and Rand, M. J.: The action of sympathomimetic amines in animals treated with reserpine, J. Physiol. 144:314, 1958.

8 Carlsson, A., and Hillarp, N. A.: On the state of the catecholamines of the adrenal medullary granules, Acta Physiol. Scand. 44:163, 1958.

9 Carr, L. A., and Moore, K. E.: Norepinephrine: release from brain by d-amphetamine in vivo, Science 164:322, 1969.

10 Costa, E., and Garattini, S., editors: International Symposium on amphetamines, New York, 1970, Raven Press.

11 Crout, J. R.: Sampling and analysis of catecholamines and metabolites, Anesthesiology 29:661, 1968.

12 Crout, J. R., Alpers, H. S., Tatum, E. L., and Shore, P. A.: Release of metaraminol (Aramine)

from the heart by sympathetic nerve stimulation, Science 145:828, 1964.

13 Crout, J. R., Pisano, J. J., and Sjoerdsma, A.: Urinary excretion of catecholamines and their metabolites in pheochromocytoma, Amer. Heart J. 61:375, 1961.

14 Crout, J. R., and Sjoerdsma, A.: Catecholamines in the localization of pheochromocytoma, Circulation 22:516, 1960.

15 Dale, H. H.: On some physiological actions of ergot, J. Physiol. 34:163, 1906.

16 Dengler, H. J., Michaelson, I. A., Spiegel, H. E., and Titus, E. O.: The uptake of labeled norepinephrine by isolated brain and other tissues of the cat, Int. J. Neuropharmacol. 1:23, 1962.

17 Dickman, S. R., Wiest, W. G., and Eik Nes, K.: Effects of epinephrine on metabolism of glucose of normal dogs, Amer. J. Physiol. 194:327, 1958.

18 Drury, D. R., and Wick, A. N.: Epinephrine and carbohydrate metabolism, Amer. J. Physiol. 194:465, 1958.

19 Engelman, K., and Sjoerdsma, A.: A new test for pheochromocytoma, J.A.M.A. 189:81, 1964.

20 Enna, S. J., Dorris, R. L., and Shore, P. A.: Specific inhibition by α-methyltyrosine of amphetamine induced amine release from brain, J. Pharmacol Exp. Ther. 184:576, 1973.

21 Espelin, D. E., and Done, A. K.: Amphetamine poisoning; effectiveness of chlorpromazine, New Eng. J. Med. 278:1361, 1968.

22 von Euler, U. S.: A specific sympathomimetic ergone in adrenergic nerve fibers (sympathin) and its relation to adrenaline and noradrenaline, Acta Physiol. Scand. 12:73, 1946.

23 von Euler, U. S.: Noradrenaline: chemistry, physiology, pharmacology, and clinical aspects, Springfield, Ill., 1956, Charles C Thomas, Publisher.

24 von Euler, U. S., and Purkhold, A.: Effect of sympathetic denervation on the noradrenaline and adrenaline content of the spleen, kidney, and salivary glands in the sheep, Acta Physiol. Scand. **24**:212, 1951.

25 Frederickson, D. S., and Gordon, R. S.: Transport of fatty acids, Physiol. Rev. **38**:585, 1958.

26 Furchgott, R. F.: The receptors for epinephrine and norepinephrine (adrenergic receptors), Pharmacol. Rev. **11**:429, 1959.

27 Goldberg, L. I., McDonald, R. H., and Zimmerman, A. M.: Sodium diuresis produced by dopamine in patients with congestive heart failure, New Eng. J. Med. **269**:1060, 1963.

28 Goldenberg, M.: Adrenal medullary function, Amer. J. Med. **10**:627, 1951.

29 Goldenberg, M., Aranow, H., Jr., Smith, A. A., and Faber, M.: Pheochromocytoma and essential hypertensive disease, Arch. Intern. Med. **86**:823, 1950.

30 Goldenberg, M., Pines, K. L., Baldwin, E. deF., Greene, D. G., and Roh, C. E.: The hemodynamic response of man to nor-epinephrine and epinephrine and its relation to the problem of hypertension, Amer. J. Med. **5**:792, 1948.

31 Govier, W. C.: A positive inotropic effect of phenylephrine mediated through alpha adrenergic receptors, Life Sci. **6**:1361, 1967.

32 Hertting, G., Axelrod, J., and Whitby, L. G.: Effect of drugs on the uptake and metabolism of H³-norepinephrine, J. Pharmacol. Exp. Ther. **134**:146, 1961.

33 Hertting, G., Kopin, I. J., and Gordon, E.: The uptake, release, and metabolism of norepinephrine-7-H³ in the isolated perfused rat heart, Fed. Proc. **21**:331, 1962.

34 Hertting, G., Potter, L. T., and Axelrod, J.: Effect of decentralization and ganglionic blocking agents on the spontaneous and reserpine-induced release of H³-norepinephrine, J. Pharmacol. Exp. Ther. **136**:289, 1962.

35 Hillarp, N. A., Hökfelt, B., and Nilson, B.: The cytology of the adrenal medullary cells with special reference to the storage and secretion of the sympathomimetic amines, Acta Anat. **21**:155, 1954.

36 Isaac, L., and Goth, A.: Interaction of antihistaminics with norepinephrine uptake: a cocaine-like effect, Life Sci. **4**:1899, 1965.

37 Iversen, L. L.: The uptake of adrenaline by the rat isolated heart, Brit. J. Pharmacol. Chemother. **24**:387, 1965.

38 Iversen, L. L.: The uptake of catecholamines at high perfusion concentrations in the rat isolated heart: a novel catecholamine uptake process, Brit. J. Pharmacol. Chemother. **25**:18, 1965.

39 James, T. N., Bear, E. S., Lang, K. F., and Green, E. W.: Evidence for adrenergic alpha receptor depressant activity in the heart, Amer. J. Physiol. **215**:1366, 1958.

40 Kasuya, Y., and Goto, K.: The mechanism of supersensitivity to norepinephrine induced by cocaine in rat isolated vas deferens, Europ. J. Pharmacol. **4**:355, 1958.

41 Lasagna, L., and McCann, W.: Effect of tranquilizing drugs on amphetamine toxicity in aggregated mice, Science **125**:1241, 1957.

42 Lewis, C. M., and Weil, M. H.: Hemodynamic spectrum of vasopressor and vasodilator drugs, J.A.M.A. **208**:1391, 1969.

43 Lockett, M. F.: A compound very closely resembling N-isopropylnoradrenaline in saline extracts of cat adrenal gland, J. Physiol. **124**:67, 1954.

44 MacCannell, K. L., McNay, J. L., Meyer, M. B., and Goldberg, L. I.: Dopamine in the treatment of hypotension and shock, New Eng. J. Med. **275**:1389, 1966.

45 Marrazzi, A. S., and Marrazzi, R. N.: Further localization and analysis of adrenergic synaptic inhibition, J. Neurophysiol. **10**:167, 1947.

46 Maxwell, R. A., Plummer, A. J., Povalski, H., and Schneider, F.: Concerning a possible action of guanethidine (SU-5864) in smooth muscle, J. Pharmacol. Exp. Ther. **129**:24, 1960.

47 Maxwell, R. A., Povalski, H., and Plummer, A. J.: A differential effect of reserpine on pressor amine activity and its relationship to other agents producing this effect, J. Pharmacol. Exp. Ther. **125**:178, 1959.

48 Mayer, S. E., and Moran, N. C.: Relation between pharmacologic augmentation of cardiac contractile force and the activation of myocardial glycogen phosphorylase, J. Pharmacol. Exp. Ther. **129**:271, 1960.

49 Meyer, M. B., McNay, J. L., and Goldberg, L. I.: Effects of dopamine on renal function and hemodynamics in the dog, J. Pharmacol. Exp. Ther. **156**:186, 1967.

50 Mohme-Lundholm, E.: The mechanism of the relaxing effect of adrenaline on smooth muscle, Acta Physiol. Scand. (supp. 108) **29**:1, 1953.

51 Moyer, J. H., and Handley, C. A.: Norepinephrine and epinephrine effect on renal hemodynamics, Circulation **5**:91, 1952.

52 Moyer, J. H., Morris, G., and Snyder, H.: A comparison of the cerebral hemodynamic response to Aramine and norepinephrine in the normotensive-hypotensive subject, Circulation **10**:265, 1954.

53 Patel, N., Mock, D. C., and Hagans, J. A.: Comparison of benzphetamine, phenmetrazine,

d-amphetamine, and placebo, Clin. Pharmacol. Ther. 4:330, 1963.

54 Rangno, R. E., Kaufmann, J. S., Cavanaugh, J. H., Island, D., Watson, J. T., and Oates, J.: Effects of a false neurotransmitter, p-hydroxy-norephedrine, on the function of adrenergic neurons in hypertensive patients, J. Clin. Invest. 52:952, 1973.

55 Schmid, P. G., Eckstein, J. W., and Abboud, F. M.: Comparison of effects of deoxycorticosterone and dexamethasone on cardiovascular responses to norepinephrine, J. Clin. Invest. 46:590, 1967.

56 Scroop, G. C., Walsh, J. A., and Whelan, R. F.: A comparison of the effects of intra-arterial and intravenous infusions of angiotensin and noradrenaline on the circulation in man, Clin. Sci. 29:315, 1965.

57 Shore, P. A., Busfield, D., and Alpers, H. S.: Binding and release of metaraminol: mechanism of norepinephrine depletion by alpha-methyl-M-tyrosine and related agents, J. Pharmacol. Exp. Ther. 146:194, 1964.

58 Sutherland, E. W.: The effect of the hyperglycemic factor and epinephrine on enzyme systems of liver and muscle, Ann. N. Y. Acad. Sci. 54:693, 1951.

59 Sutherland, E. W., and Rall, T. W.: The relation of adenosine-3',5'-phosphate to the action of catechol amines. In Adrenergic mechanisms, Ciba Foundation and Committee for Symposium on Drug Action, Boston, 1960, Little, Brown & Co.

60 Sutherland, E. W., and Rall, T. W.: The relation of adenosine-3',5'-phosphate and phosphorylase to the actions of catecholamines and other hormones, Pharmacol. Rev. 12:265, 1960.

61 Thoenen, H., and Tranzer, J. P.: Chemical sympathectomy by selective destruction of adrenergic nerve endings with 6-hydroxydopamine, Naunyn-Schmiedebergs Arch. Exp. Path. 261: 271, 1968.

Recent reviews

62 Abboud, F. M.: Clinical importance of adrenergic receptors, Arch. Intern. Med. 118:418, 1966.

63 Boura, A. L. A., and Green, A. F.: Adrenergic neuron blocking agents, Ann. Rev. Pharmacol. 5:183, 1965.

64 Burn, J. H., and Rand, M. J.: Acetylcholine in adrenergic transmission, Ann. Rev. Pharmacol. 5:163, 1965.

65 Butcher, R. W.: Role of cyclic AMP in hormone action, New Eng. J. Med. 279:1378, 1968.

66 Eckstein, J. W., and Abboud, F. M.: Circulatory

effects of sympathomimetic amines, Amer. Heart J. 63:119, 1962.

67 Engelman, K., and Sjoerdsma, A.: A new test for pheochromocytoma: pressor responsiveness to tyramine, J.A.M.A. 189:81, 1964.

68 Friend, D. G.: Drugs for peripheral vascular disease, Clin. Pharmacol. Ther. 5:666, 1964.

69 Geffen, L. B., and Livett, B. G.: Synaptic vesicles in sympathetic neurons, Physiol. Rev. 51:98, 1971.

70 Haddy, F. J., and Scott, J. B.: Cardiovascular pharmacology, Ann. Rev. Pharmacol. 6:49, 1966.

71 Hess, M. E., and Haugaard, N.: Actions of autonomic drugs on phosphorylase activity and functions, Pharmacol. Rev. 17:27, 1965.

72 Himms-Hagen, J.: Sympathetic regulation of metabolism, Pharmacol. Rev. 19:367, 1967.

73 Iversen, L. L.: The uptake and storage of noradrenaline in sympathetic nerves, New York, 1967, Cambridge University Press.

74 Koch-Weser, J.: Beta adrenergic blockade and circulating eosinophils, Arch. Intern. Med. 121: 255, 1968.

75 Kopin, I. J.: Storage and metabolism of catecholamines: the role of monamine oxidase, Pharmacol. Rev. 16:179, 1964.

76 Kopin, I. J., and others: False neurochemical transmitters and the mechanism of sympathetic blockade by monoamine oxidase inhibitors, J. Pharmacol. Exp. Ther. 147:186, 1965.

77 Lundholm, L., Mohme-Lundholm, E., and Svedmyr, N.: Metabolic effects of catecholamines. In Bittar, E. E., and Bittar, N., editors: The biological basis of medicine, vol. 2, New York, 1968, Academic Press, Inc.

78 Malmfors, T.: Histochemical studies of adrenergic neurotransmission. In Adrenergic neurotransmission, Ciba Foundation Study Group No. 33, Boston, 1968, Little, Brown & Co.

79 Marley, E.: The adrenergic system and sympathomimetic amines, Advances Pharmacol. 3:168, 1964.

80 Modell, W., and Hussar, A. E.: Failure of dextroamphetamine sulfate to influence eating and sleeping patterns in obese schizophrenic patients, J.A.M.A. 193:275, 1965.

81 Nickerson, M.: Vasoconstriction and vasodilation in shock. In Hershey, S. G., editor: Shock, Boston, 1964, Little, Brown & Co.

82 Norberg, K. A., and Hamberger, B.: The sympathetic adrenergic neuron, Acta Physiol. Scand. (supp. 238) 63:1, 1964.

83 Second symposium on catecholamines, Pharmacol. Rev. 18:1, 1966.

84 Shore, P. A.: Transport and storage of bio-

genic amines, Ann. Rev. Pharmacol. **12**:209, 1972.

85 Trendelenburg, U.: Supersensitivity and subsensitivity to sympathomimetic amines, Pharmacol. Rev. **15**:225, 1963.

86 Udenfriend, S.: Physiological regulation of nor-

adrenaline biosynthesis. In Adrenergic neurotransmission, Ciba Foundation Study Group No. 33, Boston, 1968, Little, Brown & Co.

87 Wurtman, R. J.: Catecholamines, New Eng. J. Med. **273**:637, 693, 1965.

9

Atropine group of cholinergic blocking drugs

GENERAL CONCEPT

Atropine and related drugs are important therapeutic agents and have widespread uses as pharmacologic tools. They are competitive antagonists of acetylcholine on organs innervated by postganglionic cholinergic nerves. Atropine, scopolamine, and related drugs find important applications in ophthalmology, anesthesia, and cardiac and gastrointestinal diseases. In addition to their peripheral anticholinergic effects, most of these drugs act on the central nervous system and are used in the treatment of Parkinson's disease and vestibular disorders, and as proprietary hypnotics and antidotes for the anticholinesterases. In this last instance both peripheral and central actions of the drugs are of great benefit.

ATROPINE AND SCOPOLAMINE

Atropine and scopolamine are among the oldest drugs in medicine. Many solanaceous plants have been used for centuries because of their active principles of *l*-hyoscyamine and *l*-hyoscine. The name *hyoscyamine* is derived from *Hyoscyamus niger* (henbane). It is of some toxicologic interest to know that the common jimsonweed, *Datura stramonium*, also contains these alkaloids. These drugs also are often called the belladonna alkaloids because they are found in the deadly nightshade, *Atropa belladonna*.

Chemistry

The alkaloids as they occur in the plants are *l*-hyoscyamine and *l*-hyoscine (scopolamine). Atropine is *dl*-hyoscyamine, racemization occurring during the extraction process. Just as acetylcholine is an ester of an amino alcohol, the blocking drugs of the belladonna group are esters of complex organic bases with tropic acid. Atropine and scopolamine differ only slightly in the structure of the organic base part of the molecule, as is evident from comparison of their structural formulas.

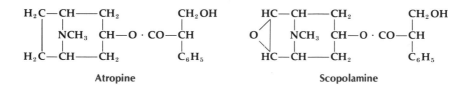

Atropine   Scopolamine

Mode of action

Atropine and scopolamine are competitive antagonists of acetylcholine at receptor sites in smooth muscles, cardiac muscle, and various glandular cells. (See Fig. 2-2, p. 11.) The effectiveness of this competition is greatest against the muscarinic effects of injected cholinergic drugs and against the tonic effect of the vagus nerve on the heart. These drugs are less effective in blocking the actions of parasympathetic nerves on the gastrointestinal tract and urinary bladder. In very large doses and with intra-arterial administration, interference with ganglionic and neuromuscular transmission may be demonstrable. These junctions, however, are so much less sensitive to the belladonna alkaloids that for practical purposes these drugs are only muscarinic blocking agents.

Clinical pharmacology

The actions of atropine and scopolamine on the cardiovascular system and on the eye are very similar. The two drugs differ mainly in their central nervous system effects. In therapeutic doses, given parenterally, scopolamine tends to produce considerable sleepiness, whereas atropine is not likely to produce this evidence of central nervous system depression. While it is generally believed that scopolamine is a central nervous system depressant and atropine is a stimulant, in reality the effect depends upon the dose. In low doses both drugs tend to cause sedation. In larger doses both cause stimulation, which may progress to delirium. Finally, after very high doses of either drug, coma may supervene.

There is a definite gradation in the sensitivity of various functions mediated by acetylcholine to inhibition by atropine and scopolamine. Therapeutic doses of 0.6 mg. of atropine or 0.3 mg. of scopolamine may cause dryness of the mouth and inhibit sweating. Blockade of the cardiac vagus requires somewhat larger doses. Gastrointestinal and urinary tract smooth muscle is even more resistant to the action of atropine and scopolamine. Finally, the inhibition of gastric secretion requires such large doses in man that side effects on the more susceptible sites would make that therapeutic objective completely impractical.

The effects of atropine and scopolamine on blood pressure are not impressive. It should be recalled that most vascular areas in the body do not receive parasympathetic innervation. It is common experience in the laboratory to inject atropine intravenously into a dog, 1 mg./kg. of body weight, without observing a significant change in the mean pressure.

The effect of atropine on the heart rate in man is complex. With large enough doses, tachycardia develops, as expected, from blockade of vagal influences on the heart. With smaller doses, paradoxical as it may seem, the heart rate may be slowed. Ablation experiments have shown that atropine stimulates vagal nuclei in the medulla, an action that results in bradycardia unless large enough doses are used to prevent such an action at the muscarinic receptors. In one study the final effect of scopolamine on heart rate was found to be the result of two separate actions, one tending to produce tachycardia, the other bradycardia.[13]

A distinctly anomalous vascular effect of atropine is its production of cutaneous dilatation. In warm environments, atropine may promote cutaneous vasodilatation because it tends to block sweating, thus causing body temperature to rise. However, atropine has an additional cutaneous vasodilator action that cannot be explained on this basis. Flushing of the skin may be very noticeable following moderately large

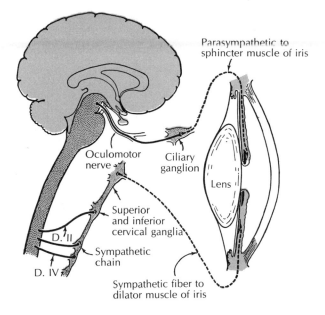

Fig. 9-1. Autonomic innervation of iris.

doses of atropine. Again, there is no known action of atropine on neural transmission to blood vessels that would explain this dilatation. It has been postulated that perhaps atropine can cause the release of some other agent, possibly histamine, which in turn causes the anomalous cutaneous vasodilatation.

Gastrointestinal effects. In large enough doses the belladonna alkaloids will reduce motility and tone of the gastrointestinal tract and may even reduce the volume of its various secretions. Motility is more easily reduced by therapeutic doses than is gastric secretion, particularly if a peptic ulcer is present.

Effect on urinary tract. Atropine has little effect on the ureters. It relaxes the fundus of the bladder but promotes contraction of the sphincter, thus favoring urinary retention.

Effect on eye. The actions of atropine on the eye are straightforward. When it is applied directly to the conjunctiva (0.5 to 1% solutions), the drug will produce mydriasis and paralysis of accommodation (cycloplegia). In addition, in patients subject to glaucoma it may precipitate an acute attack with catastrophic increases in intraocular pressure.

The circular muscle of the iris receives cholinergic innervation through fibers traveling in the third nerve. Atropine blocks the actions of acetylcholine on this sphincter muscle, and the resulting predominance of the radial fibers produces mydriasis. The atropinized pupil does not react to light. Cycloplegia is caused by paralysis of the ciliary muscles, which are normally innervated by cholinergic fibers. Increased intraocular pressure is generally attributed to impeded drainage of aqueous humor through the canals of Schlemm.

It should be recalled that the adrenergic drugs also can produce mydriasis. They act, however, by contracting the radial muscle of the iris. Accommodation is not paralyzed by the adrenergic drugs, in contrast to the atropine-like compounds.

Central nervous system effects. In atropine poisoning the central nervous system effects are very striking; patients become excited and maniacal. Large therapeutic doses stimulate respiration and may prevent death from respiratory depression in poisoning due to the alkyl phosphate cholinesterase inhibitors.

There are additional reasons for believing that the belladonna alkaloids affect the central nervous system. Scopolamine in particular is valuable in the management of Parkinson's disease and in the prevention of motion sickness.[25] When it is given by injection, the drug promotes a state of sedation and twilight sleep and may cause amnesia.

Absorption, excretion, and metabolism

Atropine and scopolamine are well absorbed from the gastrointestinal tract and following subcutaneous injection. They may even be absorbed following topical application. Accidents may occur in ophthalmologic use, particularly in children, if the drug is allowed to reach the nasal mucosa through the nasolacrimal duct after its application to the conjunctival sac.

Atropine is rapidly excreted from the body and about 50% of an injected dose appears in the urine within 4 hours. The remainder is excreted within 24 hours in the form of metabolites and also the unchanged drug.[29] The duration of the pharmacologic effects reflects the rapidity of excretion except for the dilatation of the pupils and paralysis of accommodation, which may persist for a long time, particularly when atropine is applied topically to the conjunctiva.

Preparations and clinical uses

The belladonna alkaloids are used either in galenic preparations* or in a pure form. Belladonna tincture is given orally in a dose of 0.6 ml., which is equivalent to 0.2 mg. of atropine. Atropine sulfate tablets are available in several different sizes. The usual dose is 0.6 mg. Scopolamine hydrobromide tablets are available in sizes of 0.3 and 0.6 mg. The usual dose is 0.6 mg. Solutions of atropine sulfate are available for instillation into the conjunctival sac. The usual strength of these solutions is 0.5 to 1%.

Ophthalmologic uses. The anticholinergic drugs are applied topically for producing mydriasis and cycloplegia. Atropine itself has such a long duration of action that its use in ophthalmology is impractical. Homatropine or cyclopentolate are much more commonly employed and have a much shorter duration of action.

Preoperative uses. It is customary to administer atropine or scopolamine before operative procedures and general anesthesia. The drug protects the patient from excessive salivation and bradycardia. Scopolamine is often used in obstetrics because it produces sedation and amnesia. The anticholinergics were particularly important when ether was widely employed. With the newer anesthetics, excessive tracheobronchial secretions are not produced and the need for routine preanesthetic anticholinergics is questioned by some.[29]

Cardiac uses. Atropine is being used increasingly after myocardial infarction for reversing bradycardia caused by excessive vagal activity. The drug is useful also in digitalis-induced heart block. Although many physicians will use atropine after myocardial infarction if the heart rate falls below 60,[29] there is no certainty about the need

---

*Galenic preparations contain one or several organic ingredients as contrasted with pure chemical substances.

or safety of this procedure unless hypotension or arrhythmias justify it. Large intravenous doses of atropine may cause dangerous tachycardia and ventricular arrhythmias in cardiac patients.

Uses in gastrointestinal disease. Anticholinergic drugs are used widely in the treatment of peptic ulcer. The drugs may diminish vagally mediated secretion, relieve spasm, and prolong the time during which antacids remain in the stomach by slowing down gastric emptying. To be effective, the anticholinergics must often be administered in large enough doses to cause discomfort, such as difficulty of vision and urination. Although there is no evidence for a favorable effect of anticholinergics on the long-term progress of ulcer disease, these drugs are unquestionably of considerable symptomatic benefit. The quaternary anticholinergics are preferred by many gastroenterologists. In large doses they may cause postural hypotension in addition to other predictable atropine-like effects. In addition to the usual contraindications, atropine should not be used in the presence of obstructive lesions, since it should promote retention.

Antiparkinsonism drugs. These drugs are discussed on p. 128. *Atropine-like drugs for vestibular disorders* will be discussed along with the antihistaminic drugs on p. 199. The use of scopolamine as a hypnotic in combination with antihistaminics is unimportant except from a commercial standpoint. The presence of scopolamine in such "over-the-counter" preparations should be kept in mind in relation to possible drug interactions and in cases in which atropine-like drugs are contraindicated.

Toxicity and antidotes

The belladonna alkaloids and atropine-like drugs are generally safe medications. Large doses in a normal individual may cause unpleasant effects but are not life-threatening. Blurred vision, tachycardia, dry mouth, constipation, and urinary retention are among these unpleasant effects. Patients with glaucoma and prostatic hypertrophy may have disastrous reactions even to therapeutic doses of these drugs. Normal individuals have survived doses as high as 1 Gm. taken by mouth.[1]

Full-blown atropine poisoning is characterized by excitement and maniacal tendencies, hot and dry skin, dilated pupils, and tachycardia. The subcutaneous injection of 25 mg. of methacholine will not elicit cholinergic effects in such patients.

Patients with atropine poisoning should be managed with supportive care. Sedatives such as chlordiazepoxide or diazepam may be helpful in controlling violent excitement.

Physostigmine has been found remarkably effective as an antidote in atropine poisoning. The drug may be injected subcutaneously in doses of 1 to 4 mg.[16] The injection may be repeated in an hour if necessary. Although the effectiveness of physostigmine in atropine poisoning has been known for years on the basis of animal experiments, its clinical usefulness became obvious more recently as a consequence of clinical observations made on patients with Parkinson's disease who received excessive amounts of atropine-like drugs.[16]

Problem 9-1. Why is physostigmine preferable to neostigmine in reversing the central nervous system effects of atropine? The answer undoubtedly has some connection with the relative rates of penetration of the two drugs across the blood-brain barrier. Physostigmine is not a quaternary compound but neostigmine is.

ATROPINE SUBSTITUTES

The atropine substitutes will be classified on the basis of their primary usefulness, which to a certain extent reflects their selectivity. On this basis they fall into three groups: the atropine-like mydriatics, the antispasmodics, and the antiparkinsonism drugs.

ATROPINE-LIKE MYDRIATICS

Atropine itself is a powerful mydriatic and cycloplegic, but its long duration of action is generally a disadvantage except in the treatment of iritis. For examination of the fundus and measurement of refractive errors, a number of shorter-acting agents are preferred. Some of these are homatropine, eucatropine, dibutoline, cyclopentolate, and tropicamide. In addition, adrenergic drugs such as phenylephrine (Neo-Synephrine) produce mydriasis without cycloplegia when applied topically to the eye.

Homatropine is the oldest of the atropine-like mydriatic drugs. It differs from atropine only in the fact that it is an ester of mandelic rather than of tropic acid. Homatropine is applied to the eye in solutions of 2%. It produces mydriasis fairly rapidly, but its action lasts only 1 or 2 days. It is a less potent cycloplegic than atropine and is commonly used in ophthalmology.

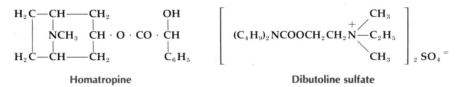

Homatropine   Dibutoline sulfate

Eucatropine (Euphthalmine) is a weaker drug than homatropine. It produces mydriasis in 30 minutes, which lasts only about 12 hours. The drug has little cycloplegic action. It is used in 2 to 5% solutions.

Dibutoline (di-n-butyl carbamylcholine) is interesting from the standpoint of structure-activity relationships. Whereas carbachol (carbamylcholine) itself is a potent cholinergic drug, the addition of two n-butyl radicals on the carbamyl nitrogen convert it into a cholinergic blocking drug.

Cyclopentolate hydrochloride (Cyclogyl) produces mydriasis in 30 to 60 minutes, with return of normal vision in less than 24 hours. It is used in 0.5 and 1% solutions, although for deeply pigmented eyes a 2% solution may be necessary.

Tropicamide (Mydriacyl) is a very rapidly acting mydriatic and cycloplegic. It produces mydriasis in less than 30 minutes, and its action lasts only 15 to 20 minutes. It is used in 0.5 and 1% solutions.

ANTICHOLINERGIC SMOOTH MUSCLE RELAXANTS

A large group of atropine substitutes have been synthesized for the purpose of obtaining some selective action on the gastrointestinal tract. The great incentive for this search is the prevalence of peptic ulcer and the belief that desirable objectives in its management are relief of smooth muscle spasm and hypersecretion.

The defects of atropine for gastrointestinal use are a lack of selectivity, systemic and central nervous system side effects, and lack of potency in ulcer patients.

Conversion of the usual tertiary atropine-like drugs to quaternary amines introduces a number of important changes into their pharmacology. (1) Quaternary amines

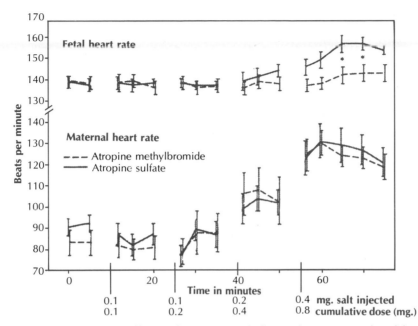

Fig. 9-2. Effect of atropine sulfate and atropine methylbromide on maternal and fetal heart rates. The lesser effect of the quaternary anticholinergic drug on fetal heart rate illustrates a basic difference between the two types of drugs as regards their passage across biologic membranes. (From dePadua, C. B., and Gravenstein, J. S.: J.A.M.A. **208:**1022, 1969.)

are less lipid soluble and do not penetrate the central nervous system. (2) The quaternary atropine-like drugs exert some ganglionic blocking effect that may reinforce their actions on the gastrointestinal tract. Thus the quaternary atropine methylbromide would not be expected to penetrate into the central nervous system as efficiently as atropine sulfate. The difference between the two in regard to penetration across biologic membranes is shown in Fig 9-2.

Quaternary anticholinergic drugs

Quaternary anticholinergic drugs used in 2 to 15 mg. doses include methscopolamine (Pamine), homatropine methylbromide (Novatran), propantheline (Pro-Banthine), oxyphenonium (Antrenyl), penthienate (Monodral), valethamate (Murel), pipenzolate (Piptal), and poldine (Nacton). Quaternary anticholinergics used in doses of 50 to 100 mg. or more include methantheline (Banthine), tridihexethyl (Pathilon), mepiperphenidol (Darstine), tricyclamol (Elorine), diphemanil (Prantal), amolanone (Amethone), and hexocyclium (Tral). The structural formulas of propantheline, methscopolamine, and tridihexethyl follow:

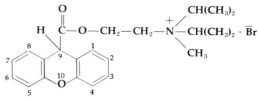

Propantheline bromide

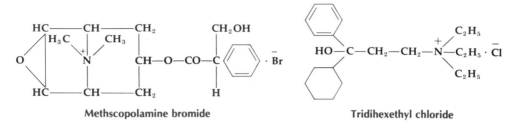

Methscopolamine bromide   Tridihexethyl chloride

Tertiary anticholinergic drugs

Among these synthetic atropine substitutes the most potent, used in doses of 10 mg., are dicyclomine (Bentyl) and oxyphencyclimine (Daricon). Drugs of this group used in doses of 50 mg. or more are piperidolate (Dactil), aminocarbofluorene (Pavatrine), and amprotropine (Syntropan). Adiphenine (Trasentine), largely obsolete, also belongs to this group. Formulas of oxyphencyclimine, piperidolate, and amprotropine are as follows:

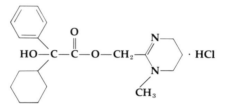

Oxyphencyclimine hydrochloride

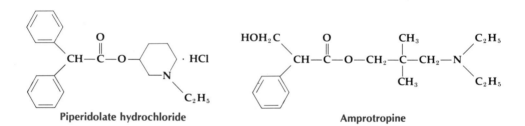

Piperidolate hydrochloride   Amprotropine

Methantheline was introduced at a time when there was a great deal of interest in surgical vagotomy for the treatment of peptic ulcer. The idea of a "chemical vagotomy" of the gastrointestinal tract was striking and received much attention. In therapeutic doses these drugs probably act in the same manner as atropine, preventing the actions of acetylcholine on the gastrointestinal smooth muscle. In larger doses they also block ganglionic transmission, and in very large experimental doses they have some blocking actions on neuromuscular transmission in skeletal muscles.

ANTIPARKINSONISM DRUGS

The pharmacology of parkinsonism has been revolutionized during the last few years by the discovery of the effectiveness of L-dopa in its treatment and the role of dopamine in extrapyramidal function. Until recently the treatment of this common and disabling condition was based on the empirical use of (1) belladonna alkaloids and

Table 9-1. Drug effects in parkinsonism

Drugs that aggravate or cause parkinsonism	Drugs that relieve parkinsonism
Reserpine	Belladonna alkaloids
Chlorpromazine (phenothiazines)	Synthetic anticholinergic drugs
Haloperidol	Antihistamines
Alpha-methyl-dopa	Drugs having both anticholinergic and antihistaminic properties
	Levodopa
	Amantadine
	Dextroamphetamine

their synthetic congeners, (2) antihistamines, (3) drugs with both anticholinergic and antihistaminic properties (benztropine), and (4) dextroamphetamine for some manifestations of postencephalitic parkinsonism, such as oculogyric crisis and rigidity.

Parkinsonism, characterized by tremor, rigidity, and akinesia, includes idiopathic paralysis agitans, postencephalitic parkinsonism, and other disturbances of the extrapyramidal system. It may also be caused by drugs. It was suggested more than a hundred years ago that the belladonna alkaloids might be useful in the management of the syndrome, and drug studies have contributed greatly to current concepts of its pathophysiology (Table 9-1).

Cholinergic and dopaminergic mechanisms in parkinsonism

The effectiveness of belladonna alkaloids in the treatment of parkinsonism called attention to the possible role of cholinergic mechanisms in its causation. It seemed reasonable to theorize that some brain centers must have become supersensitive to acetylcholine in the parkinsonian patient, perhaps as a form of denervation supersensitivity or as a consequence of removal of an inhibitory influence.

The role of cholinergic mechanisms in parkinsonism was supported by experiments which showed that *tremorine*, a cholinomimetic drug, produces a syndrome in animals resembling parkinsonism.[31] The injection of acetylcholine into the globus pallidus of patients undergoing stereotaxic surgery resulted in increased tremor contralaterally.[21] Furthermore, the anticholinesterase physostigmine was found to exacerbate the symptoms of parkinsonian patients.[26] In this last study the suggestion was made that the role of the cholinergic system may be secondary to the involvement of a dopaminergic mechanism.[26]

Dopamine, the immediate precursor of norepinephrine (p. 66), undoubtedly plays an important role in brain function in its own right. First, in several species this catecholamine represents more than 50% of the total catecholamine in the brain. Its unequal distribution in various areas suggests specialized functions also. Thus the caudate nucleus contains as much as 10 μg/gram of dopamine and only 0.1 μg/gram of norepinephrine, whereas the hypothalamus contains only 0.2 μg/gram of dopamine and 1 to 2 μg/gram of norepinephrine.

Histochemical fluorescence techniques have shown[2] that the characteristic green fluorescence of catecholamines is present in the nerve cell bodies of the *substantia nigra* and in the nerve terminals of the *striatum*, both areas being rich in dopamine. Furthermore, lesions placed in the substantia nigra of rats resulted in a decrease in dopamine in the ipsilateral striatum.[2]

The nigro-striatal dopaminergic system probably plays an important pathogenetic role in parkinsonism. In idiopathic parkinsonism the most conspicuous lesions are found in the substantia nigra, and the level of dopamine is found to be decreased in the striatum where the axonal terminations of the striatal neurons are located. The effectiveness of L-dopa in the treatment of parkinsonism suggests also that this precursor of dopamine, when administered in large doses, may overcome the deficiency of dopamine which is known to exist in the nigro-striatal dopaminergic pathway.

The proposal of antagonistic roles of cholinergic and dopaminergic pathways and loss of dopaminergic inhibitory functions at the level of the striatum serves admirably for explaining the mode of action of drugs that aggravate or relieve parkinsonism.

Drugs that aggravate parkinsonism. Both reserpine and chlorpromazine aggravate the symptoms of parkinsonism. Reserpine causes a depletion of dopamine in the striatum and thus, according to the theory, would remove an inhibitory influence on a cholinergic system. L-Dopa reverses the effect of reserpine, since it is converted to dopamine.

Chlorpromazine, and also haloperidol, have some adrenergic receptor–blocking effects and may antagonize dopamine at central receptor sites. In this instance L-dopa would not be expected to be effective because the dopamine receptors are blocked, and this appears to be the case.

Drugs that relieve parkinsonism. The anticholinergic drugs would be expected to be effective if the cholinergic system is hyperactive as a consequence of removal of dopaminergic inhibitory influences. Most of the antihistaminics also have anticholinergic actions, which may account for their effectiveness. A role in parkinsonism for histamine and also serotonin cannot be stated at present.

Dextroamphetamine has been used in the treatment of certain manifestations of postencephalitic parkinsonism, such as rigidity and oculogyric crisis. Peripherally, dextroamphetamine causes catecholamine release, and its action is antagonized by reserpine, which depletes catecholamine stores. The central effects of dextroamphetamine are not blocked by reserpine pretreatment, suggesting that within the central nervous system dextroamphetamine may act directly, perhaps on dopaminergic receptors.

Amantadine, an antiviral drug, has been reported to be beneficial in parkinsonism. Although the mode of action of this drug is uncertain, dopamine release from neuronal storage sites following its injection has been claimed on the basis of animal experiments.[15]

• • •

In summary, then, although the cholinergic-dopaminergic hypothesis about parkinsonism may turn out to be too simple, it has the great advantage of providing a unifying concept on the mode of action of all drugs that are known to influence the major manifestations of the syndrome.

Major antiparkinsonism agents

The available antiparkinsonism drugs fall into the following groups on the basis of their pharmacologic properties:

1. Belladonna alkaloids, including atropine and scopolamine
2. Synthetic anticholinergics, such as trihexyphenidyl hydrochloride (Artane), biperiden hydrochloride (Akineton), cycrimine hydrochloride (Pagitane), and procyclidine hydrochloride (Kemadrin)
3. Antihistamines, such as diphenhydramine hydrochloride (Benadryl), and orphenadrine citrate (Norflex) or orphenadrine hydrochloride (Disipal)
4. Drugs with both anticholinergic and antihistaminic properties, such as benztropine mesylate (Cogentin mesylate)
5. Phenothiazines with anticholinergic and antihistaminic actions, such as ethopropazine (Parsidol)
6. Levodopa (L-dopa), acting on dopaminergic mechanisms
7. Miscellaneous drugs probably acting on dopaminergic mechanisms, such as amantadine and dextroamphetamine

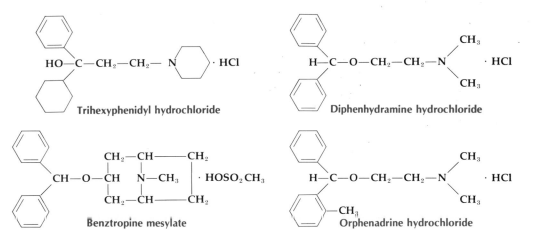

Belladonna alkaloids and synthetic anticholinergics. The naturally occurring belladonna alkaloids, atropine and scopolamine, have been used for many years in the treatment of parkinsonism. They have been replaced by the newer synthetics because the latter do not produce as powerful peripheral anticholinergic symptoms for a given amount of relief of parkinsonian disability.

The action and uses of the synthetic anticholinergics are very similar. All are chemically related to trihexyphenidyl, and all produce atropine-like untoward effects such as dryness of the mouth, blurred vision, dizziness, and dysuria.

Trihexyphenidyl hydrochloride (Artane) is available in tablets of 2 and 5 mg., timed-release capsules of 5 mg., and elixir, 2 mg./5 ml. Dosage ranges from 1 mg. initially to a maximum of 20 mg. daily.

Biperiden hydrochloride and biperiden lactate (Akineton hydrochloride and Akineton lactate): The hydrochloride is available in 2 mg. tablets for oral administration; the lactate is available as a solution, 5 mg./ml., for injection.

Cycrimine hydrochloride (Pagitane hydrochloride) is available in tablets of 1.25 and 2.5 mg.

Procyclidine hydrochloride (Kemadrin) is available in tablets of 2 and 5 mg.

Antihistamines. Diphenhydramine and the closely related orphenadrine have some usefulness in the treatment of parkinsonism including that induced by drugs such as the phenothiazines. They are not as effective as the anticholinergics but produce fewer atropine-like untoward effects. On the other hand, they produce considerable drowsiness.

Diphenhydramine hydrochloride (Benadryl) is available in 25 and 50 mg. capsules, elixirs of 12.5 mg./5 ml., and solutions for intravenous and intramuscular injections containing 10 or 50 mg./ml.

Orphenadrine citrate (Norflex) is available in tablets, 100 mg., and solutions for injection, 30 mg./ml.

Orphenadrine hydrochloride (Disipal) is available in tablets, 50 mg.

Drugs with both anticholinergic and antihistaminic properties. The major representative of this class is benztropine mesylate. An examination of its chemical structure reveals similarities to atropine and a typical antihistaminic. Its pharmacologic properties resemble those of atropine not only with regard to untoward effects but also from the standpoint of duration of action, which is long. On continued use, accumulative effect may be prominent. Benztropine is used widely to counteract the untoward parkinsonian effects of the phenothiazines. On the other hand, a phenothiazine with both anticholinergic and antihistaminic actions, ethopropazine hydrochloride, has some usefulness in the treatment of parkinsonism.

Benztropine mesylate (Cogentin mesylate) is available in tablets of 0.5, 1, and 2 mg. and in solution for intramuscular or intravenous injection, 1 mg./ml.

Ethopropazine hydrochloride (Parsidol), a phenothiazine with both anticholinergic and antihistaminic actions, may be useful as an adjunct to the anticholinergic drugs. It causes considerable drowsiness, dizziness, muscle cramps, and paresthesia and may cause agranulocytosis. It may also cause hypotension. Its preparations include tablets of 10, 50, and 100 mg.

Levodopa. Levodopa is considered the most effective medication for parkinsonism. When administered orally in increasing doses, it is likely to benefit at least half the patients, although it may take several weeks for the improvement to become manifest. Fortunately it is not necessary to discontinue the usual anticholinergic medications while the dosage is being built up. The initial daily dose is 300 mg. to 1 Gm. Dosage is built up gradually until marked improvement occurs or adverse reactions make further increases impractical.

Adverse reactions to levodopa include nausea, vomiting, orthostatic hypotension, cardiac arrhythmias, psychic disturbances, and involuntary movements.

Drug interactions during levodopa treatment may be of great importance. Monoamine oxidase inhibitors in association with levodopa may cause hypertensive crises. Large doses of pyridoxine (more than 5 mg.) may decrease the effectiveness of levodopa, probably because the vitamin favors the peripheral decarboxylation of the drug. On the other hand, some decarboxylase inhibitors are being tried experimentally, which by preventing the peripheral decarboxylation of levodopa, may allow a reduction in its dosage. These decarboxylase inhibitors do not penetrate the central nervous system and thus do not prevent the formation of dopamine in the basal ganglia.

Levodopa (Dopar, Larodopa) is available in capsules containing 100, 250, and 500 mg.

Amantadine. This antiviral agent produces clinical improvement in some patients having parkinsonian symptoms and does so more rapidly than levodopa. The mode of action of amantadine is not understood, although there is a highly suggestive experimental finding of an amantadine-dopamine interaction.[15] Small intravenous doses of amantadine caused a release of dopamine and other catecholamines from neuronal storage sites in dogs primed with dopamine. If amantadine has the same dopamine-releasing action in the central nervous system of man, its effectiveness in the treatment of parkinsonism could become understandable.

Adverse effects of amantadine include hyperexcitability, slurred speech, ataxia, insomnia, and gastrointestinal disturbances. Convulsions have occurred after the administration of excessive doses.

Amantadine hydrochloride (Symmetrel) is available in capsules of 100 mg. and as a syrup containing 50 mg./ml. Initial dose for adults is 100 mg. once daily for 5 to 7 days.

References

1 Alexander, E., Jr., Morris, D. P., and Eslick, R. L.: Atropine poisoning: report of a case, with recovery after the ingestion of one gram, New Eng. J. Med. **234**:258, 1946.

2 Anden, N. E., Carlsson, A., Dahlstrom, A., Fuxe, K., Hillarp, N. A., and Larsson, K.: Demonstration and mapping out of nigro-neostriatal dopamine neurons, Life Sci. **3**:523, 1964.

3 Calne, D. B., Laurence, D. R., and Stern, G. M.: L-Dopa in postencephalitic parkinsonism, Lancet **1**:744, 1969.

4 Cotzias, G. C., and Papavasiliou, P. S.: Blocking the negative effects of pyridoxine on patients receiving levodopa, J.A.M.A. **215**:1504, 1971.

5 Cotzias, G. C., Papavasiliou, P. S., and Gellene, R.: Modification of parkinsonism—chronic treatment with L-dopa, New Eng. J. Med. **280**:337, 1969.

6 Cotzias, G. C., Van Woert, M. H., and Schiffer, L. M.: Aromatic amino acids and modification of parkinsonism, New Eng. J. Med. **276**:374, 1967.

7 DePadua, C. B., and Gravenstein, J. S.: Atropine sulfate vs atropine methyl bromide: effect on maternal and fetal heart rate, J.A.M.A. **208**:1022, 1969.

8 Doshay, L. J., and Constable, K.: Treatment of paralysis agitans with orphenadrine (Disipal): results in one hundred seventy-six cases, J.A.M.A. **163**:1352, 1957.

9 Doshay, L. J., Constable, K., and Fromer, S.: Preliminary study of a new anti-Parkinson agent, Neurology **2**:233, 1952.

10 Doshay, L. J., Constable, K., and Zier, A.: Five-year follow-up of treatment with trihexyphenidyl (Artane), J.A.M.A. **154**:1334, 1954.

11 Gershon, S., Neubauer, H., and Sundland, D. M.: Interaction between some anticholinergic agents and phenothiazines, Clin. Pharmacol. Ther. **6**:749, 1965.

12 Gosselin, R. E., Gabourel, J. D., and Wills, J. H.: The fate of atropine in man, Clin. Pharmacol. Ther. **1**:597, 1960.

13 Gravenstein, J. S., Ariet, M., and Thornby, J. I.: Atropine on the electrocardiogram, Clin. Pharmacol. Ther. **10**:660, 1969.

14 Gravenstein, J. S., and Thornby, J. I.: Scopolamine in heart rates in man, Clin. Pharmacol. Ther. **10**:395, 1969.

15 Grelak, R. P., Clark, R., Stump, J. M., and Vernier, V. G.: Amantadine-dopamine interaction: possible mode of action in Parkinsonism, Science **169**:203, 1970.

16 Heiser, J. F., and Gillin, J. C.: The reversal of anticholinergic drug-induced delirium and coma with physostigmine, Amer. J. Psychiatry **127**:1050, 1971.

17 Hornykiewicz, O.: Die topische Lokalisation und das Verhalten von Noradrenalin and Dopamin (3-Hydroxytyramin) in der Substantia nigra der normalen und Parkinson-kranken Menschen, Wien. Klin. Wschr. **75**:309, 1963.

18 Ingelfinger, F. J.: In Symposium on clinical drug evaluation and human pharmacology. XIX. Clinical judgment in clinical research, Clin. Pharmacol. Ther. **3**:685, 1962.

19 Levine, R. M., Blair, M. R., and Clark, B. B.: Factors influencing the intestinal absorption of certain monoquaternary anticholinergic compounds with special reference to benzomethamine [N-diethylaminoethyl-N′-methyl-benzilamide methobromide (MC-3199)], J. Pharmacol. Exp. Ther. **114**:78, 1955.

20 McGreer, P. L., Boulding, J. E., Gibson, W. C., and Foulkes, R. G.: Drug-induced extrapyramidal reactions. Treatment with diphenhydramine hydrochloride and dihydroxyphenylalanine, J.A.M.A. **177**:665, 1961.

21 Nashold, B. S.: Cholinergic stimulation of glo-

bus pallidus in man, Proc. Soc. Exp. Biol. Med. **101**:68, 1959.

22 Schwab, R. S., England, A. C., Jr., Poskanzer, D. C., and Young, R. R.: Amantadine in the treatment of parkinson's disease, J.A.M.A. **208**:1168, 1969.

23 Stern, J., and Ward, A.: Inhibition of the muscle spindle discharge by ventrolateral thalamic stimulation, Arch. Neurol. Psychiat. **3**:193, 1960.

Recent reviews

24 Barbeau, A.: The pathogenesis of Parkinson's disease: a new hypothesis, Canad. Med. Ass. J. **87**:802, 1962.

25 Brand, J. J., and Perry, W. L. M.: Drugs used in motion sickness. A critical review of methods available for the study of drugs of potential value in its treatment and of the information which has been derived by these methods, Pharmacol. Rev. **18**:895, 1966.

26 Duvoisin, R. C.: Cholinergic-anticholinergic antagonism in parkinsonism, Arch. Neurol. **17**:124, 1967.

27 Eger, E. I.: Atropine, scopolamine, and related compounds, Anesthesiology **23**:365, 1962.

28 Friend, D. G.: Anti-parkinsonism drug therapy, Clin. Pharmacol. Ther. **4**:815, 1963.

29 Greenblatt, D. J., and Shader, R. I.: Anticholinergics, New Eng. J. Med. **288**:1215, 1973.

30 Hornykiewicz, O.: Dopamine (3-hydroxytyramine) and brain function, Pharmacol. Rev. **18**:925, 1966.

31 Ingelfinger, F. J.: Anticholinergic therapy of gastrointestinal disorders, New Eng. J. Med. **268**:1454, 1963.

32 Klawans, H. L., Jr.: The pharmacology of parkinsonism (a review), Dis. Nerv. Sys. **29**:805, 1968.

33 Toman, J. E. P.: Some aspects of central nervous pharmacology, Ann. Rev. Pharmacol. **3**:153, 1963.

10 Ganglionic blocking agents

GENERAL CONCEPT

Ganglionic transmission can be blocked either by compounds that prevent the depolarizing actions of acetylcholine or by drugs that produce persistent depolarization. In concentrations that have little effect at other sites, the clinically useful ganglionic blocking agents prevent the actions of acetylcholine on ganglionic neurons. In addition, other amines may exert a modulating influence on ganglionic transmission. Sympathetic ganglia contain catecholamines that may exert an inhibitory influence on ganglionic transmission. Ganglionic neurons have atropine-sensitive receptors in addition to the ones blocked by hexamethonium and related drugs.

There are few uses for ganglionic blocking agents. **Trimethaphan** (Arfonad) is of value in producing controlled hypotensive states for surgery, and **mecamylamine hydrochloride** (Inversine) is used occasionally in hypertension.

GANGLIONIC STIMULANTS

When a preganglionic fiber is stimulated, acetylcholine mediates the transmission of impulses in the ganglia. This mediator itself may be looked upon as a ganglionic stimulant, but when cholinergic drugs are injected, their actions on the cardiovascular system are so prominent that these ganglionic effects are completely obscured. If atropine is used to block the direct cardiovascular actions, a blood pressure rise following the administration of cholinergic drugs reflects stimulation of sympathetic ganglia and the adrenal medulla. Even without premedication with atropine, certain ganglionic stimulants such as tetramethylammonium, small doses of nicotine, and the experimental drug dimethylphenylpiperazinium (DMPP) will cause vasoconstriction and blood pressure elevations as a consequence of their stimulant action on ganglia. This type of drug effect has not yet found therapeutic applications. It should be remembered, however, that some of the drugs used in the diagnosis of pheochromocytoma (for example, methacholine) cause catecholamine release. This is analogous to ganglionic or adrenomedullary stimulation.

GANGLIONIC BLOCKING AGENTS
Development

The curious ability of nicotine to block ganglionic transmission following initial stimulation has been known for many years. During the latter part of the nineteenth century Langley made extensive use of the local application of nicotine for charting sympathetic ganglia in the cat and the distribution of the fibers emanating from them.

The ability of tetraethylammonium to block the effect of ganglionic stimulants was also known for many years. Such blocking agents received little attention, however, until 1946, when the mode of action of tetraethylammonium on the mammalian circulation was thoroughly investigated.[1] These studies suggested the possibility of blocking ganglionic transmission in a fairly selective manner. The great interest in hypertensive diseases and vasospastic disorders prompted many investigators to develop and expand this field. Additional interest was aroused when controlled hypotension was found to be a desirable objective in some surgical operations.

Tetraethylammonium (TEA; Etamon) has proved to be an interesting pharmacologic tool. Its general application in disease states has been impractical, however, because its poor absorption from the gastrointestinal tract and rapid excretion by the kidney result in a very brief duration of action.

A variety of ganglionic blocking agents were developed for practical use, particularly in treating hypertension and in producing controlled hypotension. Some of the most widely used compounds are hexamethonium, pentolinium, chlorisondamine, and trimethaphan camphorsulfonate. More recently, mecamylamine and pempidine have received clinical applications.

Chemistry

The chemical formulas of some of the ganglionic blocking agents are as follows:

$$(C_2H_5)_3 \overset{+}{\equiv} N - CH_2 - CH_3 \cdot \overset{-}{Cl}$$

Tetraethylammonium chloride

$$(CH_3)_3 \overset{+}{\equiv} N - CH_2 - (CH_2)_4 - CH_2 - \overset{+}{N} \equiv (CH_3)_3 \cdot 2Cl$$

Hexamethonium chloride

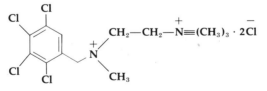

Pentolinium tartrate

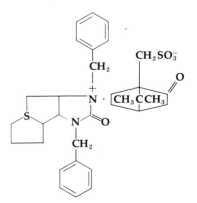

Chlorisondamine chloride

Trimethaphan camphorsulfonate

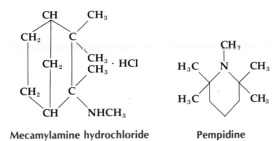

Mecamylamine hydrochloride   Pempidine

It may be seen that the majority of the ganglionic blocking drugs are quaternary ammonium compounds, just as acetylcholine has a quaternary nitrogen. Mecamylamine and pemipidine, however, are not quaternary amines.

Clinical pharmacology

The ganglionic blocking agents are used principally for decreasing the influence of the sympathetic division of the autonomic nervous system on the circulation. These compounds will also affect transmission across parasympathetic ganglia and can produce numerous side effects.

A very picturesque description of the actions of a typical ganglionic drug was given by Paton in his account of the "hexamethonium man."

> He is a pink complexioned person, except when he has stood in a queue for a long time, when he may get pale and faint. His handshake is warm and dry. He is a placid and relaxed companion; for instance he may laugh, but he can't cry because the tears cannot come. Your rudest story will not make him blush, and the most unpleasant circumstances will fail to make him turn pale. His collars and socks stay very clean and sweet. He wears corsets and may, if you meet him out, be rather fidgety (corsets to compress his splanchnic vascular pool, fidgety to keep the venous return going from his legs). He dislikes speaking much unless helped with something to moisten his dry mouth and throat. He is long sighted and easily blinded by bright light. The redness of his eyeballs may suggest irregular habits and in fact his head is rather weak. But he always behaves like a gentleman and never belches nor hiccups. He tends to get cold and keeps well wrapped up. But his health is good; he does not have chilblains and those diseases of modern civilization, hypertension and peptic ulcer, pass him by. He is thin because his appetite is modest; he never feels hunger pains and his stomach never rumbles. He gets rather constipated so that his intake of liquid paraffin is high. As old age comes on, he will suffer from retention of urine and impotence, but frequency, precipitancy, and strangury will not worry him. One is uncertain how he will end, but perhaps if he is not careful, by eating less and less and getting colder and colder, he will sink into a symptomless, hypoglycemic coma and die, as was proposed for the universe, a sort of entropy death.*

Circulatory effects. The ganglionic blocking drugs tend to lower blood pressure by decreasing sympathetic tone to various vascular areas. The intensity of this hypotensive action depends on a number of factors. First, the position of the patient has a great influence. There may be only slight lowering of the pressure while the patient is in the recumbent position. When he stands, however, the mean pressure may fall precipitously to the point of faintness. This is known as postural hypotension and undoubtedly results from pooling of blood in the extremities in the absence of compensatory vasoconstriction there. Faintness reflects the subsequent cerebral ischemia.

---

*From Paton, W. D. M.: The principles of ganglionic block. In Scientific basis of medicine, vol. 2, London, 1954, Athlone Press.

The intensity of the hypotensive effect depends also on factors that happen to influence the blood pressure level at the time of the administration of the ganglionic blocking drug. If the blood pressure is maintained at an elevated level as a result of the presence of a vasoconstrictor compound, as in pheochromocytoma, the ganglionic blocking drugs are not effective in reducing it. On the other hand, if the sympathetic tone is high or the blood vessels are very sensitive to the tonic influence of the sympathetic system, a marked fall of blood pressure may be elicited by the ganglionic blocking drugs.

Side effects and complications. In addition to the unavoidable postural hypotension reflecting decreased sympathetic outflow, the ganglionic blocking drugs may produce side effects due to blockade of parasympathetic ganglia.

The smooth muscle tone of the gastrointestinal and urinary tracts may be relaxed by the ganglionic blocking agents, resulting in constipation or difficulty in voiding. As one might expect, the pupils may dilate and there can be interference with accommodation for near vision. Salivary secretion may be inhibited, and the resulting dry mouth may be sufficiently uncomfortable to require administration of pilocarpine. Sweating is also reduced, not by an atropine-like effect, but because of decreased sympathetic activity as a consequence of the ganglionic block.

Metabolism

The quaternary ammonium ganglionic blocking agents are poorly absorbed from the gastrointestinal tract. Drugs such as tetraethylammonium or trimethaphan camphorsulfonate cannot be used by mouth because of poor absorption. Although chlorisondamine and pentolinium are given by oral administration, their absorption is far from complete. The oral-intravenous LD_{50} ratio of these drugs in mice is about 20:1. On the other hand, the secondary amine, mecamylamine, is much better absorbed, giving an oral-intravenous LD_{50} ratio of about 4:1.[4]

The ganglionic blocking agents of the quaternary ammonium group are eliminated through renal excretion. Their distribution in the body is largely extracellular.

Differences among various ganglionic blocking agents

The various ganglionic blocking drugs differ with respect to potency, oral absorption, and duration of action.

Mecamylamine hydrochloride (Inversine) is a potent drug that is well absorbed from the gastrointestinal tract and has a duration of action of 4 to 12 hours. The initial oral dose is 2.5 mg. twice daily. This dose is gradually increased until a satisfactory effect is obtained, usually at a dose level of 30 mg./day.

The drug may cause central nervous system stimulation and neuromuscular blockade in large doses.

Pempidine (Perolysen) is similar in action to mecamylamine. It is well absorbed from the gastrointestinal tract and is used in doses of 2.5 mg. twice daily by mouth. In large doses it may cause central nervous system stimulation and neuromuscular blockade.

Hexamethonium (Methium), at the other end of the spectrum, is poorly and irregularly absorbed and is now obsolete.

Pentolinium (Ansolysen) is about five times as potent as hexamethonium in lowering blood pressure. The subcutaneous injection of 3 mg. of pentolinium has about the same effect as 15 mg. of hexamethonium by the same route.

Chlorisondamine (Ecolid) appears to be a potent ganglionic blocking agent that has a long duration of action. The recommended daily dose is about 100 to 200 mg., usually given in two doses (only by intravenous infusion).

Trimethaphan camphorsulfonate (Arfonad) is a very short-acting ganglionic blocking agent. It is chiefly used for producing controlled hypotension during special surgical operations. Although it is a potent histamine-releasing agent in dogs, no adverse effects that could be attributed to histamine release have occurred in the human being. Intravenous infusion of a solution containing 1 mg./ml. will significantly lower blood pressure. When the infusion is stopped, blood pressure returns to its normal levels in about 5 minutes. Trimethaphan camsylate (Arfonad) is available as a 50 mg./ml. solution that is diluted to 1 mg./ml. for intravenous infusion.

References

1 Acheson, G. H., and Moe, G. K.: The action of tetraethylammonium ion on the mammalian circulation, J. Pharmacol. Exp. Ther. **87**:220, 1946.

2 Ford, R. V., Moyer, J. H., and Spurr, C. L.: Hexamethonium in the chronic treatment of hypertension: its effect on renal hemodynamics and on the excretion of water and electrolytes, J. Clin. Invest. **32**:1133, 1953.

3 Paton, W. D. M.: The principles of ganglionic block. In Scientific basis of medicine, vol. 2, London, 1954, Athlone Press.

4 Stone, C. A., Torchiana, M. L., Navarro, A., and Beyer, K. H.: Ganglionic blocking properties of 3-methylaminoisocamphane hydrochloride (mecamylamine): a secondary amine, J. Pharmacol. Exp. Ther. **117**:169, 1956.

5 Winbury, M. M.: Comparison of the vascular actions of 1-1-dimethyl-4-piperazinium (DMPP), a potent ganglionic stimulant, J. Physiol. **147**:1, 1959.

Recent reviews

6 Aviado, D. M.: Hemodynamic effects of ganglion blocking drugs, Circ. Res. **8**:304, 1960.

7 Volle, R. L.: Modification by drugs of synaptic mechanisms in autonomic ganglia, Pharmacol. Rev. **18**:839, 1966.

11 Neuromuscular blocking agents

GENERAL CONCEPT

The clinically useful neuromuscular blocking drugs act postsynaptically by one of two major mechanisms: (1) competition with acetylcholine for the end plate receptor (nondepolarizing blocking agents) and (2) initial depolarization followed by desensitization to the transmitter despite repolarization. An example of a nondepolarizing blocking agent is *d*-tubocurarine; succinylcholine acts by the second mechanism.

In addition to these postsynaptic influences, drugs may act on presynaptic aspects of neuromuscular transmission. Most of these effects are of only academic interest. According to current concepts, acetylcholine is contained in the synaptic vesicles. Spontaneous emptying of these vesicles results in the miniature end plate potentials. The nerve impulse causes a large increase in the number of vesicles released, leading to depolarization of the postsynaptic membrane, and the muscle end plate potential. Drugs that alter the synthesis, storage, or release of acetylcholine are known, but they have no therapeutic importance. *Hemicholinium* blocks acetylcholine synthesis by interfering with choline uptake in nerves. On the other hand, the toxin of *Clostridium botulinum* paralyzes the release mechanism in all cholinergic fibers. High magnesium or low calcium concentrations, neomycin, streptomycin, kanamycin, and local and general anesthetics may also lower the release of the transmitter. Catecholamines and high calcium concentrations tend to raise transmitter release.

Although evidence is increasing for a presynaptic as well as postsynaptic action of drugs that depress neuromuscular transmission, the relative importance of these two sites of action is not clear. Partial blockade by "nondepolarizing" relaxants is characterized by a decay in response to tetanic stimulation of the motor nerve, which could indicate a presynaptic action. On the other hand, tetanus is well maintained after partial blockade induced by the depolarizing muscle relaxants.

There are other possible ways to cause skeletal muscle relaxation. Certain drugs may act on the spinal cord and portions of the central nervous system to cause relaxation of skeletal muscles.

The use of neuromuscular blocking agents is limited largely to anesthesia, with some other minor uses. The centrally acting drugs have clinical usefulness in a variety of disorders accompanied by painful contraction of skeletal muscles.

NEUROMUSCULAR BLOCKING AGENTS
Development

Experimentation with the South American arrow poison, *curare*, was one of the earliest examples of scientific work in pharmacology. Magendie and his pupil Claude Bernard studied the effects of curare on nerve-muscle preparations in the nineteenth century. Claude Bernard was able to show that the drug prevented the response of the muscle to nerve stimulation. Surprisingly, it did not prevent the muscle from responding to direct stimulation and it failed to block conduction in the nerve. It therefore seemed to exert its effect at the junction of nerve and muscle.

The active principle of *Chondodendron tomentosum* roots is *d*-tubocurarine, which has been isolated and its structure established.[6] It is a fairly large molecule in which two quaternary ammonium structures appear to be separated by an estimated distance of 14 Å, compared with the critical distance of 7 Å in acetylcholine. The curare-like activity of quaternary ammonium compounds has been known ever since the early work of Alexander Crum Brown and Thomas Richard Fraser (1868, 1869).

The introduction of purified curare compounds into anesthesiology[11] stimulated interest in the development of synthetic curariform drugs. The guiding principle for these syntheses has been the knowledge that the compounds must be of a quaternary ammonium structure and that two of these quaternary nitrogens must be separated by a distance of about 14 Å.[3] The importance of this distance, particularly in flexible molecules, has been questioned.[8]

The resulting compounds were of two types. Gallamine, benzoquinonium, and the more recent pancuronium are nondepolarizing blocking agents. On the other hand, succinylcholine and decamethonium produce initial depolarization followed by a decreased receptor sensitivity to acetylcholine despite repolarization.

Clinical pharmacology

The intravenous injection of 5 to 10 mg. of *d*-tubocurarine produces flaccid paralysis of the extremities. Doubling these doses may produce apnea. The effects last for 10 minutes, with muscle strength returning in 40 minutes. There is a characteristic progression of effects, with the extrinsic muscles of the eye being affected first and then those of the face, the extremities, and finally the diaphragm.

The usual therapeutic doses of *d*-tubocurarine are unlikely to produce significant central nervous system action, since the blood-brain barrier represents a considerable defense against quaternary ammonium compounds. The beneficial effect on pain in certain clinical conditions is ascribed to the relaxation of contracted muscles and not to a primary analgesic or hypnotic effect.

Drug interactions with nondepolarizing muscle relaxants such as *d*-tubocurarine are of great importance. General anesthetics such as ether, halothane, cyclopropane, and methoxyflurane intensify the action of nondepolarizing agents, making a reduction of their dosage necessary. Antibiotics such as neomycin, streptomycin, polymyxin B, colistin, kanamycin, and viomycin potentiate neuromuscular blockade. Quinine and and quinidine also potentiate the action of neuromuscular blocking drugs. Anticholinesterase insecticides such as parathion, malathion, and tetraethyl pyrophosphate have some properties similar to those of the depolarizing blocking agents, and prolonged apnea may result when the patient exposed to such insecticides is treated with neuromuscular blocking drugs. Finally, patients with myasthenia gravis, acidosis, or severe renal disease react excessively to the usual doses of *d*-tubocurarine.

Adverse reactions to the nondepolarizing neuromuscular blocking drugs include prolonged apnea, bronchospasm, and hypotension, the latter two being partly a consequence of histamine release.[14, 17] Ganglionic blockade may contribute to the hypotension. Neostigmine and edrophonium (Tensilon) are antagonists of the early nondepolarizing actions of *d*-tubocurarine. Nevertheless, the most important antidotal measure is artificial respiration.

Mode of action

It is generally believed that acetylcholine is released from synaptic vesicles with passage of the nerve impulse.[7] The mediator produces a small electrical charge known as the *end plate potential*. Under normal circumstances this produces in turn the propagated *action potential*. In a partially curarized preparation the small end plate potential is clearly visible, since it is not followed by the larger action potential. The effect of curare on the end plate potential and the anticurare action of physostigmine are shown in Fig. 11-1.

The differences between the competitive and depolarizing blocking agents may now be summarized.

Neostigmine, edrophonium, and potassium tend to oppose the action of the competitive blocking agents, whereas ether anesthesia and myasthenia gravis increase the susceptibility of the patient to these drugs. On the other hand, *d*-tubocurarine and ether tend to oppose the actions of the depolarizing agents, whereas the anticholinesterases, edrophonium, and potassium have no effect on them.

The administration of the depolarizing agents results in muscle fasciculations as the initial response, whereas the competitive blocking agents do not have this effect.

Mixed block. Initial depolarization followed by block is referred to as mixed block.

When a depolarizing drug is applied to a muscle, the depolarization is not sustained but tends to fade.[23] It appears as if the acetylcholine receptors become inactive and

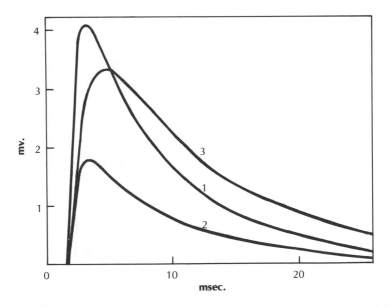

Fig. 11-1. Effect of curarine on the end plate potential of the frog sartorius and the antagonistic action of physostigmine. *1,* After 6 micromoles of curarine; *2,* after 9 micromoles of curarine; *3,* after 9 micromoles of curarine plus physostigmine 10^{-5}. (From Eccles, J. C., et al.: J. Neurophysiol. **5:**211, 1942.)

the term "receptor inactivation" has been introduced to describe this phenomenon, which is probably of great importance in the second phase of the action of succinylcholine.

Problem 11-1. What is the mechanism of "receptor inactivation"? According to an ingenious explanation,[23] prolonged endplate depolarization and consequent increase in Ca^{++} conductance lead to a combination of Ca^{++} with anionic sites that control ionic movements of sodium and potassium. This leads to a reduction of membrane depolarization.

Differences among more common neuromuscular blocking agents

The various neuromuscular blocking agents differ with respect to potency, mode of action, and the nature of their side effects.

d-**Tubocurarine** is injected intravenously in the form of solutions containing 3 or 15 mg./ml. *d*-Tubocurarine chloride (Tubarine) is available for injection in a solution, 3 mg./ml. Its action is transient. About one third of the amount administered is excreted unchanged in the urine, whereas the rest is metabolically altered. It is probably still the most important competitive neuromuscular blocking agent, although the newer **dimethyltubocurarine chloride** (Mecostrin) has a potency about three times as great. A solution of dimethyltubocurarine iodide (Metubine iodide), 2 mg./ml., is available for injection.

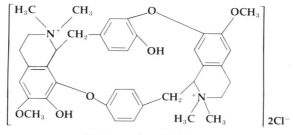

d-**Tubocurarine chloride**

Pancuronium dimethobromide is a recently introduced nondepolarizing neuromuscular blocking agent that differs from *d*-tubocurarine in its greater potency and lack of histamine-releasing or ganglionic blocking actions. As indicated in its structural formula, the drug has a steroid nucleus with two quaternary amines attached. Its potency is such that, administered intravenously, 2 mg. of pancuronium dimethobromide produce about the same effect as 10 to 15 mg. of *d*-tubocurarine.[25]

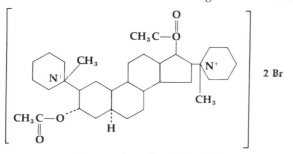

Pancuronium dimethobromide

Gallamine triethiodide (Flaxedil triethiodide) and **benzoquinonium** (Mytolon) are also neuromuscular blocking drugs of the competitive type. They have certain side effects that are not observed following the use of *d*-tubocurarine. Gallamine has an atropine-like effect on the cardiac branch of the vagus nerve and can produce considerable tachycardia.[18] Gallamine triethiodide is available in solutions for injection of 20 and 100 mg./ml. The actions of gallamine triethiodide are very similar to those of tubocurarine. It may have a slightly shorter duration of action, and it does not cause histamine release. This may be an advantage in asthmatics. On the other hand, its tendency to cause tachycardia by its vagolytic and perhaps catecholamine-releasing action may be a disadvantage in patients in whom tachycardia may represent a hazard.

Decamethonium bromide (Syncurine; C-10), one of the methonium compounds, is a depolarizing blocking agent that has been largely replaced by succinylcholine. Decamethonium bromide solution, 1 mg./ml., is available for injection.

$$Br^- \cdot (CH_3)_3 \equiv N^+ - (CH_2)_{10} - N^+ \equiv (CH_3)_3 \cdot Br^-$$

Decamethonium bromide

It is interesting to note that the difference between this drug and hexamethonium consists of four additional methylene groups in decamethonium. This change in the distance between the two quaternary ammonium groups is sufficient to change the drug from a primary ganglionic blocking agent to one that is principally active on the neuromuscular junction.

Succinylcholine (Anectine) has the following structural formula:

$$Cl^- \cdot H_3C - \overset{\overset{\displaystyle H_3C}{\diagdown}}{\underset{\underset{\displaystyle H_3C}{\diagup}}{N^+}} CH_2CH_2O\overset{\overset{\displaystyle O}{\|}}{C}CH_2CH_2\overset{\overset{\displaystyle O}{\|}}{C}OCH_2CH_2N^+\overset{\overset{\displaystyle CH_3}{\diagup}}{\underset{\underset{\displaystyle CH_3}{\diagdown}}{-CH_3}} \cdot Cl^-$$

Succinylcholine chloride

Succinylcholine is an important blocking agent of the depolarizing type.

When succinylcholine chloride, 0.5 to 1 mg./kg. of body weight, is injected intravenously, there may be considerable muscular contraction for several seconds before paralysis develops. The muscles remain paralyzed for about 5 minutes and resume their function in another 5 minutes.

The drug has a selective action on the neuromuscular receptor sites, although in large doses it may cause some effects similar to those of acetylcholine on the heart and circulation.

The actions of succinylcholine are prevented by *d*-tubocurarine, whereas neostigmine is definitely not an antidote and may even aggravate the muscle paralysis caused by succinylcholine.

The short duration of action of succinylcholine may be attributed to its rapid metabolic degradation. The compound is hydrolyzed by plasma cholinesterase to succinylmonocholine and choline. In a second step, succinylmonocholine is hydrolyzed to succinic acid and choline by the cholinesterases.[10]

In some patients, succinylcholine has produced prolonged apnea caused by quantitative or qualitative differences in cholinesterase, a genetic abnormality (p. 36).

Succinylcholine is a valuable agent for producing short periods of muscular relaxation. It may be given in single intravenous doses or by intravenous infusion. Preparations of succinylcholine chloride (Anectine chloride) for injection include powder,

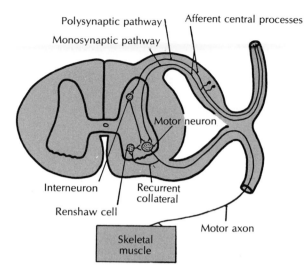

Polysynaptic pathway
Monosynaptic pathway
Afferent central processes
Motor neuron
Interneuron
Recurrent collateral
Renshaw cell
Motor axon
Skeletal muscle

Fig. 11-2. Innervation of skeletal muscle.

500 mg. and 1 Gm., and solutions of 20, 50, and 100 mg./ml. Facilities for artificial respiration are essential, since this appears to be the only effective antidotal measure to apnea.

Usefulness

The greatest usefulness of the neuromuscular blocking agents is in anesthesia, in which they contribute to muscular relaxation. They also are employed for facilitating endotracheal intubation.

Succinylcholine is employed for protecting patients against severe convulsions in electroconvulsive therapy. Curare-like drugs have also been used in the treatment of tetanus, but they are not the drugs of choice for this condition.

SKELETAL MUSCLE DEPRESSANTS THAT ACT ON THE SPINAL CORD
Centrally acting skeletal muscle relaxants

In addition to those acting at the neuromuscular junction, other drugs can cause muscle relaxation by acting on internuncial spinal neurons to depress polysynaptic pathways. (See Fig. 11-2.) These centrally acting muscle relaxants act on higher centers also and are commonly used as antianxiety agents. Although experimentally these drugs can depress the spinal cord at dose levels that do not cause sleep or anesthesia, in clinical practice it is difficult to say how much of their muscle-relaxing power is simply a consequence of the antianxiety effects. Although some drugs in this series are promoted as centrally acting muscle relaxants, others almost identical in structure are widely used for their antianxiety properties.

Indications for these drugs include the treatment of muscle spasm resulting from sprains, arthritis, myositis, and fibrositis. Drugs in this group can cause adverse effects such as drowsiness, lethargy and ataxia, allergic manifestations, and psychic dependence particularly to the meprobamate and chlordiazepoxide group of compounds.

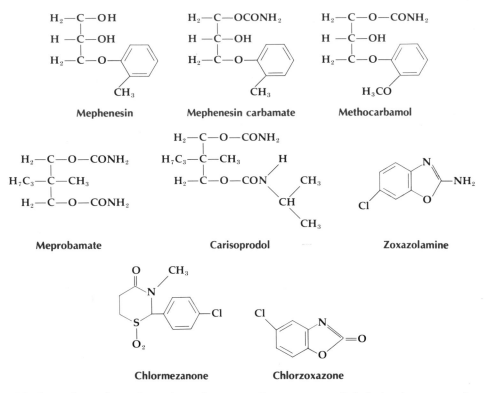

Mephenesin

Mephenesin carbamate

Methocarbamol

Meprobamate

Carisoprodol

Zoxazolamine

Chlormezanone

Chlorzoxazone

Mephenesin and mephenesin carbamate. These propanediol derivatives were the first drugs introduced as centrally acting muscle relaxants. Their selective action on spinal neurons was shown by abolition of strychnine convulsions in animals at dose levels that, in contrast to general anesthetics, did not cause sleep. These drugs are rather weak and must be given in large doses to obtain an effect. Preparations for Mephenesin (Tolserol) include tablets, 500 mg., and elixir, 500 mg./5 ml. Mephenesin carbamate (Tolseram) is available in tablets, 500 mg., and elixir, 1 Gm./5 ml.

The duration of action of mephenesin-like compounds is somewhat prolonged if the hydroxyl groups are masked by preparing the carbamate of the drug. This is the reason for the availability of a variety of drugs that are carbamates of glycerol ethers or propanediols. Even with this modification the low potency has limited the usefulness of these compounds as skeletal muscle relaxants, although they do have some clinical applications in parkinsonism, in orthopedic conditions with muscular stiffness, in strychnine poisoning, in tetanus, and in some other conditions.

Methocarbamol. Closely related to mephenesin carbamate, the drug has the same indication, uses, and limitations. Methocarbamol (Robaxin) is available in tablets, 500 and 750 mg., and, for injection, in solution of 100 mg./ml. in 50% polyethylene glycol.

Chlorphenesin carbamate. This drug is closely related to mephenesin and has the same moderate effectiveness as a centrally acting muscle relaxant. Chlorphenesin carbamate (Maolate) is available in tablets, 400 mg.

Meprobamate. Another drug closely related to mephenesin, this propanediol has become extremely popular as a so-called "minor tranquilizer." Its use and abuse will be discussed on p. 231. Preparations of meprobamate (Miltown; Equanil) include capsules and tablets containing 200 and 400 mg.

Carisoprodol. Closely related to meprobamate, this drug has some limited usefulness in the treatment of muscle spasms. Preparations of carisoprodol (Soma) include tablets, 350 mg., and capsules, 250 mg.

Benzoxazole derivatives. The centrally acting muscle relaxants zoxazolamine (Flexin) and chlorzoxazone (Paraflex) were developed on the basis of the observation that benzimidazole had depressant effects on polysynaptic pathways of the spinal cord. Zoxazolamine turned out to be hepatotoxic and was removed from the market. The closely related chlorzoxazone has some usefulness in muscle spasms caused by neurologic diseases. It also may cause jaundice in an occasional patient. It is available in tablets, 500 mg.

Metaxalone. Chemically unrelated to the propanediols, this drug is 5-[3,5,(-dimethylphenoxyl)methyl]-2-oxazolidinone. Its usefulness in spastic conditions is probably related to its sedative effect. Metaxalone (Skelaxin) is available in tablets, 400 mg.

The diazepoxides. Chlordiazepoxide (Librium) and diazepam (Valium) are generally viewed as antianxiety agents and will be discussed in Chapter 19. These drugs may be useful for reducing spasm in musculoskeletal disorders and may be considered as centrally acting skeletal muscle relaxants. They are available in tablet form and also as injectable solutions.

Clinical pharmacology

The drugs discussed in this section are widely offered and used for the relief of spasm and spasticity associated with diseases or injury of muscles, bones, and joints. Claims for their effectiveness are based on the attractive experimental evidence discussed in connection with mephenesin and on largely uncontrolled clinical trials.

Although these drugs are offered with the implication that they are fairly specific muscle relaxants, there is a growing feeling among clinical investigators that these drugs act simply as sedatives, particularly when orally administered. Significantly, barbiturates also can reduce muscle spasm.[19] Even placebos have a marked effect on pains and aches claimed to be benefited by the muscle relaxants.

Drugs in this group may be quite useful, although they should not be looked upon as specific muscle relaxants. It is no coincidence that some members of this group, such as meprobamate, are much more widely used as sedative tranquilizers than as muscle relaxants.

References

1 Beecher, H. K., and Todd, D. P.: A study of the deaths associated with anesthesia and surgery, based on a study of 599,548 anesthesias in ten institutions, Ann. Surg. 140:2, 1954.

2 Berger, F. M.: Spinal cord depressant drugs, Pharmacol. Rev. 1:243, 1949.

3 Bridenbaugh, P. O., and Churchill-Davidson, H. C.: Response to tubocurarine chloride and its reversal by neostigmine methylsulfate in man, J.A.M.A. 203:541, 1968.

4 Churchill-Davidson, H. C., and Richardson, A. T.: Neuromuscular transmission in myasthenia gravis, J. Physiol. 122:252, 1953.

5 Comroe, J. H., Jr., and Dripps, R. D.: The histamine-like action of curare and tubocurarine injected intracutaneously and intraarterially in man, Anesthesiology 7:260, 1946.

6 Dutcher, J. D.: The isolation and identification of additional physiologically active alkaloids in extracts of Chondodendron tomentosum ruiz and pavon, Ann. N. Y. Acad. Sci. 54:326, 1951.

7 Eccles, J. C.: The physiology of nerve cells, Baltimore, 1957, The Johns Hopkins Press.

8 Ehrenpreis, S.: The interaction of quaternary ammonium ions with various macromolecules, Georgetown Med. Bull. 16:148, 1963.

9 Foldes, F. F.: The mode of action of quaternary ammonium type neuromuscular blocking agents, Brit. J. Anaesth. **26**:394, 1954.

10 Foldes, F. F., Vandervort, R. S., and Shanor, S. P.: The fate of succinylcholine in man, Anesthesiology **16**:11, 1955.

11 Griffith, H. R., and Johnson, G. E.: The use of curare in general anesthesia, Anesthesiology **3**:418, 1942.

12 Henneman, E., Kaplan, A., and Unna, K.: A neuropharmacological study on the effect of myanesin (Tolserol) on motor systems, J. Pharmacol. Exp. Ther. **97**:331, 1949.

13 Kamijo, K., and Koelle, G. B.: 2-Amino-5-chlorobenzoxazole, Proc. Soc. Exp. Biol. Med. **88**:565, 1955.

14 Mongar, J. L., and Whelan, R. F.: Histamine release by adrenaline and d-tubocurarine in the human subject, J. Physiol. **120**:146, 1953.

15 Paton, W. D. M.: A theory of drug action based on the rate of drug-receptor combination, Proc. Roy. Soc. [Biol.] **154**:21, 1961.

16 Riker, W. F.: Pharmacologic considerations in a reevaluation of the neuromuscular synapse, Arch. Neurol. **3**:488, 1960.

17 Riker, W. F., and Wescoe, W. C.: The pharmacology of Flaxedil, with observations on certain analogs, Ann. N. Y. Acad. Sci. **54**:373, 1951.

18 Salem, M. R., Kim, Y., and El Etr, A. A.: Histamine release following the intravenous injection of d-tubocurarine, Anesthesiology **29**:380, 1968.

19 Shideman, F. E.: Clinical pharmacology of hypnotics and sedatives, Clin. Pharmacol. Ther. **2**:313, 1961.

20 Thesleff, S.: The mode of neuromuscular block caused by acetylcholine, nicotine, decamethonium, and succinylcholine, Acta Physiol. Scand. **34**:218, 1955.

Recent reviews

21 Friend, D. G.: Pharmacology of muscle relaxants, Clin. Pharmacol. Ther. **5**:871, 1964.

22 Galindo, A.: The role of prejunctional effects in myoneural transmission, Anesthesiology **36**:598, 1972.

23 Hubbard, J. I., and Quastel, D. M. J.: Micropharmacology of vertebrate neuromuscular transmission, Ann. Rev. Pharmacol. **13**:199, 1973.

24 Karczmar, A. G.: Neuromuscular pharmacology, Ann. Rev. Pharmacol. **7**:241, 1967.

25 Kariss, J. H., and Gissen, A. J.: Evaluation of new neuromuscular blocking agents, Anesthesiology **35**:149, 1971.

26 Riker, W. F., and Okamoto, M.: Pharmacology of motor nerve terminals, Ann. Rev. Pharmacol. **9**:173, 1969.

27 Thesleff, S., and Quastel, D. M. J.: Neuromuscular pharmacology, Ann. Rev. Pharmacol. **5**:263, 1965.

12 Adrenergic blocking agents

GENERAL CONCEPT

Adrenergic blocking agents are drugs that competitively inhibit the actions of catecholamines and other adrenergic agonists on their specific receptors. They are effective against catecholamines released from sympathetic nerve endings.

Adrenergic blocking drugs are classified as *alpha* and *beta* adrenergic blocking agents, reflecting the existence of two types of receptors. In tissues that possess both types of receptors, such as most blood vessels, alpha stimulation causes contraction and beta stimulation causes relaxation. The alpha adrenergic blocking drugs in such a tissue cause vasodilation. In organs whose receptors are almost entirely beta, such as the heart, the beta blockers oppose the excitatory effects of norepinephrine released from sympathetic nerve endings.

Drugs that deplete catecholamines or prevent their release in adrenergic nerves should be called *catecholamine depleters* and *adrenergic neuronal blocking drugs*, respectively, and should not be confused with the *adrenergic blocking agents* that act on alpha

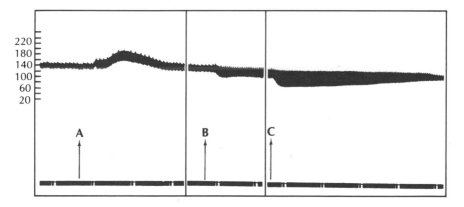

Fig. 12-1. Epinephrine reversal by phentolamine. Effect of epinephrine on blood pressure before and after injection of phentolamine. Dog was anesthetized with pentobarbital sodium. At **A,** epinephrine was injected intravenously, 1 μg/kg. At **B,** phentolamine was injected, 5 mg./kg. At **C,** epinephrine injection was repeated. Time in seconds. Note lowering of mean pressure by epinephrine following adrenergic blocking agent. Increased pulse pressure under these circumstances is an indication that adrenergic blocking agent does not prevent the cardiac stimulant effect of epinephrine.

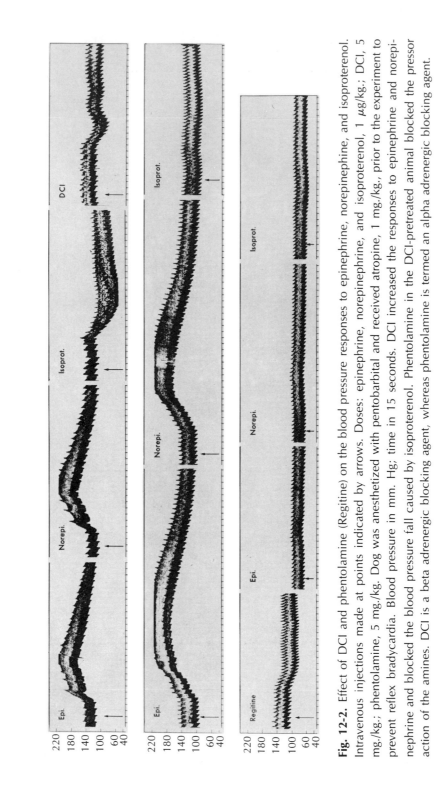

Fig. 12-2. Effect of DCI and phentolamine (Regitine) on the blood pressure responses to epinephrine, norepinephrine, and isoproterenol. Intravenous injections made at points indicated by arrows. Doses: epinephrine, norepinephrine, and isoproterenol, 1 μg/kg.; DCI, 5 mg./kg.; phentolamine, 5 mg./kg. Dog was anesthetized with pentobarbital and received atropine, 1 mg./kg., prior to the experiment to prevent reflex bradycardia. Blood pressure in mm. Hg; time in 15 seconds. DCI increased the responses to epinephrine and norepinephrine and blocked the blood pressure fall caused by isoproterenol. Phentolamine in the DCI-pretreated animal blocked the pressor action of the amines. DCI is a beta adrenergic blocking agent, whereas phentolamine is termed an alpha adrenergic blocking agent.

and beta receptors. Certain imprecise older terms such as *adrenolytic, sympatholytic,* and *sympathoplegic* should be abandoned.

CONCEPT OF EPINEPHRINE REVERSAL

The single most characteristic feature of the alpha adrenergic blocking drugs is their ability to transform the pressor effect of injected epinephrine into a depressor response. This "epinephrine reversal" was first observed by Dale in 1905 following the injection of certain ergot preparations.

The epinephrine reversal caused by phentolamine is shown in Fig. 12-1.

The facts fit the hypothesis that arteriolar smooth muscle has both alpha and beta receptors, the former mediating vasoconstriction and the latter mediating vasodilatation by adrenergic drugs. Epinephrine acts on both receptors. An alpha blocker such as phentolamine prevents access of the drug to alpha receptors and thus unmasks its action on beta receptors, the result being vasodilatation instead of the usual vasoconstriction.

Norepinephrine, on the other hand, has no effect on vascular beta receptors. Thus the alpha blockers prevent blood pressure rise by the drug without causing a norepinephrine reversal. As shown in Fig. 12-2, the epinephrine reversal is prevented by a beta blocker.

ALPHA ADRENERGIC BLOCKING AGENTS
Development

As early as 1905 some of the ergot alkaloids were shown by Dale to have adrenergic blocking properties, although they have not achieved any usefulness on this basis. Certain benzodioxans were known to have adrenergic blocking actions,[3] but these compounds were somewhat weak and produced many other effects in the body.

Great impetus was given to the study of adrenergic blocking agents when Dibenamine and the related β-haloalkylamines were shown to be specific and potent agents with a long duration in the body.[10] Phenoxybenzamine still has some usefulness.

Certain imidazoline compounds such as tolazoline and phentolamine have not only some adrenergic blocking actions but also many other effects. Additional drugs with adrenergic blocking effects are azapetine and chlorpromazine.

Current status

The alpha blocking agents are valuable investigative tools in pharmacology at both the preclinical and clinical levels. They are useful in the diagnosis of pheochromocytoma. These drugs have been generally disappointing as therapeutic agents in hypertension, peripheral vascular diseases, and other conditions. There is some research interest as well as debate about the usefulness of phenoxybenzamine in shock associated with peripheral vasoconstriction. Despite the encouraging results reported,[23,30] such treatment must be considered strictly experimental.

General features

The alpha adrenergic blocking drugs oppose the actions of norepinephrine and the effects of sympathetic stimulation. They reverse the actions of epinephrine on blood pressure but do not oppose vasodilatation or cardioacceleration produced by adrenergic drugs.

The most striking effects of the adrenergic blocking agents, then, are inhibition of the effects of norepinephrine on blood vessels, unmasking of the dilator action of epinephrine, and failure to influence the cardiac actions of catecholamines.

Differences among various alpha adrenergic blocking agents

The various drugs in this group differ from each other in potency and duration of action. They may also possess pharmacologic properties entirely unrelated to adrenergic blockade.

Dibenamine is a long-acting blocking agent that has been replaced by its close relative phenoxybenzamine.

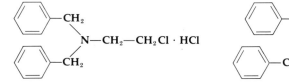

Dibenamine hydrochloride   Phenoxybenzamine hydrochloride

Phenoxybenzamine (Dibenzyline), when administered in doses of 20 to 100 mg., produces lowering of blood pressure and orthostatic hypotension. The effects of the drug last more than 24 hours. It is available in capsules of 10 mg.

The long duration of action of phenoxybenzamine is probably a consequence of a stable combination between the drug and the alpha receptor. In this case, although competition exists between the drug and catecholamines for the receptor during the early stages of blockade, such competition becomes ineffective as the blockade develops fully. The term *nonequilibrium blockade*[9] has been applied to such an interaction between agonist and antagonist.

Occasional indications for the use of phenoxybenzamine include peripheral vascular diseases in which vasospasm is an important feature, such as Raynaud's disease, and the management of pheochromocytoma both prior to, and during, the operation.

Among the many adverse effects that may be caused by phenoxybenzamine, orthostatic hypotension, tachycardia, nasal congestion, and miosis are common and predictable. Some of these adverse effects may be treated with nonadrenergic vasopressors such as angiotensin amide or with adrenergic drugs that do not have prominent beta effects, such as methoxamine. Epinephrine would aggravate the hypotension caused by phenoxybenzamine, an example of epinephrine reversal by alpha blockers.

Tolazoline hydrochloride (Priscoline), a weak alpha blocker, causes peripheral vasodilatation largely by a direct relaxant effect on vascular smooth muscle. In addition, the drug is a direct cardiac stimulant and its use is often accompanied by tachycardia.

Tolazoline is used in the treatment of peripheral vascular diseases for the relief of vasospasm. It is available in tablets, 25 mg., timed-release tablets, 80 mg., and solution for injection, 25 mg./ml.

Adverse effects to the drug include pilomotor stimulation (gooseflesh), tachycardia, and increased gastrointestinal motility and hydrochloric acid secretion. Tolazoline is related structurally to histamine.

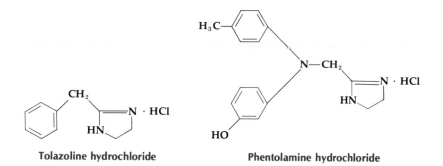

Tolazoline hydrochloride   **Phentolamine hydrochloride**

Phentolamine is an alpha blocker used almost exclusively for the diagnosis of pheochromocytoma and for the prevention of hypertension during operative removal of the tumor. Preparations include phentolamine hydrochloride (Regitine hydrochloride) in tablets, 50 mg., and phentolamine mesylate (Regitine mesylate) in powder for injection, 5 mg. In addition to its blocking action on receptors, the drug has other pharmacologic actions similar to those of tolazoline, to which it is chemically related.

Adverse effects include orthostatic hypotension, tachycardia, nasal stuffiness, and gastrointestinal disturbances such as nausea, vomiting, and diarrhea. The antidote to the hypotensive action of phentolamine should be angiotensin amide or levarterenol. Epinephrine after phentolamine would elicit the reversal phenomenon and could further aggravate the hypotension.

In patients having an adrenal medullary tumor, the intravenous injection of 5 mg. of phentolamine generally causes a rapid fall of blood pressure, 25 mm. Hg diastolic and 33 mm. Hg systolic. False positive reactions and false negative reactions may occur, however, and the pharmacologic tests for pheochromocytoma are being replaced by the more reliable chemical tests (p. 106).

Azapetine phosphate (Ilidar), an alpha adrenergic blocking drug with additional smooth muscle–relaxing actions on the peripheral vasculature, is used in vasospastic diseases. It is available in tablets, 25 mg., and has the following structural formula:

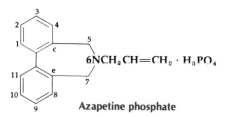

Azapetine phosphate

Ergot alkaloids. Certain alkaloids of ergot, such as ergotamine, have some alpha adrenergic blocking action, and the original observation of the epinephrine reversal by Dale was based on the ability of ergot extracts to elicit this remarkable phenomenon. Ergot alkaloids, however, are never used therapeutically as alpha receptor blocking drugs. Their pharmacology is related more to direct smooth muscle stimulation, and they are used largely as oxytocics and in the treatment of migraine. Since ergot alkaloids are lysergic acid derivatives and in many instances possess powerful antiserotonin properties, they will be discussed in Chapter 17 dealing with serotonin and antiserotonins.

BETA ADRENERGIC BLOCKING AGENTS

The beta adrenergic blocking agents competitively inhibit the actions of adrenergic agonists on beta receptors.

Development

It was observed by Dale in 1906[8] that ergot reversed the pressor effect to epinephrine but did not prevent the cardiac stimulant effect of the drug. Ahlquist suggested in 1948 that there must be two types of receptors, alpha and beta, for adrenergic drugs. Norepinephrine generally has a greater effect on alpha receptors, epinephrine acts on both, and isoproterenol acts only on beta receptors. The experimental drug dichloro-isoproterenol (DCI)[13] was the first beta blocker, but it had some sympathomimetic effects of its own and failed to become clinically useful.

Subsequent research led to a large number of beta blockers of great clinical usefulness. Pronethalol (Alderlin) received extensive clinical trial but was abandoned because it produced tumors in experimental animals. Propranolol (Inderal) is the only beta blocker used generally in the United States, although many newer ones such as practolol are widely employed in other countries. The stimulus for the production of newer beta blockers is the production of compounds having a greater selectivity. It would be advantageous to have beta blockers that act only on the heart but not on the bronchial muscle or blood vessels. Indications are that such a selectivity can be achieved.

The formulas of dichloroisoproterenol (DCI), pronethalol, and propranolol contrasted with that of isoproterenol are as follows:

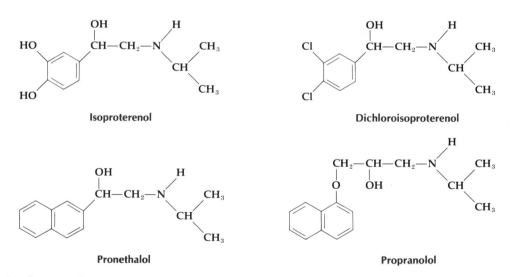

Isoproterenol

Dichloroisoproterenol

Pronethalol

Propranolol

Basic pharmacology

Blockade of the beta receptors produces the effects listed in Table 12-1. The beta blockers reduce catecholamine-mediated increases in chronotropic and inotropic activity. They decrease the rate of impulse generation in the sinoatrial node, decrease conduction velocity and increase the refractory period in the atrioventricular node,

Table 12-1. Effects of beta adrenergic receptor blockade

Heart rate	Decreased
Myocardial contractility	Decreased
Cardiac output	Decreased
Arterial blood pressure	Unaffected or decreased
Effect of exercise on heart rate and cardiac output	Decreased
Effects of isoproterenol	Blocked
Beta adrenergic drug effects (myocardial, arterial, bronchial, metabolic)	Blocked

decrease cardiac contractility, and reduce automaticity by inhibiting sympathetic influences on the heart.

In addition to the effects listed in Table 12-1, beta blockers may cause bronchial constriction, decrease muscle glycogenolysis and catecholamine-induced lipolysis, and have some effects on the central nervous system. There is suggestive evidence also for inhibition of insulin secretion and renin release[11,25] by beta blockers.

Propranolol has pharmacologic effects in addition to beta blockade. It has direct antiarrhythmic properties and is also a local anesthetic.

The direct antiarrhythmic actions of propranolol and some other beta blockers are shown clearly by experimental studies on the prevention of digitalis-induced arrhythmias. The dextro-isomer of propranolol has only about one fortieth of the beta blocking potency of the racemate. Nevertheless, it is as effective as the racemate against digitalis-induced arrhythmias.[25]

There has been a recent tendency to subdivide the beta receptors into beta$_1$ and beta$_2$.[25] Beta$_1$ receptors are responsible for cardiac stimulation and lipolysis, whereas those responsible for bronchodilatation and vasodepression are termed beta$_2$. Some of the newer beta blockers reflect this difference between beta receptors in various tissues. For example, practolol blocks the cardiac effects of isoproterenol without blocking its vascular actions. It does not cause bronchial constriction.

CLINICAL PHARMACOLOGY AND THERAPEUTIC USES OF PROPRANOLOL

The clinical applications of propranolol include cardiac arrhythmias, hypertrophic subaortic stenosis, and pheochromocytoma. In addition, propranolol is employed sometimes in the management of angina pectoris and as an adjuvant in the treatment of hypertension.

Cardiac arrhythmias. A variety of arrhythmias are treated with propranolol. These include arrhythmias of thyrotoxicosis, pheochromocytoma, surgical procedures, and digitalis intoxication. Propranolol slows the heart rate and reduces the tachycardia of exercise. It slows conduction at the atrioventricular node. It may prevent ectopic rhythms, both atrial and those originating in the ventricles. The drug is hazardous, particularly when given intravenously. Patients with atrioventricular block, impending heart failure, and bradycardia are especially at risk.

Hypertrophic subaortic stenosis. In this condition beta receptor stimulation aggravates the elevated intraventricular pressure gradient. Propranolol may improve some of the symptoms and signs of the disease.

Pheochromocytoma. This condition is an indication for the use of propranolol, both before and during the surgical intervention. Propranolol should be used in con-

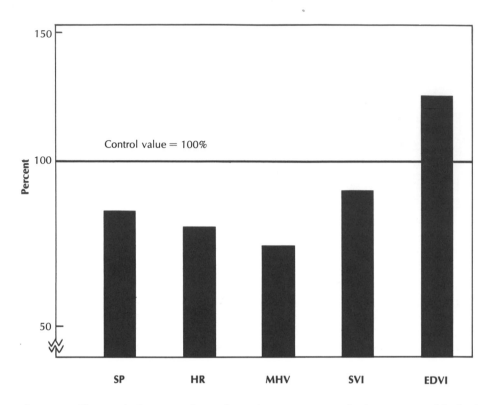

Fig. 12-3. Changes in important hemodynamic parameters under beta receptor blockade in dog. Percentage changes in systolic rise in ventricular pressure **(SP)**, heart rate **(HR)**, cardiac output **(MHV)**, stroke volume index **(SVI)**, and end diastolic ventricular volume index **(EDVI)** after beta receptor blockade by propranolol (0.5 mg./kg.). (From Gander, M., Veragut, U., Köhler, R., and Lüthy, E.: Cardiologia **49:**19, 1966.)

junction with an alpha blocker to prevent the excessive rise of blood pressure aggravated by the beta blockade.

Angina pectoris. The use of propranolol in angina rests on the following considerations: exercise, emotions, and catecholamines are known to increase cardiac work and oxygen consumption and tend to precipitate anginal attacks. The beta blockers reduce this possibility and propranolol has been shown to improve exercise tolerance in angina.[4, 17]

Hypertension. Propranolol and other beta blockers surprisingly cause some lowering of the blood pressure in hypertensive patients. These drugs are especially effective with the concurrent use of a direct vasodilator, such as hydralazine or minoxidil. When the blood pressure is lowered by a direct vasodilator drug, there is a compensatory sympathetic discharge that may result in tachycardia and arrhythmias. The concurrent use of the beta blockers tends to eliminate these secondary cardiac effects.[12]

The antihypertensive action of the beta blockers is not completely understood. There are those who believe that renin release is a beta function.[11] The problem is complicated, however, by the possible cardiac and central nervous system actions of the beta blockers.

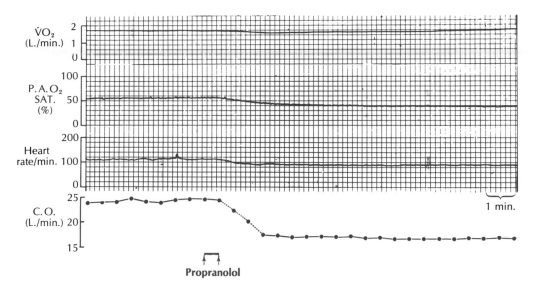

Fig. 12-4. Circulatory effects of acute induction of beta adrenergic blockade during steady submaximal exercise. From above downward: oxygen uptake (tracing has been shifted 1 minute to the left to allow for instrumental delay); pulmonary arterial O_2 saturation; heart rate; cardiac output (calculated by Fick principle). (From Epstein, S. E., Robinson, B. F., Köhler, R. L., and Braunwald, E.: J. Clin. Invest. **44:**1745, 1965.)

Adverse effects. Propranolol may precipitate congestive failure and is dangerous in patients whose cardiac reserve is low as a consequence of disease or drugs such as anesthetics that depress the myocardium. It may cause bradycardia, gastrointestinal disturbances, and hypoglycemia particularly in patients on insulin. Bronchial constriction is an expected adverse effect of a beta blocker, and the drug is contraindicated in bronchial asthma.

Preparations. Propranolol hydrochloride (Inderal) is available in tablets of 10 and 40 mg. Dosage should be individualized because of the great variation in susceptibility to the drug. It is also available for injection in a solution of 1 mg./ml. The drug should be well diluted and given slowly at 3-minute intervals in a dose of 0.5 to 1 mg. The total intravenous dose should not exceed 0.1 mg./kg. of body weight.

Newer beta blockers

In addition to propranolol, a large number of beta blockers have been synthesized and tested. The incentive is the finding of agents more selective than propranolol.

Practolol has several advantages over propranolol: (1) It is relatively cardioselective in its blockade of receptors with much less effect on the bronchial muscle. (2) It lacks the "quinidine-like" activity of propranolol. (3) Its half-life (10 to 12 hours) is much longer than that of propranolol (2 to 4 hours). Unfortunately, the drug has caused some tumors in animals.[20]

Oxyprenolol has fewer cardiac depressant actions than propranolol. **Sotalol** resembles oxyprenolol in having few direct cardiac depressant properties. **Butoxamine** is of experimental interest only. It antagonizes the metabolic effects of epinephrine but not its effects on the heart.

Pindolol is an indole derivative of isoproterenol. It has much weaker "quinidine-like" effects on the heart than propranolol and has a slight intrinsic sympathomimetic activity. It has been used successfully in reducing tachycardia in hyperthyroidism.[16]

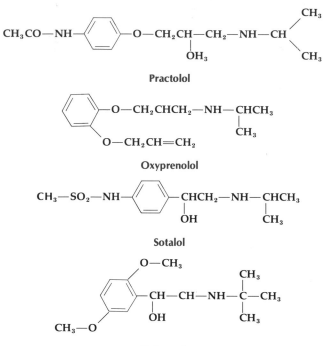

Practolol

Oxyprenolol

Sotalol

Butoxamine

References

1 Antonis, A., Clark, M. L., Hodge, R. L., Molony, M., and Pilkington, T. R.: Receptor mechanisms in the hyperglycaemic response to adrenaline in man, Lancet 1:1135, 1967.

2 Cohen, L. S., and Braunwald, E.: Amelioration of angina pectoris in idiopathic hypertrophic subaortic stenosis with beta-adrenergic blockade, Circulation 35:847, 1967.

3 Fourneau, E., and Bovet, D.: Récherches sur l'action sympathicolytique d'un nouveau dérivé du dioxane, Arch. Int. Pharmacodyn. 46:178, 1933.

4 Hamer, J., Grandjean, T., Melendez, L., and Sowton, G. E.: Effect of propranolol (Inderal) in angina pectoris: preliminary report, Brit. Med. J. 2:720, 1964.

5 Irons, G. V., Ginn, W. N., and Orgain, E. S.: Use of a beta adrenergic receptor blocking agent (propranolol) in the treatment of cardiac arrhythmias, Amer. J. Med. 43:161, 1967.

6 Kelliher, G. J., and Roberts, J.: The effect of d (+) and l (−) practolol on ouabain-induced arrhythmia, Europ. J. Pharmacol. 20:243, 1972.

7 Levy, B.: Adrenergic blocking activity of N-tertiary-butylmethoxamine (butoxamine), J. Pharmacol. Exp. Ther. 151:413, 1966.

8 Nickerson, M.: The pharmacology of adrenergic blockade, Pharmacol. Rev. 1:27, 1949.

9 Nickerson, M.: Nonequilibrium drug antagonism, Pharmacol. Rev. 9:246, 1957.

10 Nickerson, M., and Goodman, L. S.: Pharmacological properties of a new adrenergic blocking agent; N,N-dibenzyl-β-chloroethylamine (Dibenamine), J. Pharmacol. Exp. Ther. 89:167, 1947.

11 Pettinger, W. A., Campbell, W. B., and Keeton, K.: The adrenergic component of renin release induced by vasodilating antihypertensive drugs in the rat, Circ. Res. 33:82, 1973.

12 Pettinger, W. A., and Mitchell, H. C.: Minoxidil: a possible alternative to nephrectomy for hypertension, New Eng. J. Med. 289:167, 1973.

13 Powell, C. E., and Slater, I. H.: Blocking of inhibitory adrenergic receptors by a dichloro analog of isoproterenol, J. Pharmacol. Exp. Ther. 122:480, 1958.

14 Prichard, B. N. C., and Gillam, P. M. S.: Use of propranolol (Inderal) in treatment of hypertension, Brit. Med. J. **2**:725, 1964.

15 Sandler, G., and Clayton, G. A.: Clinical evaluation of practolol, a new cardioselective beta-blocking agent in angina pectoris, Brit. Med. J.: **1**:399, 1970.

16 Schelling, J. L., Scazziga, B., Dufour, R. J., Milinkovic, N., and Weber, A. A.: Effect of pindolol, a beta receptor antagonist, in hyperthyroidism, Clin. Pharmacol. Ther. **14**:158, 1973.

17 Srivastava, S. C., Dewar, H. A., and Newell, D. J.: Double-blind trial of propranolol (Inderal) in angina of effort, Brit. Med. J. **2**:724, 1964.

18 Stallworth, J. M., and Jeffords, J. V.: Clinical effects of azapetine (Ilidar) on peripheral vascular disease, J.A.M.A. **161**:840, 1956.

19 Taylor, R. R., Johnston, C. I., and José, A. D.: Reversal of digitalis intoxication by beta adrenergic blockade with pronethalol, New Eng. J. Med. **271**:877, 1964.

20 Traub, Y., Shaver, J. A., McDonald, R. H., and Shapiro, A. P.: Effects of practolol on pressor responses to noxious stimuli in hypertensive patients, Clin. Pharmacol. Ther. **14**:165, 1973.

21 Westfall, T. C., Cipolloni, P. B., and Edmundowicz, A. C.: Influence of propranolol on hemodynamic changes and plasma catecholamine levels following cigarette smoking and nicotine, Proc. Soc. Exp. Biol. Med. **123**:174, 1966.

Recent reviews

22 Belleau, B.: Relationships between antagonists and receptor sites. In Adrenergic mechanisms, Ciba Foundation and Committee on Drug Action, Boston, 1960, Little, Brown & Co.

23 Bloch, J. H., Pierce, C. H., and Lillehei, R. C.: Adrenergic blocking agents in the treatment of shock, Ann. Rev. Med. **17**:483, 1966.

24 Cotten, M. D., and Moran, N. C.: Cardiovascular pharmacology, Ann. Rev. Pharmacol. **1**:261, 1961.

25 Dollery, C. T., Paterson, J. W., and Conolly, M. E.: Clinical pharmacology of beta-receptor-blocking drugs, Clin. Pharmacol. Ther. **10**:765, 1969.

26 Dornhorst, A. C., and Robinson, B. F.: Clinical pharmacology of a beta-adrenergic blocking agent (nethalide), Lancet **2**:413, 1962.

27 Epstein, S. E., and Braunwald, E.: Beta-adrenergic receptor blocking drugs, New Eng. J. Med. **275**:1106, 1175, 1966.

28 Frohlich, E. D., and Page, I. H.: The clinical meaning of cardiovascular beta-adrenergic receptors, Physiol. Pharmacol. Physicians **1**(11): 1, 1966.

29 Lands, A. M., Arnold, A., and McAnliff, J. P.: Differentiation of receptor systems activated by sympathomimetic amines, Nature **214**:597, 1967.

30 Nickerson, M.: Vasoconstriction and vasodilation in shock. In Hershey, S. G., editor: Shock, Boston, 1964, Little, Brown & Co.

13 Drugs affecting catecholamine binding and release

GENERAL CONCEPT

Drugs can influence sympathetic functions by the remarkable mechanism of affecting the binding and release of catecholamines, thus providing tools for an entirely new pharmacologic approach to the nervous system. Such drugs have found wide application as *antihypertensive agents* and in the field of *psychopharmacology.*

This field was opened up by the discovery that reserpine, a *Rauwolfia* alkaloid, caused a release of serotonin (5-hydroxytryptamine) from its binding sites in various tissues.[26] Subsequently it was shown that reserpine also releases norepinephrine and dopamine.[13] Decreased sympathetic functions induced by reserpine, such as hypotension and bradycardia, are now generally attributed to the catecholamine depletion at the adrenergic nerve endings.

Other drugs can influence catecholamine stores also. Guanethidine causes depletion of peripheral amine stores. Such decarboxylase inhibitors as methyldopa produce their prolonged effect on catecholamine stores by a release mechanism attributable to their metabolic product, methyldopamine.[28] On the other hand, bretylium blocks adrenergic fibers without depleting their catecholamine content.

The monoamine oxidase (MAO) inhibitors raise the catecholamine content of neural tissues in several species. This finding suggests that the enzyme may have a regulatory function on the concentration of bound catecholamines. Hypotension that follows the use of MAO inhibitors may be related to the accumulation of norepinephrine or some other amine in ganglia and adrenergic fibers.[33]

Studies on the catecholamine-depleting agents led to the concept that tyramine and many sympathomimetic amines act indirectly by releasing catecholamines in the body. These studies led to the discovery that certain amines such as metaraminol are taken up by adrenergic nerves, where they may function as false transmitters.[24]

MECHANISMS OF CATECHOLAMINE RELEASE

The complex drug effects on catecholamine release may be understood by formulating some hypotheses based largely on experimental work.[25, 35]

According to the best evidence, drugs may release catecholamines by one of two mechanisms, and these mechanisms may be further influenced by at least three additional pharmacologic actions.

The *two basic mechanisms* of release and the drugs that illustrate them are as follows:

Interference with granular storage mechanism
  Reserpine
  Guanethidine

Displacement of catecholamines
   Tyramine
   Amphetamine
   Metaraminol
   Methyldopa (through its metabolite alpha-methylnorepinephrine)

1. *Interference with granular storage mechanism.* As shown in Fig. 13-1, when cate-cholamines are released physiologically, a small granule is extruded and its amine acts on the receptor. On the other hand, when the amine is released by drugs such as re-serpine or guanethidine, it is freed from the granule within the axoplasm, making it subject to attack by MAO. Instead of the active amine, mostly its inactivated products appear outside the nerve. This is likely the reason why the injection of reserpine, although causing massive depletion of catecholamines, does not result in an elevation of blood pressure.

2. *Displacement of catecholamines.* The indirectly acting sympathomimetic drugs such as tyramine and amphetamine can cause release of catecholamines. Other amines not only displace catecholamines but also are incorporated into the granule. These include metaraminol[28] and alpha-methylnorepinephrine. The latter is a metabolite of methyl-dopa, which undoubtedly causes amine depletion by this indirect mechanism.

The basic mechanisms of catecholamine release can be modified by at least four pharmacologic influences.

The *MAO inhibitors* protect the intraneuronally released catecholamines from inactivation. They do not, however, block drug-induced release. On the other hand, the MAO inhibitors undoubtedly cause an increase in the catecholamine content of adrenergic fibers, and they lead to decreased sympathetic activity clinically. It is likely that they have some inhibitory action on the physiologic release of catecholamines.

Certain drugs, the *adrenergic neuronal blocking agents*, prevent catecholamine release induced by nerve stimulation or by the indirectly acting amines such as tyramine. The best known example of such drugs is bretylium. Conceptually, these drugs behave as if they anesthetized the adrenergic fibers. Indeed, they have local anesthetic prop-erties and they concentrate in adrenergic fibers.

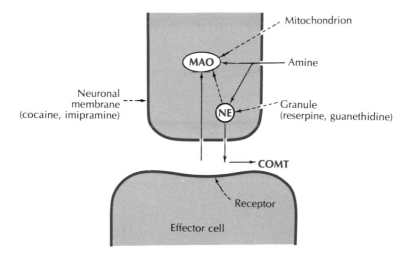

Fig. 13-1. Schematic representation of nerve ending and effector cell. (For details see text.)

Drugs that act at the neuronal membrane (Fig. 13-1) such as cocaine and imipramine have several important actions on catecholamine release. They block the action of tyramine and other indirectly acting amines. They do not block the action of reserpine, a point in favor of a difference in the site of action of tyramine and reserpine. Cocaine and other drugs that inhibit the membrane pump for amines cause an apparent "sensitization" of the receptor by allowing the local accumulation of catecholamine.

Drugs may act on presynaptic alpha receptors that modify catecholamine release. For details, see Langer, S. Z.: Presynaptic regulation of catecholamine release, Biochem. Pharmacol. (In press.)

BASIC DIFFERENCES BETWEEN THE ACTIONS OF RESERPINE AND GUANETHIDINE

While both drugs deplete nerves of their catecholamine by acting on the granular storage mechanism, guanethidine has additional effects. Its intravenous injection regularly leads to a transient elevation of blood pressure, caused by a *tyramine-like* effect that can be blocked by cocaine. To make matters more complex, guanethidine has an early *bretylium-like* effect that somehow interferes with norepinephrine release after nerve stimulation.

An additional difference between reserpine and guanethidine is of great importance. Reserpine depletes catecholamines and serotonin from many sites, including the brain. Guanethidine apparently fails to cross the blood-brain barrier and thus has no effect on brain amines.

MECHANISM OF DECREASED SYMPATHETIC ACTIVITY INDUCED BY CATECHOLAMINE DEPLETION

Since norepinephrine is the sympathetic mediator, it is not surprising that its depletion at adrenergic nerve endings should lead to lessened sympathetic activity. The quantitative relations between catecholamine depletion and decreased sympathetic activity are of great interest.

When the catecholamine content of a nerve is decreased to below 50%, stimulation of the nerve results in a lessened response. The rate of depletion varies in different organs. Cardiac catecholamine declines rapidly, and adrenal stores are most resistant. The rate of depletion is a function not only of the dose of reserpine but also of the rate of turnover of the amine at the various sites.[21, 29] It has been estimated that the half-time of catecholamines in the heart is 4 to 8 hours, in contrast with their half-time of 7 days in the adrenal medulla.[8] Depletion must be rapid in arterioles and venules. This is why reserpine is useful as an antihypertensive drug.

CATECHOLAMINE UPTAKE

Several experiments suggest that catecholamines are taken up by adrenergic nerves.[2] It has been shown that in a reserpinized animal neither sympathetic stimulation nor injected tyramine will cause a pressor response.[9] After an infusion of norepinephrine, the pressor response to nerve stimulation and tyramine is restored, although only a small fraction of the catecholamine stores is replenished.

It appears, then, that there must be a pool of available norepinephrine[36] that is essential for function of the sympathetic endings. It has been shown that the ³H-norepinephrine taken up by the pool is actually released by sympathetic nerve stimulation and appears in the venous effluent blood.[2]

RESERPINE

Alkaloids of *Rauwolfia serpentina* have antihypertensive and tranquilizing properties. Reserpine and some other *Rauwolfia* alkaloids produce depletion of norepinephrine, dopamine, and also serotonin from various binding sites in the brain and peripheral nerves. The drug not only causes a release of amines but also blocks their granular uptake. It does not, however, block the action of catecholamines. It may have some blocking effects on catecholamine synthesis by preventing granular uptake of dopamine in neurons.[37]

Reserpine was at first widely used as a tranquilizer. It is much more commonly employed now as an antihypertensive drug.

GUANETHIDINE

The antihypertensive drug guanethidine (Ismelin)[16,22] causes decreased sympathetic activity by a dual mechanism, depleting norepinephrine at peripheral nerve endings in the manner of reserpine and also causing early sympathetic neuronal blockade at a time when catecholamines are not yet depleted in the nerve. It is not a ganglionic blocking agent and does not prevent the action of injected catecholamines (p. 172).

DEBRISOQUIN

Debrisoquin (Declinax) is structurally related to guanethidine, but it produces adrenergic neuronal blockade by the same mechanisms as bretylium. It is a potent antihypertensive agent when used in the same dosage as guanethidine.[34]

The studies showing that debrisoquin as well as bretylium inhibits MAO and is apparently concentrated in the adrenergic neurons throw new light on the mode of action of these drugs.[20]

BRETYLIUM

Bretylium (Darenthin) was first described in 1959. Boura and co-workers[3] showed that this drug produces a selective block on the peripheral sympathetic nervous system without opposing the action of injected or released catecholamines.

Later work on bretylium[1] showed that the drug can cause immediate blockade of cardiac sympathetic nerves. Injected norepinephrine (levarterenol) still exerted its effect, so that bretylium is obviously not an adrenergic blocking agent in the usual sense. The drug also failed to block the effects of vagal stimulation on the heart, which indicates that it is not a ganglionic blocking agent. The immediate effects of the drug on blood pressure in dogs was variable. It could cause a fall of blood pressure or an initial rise followed by a fall. There was consistent initial strengthening of myocardial contractile force.

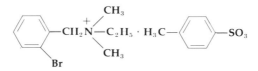

Bretylium sulfite

Bretylium blocks the adrenergic fiber without depleting its catecholamine content and may act as a local anesthetic that concentrates in adrenergic fibers.[3] However, the mode of action of bretylium is not known with certainty. Since bretylium is a quaternary amine, it has been suggested that perhaps it blocks the action of acetylcholine in the nerve fiber,[9] assuming that acetylcholine plays a role in nerve conduction or catecholamine release. The objections to this theory have been summarized by Boura and Green.[28]

The MAO inhibitory action of bretylium is of great interest.[20]

Although bretylium is basically a very interesting drug, its clinical use has been attended by so many toxic effects, including muscular weakness and mental confusion, that it is no longer available.

METHYLDOPA

Methyldopa (Aldomet), an analog of dihydroxyphenylalanine, competes with this precursor of norepinephrine for the enzyme that decarboxylates aromatic L-amino acids. Although it inhibits the synthesis of both norepinephrine and serotonin, nor-

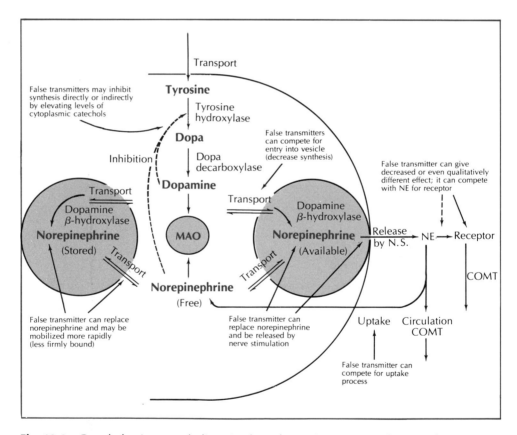

Fig. 13-2. Catecholamine metabolism in the adrenergic neuron, indicating the possible role of false transmitters. (From Kopin, I. J.: In Adrenergic neurotransmission, Ciba Foundation Study Group No. 33, Boston, 1968, Little, Brown & Co.)

epinephrine levels in the brain remain low for a much longer time than serotonin levels.[28] This and other evidence suggest that much of the catecholamine depletion induced by methyldopa is due to the drug's being decarboxylated to form α-methylnorepinephrine that replaces norepinephrine and acts as a "false transmitter."[35] The various consequences of the presence of false transmitters are summarized in Fig. 13-2.

MAO INHIBITORS

MAO inhibitors were introduced as antidepressants. One of their surprising side effects was orthostatic hypotension, which suggested interference with sympathetic functions.

Experimentally, the MAO inhibitors elevate the levels of norepinephrine and serotonin in the brain and ganglia and other peripheral tissues.[15] In addition, they prevent many of the actions of reserpine, including its ability to lower amine levels.

Although it has been suggested that the MAO inhibitors block the amine release phenomenon directly, it is more likely that they prevent the metabolic degradation of endogenous amines released from subcellular structures, thus causing elevation of their levels in the axoplasm of adrenergic neurons. MAO inhibitors may also promote the formation of false transmitters such as octopamine.[31] False transmitters, in turn, may block norepinephrine release (Fig. 13-2).

One of the serious disadvantages of the MAO inhibitors is the increased likelihood of adverse reactions to ingested foods and to drugs that may release monoamines in the body.[30,38] The ingestion of aged cheese, beer, or certain wines has caused hypertensive emergencies in patients who were being treated with MAO inhibitors. These serious reactions have been traced to the presence of tyramine in these foods and beverages. Tyramine would normally be deaminated by MAO. When its deamination is inhibited by drugs, it releases catecholamines in the body. Adverse reactions to indirectly acting sympathomimetic drugs have also occurred under similar circumstances.

Although most MAO inhibitors are used as antidepressants, one of these, pargyline (Eutonyl), was introduced as an antihypertensive agent.[7]

References

1 Aviado, D. M., and Dil, A H.: The effects of a new sympathetic blocking drug (bretylium) on cardiovascular control, J. Pharmacol. Exp. Ther. 129:328, 1960.

2 Axelrod, J., Whitby, L. G., and Hertting, G.: Effect of psychotropic drugs on the uptake of H³-norepinephrine by tissues, Science 133:383, 1961.

3 Boura, A. L., Green, A. F., McCoubrey, A., Laurence, D. R., Moulton, R., and Rosenheim, M. L.: Darenthin: hypotensive agent of new type, Lancet 2:17, 1959.

4 Brodie, B. B., and Kuntzman, R.: Pharmacological consequences of selective depletion of catechol amines by antihypertensive agents, Ann. N. Y. Acad. Sci. 88:939, 1960.

5 Brodie, B. B., Olin, J. S., Kuntzman, R. G., and Shore, P. A.: Possible interrelationships between release of brain norepinephrine and serotonin by reserpine, Science 125:1293, 1957.

6 Brooks, V. B.: The action of botulinum toxin on motor-nerve filaments, J. Physiol. 123:501, 1954.

7 Bryant, J. M., Torosdag, S., Schvartz, N., Fletcher, L., Fertig, H., Schwartz, S., and Quan, R. B. F.: Antihypertensive properties of pargyline hydrochloride, J. A. M. A. 178:406, 1961.

8 Burack, W. R., and Draskoczy, P. R.: The turnover of endogenously labeled catecholamines in several regions of the sympathetic nervous system, J. Pharmacol. Exp. Ther. 144:66, 1964.

9 Burn, J. H., and Rand, M. J.: A new interpreta-

tion of the adrenergic nerve fiber, Advances Pharmacol. **1**:1, 1962.

10 Butterfield, J. L., and Richardson, J. A.: Acute effects of guanethidine on myocardial contractility and catecholamine levels, Proc. Soc. Exp. Biol. Med. **106**:259, 1961.

11 Carlsson, A., and Lindquist, M.: In vivo decarboxylation of α-methylDOPA and α-methyl metatyrosine, Acta Physiol. Scand. **54**:87, 1962.

12 Carlsson, A., Lindquist, M., Magnusson, T., and Waldeck, B.: On the presence of 3-hydroxytyramine in brain, Science **127**:471, 1958.

13 Carlsson, A., Rosengren, E., Bertler, A., and Nilsson, J.: Effect of reserpine on the metabolism of catecholamines. In Garattini, S., and Ghetti, U., editors: Psychotropic drugs, Amsterdam, 1957, Elsevier Publishing Co.

14 Cass, R., and Spriggs, T. L. B.: Tissue amine levels and sympathetic blockade after guanethidine and bretylium, Brit. J. Pharmacol. **17**:442, 1961.

15 Chessin, M., Kramer, E. R., and Scott, C. C.: Modifications of the pharmacology of reserpine and serotonin by iproniazid, J. Pharmacol. **119**:453, 1957.

16 Cohn, J. N., Liptak, T. E., and Freis, E. D.: Hemodynamic effects of guanethidine in man, Circ. Res. **12**:298, 1963.

17 Costa, E., and Brodie, B. B.: A role for norepinephrine in ganglionic transmission, J. Amer. Geriat. Soc. **9**:119, 1961.

18 Eccles, J. C.: The physiology of nerve cells, Baltimore, 1957, The Johns Hopkins Press.

19 Fleming, W. W., and Trendelenburg, U.: Development of supersensitivity to norepinephrine after pretreatment with reserpine, J. Pharmacol. Exp. Ther. **133**: 41, 1961.

20 Giachetti, A., and Shore, P. A.: Monoamine oxidase inhibition in the adrenergic neuron by bretylium, debrisoquin, and other adrenergic neuronal blocking agents, Biochem. Pharmacol. **16**:237, 1967.

21 Lee, F. L.: The relation between norepinephrine content and response to sympathetic nerve stimulation of various organs of cats pretreated with reserpine, J. Pharmacol. Exp. Ther. **156**:137, 1967.

22 Maxwell, R. A., Plummer, A. J., Schneider, F., Povalski, H., and Daniel, A. I.: Pharmacology of [2-(octahydro-1-azocinyl)ethyl] guanethidine sulfate (SU-5864), J. Pharmacol. Exp. Ther. **128**: 22, 1960.

23 Richardson, D. W., and Wyso, E. M.: Effective reduction in blood pressure without ganglionic blockade, Virginia Med. Monthly **86**:377, 1959.

24 Shore, P. A., Busfield, D., and Alpers, H. S.: Binding and release of metaraminol: mechanism of norepinephrine depletion by α-methyl-M tyrosine and related agents, J. Pharmacol. Exp. Ther. **146**:194, 1964.

25 Shore, P. A., and Giachetti, A.: Dual actions of guanethidine on amine uptake mechanisms in adrenergic neurons, Biochem. Pharmacol. **15**: 899, 1966.

26 Shore, P. A., Silver, S. L., and Brodie, B. B.: Interaction of reserpine, serotonin, and lysergic acid diethylamide in brain, Science **122**:284, 1955.

27 Udenfriend, S., Connamacher, R., and Hess, S. M.: On the mechanism of release of norephinephrine by alpha-methyl-M-tyrosine and alpha-methyl-M-tyramine, Biochem. Pharmacol. **8**:419, 1962.

Recent reviews

28 Boura, A. L., and Green, A. F.: Adrenergic neurone blocking agents, Ann. Rev. Pharmacol. **5**:183, 1965.

29 Carlsson, A.: Physiological and pharmacological release of monoamines in the central nervous system. In von Euler, U. S., Rosell, S., and Uvnas, B., editors: Mechanisms of release of biogenic amines, New York, 1966, Pergamon Press, Inc.

30 Editorial: Hypertensive reactions to monoamine oxidase inhibitors, Brit. Med. J. **1**:578, 1964.

31 Kopin, I. J.: False adrenergic transmitters, Ann. Rev. Pharmacol. **8**:377, 1968.

32 Kopin, I. J.: The influence of false adrenergic transmitters on adrenergic neurotransmission. In Adrenergic neurotransmission, Ciba Foundation Study Group No. 33, Boston, 1968, Little, Brown & Co.

33 Kopin, I. J., Fischer, J. E., Musacchio, J. M., Horst, W. D., and Weise, V. K.: False neurochemical transmitters and the mechanism of sympathetic blockade by monamine oxidase inhibitors, J. Pharmacol. Exp. Ther. **147**:186, 1965.

34 Moe, R. A., et al.: Cardiovascular effects of 3, 4,-dihydro-2(1H) isoquinoline carboxamidine (Declinax), Curr. Ther. Res. **6**:299, 1964.

35 Muscholl, E.: Effect of drugs on smooth muscle: newer mechanisms of adrenergic blockade, Ann. Rev. Pharmacol. **6**:107, 1966.

36 Shore, P. A.: Release of serotonin and catecholamines by drugs, Pharmacol. Rev. **14**:531, 1962.

37 Shore, P. A.: Transport and storage of biogenic amines, Ann. Rev. Pharmacol. **12**:209, 1972.

38 Thomas, J. C. S.: Monoamine oxidase inhibitors and cheese, Brit. Med. J. **2**:1406, 1963.

14 Antihypertensive drugs

GENERAL CONCEPT

The treatment of hypertension has been revolutionized during the last few years by the introduction of drugs that can cause sustained lowering of the blood pressure without intolerable side effects. A most significant consequence of this development is the proof based on controlled clinical trials[90,91] of a favorable effect of antihypertensive therapy on life expectancy and complications resulting from hypertension.

The antihypertensive drugs act by many different mechanisms summarized in Table 14-1. In most instances the therapeutic efforts are directed at promoting sodium excretion with a simultaneous reduction of sympathetic activity. A diagrammatic representation of blood pressure–regulating mechanisms is shown in Fig. 14-1.

Table 14-1. Site of action of antihypertensive drugs

Site of action	Mode of action	Drug	Trade name
Arteriolar smooth muscle	Direct vasodilation	Hydralazine Diazoxide Minoxidil	Apresoline Hyperstat
Alpha adrenergic receptors	Receptor blockade	Phentolamine Phenoxybenzamine	Regitine Dibenzyline
Sympathetic fibers	Blockade of NE release (also depletion) Inhibition of MAO	Guanethidine Pargyline	Ismelin Eutonyl
Paravertebral Ganglia	Ganglionic blockade	Chlorisondamine Hexamethonium Mecamylamine Pentolinium Trimethaphan	Ecolid Inversine Ansolysen Arfonad
Central nervous system	Depression of C-V control center False neurotransmitter NE depletion	Clonidine Methyldopa Reserpine	Catapres Aldomet Many
Carotid sinus	Reflex sympathetic depression	Veratrum Electrical stimulation	
Beta adrenergic receptors	CNS effect Myocardial depression Renin release inhibition	Propranolol	Inderal
Kidney	Sodium excretion Volume depletion	Many diuretics	

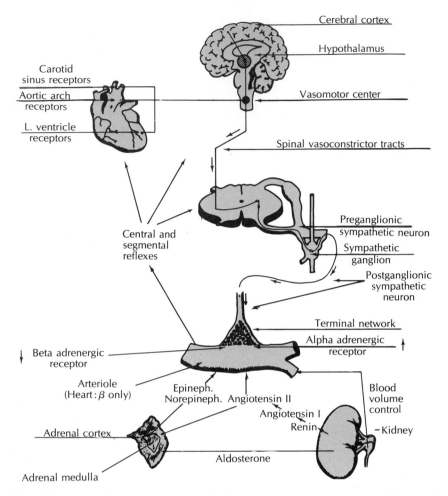

Fig. 14-1. Diagrammatic representation of blood pressure–regulating mechanisms. (From Abrams, W. B.: Dis. Chest **55:**148, 1969.)

RELATION OF ANGIOTENSIN AND ALDOSTERONE TO HYPERTENSION

The demonstration that renal ischemia leads to hypertension[24] resulted in the discovery of a kidney enzyme, renin, which is probably in the granules of the juxtaglomerular apparatus.[25] When this enzyme is released by ischemia or perhaps by a decreased caliber of the afferent arteriole, it acts on a substrate in blood and eventually yields angiotensin, a potent vasopressor polypeptide. This sequence of events is as follows:

Renin substrate → **Renin** → **Angiotensin I** → **Converting enzyme** → **Angiotensin II**
   in blood   **(decapeptide)**   **(octapeptide)**

Angiotensin II is a potent vasoconstrictor.[67] Its amide has been introduced into therapeutics under the trade name of Hypertensin. It can cause significant elevation of blood pressure in man when infused intravenously in doses as low as 1µg/min. Subcutaneous injections of 50 µg are effective also.

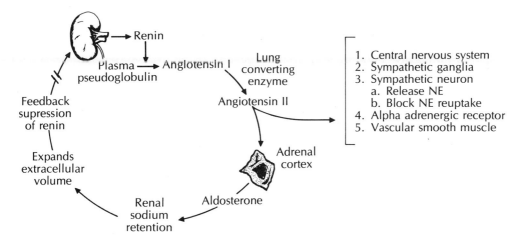

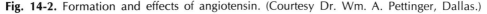

Fig. 14-2. Formation and effects of angiotensin. (Courtesy Dr. Wm. A. Pettinger, Dallas.)

The amino acid composition of angiotensin I is as follows:

Asp-Arg-Val-Tyr-Ileu-His-Pro-Phe-His-Leu

The converting enzyme removes the terminal histidyl-leucine to form angiotensin II. Angiotensin II is removed and destroyed by the tissues.[68] Angiotensin I has little or no biologic activity, although it may have some effect on aldosterone release.

The release of renin from the juxtaglomerular apparatus of the kidney is under intensive investigation. Lowering of blood pressure and renal perfusion pressure promotes the release of the enzyme.[89] Some of the effect of lowered blood pressure on renin release may be mediated through sympathetic fibers. In fact, catecholamines can cause renin release. They do this apparently by acting on beta receptors, since propranolol blocks catecholamine-induced renin release.[92]

The pharmacologic effects of angiotensin II (hereafter referred to as angiotensin) are as follows: (1) elevation of blood pressure, (2) contraction of isolated smooth muscle preparations, (3) release of aldosterone, and (4) release of catecholamines from adrenal medulla and adrenergic nerves.[18,56] Not only does angiotensin release catecholamines but it also prevents their reuptake by adrenergic nerves.[94]

The vasopressor effects of angiotensin are exerted primarily on peripheral resistance vessels in the skin, splanchnic area, and the kidney. It has little cardiac stimulant action. The capacitance vessels are not greatly affected by it, differing in this respect from the response to catecholamines.

Several features of the action of angiotensin are of great interest in research on hypertension. This polypeptide has a central effect on the vasomotor centers, resulting in increased sympathetic activity. It also potentiates the actions of catecholamines. It causes sodium retention by promoting the release of aldosterone from the adrenal cortex. It is of great interest also that infusions of angiotensin in sub-pressor doses lead to *autopotentiation* after several hours, so that the initial sub-pressor doses become effective in raising the blood pressure.[17] It is easy to see that angiotensin could be an important factor in the pathogenesis of certain forms of hypertension.[70]

There is little doubt about the role of the renin-angiotensin system in several hypertensive states. In addition, oral contraceptives increase the renin substrate level and possibly promote angiotensin formation.[52]

CLASSIFICATION OF ANTIHYPERTENSIVE DRUGS

The various antihypertensive drugs may be classified according to their mode of action as shown in Table 14-1. They will be discussed under the headings of direct vasodilators, alpha adrenergic blocking drugs, adrenergic neuronal blocking drugs, ganglionic blocking agents, central depressants of sympathetic functions, reflex inhibitors of central sympathetic function, beta adrenergic blocking drugs, and antihypertensive drugs that promote salt excretion.

DIRECT VASODILATORS

Among the antihypertensive drugs that act directly on the vascular smooth muscle, hydralazine is in common use, diazoxide has been introduced more recently for the management of hypertensive emergencies, and minoxidil is an experimental preparation of some promise. The obsolete drug sodium nitroprusside is effective also when given by intravenous injection.

HYDRALAZINE IN HYPERTENSION

Hydralazine hydrochloride (1-hydrazinophthalazine hydrochloride) (Apresoline) is a direct relaxant of the vascular smooth muscle, which is used commonly in chronic hypertension and also in hypertensive emergencies. Although the drug relaxes the vascular smooth muscle, it often produces considerable cardiac stimulation, perhaps through reflex mechanisms. The cardiac effects may be prevented experimentally by ganglionic blocking agents[50] and, according to recent clinical studies, by beta adrenergic blocking agents.[13]

Adverse effects caused by hydralazine are many. Headache, palpitations, and gastrointestinal disturbances are common after taking the drug. A unique and more serious adverse effect is seen frequently when doses larger than 200 mg. daily are administered.

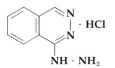

Hydralazine hydrochloride

Many such patients develop a syndrome resembling systemic lupus erythematosus. Although this syndrome is reversible in most cases, its occurrence in a fairly high percentage of patients taking large doses of the drug limits the usefulness of hydralazine.

Preparations

Hydralazine hydrochloride (Apresoline) is obtainable in tablets of 10, 25, 50, and 100 mg. and in a solution for injection, 20 mg./ml.

DIAZOXIDE

Diazoxide, a nondiuretic congener of the thiazide drugs, has been recently introduced as an antihypertensive agent under the trade name Hyperstat. It is suitable especially for the emergency reduction of blood pressure in malignant hypertension when administered by intravenous injection.

Animal experiments have shown that diazoxide causes rapid lowering of blood pressure and some unusual side effects, among which hyperglycemia is prominent. The elevation of blood glucose levels is generally attributed to inhibition of insulin release from the beta cells. Because of this effect, the drug has been used experimentally in hypoglycemic states, such as insulin-producing tumors.

Preparation and dosage

Diazoxide (Hyperstat) is supplied in a 20 ml. ampule containing 300 mg. of the drug. The preparation is injected intravenously and rapidly. Blood pressure decreases within 2 minutes to its lowest level. Then it increases fairly rapidly for 30 minutes and more slowly for the next 2 to 12 hours.

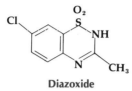

Diazoxide

MINOXIDIL

Minoxidil is an investigational antihypertensive agent of long duration of action. Chemically it is 6-imino-1,2-dihydroxy-2-imino-4-piperidinopyrimidine. It is a direct dilator of vascular smooth muscle.[75] In a comparative study on hypertensive patients, minoxidil was more potent than hydralazine in lowering the blood pressure.[75] Not only was minoxidil more potent, but it also appeared to have a greater efficacy or power than hydralazine. Sodium retention and tachycardia occur in minoxidil-treated patients, but these effects can be controlled with the concomitant use of diuretics and beta blockers. The combined use of minoxidil and beta blockers appears promising in the treatment of severe hypertension that fails to respond to other forms of treatment.[85a]

ALPHA ADRENERGIC BLOCKING DRUGS

The experience with the alpha adrenergic blocking drugs in the treatment of hypertension has been disappointing. Phenoxybenzamine (Dibenzyline) is an example of this type of drug (Chapter 12). Orthostatic hypotension, tachycardia, and many other side effects have made this approach unpromising. The alpha adrenergic blocking drugs may be used during the removal of an adrenal medullary tumor, particularly when a beta blocker is employed to prevent cardiac arrhythmias.

Problem 14-1. Why is it necessary to use an alpha blocker during the operation for pheochromocytoma when a beta blocker is being administered? Manipulation of the tumor results in the release of norepinephrine and epinephrine from the tumor. These catecholamines would produce excessive hypertension in the presence of a beta blocker. Thus an alpha blocker must be added.

ADRENERGIC NEURONAL BLOCKING DRUGS

A number of drugs, such as guanethidine, other guanidine compounds, and bretylium can block the release of catecholamines from adrenergic nerve fibers. Among these drugs, guanethidine (Ismelin) has become the most widely used antihypertensive drug.

GUANETHIDINE

Guanethidine is effective in the treatment of hypertension. Its blocking effect on the adrenergic nerve terminal is associated with catecholamine release, and in this respect it resembles the action of reserpine.

Guanethidine was actually discovered by screening various drugs for a special reserpine-like effect. Reserpine pretreatment of animals prevents the pressor response to indirectly acting sympathomimetic drugs such as amphetamine. Guanethidine was found to block the effect of amphetamine on the blood pressure.[47]

Mode of action

Guanethidine is commonly referred to as an adrenergic neuronal blocking drug. It has very complex effects on the adrenergic neuron. Experimental intravenous injection of the drug causes, first, a transient rise of blood pressure, a *tyramine-like effect*. Following this event there is interference with conduction of the nerve impulse and a defective catecholamine release, a *bretylium-like effect*. Finally, there is a depletion of catecholamines in the nerve fiber, a *reserpine-like effect*. To make matters even more complex, the drug blocks neuronal catecholamine uptake, a *cocainelike effect*.

Clinical pharmacology

The onset of action of guanethidine is slow. Maximal effects may not develop for 2 or 3 days after initiation of treatment. For this reason patients are started on small doses such as 10 mg. once daily, which are maintained for 5 to 7 days before the amount of drug administered is increased. Guanethidine is a drug with long duration of action. Its effect may persist for 7 days after its administration has been discontinued.

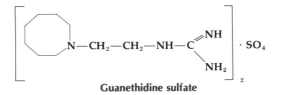

Guanethidine sulfate

The absorption of guanethidine is only about 50% of the orally administered dose. The drug is largely excreted by the kidney.

In contrast to reserpine, guanethidine causes postural hypotension with some frequency. The reason for this difference is probably related to the adrenergic neuronal blocking properties of guanethidine. In addition to postural hypotension, guanethidine causes the usual consequences of reduced sympathetic activity, such as diarrhea, bradycardia, weakness, and nasal stuffiness.

Guanethidine has a great advantage over reserpine in that it does not cross the blood-brain barrier and thus does not cause sedation and depression. It has replaced the ganglionic blocking agents because it does not inhibit parasympathetic ganglia. It has a strange effect on male sexual function, preventing ejaculation without affecting erection.

Drug interactions

Guanethidine and related adrenergic neuronal blocking guanidiniums are accumulated in the adrenergic neurons by the same transport system that carries norepineph-

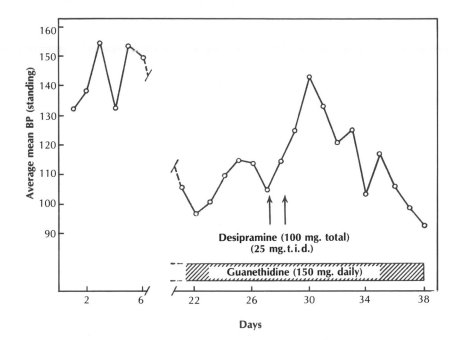

Fig. 14-3. Antagonism of guanethidine by desipramine. Guanethidine was given in increasing doses between days 6 and 21 until blood pressure was controlled (150 mg. daily). Dose was maintained during experimental period. Desipramine was administered between arrows. (From Mitchell, J. R., Arias, L., and Oates, J. A.: J.A.M.A. **202**:973, 1967.)

rine to its storage site.[49] Desipramine and related tricyclic antidepressants block the membrane transport system and prevent the accumulation of guanethidine in the adrenergic neuron. As a consequence the tricyclic antidepressants block the antihypertensive effect of the drug, as shown in Fig. 14-3.

Amphetamine also blocks the antihypertensive action of guanethidine by releasing the drug from the adrenergic neuron. As an additional drug interaction, it should be mentioned that guanethidine increases the response to injected catecholamines,[43] probably because it blocks their neuronal membrane uptake, an important factor in their termination of action.

Preparations

Guanethidine sulfate is available in tablets containing 10 and 20 mg. No parenteral forms are available because the drug is not useful for the treatment of hypertensive emergencies. In fact, it could aggravate them.

MAO INHIBITORS

One of the common side effects of MAO inhibitors is postural hypotension (p. 236). Although the mechanism of this is not well understood, at least one member of the series has been introduced as an antihypertensive agent.

Pargyline (Eutonyl) is administered orally in doses of 25 to 50 mg. once daily.

Side effects consist of orthostatic hypotension, gastrointestinal disturbances, insomnia, and headaches.

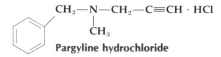

Pargyline hydrochloride

Probably the greatest disadvantage of the MAO inhibitors is their incompatibility with a large variety of drugs. Thus in patients receiving pargyline the indirect sympathomimetics would be contraindicated, as shown by the violent reaction to tyramine-containing foods in such patients. Also, combinations of antidepressants are strictly contraindicated (p. 239). It is difficult to see why the drug should be used in the face of so many dangers.

Pargyline comes in tablets containing 10, 25, and 50 mg. of the drug.

GANGLIONIC BLOCKING AGENTS

The ganglionic blocking agents (Chapter 10) such as hexamethonium, pentolinium, and mecamylamine have received extensive trial in hypertensive diseases. Reductions of blood pressure, particularly in the standing position, can be achieved, but again the inevitable side effects of orthostatic hypotension and parasympathetic ganglionic blockade complicate this approach to the management of hypertension.

CENTRAL DEPRESSANTS OF SYMPATHETIC FUNCTIONS
CLONIDINE

Clonidine hydrochloride (Catapres) is an experimental antihypertensive drug, which is unique in having an imidazoline structure and in its mode of action. Chemically clonidine is 2-2,6-dichlorophenyl-amino-2-imidazoline.

The antihypertensive potency of clonidine is quite remarkable. Administration of 0.15 to 0.9 mg. daily to patients with essential hypertension resulted in a significant reduction of their mean blood pressure.[74] The mode of action of the drug is quite complex. It reduces sympathetic activity by a central action, but it also reduces the vascular effects of both vasoconstrictors and vasodilators. Common side effects caused by clonidine are drowsiness, dryness of the mouth, and orthostasis. Tolerance may develop to its antihypertensive action. The drug is still experimental, and its ultimate usefulness remains to be established.

Recent studies indicate that clonidine is an alpha receptor agonist that inhibits norepinephrine release. The hypotensive effect of clonidine appears to be exerted on inhibitory alpha receptors in the central nervous system and in the periphery.[81a]

METHYLDOPA

Methyldopa (Aldomet) was introduced as an antihypertensive drug on the theory that, being an inhibitor of aromatic amino acid decarboxylase, it would lower catecholamine concentrations in the body by that mechanism. It was found, however, that the drug is taken up and metabolized to alpha-methylnorepinephrine, which then acts as a catecholamine depleter in the central nervous system and adrenergic fibers. The metabolic product may function as a false transmitter, and since its potency is lower than that of norepinephrine, decreased sympathetic activity results.

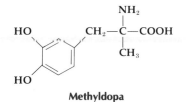

Methyldopa

Methyldopa is recommended for the treatment of most types of hypertension. It is preferred by some for patients with chronic renal disease and in hypertensive emergencies. For the latter, the drug may be injected intravenously — in contrast with guanethidine, which is used orally only. Methyldopa causes much less orthostatic hypotension than guanethidine, ganglionic blocking drugs, or monoamine oxidase inhibitors. The reason for this difference is not clear, but it is quite likely that much of the hypotensive action of the drug is a consequence of its influence on central adrenergic mechanisms rather than its peripheral catecholamine depletion.

Adverse reactions to methyldopa include marked drowsiness in many patients, depression, and nightmares. In some individuals the administration of methyldopa is followed in about a week by an influenza-like reaction that may be caused by sensitization to the drug. In some of these individuals, subsequent administration of small doses of methyldopa will elicit the same reaction. This syndrome is accompanied rarely by alterations in serum glutamic oxaloacetic transaminase levels and mild hepatitis.

The main route of excretion of methyldopa is glomerular filtration, and the drug may accumulate in severe renal disease. Its antihypertensive action is reinforced by the oral diuretics, which is the case for all antihypertensive drugs.

Preparations

Methyldopa (Aldomet) is available in tablets containing 250 mg. of the drug. Methyldopate hydrochloride (Aldomet ester hydrochloride) is available as a solution for intravenous injection, 250 mg./5 ml.

RESERPINE

Reserpine is the prototype of several alkaloids present in *Rauwolfia serpentina*, or Indian snakeroot. Used in India for centuries, it was introduced into Western medicine in the 1950's.[4] At first reserpine seemed as important for its tranquilizing properties as for its usefulness in the treatment of hypertension. It was gradually replaced as an antipsychotic drug by the phenothiazines. It is still important as an antihypertensive drug and as a fascinating pharmacologic tool.

Basic action and effects

Reserpine has one basic action responsible for most, if not all, of its pharmacologic effects. The drug causes a depletion of catecholamines and serotonin in the central and peripheral nervous system and some other sites. Depletion is a consequence of amine release. Not only are the amines released from their binding sites, but their reaccumulation is also prevented. Some interference by reserpine with catecholamine synthesis has been reported.[61]

What is the mechanism of amine release induced by reserpine? It was thought at first that reserpine must destroy the binding sites for the amines, since its depleting action lasted for a long time although its half-life in the body was only about 2 hours.[31] Most recent studies indicate, however, that a small fraction of the administered reserpine clings tenaciously to tissue elements. It is quite likely that reserpine is not a "hit-and-run" drug. Rather, a small fraction of the administered dose interfers with granular uptake of catecholamines in neural structures.[1]

A puzzling aspect of the blood pressure–lowering effect of reserpine can now be explained. When reserpine is injected intramuscularly (2.5 mg.) in a patient with severe hypertension, the blood pressure may fall significantly within 2 hours. During that time there is massive release of norepinephrine from adrenergic fibers, as shown by the appearance of catecholamine metabolites in the urine. Despite this massive release of catecholamines, there is a fall of blood pressure. Similarly, in animal experiments not even transient elevations of blood pressure are observed following the intravenous injection of large doses of the drug. This apparent paradox becomes understandable once it is recognized that reserpine releases norepinephrine from the storage granules into the axoplasm, where it is rapidly metabolized by MAO.

Although reserpine interferes with the granular uptake of catecholamines, it does not block the membrane uptake mechanism as does cocaine.[12,43] As a consequence, reserpine does not produce significant sensitization to the action of catecholamines. What little sensitization is observed may be explained on the basis of prolonged inactivity of effectors, which generally leads to a nonspecific increase in reponse to a variety of drugs.[66]

Parasympathetic effects of reserpine are undoubtedly a result of decreased sympathetic activity. Bradycardia, aggravation of peptic ulcer, increased gastrointestinal motility, and miosis may all be explained as results of parasympathetic predominance.

The *central nervous system effects* of the drug are among its greatest disadvantages in the treatment of hypertension. An unpleasant type of drowsiness and lethargy is particularly disliked by individuals who must be intellectually alert and creative. Depression and suicides have occurred during chronic reserpine administration. Reserpine increases the central nervous system depressant actions of other drugs such as barbiturates and alcohol. It predisposes patients to severe hypotension during surgery and anesthesia.

Various derivatives of reserpine are very similar in action to the parent compound. Syrosingopine produces fewer central effects in relation to its antihypertensive action. This selectivity has been attributed to the fact that its norepinephrine-depleting action is largely limited to the peripheral nervous system. It is also much less potent.

The formulas of reserpine (Serpasil) and syrosingopine (Singoserp) are as follows:

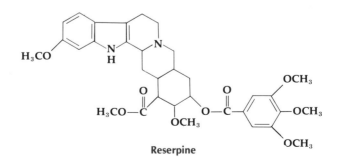

Reserpine

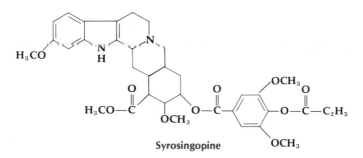

Syrosingopine

Preparations

The dried root of *Rauwolfia serpentina* Benth (Raudixin) is available in tablets containing 50 and 100 mg. Preparations of *reserpine* include tablets of 0.1, 0.25, and 1 mg.; an elixir containing 0.25 mg./4 ml.; and solution for injection, 2.5 mg./ml.

Syrosingopine (Singoserp) is available in tablets of 1 mg.

REFLEX INHIBITORS OF CENTRAL SYMPATHETIC FUNCTION

The veratrum alkaloids, protoveratrines A and B, act through the remarkable mechanism of promoting the activity of afferent nerves from the carotid sinus and aortic arch and thereby causing a reflex inhibition of central sympathetic activity with subsequent parasympathetic predominance. Unfortunately, the protoveratrines cause considerable nausea in many patients, and their dosage must be carefully adjusted in order to obtain a good hypotensive effect. These disadvantages have limited the usefulness of these compounds, but their pharmacology illustrates some unique mechanisms of drug action.

A number of alkaloids occur in plants of the species *Veratrum viride* and *Veratrum album*. They are classified as (1) tertiary amine esters and (2) secondary amines and their glycosides. The various alkaloids are polycyclic ring structures showing some resemblance to the cardiac glycosides.

Effects of protoveratrines A and B

If a small dose of less than 2 mg. of a mixture of protoveratrines A and B (Veralba) is injected intravenously into a human being, the characteristic effect consists of bradycardia and fall of blood pressure. When proportionately larger doses are given to animals, temporary apnea is produced in addition to the circulatory effects.

The mechanism of these circulatory actions is quite unusual and is related to what is known as the Bezold-Jarisch effect. It was suggested many years ago on the basis of investigations of the effect of veratrine in rabbits[5] that the cardiovascular actions of the preparation were due to stimulation of afferent nerve fibers within the thorax and probably within the heart itself. Later investigations indicate that the conclusions of Bezold were essentially correct.[35, 58]

It has been suggested that these veratrum alkaloids may sensitize the afferent endings in the baroreceptors of the carotid sinus and other areas, so that they have greater response to the normally effective stretch stimulus.[58]

An elegant direct demonstration of this mechanism of action was provided[32, 33] and is shown in Fig. 14-4.

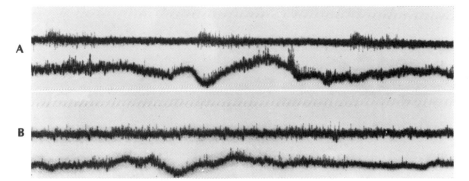

Fig. 14-4. Effect of protoveratrine in increasing afferent discharges and decreasing efferent outflow through splanchnic nerve. Upper half of each tracing is taken from carotid sinus nerve of cat; lower half from right major splanchnic nerve. **A,** Note burst of pressoreceptor activity of carotid sinus nerve, synchronous with systole, and irregular activity of splanchnic nerve. **B,** After 3 μg/kg. protoveratrine, note intensified and more or less continuous discharge of carotid sinus afferent fibers resulting in inhibition of splanchnic efferent impulses. (Courtesy Dr. A. S. Dontas; from Hoobler, S. W.: Amer. J. Med. **17**:259, 1954.)

The *veratrinic* response of striated muscle consists of repeated contractions following single nerve stimulation. It has been suggested that in myotonia congenita the skeletal muscle reacts with the veratrinic response. These effects on skeletal muscle require large doses and are not seen in the therapeutic usage of the veratrum alkaloids.

Germine is a veratrum alkaloid that has been used experimentally in the treatment of *myasthenia gravis* because of the veratrinic response it elicits in skeletal muscle.[20] This novel approach is still in the experimental stage.

BETA ADRENERGIC BLOCKING DRUGS

Beta adrenergic blocking drugs, discussed in detail in Chapter 12, are not useful by themselves as antihypertensive agents, although their administration over a period of months results in some lowering of blood pressure. The mechanism of their hypotensive action is not clear, but it may be related to a combination of pharmacologic effects such as an influence on central autonomic regulations, myocardial depression, and inhibition of renin release.

The main usefulness of the beta blockers in the treatment of hypertension is in combination with hydralazine or minoxidil.[28,75] The direct vasodilators bring out reflex cardiac stimulation. The beta blockers prevent these adverse effects.[28]

ANTIHYPERTENSIVE DRUGS THAT PROMOTE SALT EXCRETION

Drugs that promote salt secretion, such as the thiazides, are important in the treatment of hypertension because sodium is involved in some way in the pathogenesis of the disease.

Rats on a high salt intake develop hypertension.[48] Also, the hypertensive effect of deoxycorticosterone and aldosterone[40,41,57] is probably attributable to salt retention.

Conversely, the antihypertensive action of a low salt diet is generally accepted at present. The mechanism whereby an excess of salt in the body contributes to hypertension is not definitely known. Expansion of extracellular fluid volume and alterations in the salt concentration in arteriolar walls have been suggested as important factors.[64,65]

CHLOROTHIAZIDE AND RELATED DRUGS

Although some relationship was known to exist between experimental hypertension and salt intake or retention, it came as a surprise that chlorothiazide caused some lowering of the blood pressure of hypertensive patients and contributed to the antihypertensive action of other drugs.[21,72,73]

Most investigators believe that thiazide diuretics exert their antihypertensive action through salt depletion. Isolated observations suggest that these drugs may have extrarenal effects also. In any case, they have been a welcome addition to antihypertensive therapy because it is much easier to accomplish salt depletion through this means than by strict limitation of salt intake.

The most useful oral diuretics, discussed in greater detail in Chapter 33, are the thiazides and the related drugs chlorthalidone (Hygroton) and quinethazone (Hydromox). They are widely used in the treatment of hypertension because of their safety and effectiveness and their ability to increase the antihypertensive action of other unrelated drugs. Furosemide (Lasix) is being used increasingly also. On the other hand, although ethacrynic acid (Edecrin) is effective in hypertensive emergencies, it has no indications in the management of chronic hypertension.

The aldosterone antagonist spironolactone is sometimes combined with the thiazide diuretics, mainly to reduce potassium loss. The same is true for triamterene (Dyrenium). Both of these potassium-sparing diuretics have some antihypertensive action of their own.

The adverse effects of the thiazide diuretics, such as hypokalemia, hyperuricemia, and aggravation of diabetes are discussed in Chapter 33. On the whole, these drugs are very useful in the treatment of hypertension, although their mechanism of antihypertensive action is not completely understood.

ANTIHYPERTENSIVE DRUG COMBINATIONS

Since the treatment of chronic hypertension often requires the use of more than one drug, many fixed combinations of antihypertensive medications are available. They commonly contain a thiazide diuretic and reserpine or some other compound that reduces sympathetic function. As a rule, fixed combinations are undesirable because they eliminate the possibility of careful adjustment of the dosage of the individual components. Also, the use of mixtures in fixed combination promotes an attitude of not thinking in terms of the individual components with all their separate and combined adverse effects.

References

1 Alpers, H. S., and Shore, P. A.: Specific binding of reserpine—association with norepinephrine depletion, Biochem. Pharmacol. 18:1363, 1969.

2 Baker, D. R., Schrader, W. H., and Hitchcock, C. R.: Small bowel ulceration apparently associated with thiazide and potassium therapy, J.A.M.A. 190:586, 1964.

3 Baum, T., Shropshire, A. T., and Varner, L. L.: Contribution of the central nervous system to the action of several antihypertensive agents (methyldopa, hydralazine and guanethidine), J. Pharmacol. Exp. Ther. 182:135, 1972.

4 Bein, H. J.: The pharmacology of Rauwolfia, Pharmacol. Rev. 8:435, 1956.

5 von Bezold, A., and Hirt, L.: Ueber die physiologischen Wirkungen des essigsauren Veratrins, Untersuchungen Physiol. Lab. Würzburg 1:73, 1867.

6 Biron, P., Kolw, E., Nowaczynski, W., Brouillet, J., and Genest, J.: The effects of intravenous infusions of valine-5 angiotensin II and other pressor agents on urinary electrolytes and corticosteroids, including aldosterone, J. Clin. Invest. 40:338, 1960.

7 Borison, H. L., and Wang, S. C.: Physiology and pharmacology of vomiting, Pharmacol. Rev. 5:193, 1953.

8 Bowlus, W. E., and Langford, H. G.: A comparison of the antihypertensive effect of chlorthalidone and hydrochlorothiazide, Clin. Pharmacol. Ther. 5:708, 1964.

9 Brunjes, S.: Catecholamine metabolism in essential hypertension, New Eng. J. Med. 271:120, 1964.

10 Colwill, J. M., Dutton, A. M., Morrissey, J., and Yu, P. N.: Alpha-methyldopa and hydrochlorothiazide. A controlled study of their comparative effectiveness as antihypertensive agents, New Eng. J. Med. 71:696, 1964.

11 Conn, J. W.: Aldosteronism and hypertension, Arch. Intern. Med. 107:813, 1961.

12 Dahlström, A., Fuxe, K., and Hillarp, N-A: Site of action of reserpine, Acta Pharmacol. 22:277, 1965.

13 Dahr, A. S., George, C. F., and Dollery, C. T.: The effect of selective adrenergic β-blockade on the hypotensive effect of hydralazine, Experientia 27:545, 1971.

14 Davis, J. O.: The control of aldosterone secretion, Physiologist 5:65, 1962.

15 Dawes, G. S., and Comroe, J. H., Jr.: Chemoreflexes from the heart and lungs, Physiol. Rev. 34:167, 1954.

16 DeCharme, D. W., Freyburger, W. A., Graham, B. E., and Carlson, R. G.: Pharmacologic properties of minoxidil: a new hypotensive agent, J. Pharmacol. Exp. Ther. 184:662, 1973.

17 Dickinson, C. J., and Lawrence, J. R.: A slowly developing pressor response to small concentrations of angiotensin. Its bearing on the pathogenesis of chronic renal hypertension, Lancet 1:1354, 1963.

18 Feldberg, W., and Lewis, G. P.: The action of peptides on the adrenal medulla. Release of adrenalin by bradykinin and angiotensin, J. Physiol. (London) 171:98, 1964.

19 Finnerty, F. A.: Drug choice in hypertensive emergencies, Amer. J. Cardiol. 17:652, 1966.

20 Flacke, W., Caviness, V. S., Jr., and Samaha, F. G.: Treatment of myasthenia gravis with germine diacetate, New Eng. J. Med. 275:1207, 1966.

21 Freis, E. D., Wanko, A., Wilson, I. M., and Parrish, A. E.: Chlorothiazide in hypertensive and normotensive patients, Ann. N. Y. Acad. Sci. 7:450, 1958.

22 Gifford, R. W., Jr.: Bethanidine sulfate: a new antihypertensive agent, J.A.M.A. 193:901, 1965.

23 Gilmore, E., Weil, J., and Chidsey, C.: Treatment of essential hypertension with a new vasodilator in combination with beta-adrenergic blockade, New Eng. J. Med. 282:521, 1970.

24 Goldblatt, H.: The renal origin of hypertension, Springfield, Ill., 1948, Charles C Thomas, Publisher.

25 Goormaghtigh, N.: Existence of an endocrine gland in the media of the renal arterioles, Proc. Soc. Exp. Biol. Med. 42:688, 1939.

26 Gordon, R. D., Küchel, O., Liddle, G. W., and Island, D. P.: Role of the sympathetic nervous system in regulating renin and aldosterone production in man, J. Clin. Invest. 46:599, 1967.

27 Goth, A., and Harrison, F. L.: Influence of protoveratrine on effect of vasoactive drugs, Proc. Soc. Exp. Biol. Med. 87:437, 1954.

28 Gottlieb, T. B., Katz, F. H., and Chidsey, C. A.: Combined therapy with vasodilator drugs and beta-adrenergic blockade in hypertension: a comparative study of hydralazine and minoxidil, Circulation 45:571, 1972.

29 Gross, F., Druey, J., and Meier, R.: Eine neue Gruppe blutdrucksenkender Substanzen von besonderem Wirkungscharacter, Experientia 6:19, 1950.

30 Heath, W. C., and Freis, E. D.: Triamterene with hydrochlorothiazide in the treatment of hypertension, J.A.M.A. 186:119, 1963.

31 Hess, S. M., Shore, P. A., and Brodie, B. B.: Persistence of reserpine action after the disappearance of drug from brain: effect on serotonin, J. Pharmacol. Exp. Ther. 118:84, 1956.

32 Hoobler, S. W.: Treatment of hypertension, Amer. J. Med. 17:259, 1954.

33 Hoobler, S. W., and Dontas, A. S.: Drug treatment of hypertension, Pharmacol. Rev. 5:135, 1953.

34 Igloe, M. C.: Effects of methyldopa in hypertension, J.A.M.A. 189:188, 1964.

35 Jarisch, A., and Richter, H.: Die afferenten Bahnen des Veratrineffektes in den Herznerven, Arch. Exp. Path. Pharmakol. 193:355, 1939.

36 Johnsson, G., Henning, M., and Ablad, B.: Studies on the mechanism of the vasoconstrictor effect of angiotensin II in man, Life Sci. 4:1549, 1965.

37 Johnston, L. C., and Grieble, H. G.: Treatment of arterial hypertensive disease with diuretics, Arch. Intern. Med. 119:225, 1967.

38 Kopin, I. J., Fischer, J. E., Musacchio, J. M., Horst, W. D., and Weise, V. K.: "False neurochemical transmitters" and the mechanism of sympathomimetic blockade by monoamine oxidase inhibitors, J. Pharmacol. Exp. Ther. 147:186, 1965.

39 Krayer, O.: Antiaccelerator cardiac agents, J. Mount Sinai Hosp., N. Y. 19:53, 1952.

40 Laragh, J. H.: Aldosterone in fluid and electrolyte disorders: hyper- and hypoaldosteronism, J. Chronic Dis. 11:292, 1960.

41 Laragh, J. H., Angers, M., Kelly, W. G., and Lieberman, S.: Hypotensive agents and pressor substances: effect of epinephrine, norepinephrine, angiotension II, and others on the secretory rate of aldosterone in man, J.A.M.A. 174:234, 1960.

42 Laragh, J. H., Ulick, S., Januszewicz, V., Deming, Q. B., Kelly, W. G., and Lieberman, S.: Aldosterone secretion and primary and malignant hypertension, J. Clin. Invest. 39:1091, 1960.

43 Lindmar, R., and Muscholl, E.: Die Wirkung von Bharmaka auf die Elimination von Noradrenalin aus der Perfusionsflüssigkeit und die Noradrenalinaufnahme in das isolierte Herz, Arch. Exp. Path. Pharmakol. 247:469, 1964.

44 Luria, M. H., and Freis, E. D.: Treatment of hypertension with debrisoquin sulfate (Declinax), Curr. Ther. Res. 7:289, 1965.

45 McCormack, L. J., Beland, J. E., Schneckloth, R. E., and Corcoran, A. C.: Effects of antihypertensive treatment on evolution of renal lesions in malignant nephrosclerosis, Amer. J. Path. 34:1011, 1958.

46 Mason, D. T., and Braunwald, E.: Effects of guanethidine, reserpine, and methyldopa on reflex venous and arterial constriction in man, J. Clin. Invest. 43:1449, 1964.

47 Maxwell, R. A., Povalski, H., and Plummer, A. J.: A differential effect of reserpine on pressor amine activity and its relationship to other agents producing this effect, J. Pharmacol. Exp. Ther. 125:178, 1959.

48 Meneely, G. R., Tucker, R. G., Darby, J., and Auerbach, S. H.: Chronic sodium chloride toxicity: hypertension, renal and vascular lesions, Ann. Intern. Med. 39:991, 1953.

49 Mitchell, J. R., and Oates, J. A.: Guanethidine and related agents. I. Mechanism of the selective blockade of adrenergic neurons and its antagonism by drugs, J. Pharmacol. Exp. Ther. 172:100, 1970.

50 Moyer, J. H., Huggins, R. A., and Handley, C. A.: Further cardiovascular and renal hemodynamic studies following the administration of hydralazine (1-hydrazinophthalazine) and the effect of ganglionic blockade with hexamethonium on these responses, J. Pharmacol. Exp. Ther. 109:175, 1953.

51 Muelheims, G. H., Entrup, R. W., Paiewonsky, D., and Mierzwiak, D. S.: Increased sensitivity of the heart to catecholamine-induced arrhythmias following guanethidine, Clin. Pharmacol. Ther. 6:757, 1965.

52 Newton, M. A., Sealy, J. E., Ledingham, J. G. G., and Laragh, J. H.: High blood pressure and oral contraceptives, Amer. J. Obstet. Gynec. 101:1037, 1968.

53 Onesti, G., Schiazza, D., Brest, A. N., and Moyer, J. H.: Cardiac and renal hemodynamic effects of debrisoquin sulfate in hypertensive patients, Clin. Pharmacol. Ther. 7:17, 1966.

54 Page, I. H., Corcoran, A. C., Dustan, H. P., and Koppanyi, T.: Cardiovascular actions of sodium nitroprusside in animals and hypertensive patients, Circulation 11:188, 1955.

55 Page, I. H., and Dustan, H. P.: A new, potent, antihypertensive drug: preliminary study of [2-(octahydro-1-azocinyl)-ethyl] guanidine sulfate (guanethidine), J.A.M.A. 170:1265, 1959.

56 Panisset, J. C., and Bourdois, P.: Effect of angiotensin on the response to noradrenaline and sympathetic nerve stimulation, and on the 3H-noradrenaline uptake in cat mesenteric blood vessels, Canad. J. Physiol. Pharmacol. 46:125, 1968.

57 Perera, G. A., and Blood, D. W.: Pressor activity of desoxycorticosterone acetate in normotensive and hypertensive subjects, Ann. Intern. Med. 27:401, 1947.

58 Richardson, A. P., Walker, H. A., Farrar, C. B., Griffith, W., Pound, E., and Davidson, J. R.: The mechanism of the hypotensive action of veratrum alkaloids, Proc. Soc. Exp. Biol. Med. 79:79, 1952.

59 Rubin, A. A., Roth, F. E., Taylor, R. M., and Rosenkilde, H.: Pharmacology of diazoxide, an antihypertensive, nondiuretic benzothiadiazine, J. Pharmacol. Exp. Ther. 136:344, 1962.

60 Ruedy, J.: A comparative clinical trial of guanoxan and guanethidine in essential hypertension, Clin. Pharmacol. Ther. 8:38, 1967.

61 Rutledge, C. O., and Weiner, N.: The effect of reserpine upon the synthesis of norepinephrine in the isolated rabbit heart, J. Pharmacol. Exp. Ther. 157:290, 1967.

62 Schroeder, H. A.: Hydralazine in the control of severe hypertension, Practitioner **173**:195, 1954.

63 Sellers, E. M., and Koch—Weser, J.: Protein binding and vascular activity of diazoxide, New Eng. J. Med. **281**:1141, 1969.

64 Tobian, L.: Interrelationships of electrolytes, juxtaglomerular cells and hypertension, Physiol. Rev. **40**:280, 1960.

65 Tobian, L., Jr., and Binion, J.: Artery wall electrolytes in renal and DCA hypertension, J. Clin. Invest. **33**:1407, 1954.

66 Trendelenburg, U.: Supersensitivity and subsensitivity to sympathomimetic amines, Pharmacol. Rev. **15**:225, 1963.

67 Udhoji, V. N., and Weil, M. H.: Circulatory effects of angiotensin, levarterenol and metaraminol in the treatment of shock, New Eng. J. Med. **270**:501, 1964.

68 Vane, J. R.: The release and fate of vaso-active hormones in the circulation, Brit. J. Pharmacol. **35**:209, 1969.

69 Veterans Administration Cooperative Study on Antihypertensive Agents: I A double-blind control study of antihypertensive agents; comparative effectiveness of reserpine, reserpine and hydralazine, and three ganglionic blocking agents, chlorisondamine, mecamylamine, and pentolinium tartrate, Arch. Intern. Med. **106**:81, 1960.

70 Weidmann, P., Maxwell, M. H., Lupu, A. N., Lewin, A. J., and Massry, S. G.: Plasma renin activity and blood pressure in terminal renal failure, New Eng. J. Med. **285**:757, 1971.

71 Weiss, S., and Ellis, L. B.: Influence of sodium nitrite on cardiovascular system and on renal activity in health, in arterial hypertension, and in renal disease, Arch. Med. **52**:105, 1933.

72 Wilkins, R. W.: Studies on antihypertensive action of chlorothiazide, Clin. Res. **6**:831, 1958. (Abstract.)

73 Wilkins, R. W., Hollander, W., and Chobanian, A. V.: Chlorothiazide in hypertension: studies on its mode of action, Ann. N. Y. Acad. Sci. **71**:465, 1958.

74 Yeh, B. K., Nantel, A., and Goldberg, L. I.: Antihypertensive effect of clonidine, Arch. Intern. Med. **127**:233, 1971.

75 Zacest, R., Gilmore, E., and Koch-Weser, J.: Treatment of essential hypertension with combined vasodilation and beta-adrenergic blockade, New Eng. J. Med. **286**:617, 1972.

Recent reviews

76 Davis, J. O.: Aldosterone and angiotensin, J.A.M.A. **188**:1062, 1964.

77 Davis, J. O.: What signals the kidney to release renin? Circ. Res. **28**:301, 1971.

78 Ehrlich, E. N.: Aldosterone, the adrenal cortex, and hypertension, Ann. Rev. Med. **19**:373, 1968.

79 Friend, D. G.: Antihypertensive drugs, Clin. Pharmacol. Ther. **3**:269, 1962.

80 Green, A. F.: Antihypertensive drugs, Advances Pharmacol. **1**:162, 1962.

81 Gross, F., editor: Antihypertensive therapy, an international symposium, Berlin, 1966, Springer-Verlag.

81a Langer, S. Z.: Presynaptic regulation of catecholamine release, Biochem. Pharmacol. (In press.)

82 Oates, J. A.: Antihypertensive drugs that impair adrenergic neuron function, Pharmacol. Physicians **1**(6):1, 1967.

83 Oates, J. A., Seligmann, A. W., Clark, M. A., Rousseau, P., and Lee, R. E.: The relative efficacy of guanethidine, methyldopa and pargyline as antihypertensive agents, New Eng. J. Med. **273**:729, 1965.

84 Page, I. H.: A new hormone, angiotensin, Clin. Pharmacol. Ther. **3**:758, 1962.

85 Pardo, E. G., Vargas, R., and Vidrio, H.: Antihypertensive drug action, Ann. Rev. Pharmacol. **5**:77, 1965.

85a Pettinger, W. A., and Mitchell, H. C.: Minoxidil—an alternative to nephrectomy for refractory hypertension, New Eng. J. Med. **289**:167, 1973.

86 Proger, S.: Antihypertensive drugs: praise and restraint (editorial), New Eng. J. Med. **286**:155, 1972.

87 Staff Report: Recent advances in hypertension, Amer. J. Med. **39**:616, 1965.

88 Tobian, L.: Why do thiazide diuretics lower blood pressure in essential hypertension? Ann. Rev. Pharmacol. **7**:399, 1967.

89 Vander, A. J.: Control of renin release, Physiol. Rev. **47**:359, 1967.

90 Veterans Administration Cooperative Study Group on Antihypertensive Agents: Effects of treatment on morbidity in hypertension. II. Results in patients with diastolic blood pressure averaging 90 through 114 mm. Hg, J.A.M.A. **213**:1143, 1970.

91 Veterans Administration Cooperative Study of Antihypertensive Agents: III. Chlorothiazide alone and in combination with other agents: preliminary results, Arch. Intern. Med. **110**:134, 1962.

92 Winer, N., Chokshi, D. S., and Freedman, A. D.: Adrenergic receptor mediation of renin secretion, J. Clin. Endocr. **29**:1168, 1969.

93 Zbinden, G.: The antihypertensive effect of the

monoamine oxidase inhibitors — mechanism of action. In Brest, A. N., and Moyer, J. H., editors: Hypertension: recent advances, Philadelphia, 1961, Lea & Febiger.

94 Zimmerman, B. G., and Gisslen, J.: Pattern of renal vasoconstriction and transmitter release during sympathetic stimulation in presence of angiotensin and cocaine, J. Pharmacol. Exp. Ther. **163**:320, 1968.

15 Histamine

Histamine is of interest in pharmacology and medicine because of its potent pharmacologic activity and its wide distribution in tissues. When released from its binding sites, histamine can elicit reactions that range in intensity from mild itching to shock and death.

It would seem that such a potent and easily released endogenous compound would have important functions in the body. There is indeed evidence for a local role of histamine in inflammation. It is also quite certain that the amine plays a role in anaphylaxis, allergies, and drug reactions. Its role in normal physiology remains mysterious: a neurotransmitter role and additional extraneural "local hormonal" functions are attributed to it on the basis of evidence that up to now is inadequate.

HISTAMINE RECEPTORS

Histamine appears to act on two separate and distinct receptors, termed H_1 and H_2 receptors. Contraction of the smooth muscle of the bronchi and intestine is mediated by H_1 receptors and is antagonized by a typical antihistamine. On the other hand, H_2 receptors mediate the actions of histamine or gastric secretion, cardiac acceleration, and inhibition of the contractions of the rat uterus. These actions are antagonized by a new type of antihistamine exemplified by burimamide[64] and the related drug metiamide.

DEVELOPMENT OF CONCEPTS

Histamine was first synthesized in 1906 by Windaus. It was also found to occur naturally in ergot as the product of bacterial contamination. The pharmacologic properties of histamine were extensively studied by Sir Henry Dale, who was impressed with the similarities in the actions of histamine and the manifestations of anaphylaxis in several species such as the guinea pig, rabbit, and dog. Once histamine was found widely distributed in mammalian tissues, numerous roles were assigned to it, often uncritically. Studies by Thomas Lewis on the release of "H substance" from the skin in response to injury had a great influence.

When the antihistaminic drugs were developed in the 1940's, many of the histaminic theories of various physiologic functions and pathologic processes were abandoned because of the inability of these drugs to modify them.

The demonstration in the 1950's of a close association between mast cells and histamine created much interest, and research concerning histamine focused on mechanisms of its release from mast cells. It was soon realized, however, that there is also an important non-mast cell pool of histamine, the function of which is still being investigated.

In addition to the interest in preformed histamine in the tissues and its release, there has also been a great interest in newly formed histamine as a consequence of activation of histidine decarboxylase.[47] The role of this nascent histamine is uncertain.

TISSUE DISTRIBUTION AND FORMATION

Histamine is widely distributed in the body. Its concentration varies in different species; in man the highest concentrations are found in the lungs, skin, and stomach. Details of its distribution are given in Table 15-1.

It is generally believed that most of the histamine present in tissues arises locally as a consequence of decarboxylation of histidine. Various foods may contain histamine and intestinal bacteria may form large amounts, but whatever histamine is absorbed is rapidly altered and does not contribute to the body's stores of this amine.

With the availability of experimental drugs that destroy mast cells, such as compound 48/80, it has become possible to identify two pools of histamine in the body. The mast cell pool is widely distributed in the connective tissue and is depleted experimentally by the mast cell–destroying agents.

The circulating basophils behave like the mast cells and contain very high concentrations of histamine. The non-mast cell pool includes the gastric mucosa and the small amounts present in the brain, heart, and other organs. It is not known with certainty what the cellular localization of non-mast cell histamine is, but it is suspected that with the exception of the gastric mucosa, it is present in neural elements.[28] It differs from mast cell histamine in its more rapid turnover rate and its resistance to the usual histamine releasers such as compound 48/80.

Table 15-1. Histamine content of human tissues*

Tissue	Histamine content
Lung	33 ± 10 μg/gram[†]
Mucous membrane (nasal)	15.6 μg/gram
Stomach	14 ± 4.0 μg/gram[†]
Duodenum	14 ± 0.9 μg/gram[†]
Skin	6.6 μg/gram (abdomen)
	30.4 μg/gram (face)
Spleen	3.4 ± 0.97 μg/gram[†]
Kidney	2.5 ± 1.2 μg/gram[†]
Liver	2.2 ± 0.76 μg/gram[†]
Heart	1.6 ± 0.07 μg/gram[†]
Thyroid	1.0 ± 0.13 μg/gram[†]
Skeletal muscle	0.97 ± 0.13 μg/gram[†]
Central nervous tissue	0–0.2 μg/gram
Plasma	2.6 μg/L.
Basophils	1,080 μg/10^9 cells
Eosinophils	160 μg/10^9 cells
Neutrophils	3.0 μg/10^9 cells
Lymphocytes	0.6 μg/10^9 cells
Platelets	0.009 μg/10^9 platelets
Whole blood	16–89 μg/L.

* Based on data from Van Arsdel, P. P., Jr., and Beall, G. N.: Arch. Intern. Med. **106**:192, 1960.
† Mean ± Standard error.

The reason for the unequal distribution of mast cells is obscure. It has been suggested that selective localization of mast cell histamine in the skin and lungs would permit these sites, which are exposed to the environment, to respond readily via vasodilatation when bacterial invasion or injury makes local inflammation teleologically desirable. The presence of histamine in mast cells of the adipose tissue and its effect on fatty acid release from adipose tissue[10] may provide another reason for its special localization.

HISTIDINE DECARBOXYLASES

Chemically, histamine is 2(4-imidazolyl) ethylamine. Its structure is as follows:

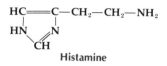

Histamine

Histamine is derived from the decarboxylation of histidine. It represents another example of a powerful pharmacologic agent resulting from the decarboxylation of an amino acid.

Mammalian tissues contain two different histidine decarboxylases. The one known as specific histidine decarboxylase, present in mast cells, is inhibited by methylhistidine and the hydrazine analog of histidine, but not by methyldopa. The other enzyme, also known as aromatic L-amino acid decarboxylase, decarboxylates several aromatic L-amino acids (dopa, for example). It is inhibited by methyldopa. There is every reason to believe that specific histidine decarboxylase is more important physiologically. Histamine appears to exist in more than one metabolic pool. In the rat, administration of an inhibitor of specific decarboxylase caused a decrease of 30 to 50% in the histamine content of the heart, stomach, and urine without having much effect on the amine content of peritoneal mast cells.[28]

DEGRADATION OF HISTAMINE IN THE BODY

The degradation of histamine in the body takes place through two main pathways, with considerable species variation in their relative importance. In man, histamine is primarily methylated to 1-methylhistamine.[46] This product is converted to 1-methyl-imidazole-4-acetic acid by the enzyme MAO. In the other pathway, which also occurs in man, histamine is oxidized by diamine oxidase to imidazole-4-acetic acid, much of which is conjugated with ribose and is excreted as the riboside. The known pathways are shown in Fig. 15-1.

In addition to these compounds, some N-acetylhistamine also appears in the urine. The acetyl compound appears to reflect orally ingested histamine and amine formed by intestinal bacteria. The exact site of acetylation is still in doubt. There are suggestions that intestinal bacteria can acetylate histamine,[59] and some investigators feel that no acetylation occurs outside the gastrointestinal tract.

It has been estimated that about 1% of histamine slowly injected intravenously appears in the urine in the free form, whereas most orally ingested histamine is found in the conjugated form in the urine. It has been estimated that in a normal person 2 to 3 mg. of histamine may be released daily from the tissues. Urticaria in man or the injection of histamine-releasing agents into animals causes an increase in the urinary excretion of histamine.[63]

BINDING AND RELEASE OF MAST CELL HISTAMINE

Histamine is highly concentrated in the granules of the mast cell. These granules also contain large amounts of heparin, proteolytic enzymes, and in some species (rats and mice), serotonin. Histamine release is visualized as a two-step process. In the first step the granules are suddenly extruded; in the second, as the granules are

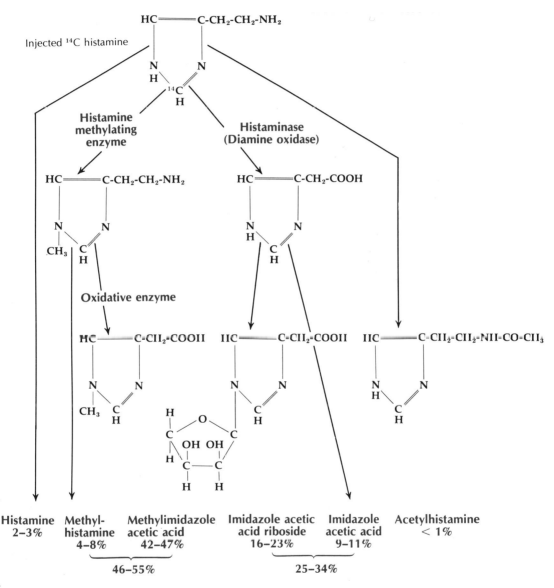

Fig. 15-1. Known pathways of histamine metabolism. Relative importance of the different pathways in human males is indicated by figures at bottom, which are expressed as percent of the total ^{14}C excreted in the urine during 12 hours after intradermal injection of ^{14}C histamine. Of the injected ^{14}C, 74 to 93% was excreted in 12 hours. (From Nilsson, K., Lindell, S.-E., Schayer, R. W., and Westling, H.: Clin. Sci. **18**:313, 1959.)

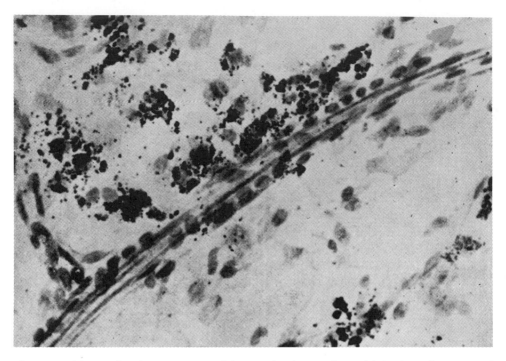

Fig. 15-2. Mast cells of rat mesentery 3 hours after intraperitoneal injection of compound 48/80. (From Riley, J. F., and West, A. B.: J. Path. Bact. **69**:269, 1955.)

exposed to the cations in the extracellular environment, histamine is relased by ion exchange. The amine is held within the granule by electrostatic forces.

Although granule release generally accompanies histamine release, it is possible that release of the amine could occur within the cell also. The appearance of granules within the mast cell is shown in Fig. 15-2.

Histamine is released from mast cells by physical and chemical agents, antigen-antibody reactions, and a variety of drugs.

Release by chemicals and drugs

Many early isolated observations suggested that simple chemicals can cause release of histamine in the body. Intracutaneous morphine injection in man produces the "triple response of Lewis" consisting of localized redness, localized edema, and a diffuse redness. This was suspected of being an example of a chemical causing release of H substance.[29] It has also been shown that curare alkaloids can liberate histamine, and this was thought to explain the episodes of bronchial constriction accompanying intravenous curare injections. With the discovery of adverse reactions to certain diamidines and polypeptide antibiotics (licheniformin, polymyxin), interest in this problem increased greatly.

The chemical histamine-releasing agents may be divided into two classes: small-molecule amines and certain large-molecule compounds such as dextran, polyvinylpyrrolidone, and ovomucoid, which are active only in some species.

A variety of organic bases can cause release of histamine from mast cells. The most active compound known is compound 48/80, a condensation product of p-methoxymethylphenylethylamine with formaldehyde (Fig. 15-2).

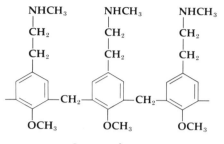

Compound 48/80

Many other amines can cause histamine release, but this action of commonly employed drugs may become manifest only if they are injected intravenously. It is a common experience in experimental studies that histamine-releasing agents may be fairly innocuous if they are administered in such a way that no high blood levels are reached at any time. High levels in the circulation are associated with greater incidence of adverse reactions of the anaphylactoid type.

It has been suggested that histamine release may be caused not only by the curare alkaloids but also by such commonly used drugs as morphine, codeine, papaverine, meperidine, atropine, hydralazine, and even sympathomimetic amines.[38] Histamine release by these drugs may not be significant unless they are administered intravenously in fairly large doses.

The histamine-releasing agents of small molecular size exert their effect in most species. On the other hand, there are a number of large-molecule compounds whose action appears to be limited to one species or family of animals. Dextran and ovomucoid (from egg white) produce a condition resembling angioneurotic edema in rats[52] and release histamine in this species[13] but do not have this effect in dogs or in man. Large-molecule dextran can cause reactions in man also. Curiously, polyvinylpyrrolidone and polysorbate 80 (Tween 80) exert similar effects in the dog but not in the rat.[17,26] The reason for this species-specific action of certain polymers has not been elucidated.[65]

A characteristic feature of histamine release by chemical compounds is the development of tachyphylaxis to subsequent injections. When one obtains a marked fall of blood pressure following intravenous injection of 100 to 200 μg/kg. of compound 48/80 in a dog, a second injection of the drug may have no effect whatever for several hours. Tachyphylaxis to Tween 20 or polyvinylpyrrolidone may last 14 to 20 hours.

Many investigators believe that the mechanism of tachyphylaxis is related to the fact that the easily releasable histamine has been exhausted by the first injection of the releasing agent.

Release in anaphylaxis and allergy

Histamine release plays an important role in the symptomatology of experimental anaphylactic shock in several species. In 1910 Dale and Laidlaw[2] observed that the symptoms elicited by histamine in guinea pigs, dogs, and rabbits were very similar to the manifestations of anaphylactic shock in these species. In guinea pigs the dominant symptom is bronchial constriction and asphyxial death from intravenous doses as small as 0.4 mg./kg. In dogs, profound hypotension and acute enlargement of the liver are caused by both histamine and anaphylaxis. In the rabbit the pulmonary arterioles are constricted and acute dilatation of the right side of the heart ensues when either histamine is injected or antigen is administered to the previously sensitized animal.

In addition, in the dog the blood may become incoagulable in anaphylaxis but not after histamine injection. Much was made of this difference until it was demonstrated that anaphylaxis in the dog also releases heparin,[4] presumably from the mast cells, which are abundant in the dog's liver.

The release of histamine by injecting antigens into the sensitized animal has been demonstrated also by perfusion experiments of the skin[7] and on addition of the antigen in vitro to sensitized minced tissues.[34]

In acute anaphylactic reactions in man, histamine probably plays an important role. In anaphylaxis the human being reacts similarly to the dog and the guinea pig, exhibiting profound hypotension, bronchial constriction, or laryngeal edema.[23]

To summarize the present consensus on the role of histamine in human allergic disease, antigen-antibody reactions are thought to damage cells by mechanisms that are not understood. One consequence of this damage may be the release of histamine, which contributes significantly to the clinical picture in urticaria and hay fever. Histamine may play a lesser role in bronchial asthma and many other disease states attributed to an allergic mechanism.

Important new observations have been made on histamine release from human leukocytes by specific antigens such as ragweed extract.[31,32] These studies suggest that the cyclic AMP and drugs that activate adenyl cyclase have an inhibitory action on histamine release. There is a possibility that drugs widely used in allergic diseases, such as the catecholamines and theophylline, may exert an inhibitory effect on histamine release in addition to their well-known antagonism to many of its pharmacologic actions. Anaphylactically induced histamine release is inhibited by the new drug disodium cromoglycate (Intal) in vitro (p. 660).[27] It is enhanced by phosphatidylserine.[12]

PHARMACOLOGIC EFFECTS

The actions of histamine vary greatly in different species, and it is erroneous to apply uncritically to man information obtained in animals such as the rabbit. Most of the effects of histamine in man, however, seem very similar to those obtained in the dog.

Histamine taken by mouth has essentially no effect because it is altered by the intestinal bacteria, the gastrointestinal wall, and also the liver.

If injected intravenously, however, as little as 0.1 mg. of histamine phosphate causes a sharp decline in the blood pressure, acceleration of the heart rate, elevation of the cerebrospinal fluid pressure, flushing of the face, and headache. There is also stimulation of gastric hydrochloric acid secretion. All these effects last only a few minutes. If a similar injection is given to an asthmatic subject, even while he is free of demonstrable breathing difficulty, there will be a marked decrease in vital capacity, and a severe attack of asthma may be precipitated.

When larger doses of histamine are administered intravenously, which can be done only in animals, the blood pressure remains low for a considerable length of time, and there is marked elevation of the hematocrit reading. Histamine shock may ensue, with possibly fatal termination. The lethal dose in species such as the dog, in which the circulatory action of histamine predominates, may be as high as several milligrams per kilogram of body weight.

Circulatory effects

The two factors involved in the circulatory actions of histamine are arteriolar dilatation and increased capillary permeability. These cause loss of plasma from the circulation. It is generally stated that histamine dilates the capillaries directly, but there is a possibility that this capillary action is a consequence of constriction of small venules.[14] Such a view, however, has been questioned.[3] The effects of histamine on veins are particularly marked on the hepatic vein of the dog, where it causes constriction of the sphincterlike smooth muscle and enlargement of the liver by pooling of the blood at that organ.

A striking demonstration of the histamine effect on capillaries is seen when very low concentrations are injected intracutaneously in man. The injection of as little as 10 μg of the drug produces the "triple response of Lewis."[30] The sequence of events consists of localized redness, localized edema or wheal, and diffuse redness or flare.

The localized redness and wheal are the consequences of vasodilatation and increased capillary permeability. The diffuse flare involves neural mechanisms, perhaps axon reflexes, since it can be abolished by previous sectioning of sensory nerves.

The triple response is interesting because human skin seems to respond to a variety of injuries in the same manner as it does to histamine injections. This similarity led Sir Thomas Lewis to suggest that perhaps various injuries may cause release of a histamine-like substance, or H substance, from the skin; this substance then mediates the manifestations of evanescent skin inflammations.

The effects of histamine on the heart are slight compared with its vascular actions. Nevertheless, histamine can cause an increase in heart rate, which is blocked by the H_2-receptor antagonist, burimamide. Large doses of histamine can cause norepinephrine release from the heart, which contributes to cardioacceleration and a positive inotropic effect.[9]

Other smooth muscle effects

Man and the guinea pig are very susceptible to the bronchoconstrictor action of histamine. Persons with a previous history of asthma are particularly vulnerable and may respond with an acute asthmatic attack to a dose of histamine that would only cause minor decreases in vital capacity in a normal person. This is generally interpreted as increased susceptibility to histamine of the bronchial smooth muscle in asthmatic persons. Asthmatics are highly susceptible not only to histamine but also to methacholine.

Effect on secretions

Histamine is a potent stimulant of gastric hydrochloric acid secretion. As little as 0.025 mg. of the drug injected subcutaneously in man will cause marked increase in hydrochloric acid secretion but has few other effects in the body. This response to histamine is utilized in tests for complete achlorhydria. Histamine-resistant achlorhydria has diagnostic importance in such conditions as addisonian pernicious anemia.

The polypeptide gastrin is an extremely potent stimulant of gastric acid secretion, being 500 times as potent as histamine.[70] The presence of both gastrin and histamine in the gastric mucosa is intriguing.

Histamine stimulates to a slight extent the secretory activities of many other glandular cells. Effects on salivary and bronchial secretions can be demonstrated, but these actions are not important in a normal person. Its effect on catecholamine secretion has been mentioned before.

ROLE IN HEALTH AND DISEASE

Very little is known about the possible physiologic roles of histamine. The presence of this potent capillary and arteriolar dilator in mast cells, which are in intimate contact with blood vessels, suggests some role more significant than causation of hives. Just what this role may be cannot be stated at present. It is probable that histamine mediates the reactions of the skin to injury.

In one interesting experiment,[8] normal rats exposed to ultraviolet light, after having been injected previously with hematoporphyrin, reacted in about a day with edema of the skin. When these rats were pretreated for a week with the histamine-releasing agent compound 48/80 in order to deplete the histamine content of their skin, they did not react to the ultraviolet light.

There may be some relationship between gastrin and histamine. Histamine is an extremely potent stimulant of gastric hydrochloric acid secretion. It has been postulated that the intrinsic local hormone *gastrin* may in fact be identical with histamine. This has been denied by workers who were able to isolate potent preparations of gastrin that did not contain histamine. It is possible that gastrin, a polypeptide, can cause release or increased synthesis of histamine.[55] Thus the latter may still be the final mediator of gastrin action.[18] Inhibition of the effect of pentagastrin on gastric secretion by the H_2 receptor antagonist burimamide adds further evidence to histamine being the final mediator of the action of gastrin.[64]

A role of histamine in neural function is suggested by the fact that the compound is present in brain and in some nerve fibers. A ganglionic stimulant action of histamine has been demonstrated following close intra-arterial injection.[57] Catecholamine release by histamine in animals and in patients with pheochromocytoma has also been demonstrated. Despite these suggestive facts, the true role of histamine in neurophysiology is still speculative.

It has also been suggested that certain types of vascular headaches may be due to histamine.[21, 22] The evidence for the histaminic etiology in this instance is largely indirect. It is based on the facts that injected histamine can reproduce the symptoms and repeated administration produces "desensitization" and symptomatic improvement.

The possible relationship of histamine to various types of shock has received much attention. It was suggested at one time that histamine may play a role in traumatic shock, but this view has now been largely abandoned. Evidence has recently been offered for the role of histamine in shock induced by endotoxin. Histamine seems to be involved in the first phase of endotoxin shock in dogs, and catecholamines in the second hypotensive phase.[72]

The recently reported lipolysis from adipose tissue by exogenous or endogenous histamine[10] is of great interest, since it suggests that by virtue of their histamine content, adipose tissue mast cells may be of importance in the regulation of lipid mobilization.[10]

MEDICAL USES

Histamine is useful as a diagnostic adjunct for differentiating pernicious anemia from other diseases of the stomach on the basis of achlorhydria. It is also used occasionally in the diagnosis of pheochromocytoma, since it stimulates the output of catecholamines from the adrenal medullary tumor. Intracutaneous injections of histamine may be used for revealing the integrity of blood supply and innervation to an area. Other medical uses based on its vasodilator action are obsolete.

Although histamine is an excellent vasodilator, it has too many adverse effects. Its use is dangerous in asthmatics and in individuals in whom sudden hypotension may cause serious effects. Its effect on gastric secretion, not antagonized by the antihistamines, is a serious disadvantage also. In animals, gastric ulcerations can be induced by slowly absorbed histamine preparations injected intramuscularly.

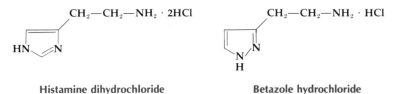

Histamine dihydrochloride   Betazole hydrochloride

Betazole is an isomer of histamine that stimulates gastric secretion but has only one-fiftieth the potency of histamine. Furthermore, it has relatively less effect than histamine on the cardiovascular system and may be safer for determination of gastric acidity. However, the drug may be dangerous in asthmatics.

Histamine preparations include histamine phosphate solutions for injection, containing 0.275, 0.55, and 2.75 mg./ml. Betazole hydrochloride (Histalog) is available as a solution for injection, 50 mg. in 1 ml.

References

1 Copenhaver, J. H., Jr., Nagler, M. E., and Goth, A.: The intracellular distribution of histamine, J. Pharmacol. Exp. Ther. 109:401, 1953.

2 Dale, H. H., and Laidlaw, P. P.: The physiological action of β-iminozolylethylamine, J. Physiol. 41:318, 1910.

3 Diana, J. N., and Kaiser, R. S.: Pre- and postcapillary resistance during histamine infusion in isolated dog hindlimb, Amer. J. Physiol. 218:132, 1970.

4 Dragstedt, C. A.: Anaphylaxis, Physiol. Rev. 21:563, 1941.

5 Dragstedt, C. A.: The role of histamine and other metabolites in anaphylaxis, Ann. N.Y. Acad. Sci. 50:1039, 1950.

6 Feldberg, W., and Loeser, A. A.: Histamine content of human skin in different clinical disorders, J. Physiol. 126:286, 1954.

7 Feldberg, W., and Schachter, M.: Histamine release by horse serum from skin of the sensitized dog and the nonsensitized cat, J. Physiol. 188:124, 1952.

8 Feldberg, W., and Talesnik, J.: Reduction of tissue histamine by compound 48/80, J. Physiol. 120:550, 1953.

9 Flacke, W., Atamackovic, D., Gillis, R. A., and Alper, M. H.: The actions of histamine on the mammalian heart, J. Pharmacol. Exp. Ther. 155:271, 1967.

10 Fredholm, B. B., and Frisk-Holmberg, M.: Lipolysis in canine subcutaneous tissue following release of endogenous histamine, Europ. J. Pharmacol. 13:254, 1971.

11 Goth, A.: Inhibition of anaphylactoid edema in the rat by 2-deoxyglucose, Amer. J. Physiol. 197:1056, 1959.

12 Goth, A., Adams, H. R., and Knoohuizen, M.: Phosphatidylserine: selective enhancer of histamine release, Science 173:1034, 1971.

13 Goth, A., Nash, W. L., Nagler, M., and Holman, J.: Inhibition of histamine release in experimental diabetes, Amer. J. Physiol. 199:25, 1957.

14 Haddy, F.: Effect of histamine on small and large vessel pressures in the dog foreleg, Amer. J. Physiol. 198:161, 1960.

15 Halpern, B. N.: Histamine release by long chain

molecules. In Ciba Foundation Symposium on Histamine, Boston, 1956, Little, Brown & Co.

16 Halpern, B. N., and Briot, M.: Étude pathogérapeutique et thérapeutique du syndrome oedèmateux provoqué chez le rat par l'ovalbumine. Arch. Int. Pharmacodyn. 82:247, 1950.

17 Halpern, B. N., and Briot, M.: Mecanisme histaminique de l'action de la polyvinylpyrrolidone chez le chien, C. R. Soc. Biol. 147:643, 1953.

18 Haverback, B. J., Tecimer, L. B., Tyce, B. J., Cohen, M., Stubrin, M. L., and Santa Ana, A. D.: The effect of gastrin on stomach histamine in the rat, Life Sci. 3:637, 1964.

19 Högberg, B., and Uvnas, B.: The mechanism of the disruption of mast cells produced by compound 48/80, Acta Physiol. Scand. 41:344, 1957.

20 Högberg, B., and Uvnas, B.: Further observations on the disruption of rat mesentery mast cells caused by compound 48/80, antigen-antibody reaction, lecithinase A and decylamine, Acta Physiol. Scand. 48:133, 1960.

21 Horton, B. T.: Use of histamine in the treatment of specific types of headache, J.A.M.A. 116:377, 1941.

22 Horton, B. T.: Management of vascular headache, Angiology 10:43, 1959.

23 James, L. P., and Austen, K. F.: Fatal systemic anaphylaxis in man, New Eng. J. Med. 270:597, 1964.

24 Kahlson, G.: A place for histamine in normal physiology, Lancet 1:67, 1960.

25 Kim, K. S., and Shore, P. A.: Mechanism of action of reserpine and insulin on gastric amines and gastric acid secretion, and the effect of monoamine oxidase inhibition, J. Pharmacol. Exp. Ther. 141:321, 1963.

26 Krantz, J. C., Jr., Carr, C. J., Bird, J. G., and Cook, S.: Sugar alcohols: pharmacodynamic studies of polyoxyalkylene derivatives of hexitol anhydride partial fatty acid esters, J. Pharmacol. Exp. Ther. 93:188, 1948.

27 Kusner, E. J., Dunnick, B., and Herzog, D. J.: The inhibition by disodium cromoglycate in vitro of anaphylactically induced histamine release from rat peritoneal mast cells, J. Pharmacol. Exp. Ther. 184:41, 1973.

28 Levine, R. J., Sato, T. L., and Sjoerdsma, A.: Inhibition of histamine synthesis in the rat by hydrazino analog of histidine and 4-bromo-3-hydroxy benzyloxyamine, Biochem. Pharmacol. 14:139, 1965.

29 Lewis, T.: The blood vessels of the human skin and their responses, London, 1927, Shaw & Sons, Ltd.

30 Lewis, T., and Grant, R. T.: Vascular reactions of the skin to injury: the liberation of histamine-like substance in injured skin; the underlying cause of factitious urticaria and of wheals produced by burning; and observations upon the nervous control of certain skin reactions, Heart 11:209, 1924.

31 Lichtenstein, L. M., Henney, C. S., Bourne, H. R., and Greenough, W. B.: Effects of cholera toxin on in vitro models of immediate and delayed hypersensitivity, J. Clin. Invest. 52:691, 1973.

32 Lichtenstein, L. M., and Margolis, S.: Histamine release in vitro: inhibition by catecholamines and methylxanthines, Science 161:902, 1968.

33 MacMillan, W. H., and Vane, J. R.: The effects of histamine on the plasma potassium levels of cats, J. Pharmacol. Exp. Ther. 118:182, 1956.

34 Mongar, J. L., and Schild, H. O.: A comparison of the effects of anaphylactic shock and of chemical histamine releasers, J. Physiol. 118:461, 1952.

35 Mongar, J. L., and Schild, H. O.: Effect of antigen and organic bases on intracellular histamine in guinea-pig lung, J. Physiol. 131:207, 1956.

36 Norton, S., and de Beer, E. J.: Effect of some antibiotics on rat mast cells in vitro, Arch. Int. Pharmacodyn. 102:352, 1955.

37 Orange, R. P., Valentine, M. D., and Austen, K. F.: Release of slow reacting substance of anaphylaxis in the rat; polymorphonuclear leukocyte, Science 157:318, 1967.

38 Paton, W. D. M.: Histamine release by compounds of simple chemical structure, Pharmacol. Rev. 9:269, 1957.

39 Piper, P. J., and Vane, J. R.: Release of additional factors in anaphylaxis and its antagonism by anti-inflammatory drugs, Nature 223:29, 1969.

40 Riley, J. F.: The effects of histamine-liberators on the mast cells of the rat, J. Path. Bact. 65:471, 1953.

41 Rocha e Silva, M., subeditor: Histamine and anti-histaminics. Encyclopedia of experimental pharmacology, vol. 18, Berlin, 1966, Springer-Verlag.

42 Rowley, D. A., and Benditt, E. P.: 5-Hydroxytryptamine and histamine as mediators of the vascular injury produced by agents which damage mast cells in rats, J. Exp. Med. 103:399, 1956.

43 Schayer, R. W.: Biogenesis of histamine, J. Biol. Chem. 199:245, 1952.

44 Schayer, R. W.: Studies on histamine-metabolizing enzymes in intact animals, J. Biol. Chem. 203:787, 1953.

45 Schayer, R. W.: Catabolism of physiological quantities of histamine in vivo, Physiol. Rev. 39:116, 1959.

46 Schayer, R. W., and Cooper, J. A. D.: Metabolism of C^{14} histamine in man, J. Appl. Physiol. 9:481, 1956.

47 Schayer, R. W., and Ganley, O. H.: Adaptive increase in mammalian histidine decarboxylase activity in response to nonspecific stress, Amer. J. Physiol. 197:721, 1959.

48 Schayer, R. W., and Karjala, S. A.: Ring N methylation: a major route of histamine metabolism, J. Biol. Chem. 221:307, 1956.

49 Schayer, R. W., Kennedy, J., and Smiley, R. L.: Studies on histamine-metabolizing enzymes in intact animals, J. Biol. Chem. 205:739, 1953.

50 Schayer, R. W., and Smiley, R. L.: Binding and release of radioactive histamine in intact rats, Amer. J. Physiol. 177:401, 1954.

51 Selye, H.: Studies on adaptation, Endocrinology 21:169, 1937.

52 Selye, H.: Effect of ACTH and cortisone upon an "anaphylactoid reaction," Canad. Med. Ass. J. 61:553, 1949.

53 Shore, P. A., Burkhalter, A., and Cohn, V. H., Jr.: A method for the fluorometric assay of histamine in tissues, J. Pharmacol. Exp. Ther. 127:182, 1959.

54 Smith, D. E.: Nature of the secretory activity of the mast cell, Amer. J. Physiol. 193:573, 1958.

55 Synder, S. H., and Epps, L.: Regulation of histidine decarboxylase in rat stomach by gastrin: the effect of inhibitors of protein synthesis, Molec. Pharmacol. 4:187, 1968.

56 Tabor, H.: Metabolic studies on histidine, histamine, and related imidazoles, Pharmacol. Rev. 6:299, 1954.

57 Trendelenburg, U.: Non-nicotinic ganglion-stimulating substances, Fed. Proc. 18:1001, 1959.

58 Ungar, G., and Damgaard, E.: Tissue reactions to anaphylactic and anaphylactoid stimuli: proteolysis and release of histamine and heparin, J. Exp. Med. 101:1, 1955.

59 Urbach, K. F.: Nature and probable origin of conjugated histamine excreted after ingestion of histamine, Proc. Soc. Exp. Biol. Med. 70:146, 1949.

60 Uvnas, B.: The mechanism of histamine liberation, J. Pharm. Pharmacol. 10:1, 1958.

61 Van Arsdel, P. P., Jr., and Beall, G. N.: The metabolism and functions of histamine, Arch. Intern. Med. 106:192, 1960.

62 Walton, R. P., Richardson, J. A., and Thompson, W. L.: Hypotension and histamine release following intravenous injection of plasma substitutes, J. Pharmacol. Exp. Ther. 127:39, 1959.

63 Wilson, C. W. M.: Factors influencing the urinary excretion of histamine in the rat, J. Physiol. 126:141, 1954.

Recent reviews

64 Black, J. W., Duncan, W. A. M., Durant, C. J., Ganellin, C. R., and Parsons, E. M.: Definition and antagonism of histamine H$_2$-receptors, Nature 236:385, 1972.

65 Goth, A.: Histamine release by drugs and chemicals. In Schachter, M., editor: International encyclopedia of pharmacology and therapy: histamine and antihistamines, vol. 1. New York, 1973, Pergamon Press.

66 Green, J. P.: Binding of some biogenic amines in tissues, Advances Pharmacol. 1:349, 1962.

67 Haverback, B. J., and Wirtschafter, S. K.: The gastrointestinal tract and naturally occurring pharmacologically active amines, Advances Pharmacol. 1:309, 1962.

68 Kahlson, G., and Rosengren, E.: Histamine, Ann. Rev. Pharmacol. 5:305, 1965.

69 Mongar, J. L., and Schild, H. O.: Cellular mechanisms in anaphylaxis, Physiol. Rev. 42:226, 1962.

70 Silen, W. B.: Advances in gastric physiology, New Eng. J. Med. 277:864, 1968.

71 Thompson, J. C.: Gastrin and gastric secretion, Ann. Rev. Med. 20:291, 1969.

72 Vick, J. A.: Bioassay of the prominent humoral agents involved in endotoxin shock. Amer. J. Physiol. 209:75, 1965.

73 West, G. B.: Studies on the mechanism of anaphylaxis: a possible basis for the pharmacologic approach to allergy. Clin. Pharmacol. Ther. 4:749, 1963.

16 Antihistaminic drugs

Drugs that block the effects of histamine competitively at various receptor sites are referred to as antihistaminic drugs. The actions of histamine on bronchial and intestinal smooth muscles can be blocked by the conventional antihistamines exemplified by mepyramine. On the other hand, the effects of histamine on gastric secretion are not blocked by the usual antihistamines but are prevented by the newer type of competitor, exemplified by burimamide.

The antihistaminics should be classified as H_1 receptor antagonists and H_2 receptor antagonists. The commonly available antihistaminics are H_1 receptor antagonists. The H_2 receptor antagonists are still experimental but are of great theoretical and possibly practical interest. Burimamide and metiamide are H_2 receptor antagonists.[12]

Some antihistaminic drugs are useful not only in allergic diseases but also for the prevention of motion sickness and in the treatment of parkinsonism. Also, their sedative effect may be of some benefit. Finally, the phenothiazine tranquilizers were developed as an outgrowth of studies on promethazine, a sedative phenothiazine antihistaminic.

DEVELOPMENT

Until about 1937 the only way to antagonize the actions of histamine consisted in administering some drug such as epinephrine that had many opposing pharmacologic actions on blood vessels and bronchial smooth muscle. The field of antihistaminics was opened up by the discovery that certain phenolic ethers could protect guinea pigs against anaphylactic shock and histamine. The response of the guinea pig to the inhalation of histamine aerosol has been used widely in subsequent development of new antihistaminics. With the recognition of the structural requirements for antihistaminic action, compounds of considerable potency and low toxicity were synthesized. Such compounds as N-benzyl-N',N'-dimethyl-N-phenylethylenediamine (Antergan), diphenhydramine, and tripelennamine were found to protect guinea pigs against as many as fifty lethal doses of histamine. These were introduced into therapeutics and were followed by an enormous number of other antihistaminics. The phenothiazine compound promethazine seemed almost the ultimate in antihistaminic action, since it could protect guinea pigs against 1,500 lethal doses of histamine. It is dangerous, however, to generalize from the results obtained in one species of animals, and the clinical results soon indicated that there was no strict correlation between these potency figures obtained in guinea pigs and effectiveness in man.

CHEMISTRY

The basic structure of the antihistaminics may be represented as a substituted ethylamine:

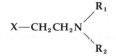

If it is recalled that histamine is 2-(4-imidazolyl)ethylamine, it is apparent that some relationship may exist between the ethylamine portion of the histamine molecule and the fact that the antihistaminics are substituted ethylamines. Perhaps this portion of the histamine molecule is essential for its attachment to some of the receptor structures.

The R groups in the ethylamine structure are in most cases CH_3. If the X in the basic structure is nitrogen, the compound may be looked on as a substituted ethylenediamine. Examples of this type of antihistaminic drugs are tripelennamine (Pyribenzamine; PBZ), methapyrilene (Thenylene; Histadyl), thonzylamine (Neohetramine), pyrilamine (Neo-Antergan), and many others. The structural formulas of tripelennamine and methapyrilene are given below.

Diphenhydramine (Benadryl), being a dimethylaminoethoxy compound, is an example of an antihistaminic in which the X of the basic structure is represented by oxygen. Its structural formula is shown below.

Dimenhydrinate (Dramamine) is a combination of diphenhydramine and 8-chlorotheophylline.

An example of an antihistaminic in which the X is carbon is chlorpheniramine (Chlor-Trimeton) (p. 198).

Promethazine (Phenergan) contains the phenothiazine structure (p. 198).

In some antihistaminics the ethylamine structure is within a heterocyclic ring. For example, cyclizine (Marezine) is 1-diphenylmethyl-4-methylpiperazine (p. 198).

Cyclizine and another piperazine derivative, meclizine (Bonamine), have been recommended particularly for the prevention of motion sickness.

Other useful antihistaminics and their average oral adult doses are methdilazine (Tacaryl), 8 mg.; carbinoxamine (Clistin), 4 mg.; triprolidine (Actidil), 2.5 mg.; dimethindene (Forhistal), 1 mg.; the dextro isomer of chlorpheniramine (Polaramine), 2 to 4 mg.; and the bromo analog of chlorpheniramine, brompheniramine (Dimetane), 4 mg. Some of the antihistaminics are also available in solution for injection. Diphenhydramine by intravenous injection may be useful in the treatment of rigidity induced by phenothiazine drugs.

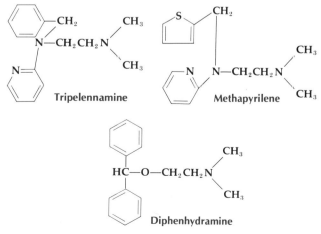

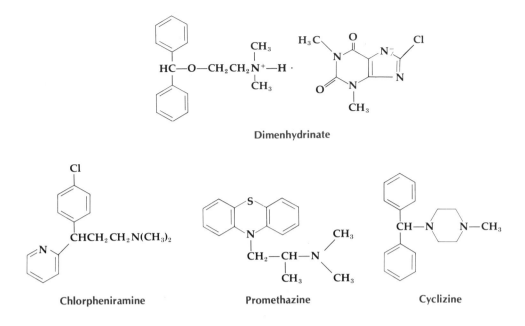

Dimenhydrinate

Chlorpheniramine   Promethazine   Cyclizine

CLINICAL PHARMACOLOGY

If a recommended dose of one of the antihistaminics is taken orally by a normal person, the only noticeable effects will be on the central nervous system. Drowsiness is quite common, and barbiturates taken simultaneously appear to be synergistic in causing sleepiness. There is no relationship between the antihistaminic potency of these drugs and their central depressant action. Chlorpheniramine produces less sedation for an equivalent antihistaminic action than diphenhydramine. An unusual antihistaminic, phenindamine (Thephorin), may even have central nervous system stimulant properties.

If the patient suffers from urticaria or hay fever, the various antihistaminics will produce considerable relief with variable sedation. Surprisingly, these drugs have very little benefit in the treatment of asthma, and this ineffectiveness has led to some doubt concerning the role of histamine in asthma.

It is important to recall that even in animal experiments the antihistaminics are more effective against exogenously administered histamine, particularly when the antihistaminic precedes the administration of histamine. In other words, the antihistaminics are more potent in preventing the actions of histamine than in reversing these actions once they develop. Another important fact that is not always appreciated is that the effectiveness of the antihistaminics against the circulatory actions of histamine is less than their ability to block bronchoconstriction induced by the amine (Fig. 16-1).

With the recognition of two separate receptors for histamine and the discovery of H_2 receptor antagonists, many puzzling aspects of the pharmacology of antihistamines can be clarified. Gastric secretion is mediated by H_2 receptors and is not blocked by the commonly available antihistamines, which are H_1 receptor antagonists.[12] It appears also that vasodilatation and increased capillary permeability are mediated by both types of receptors and such actions of histamine can be blocked completely only by a combination of H_1 and H_2 receptor antagonists.[12]

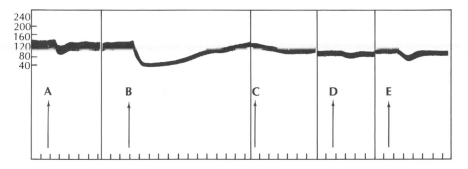

Fig. 16-1. Effect of histamine on blood pressure and its antagonism by an antihistaminic drug. **A,** Histamine, 1 μg/kg. I.V. **B,** Histamine, 5 μg/kg. I.V. **C,** Diphenhydramine, 5 mg./kg. I.V. **D,** Histamine, 1 μg/kg. I.V. **E,** Histamine, 5 μg/kg. I.V. Blood pressure recording of dog anesthetized with pentobarbital sodium. Time in 15 seconds. Note that the antihistaminic drug, while exerting considerable protection against vasodepressor action of histamine, failed to eliminate it completely.

The antihistaminics are symptomatic drugs, and there is no good evidence to indicate that they block antigen-antibody reactions or histamine release. There is some evidence from in vitro experiments that antihistaminics can block histamine release from rat peritoneal mast cells. The significance of this effect under in vivo conditions is not clear.[11]

Antihistaminics are often applied topically to obtain symptomatic improvement in itching skin conditions, but in several cases contact dermatitis developed as a consequence of sensitization of the patient to the topically applied antihistaminics. It may seem paradoxical that an antihistamine could sensitize an individual, but actually there is no reason why these drugs could not produce allergic sensitization in the same manner as many other small-molecule compounds such as the sulfonamides.

MISCELLANEOUS ACTIONS

Besides being competitive antagonists of histamine, the antihistaminics have a number of additional actions. These are (1) central nervous system effect, (2) anticholinergic effect, (3) local anesthetic properties, (4) antiserotonin action, and (5) cocaine-like effect on catecholamine uptake.

Antihistaminics produce a *sedative CNS effect* different from the actions of barbiturates and other sedative-hypnotics. The sedative effect of the antihistaminics is not pleasant. Furthermore, if the dose of the antihistamine is increased, sedation is replaced by marked irritability, leading to convulsions, hyperpyrexia, and even death. Toxic doses are likely to produce excitation in children. Additional CNS effects are probably related to anticholinergic properties.

The *anticholinergic effect* manifests itself as a drying of salivary and bronchial secretions, similar to the effect of atropine. For the same reason these drugs may have adverse effects in the treatment of bronchial asthma by increasing the viscosity of secretions in the respiratory tract.

The anticholinergic effect of the antihistaminics may be related to their usefulness in the prevention of motion sickness.[2,3] Dimenhydrinate is widely used for this. There is good indication from clinical studies that the drug owes its anti-motion sickness properties to diphenhydramine, one of its components. Certain antihistaminics such as cyclizine and meclizine are especially recommended for the prevention of motion sickness. The effectiveness of diphenhydramine in Parkinson's disease may also be due to its anticholinergic properties.

The *local anesthetic properties* of antihistaminics make them suitable as antipruritic agents in topical applications. Unfortunately they may cause sensitization, and their use as topical agents is best avoided.

Antiserotonin properties are quite common in antihistaminic drugs. At least one, cyproheptadine (Periactin), is generally viewed as a combined antihistamine-antiserotonin. There is no reason to believe, however, that antagonism to serotonin confers any special advantages in an antihistaminic.

The *cocainelike effect* of most antihistaminics[6] may only be a curiosity and has no practical importance at present.

THERAPEUTIC USES

There are many conditions in which antihistaminics are helpful. There are others in which they are used but perhaps should not be.[15]

Conditions in which the antihistaminics are helpful include allergic rhinitis, urticaria, some types of asthma, and motion sickness. Conditions in which antihistaminics are either not the drugs of choice or should not be used include acute anaphylactic emergencies (epinephrine is much more useful), most cases of asthma, diseases of the skin, eyes, and nose, and the common cold.

In the selection of antihistaminics, their sedative action is a major consideration.

Table 16-1. Doses and sedative properties of various antihistamines*

Generic name	Trade name	Usual adult dose (mg.)	Degree of sedation
Carbinoxamine	Clistin	4	+
Chlorothen	Tagathen	25	+
Phenindamine	Thephorin	25	+†
Chlorpheniramine	Chlor-Trimeton	4	++
Brompheniramine	Dimetane	4	++
Triprolidine	Actidil	2.5	++
Doxylamine	Decapryn	12.5	++
Chlorcyclizine	Di-Paralene	50	++
Methapyriline	Histadyl	25	++
Dimethindine	Forhistal	1	++
Pyrilamine	Neo-Antergan	25	++
Cyproheptadine	Periactin	4	++
Tripelennamine	Pyribenzamine	50	++
Diphenhydramine	Benadryl	50	+++
Promethazine	Phenergan	12.5	+++

* Based on data from Feinberg, S. M.: Pharmacol. Physicians **1**(12):1, 1967.
† Stimulation possible.

Potency is not so important, since it only influences the size of the tablets used. The duration of action of most antihistamines when given in a therapeutic dose is about 4 hours and is greatly influenced by the dose. The usual adult doses and sedative potencies of a number of antihistamines are shown in Table 16-1.

ABSORPTION AND METABOLISM

The antihistaminics are well absorbed from the gastrointestinal tract. The fate of the drugs following absorption has been studied only in some cases. Diphenhydramine has been shown to leave the bloodstream rapidly and become concentrated in the tissue, particularly the lungs, kidneys, liver, and brain. Practically all the drug is metabolically altered and is excreted in less than 24 hours.

TOXICITY

On the whole the antihistaminics are remarkably nontoxic compounds when used in the recommended doses. It is possible that the widespread use of these drugs may contribute to automobile accidents because of their sedative properties. It is also likely that the simultaneous use of antihistaminics and other depressant drugs such as barbiturates or alcohol may exert synergistic depressant actions.[5] A few cases of skin sensitization have been reported following topical use of antihistaminics.

Acute poisoning has occurred following ingestion of very large doses of the antihistaminics, particularly in children. Surprisingly, the symptoms consisted of central nervous system excitation and convulsive phenomena. The management of acute poisoning is purely symptomatic. The anticonvulsant barbiturates must be tried very cautiously because there is experimental evidence that their toxicity may be additive to that of the antihistaminics.

Some of the antihistaminics commonly used for the prevention of motion sickness have been found to be teratogenic in rats. As a consequence, meclizine, cyclizine, and chlorcyclizine should not be used in pregnant women and preparations offered for self-medication must bear a warning to that effect.[16] The teratogenic effect is not related to an antihistaminic effect but seems related to a structural feature, all of these drugs being piperazines.

ANTIHISTAMINICS WITH ANTISEROTONIN ACTION

Among the antihistaminic drugs, promethazine has considerable antiserotonin action on smooth muscles, approaching LSD in this activity. Chlorpromazine, a tranquilizer, is about half as active. A relatively new antihistaminic, cyproheptadine hydrochloride, is a potent antiserotonin drug as well.

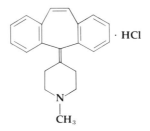

Cyproheptadine hydrochloride

Administered in doses of 4 to 20 mg. daily, cyproheptadine is available for the same indications as other antihistaminics. In addition, there are claims for its effectiveness in the postgastrectomy dumping syndrome and other conditions, but further experience is needed for evaluating these claims.

H₂ RECEPTOR ANTAGONISTS: BURIMAMIDE AND METIAMIDE

The new antihistaminic burimamide[12] and derivatives have been defined as H_2 receptor antagonists. They antagonize those responses to histamine, such as gastric secretory effect, that are uninfluenced by the previously discussed H_1 receptor antagonists.

Burimamide not only antagonizes the gastric secretory effect of histamine but also that of pentagastrin,[12] indicating a relationship between the action of gastrin and histamine. It is of great interest also that the vasodilator and capillary permeability increasing actions of histamine can be antagonized by a combination of burimamide and an H_1 receptor antagonist.

The discovery of potent H_2 receptor antagonists may have far-reaching consequences. The role of histamine in physiologic and pathologic states will have to be reexamined with the availability of this new tool.

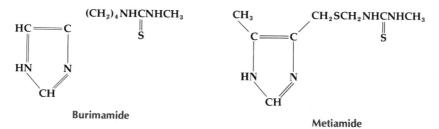

Burimamide

Metiamide

Metiamide is closely related to burimamide but has a much greater potency as an H_2 receptor antagonist. Its effect in reducing gastric hydrochloric acid secretion in man is impressive.

References

1 Bovet, D., and Staub, A.: Action protrectrice des éthers phénoliques au cours de l'intoxication histaminique, C. R. Soc. Biol. **124**:547, 1937.

2 Chinn, H. I., and Milch, L. J.: Comparison of airsickness preventives, J. Appl. Physiol. **5**:162, 1952.

3 Chinn, H. I., and Oberst, F. W.: Effectiveness of various drugs in prevention of airsickness, Proc. Soc. Exp. Biol. Med. **73**:218, 1950.

4 Glazko, A. J., and Dill, W. A.: Biochemical studies on diphenhydramine (Benadryl): distribution in tissues and urinary excretion, J. Biol. Chem. **179**:403, 1949.

5 Hughes, F. W., and Forney, R. B.: Comparative effects of three antihistaminics and ethanol on mental and motor performance, Clin. Pharmacol. Ther. **5**:414, 1964.

6 Isaac, L., and Goth, A.: Interaction of antihistaminics with norepinephrine uptake: a cocaine-like effect, Life Sci. **4**:1899, 1965.

7 Isaac, L., and Goth, A.: The mechanism of the potentiation of norepinephrine by antihistaminics, J. Pharmacol. Exp. Ther. **156**:463, 1967.

8 Stone, C. A., Wenger, H. C., Ludden, C. T., Stavorski, J. M., and Ross, C. A.: Anti-serotonin-antihistaminic properties of cyproheptadine, J. Pharmacol. Exp. Ther. **131**:73, 1961.

9 Weinman, E. O., and Geissman, T. A.: The distribution, excretion, and metabolism of C¹⁴-labeled tripelennamine (Pyribenzamine) by guinea pigs, J. Pharmacol. Exp. Ther. **125**:1, 1959.

10 Winbury, M. M., and Alworth, B. L.: Suppression of experimental atrial arrhythmias by several antihistamines, Arch. Int. Pharmacodyn. **122**:318, 1959.

11 Zeppa, R., and Hemingway, G. C.: Inhibition of histamine release from mast cells, Surg. Forum **14**:56, 1963.

Recent reviews

12 Black, J. W., Duncan, W. A. M., Durant, C. J., Ganellin, C. R., and Parsons, E. M.: Definition and antagonism of histamine receptors, Nature **236**:385, 1972.

13 Brand, J. J.: The pharmacologic basis for the control of motion sickness by drugs, Pharmacol. Physicians 2(3):1, 1968.

14 Brand, J. J., and Perry, W. L. M.: Drugs used in motion sickness, Pharmacol. Rev. **18**:895, 1966.

15 Feinberg, S. M.: The antihistamines: pharmacologic principles in their use, Pharmacol. Physicians. **1**(12):1, 1967.

16 Sadusk, J. F., and Palmisano, P. A.: Teratogenic effect of meclizine, cyclizine and chlorcyclizine, J.A.M.A. **194**:139, 1965.

17

Serotonin and antiserotonins

Serotonin, or 5-hydroxytryptamine, occupies a surprisingly prominent position in the medical literature, considering the ignorance that surrounds its functions in the body. The reasons for this paradox are many. This endogenously produced amine is almost certainly one of the central neurotransmitters. It is also present in large quantities in the enterochromaffin system of the intestine and in platelets, where its functions are unknown. Moreover, studies on serotonin have contributed greatly to theories on biochemical mechanisms in disease states ranging from mental disease to migraine. The relationships between LSD and serotonin and the release of the amine by reserpine provided potent stimuli for psychopharmacologic research. The same can be said of the hallucinogenic properties of many serotonin derivatives.

In addition to serotonin, some of its therapeutically useful antagonists will be discussed in this chapter. Furthermore, the pharmacology of ergot alkaloids, lysergic acid derivatives that are generally serotonin antagonists, will also be considered at this point.

SEROTONIN

The discovery of serotonin (5-hydroxytryptamine; 5-HT) as a normally occurring amine resulted from independent studies on the vasoconstrictor substance in serum[15] at the Cleveland Clinic and the active substance in intestinal enterochromaffin cells[21] named *enteramine* by investigators in Italy. The compound investigated by both groups was eventually shown to be 5-HT.

Occurrence and distribution

Serotonin is widely distributed in the animal and plant kingdom. Some fruits such as bananas contain high concentration but represent no threat of causing serotonin poisoning because the amine is not well absorbed from the gastrointestinal tract and is rapidly metabolized. Ingestion of such fruits, however, may increase the urinary excretion of serotonin metabolites, giving false positive tests in the diagnosis of carcinoid tumor.

In mammals about 90% of the total serotonin is in the enterochromaffin cells of the intestine, about 8% in platelets, and 2% in the central nervous system, particularly in the pineal gland and the hypothalamus. In rats and mice serotonin is also present in mast cells along with histamine. Human mast cells probably do not contain serotonin, since in mastocytosis the excretion of the serotonin metabolite 5-hydroxyindoleacetic acid in the urine is not increased.

At the various sites mentioned except the platelets, which actively concentrate the amine but do not make it, serotonin is synthesized from tryptophan.

Biosynthesis and metabolic degradation

Serotonin is made from tryptophan. Normally only a small fraction of the dietary tryptophan is utilized for serotonin synthesis. In patients with carcinoid tumors this fraction may increase so greatly that pellagra may result. *niacin?*

The various steps in the biosynthesis and biodegradation of serotonin are as follows:

Tryptophan → 5-Hydroxytryptophan → 5-Hydroxytryptamine → 5-Hydroxyindoleacetic acid

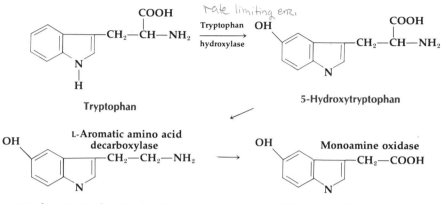

In addition, serotonin is converted in the pineal gland to *N*-acetyl serotonin and its *O*-methyl derivative, *melatonin*.

The biosynthesis of serotonin is blocked by *p-chlorophenylalanine*, which inhibits tryptophan hydroxylase, the rate-limiting enzyme. Degradation of serotonin is blocked by the MAO inhibitors. Turnover of serotonin is quite rapid in the central nervous system and also in the intestine. MAO inhibitors can double the serotonin content of brain in less than an hour.

The daily excretion of 5-hydroxyindoleacetic acid in the urine is 3 to 10 mg. in a normal adult. It increases greatly in the presence of a carcinoid tumor and also with the ingestion of bananas and the administration of reserpine, which releases serotonin from its binding sites. Excretion of 5-hydroxyindoleacetic acid is decreased by MAO inhibitors.[21]

Pharmacologic effects

The actions of serotonin are exerted on smooth muscles and on nerve elements including afferent nerve endings. The smooth muscle effects are prominent in the cardiovascular system and the gastrointestinal tract.

Intravenous injection of a few micrograms of serotonin as the creatinine sulfate complex produces a *triphasic* response: (1) a transient fall of blood pressure, (2) a brief period of hypertension, and (3) a more prolonged period of pressure lowering. The early depressor phase is probably caused by a reflex elicited by stimulation of chemoreceptors (Bezold-Jarisch effect). The blood pressure elevation is a consequence of constriction of blood vessels in many areas. Finally, the late depressor phase is attributed to the vasodilator action of serotonin in areas such as the skeletal muscle. Continuous intravenous infusion of serotonin produces only the prolonged lowering of peripheral resistance, with lowering of mean blood pressure.

In addition to its effect on the cardiovascular system, serotonin stimulates the gastro-intestinal and bronchial smooth muscles. The gastrointestinal effects are both direct and also a consequence of excitation of ganglion cells. The direct effects are blocked by serotonin antagonists such as LSD; the ganglionic action is, interestingly, blocked by morphine. The bronchial stimulant action of the drug is probably unimportant in man, although asthmatics may be unduly responsive to it.

Serotonin can stimulate afferent nerve endings, ganglion cells, and adrenal medullary cells. It does not cross the blood-brain barrier but exerts striking effects when injected into the lateral ventricles of cats.[8] Sleep, catatonia, and fever have been elicited by such injections.

Role in health and disease

Serotonin is almost certainly one of the central neurotransmitters. Normal functions have been attributed to it in sleep and in temperature regulation. p-Chlorophenylala-nine, which depletes brain serotonin, tends to decrease rapid eye movement—sleep in man.

The possible role of serotonin in mood and behavior and in mental disease comes from speculations based on several lines of evidence. First, the powerful psychotomi-metic drug LSD was early found to inhibit the actions of serotonin on smooth muscles. The simple hypothesis based on these facts found little support, however, when it was shown that other antiserotonins, even the closely related D-2-bromolysergic acid diethylamide, were not psychotomimetic. When reserpine, the powerful tranquilizer, was shown to release serotonin from the central nervous system, hopes were again aroused for finding a simple chemical theory of the basis of mood and behavior. It was shown subsequently, however, that reserpine depletes catecholamines also from the brain. Furthermore, p-chlorophenylalanine, which depletes serotonin by inhibiting its synthesis, does not cause the same effects as reserpine.

The final remaining speculation in regard to a link between serotonin and mental disease is the demonstrated hallucinogenic effect of a variety of compounds structually related to the amine. For example, bufotenine is 5-hydroxy-dimethyltryptamine, and psilocin is 4-hydroxy-dimethyltryptamine. Bufotenine is present in some plants and in toads. Psilocin and its phosphoryl ester psilocybin are very potent LSD-like hallu-cinogens. Many other tryptamine derivatives have psychotomimetic effects, and it is intriguing to speculate on biochemical explanations of schizophrenia. A critical review of this problem[10] concluded that all such speculations are interesting but up to then, at least, not convincing.

Serotonin probably plays a role in intestinal motility, since there is an abundance of this amine in the enterochromaffin cells that can be released by distention and other mechanical stimuli. Morphine blocks the effects of serotonin on intramural ganglion cells.

Serotonin probably plays a role in the causation of symptoms in the *carcinoid syn-drome*. Flushing and increased intestinal motility have been attributed to serotonin release. However, the flush that occurs in carcinoid patients cannot be elicited by the injection of serotonin but will occur, on the other hand, after the administration of epinephrine or bradykinin.[14] It has been shown that kinin-producing enzymes are released from the carcinoid tumor. In addition, in the gastric carcinoid syndrome his-tamine plays an important role. The ameliorating effect of p-chlorophenylalanine on intestinal motility of carcinoid patients suggests a role for serotonin in its causation.[6]

The role of serotonin in platelets is completely unknown, although for years it was believed to play a role in hemostasis as the vasoconstrictor of serum. This hypothesis was put to a test when reserpine became available as a serotonin depletor.[9] Reserpine was administered to patients in sufficient dosage to reduce serotonin levels to negligible amounts. This procedure had no effect on bleeding time or clotting time, a result that casts doubt on the role of serotonin in hemostasis.

Because of the effectiveness of several serotonin antagonists in the prevention of *migraine,* a role for the amine in the causation of vascular headaches has been suggested. The evidence for this is poor. Intravenous infusions of small doses of serotonin in man do not produce migrainelike headaches but rather the following symptoms: facial flush, intestinal hypermotility, mild epigastric pain, heaviness in the legs and arms, nausea, and tightness across the chest. In an occasional individual there may be a sudden fall of blood pressure, bradycardia, or tachycardia.

The unique features of serotonin metabolism in the pineal gland and its relationship to melatonin have been commented on (p. 72).

SEROTONIN ANTAGONISTS, OR ANTISEROTONINS

There are numerous pharmacologic antagonists of serotonin. Many of these drugs have important applications in medicine, although their therapeutic usefulness generally has nothing to do with antiserotonin action.

Serotonin antagonists include numerous *lysergic acid derivatives,* many of which are naturally occurring ergot alkaloids. Methysergide (Sansert) is a potent antiserotonin of clinical usefulness in the prevention of vascular headaches. Other lysergic acid derivatives that are potent antiserotonins include LSD and D-2-bromolysergic acid diethylamide. Many *antihistamines* have antiserotonin effects also. Among these *cyproheptadine* (Periactin) is potent and has been discussed among the antihistamines (p. 201). *Chlorpromazine,* other *phenothiazines,* and *alpha adrenergic blocking agents* such as *phenoxybenzamine* also block the effects of serotonin.

For practical purposes methysergide (Sansert) and cyproheptadine (Periactin) are the only two drugs available for antagonizing symptoms that might be attributed to serotonin clinically.

Methysergide maleate

Methysergide is closely related to the ergot alkaloid methyl-ergonovine, which is used as an oxytocic drug. It is 1-methyl-*d*-lysergic acid butanolamide and was introduced specifically as a prophylactic agent for migraine headaches. It is a potent serotonin antagonist, even more potent than ergotamine or LSD. The drug is useful only for the prevention and not for the treatment of migraine. Its mode of action is not well understood, since connections between migraine and serotonin are in the realm of speculation.

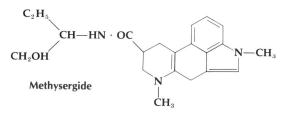

Methysergide

Adverse reactions to methysergide are many and include nausea, dizziness, insomnia, behavioral changes (reminiscent of mild LSD reactions), gastrointestinal disturbances, and others. A serious complication seen in several patients after long-term use of methysergide was retroperitoneal fibrosis and pleural pulmonary fibrosis. Retroperitoneal fibrosis may lead to urinary tract obstruction.

Contraindications to the use of methysergide are peripheral vascular disease, hypertension, peptic ulcer, coronary artery disease, and pregnancy.

Methysergide maleate (Sansert) is available in tablets containing 2 mg.

Cyproheptadine hydrochloride

Cyproheptadine hydrochloride is an antihistaminic drug with also potent antiserotonin properties. It has been proposed for some indications that are different from those requiring the usual antihistamines. The drug is effective in the treatment of allergic rhinitis and for the relief of pruritus in a variety of skin disorders. In addition, it is claimed to be effective in promoting weight gain in children by mechanisms that are not understood.

The main untoward effect seen after the administration of cyproheptadine is drowsiness. Preparations of cyproheptadine hydrochloride (Periactin hydrochloride) include tablets, 4 mg., and syrup, 2 mg./5 ml.

ERGOT ALKALOIDS

Some of the ergot alkaloids are quite useful in treating vascular headaches, some are employed for stimulating the uterine smooth muscle, and still others have been tried as hypotensive agents. The work on lysergic acid diethylamide (LSD) is an outgrowth of pharmacologic studies on ergot alkaloids.

Historical aspects of pharmacology

It has been known for centuries that ingestion of diseased rye can cause poisoning characterized by gangrene, abortion, and sometimes convulsions. The fungus that causes this disease of rye is *Claviceps purpurea*, often called *ergot*. It contains a large variety of potent pharmacologic agents referred to as the ergot alkaloids, many of which are derivatives of lysergic acid. The structural formulas of lysergic acid and ergonovine, one of the ergot alkaloids, are shown below.

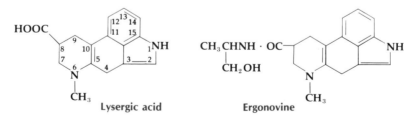

Lysergic acid   Ergonovine

The isolation of ergotamine and ergotoxine, a mixture of ergot alkaloids, led to the belief that most of the pharmacologic properties of ergot were due to these compounds. It was later shown, however, that crude ergot extracts had a greater effect on the uterus than did ergotamine or ergotoxine.[5] Soon the alkaloid ergonovine was also isolated, and this unsuspected new compound served to explain the greater activity of the crude extracts.

Chemistry

The important alkaloids of ergot are ergotamine, ergotoxine, and ergonovine. In addition, ergotoxine has been shown to be a mixture of three compounds, ergocristine, ergocryptine, and ergocornine.

From a chemical standpoint, ergonovine is the simplest compound. Its structural formula indicates that it is a combination of lysergic acid with d-2-aminopropanol.

In contrast to ergonovine, ergotamine and the ergotoxine group yield amino acids on hydrolysis and have a considerably higher molecular weight than ergonovine, although they also are lysergic acid derivatives.

Pharmacologic effects

The ergot alkaloids have three major actions in the body: smooth muscle contraction, particularly evident on blood vessels and the uterus, adrenergic blocking effect, and central nervous system effects leading to hypotension. These actions are present to a varying extent in the different alkaloids. Ergonovine has powerful smooth muscle effects without the other properties characteristic of many of the other alkaloids. Ergotamine and the ergotoxine group have smooth muscle actions and can also block norepinephrine and epinephrine.

The two most commonly used ergot alkaloids in therapeutics are ergotamine (Gynergen) and ergonovine (Ergotrate). Ergotamine is extensively employed in the treatment of vascular headaches such as migraine, whereas ergonovine finds its greatest usefulness in obstetrics for its stimulant effect on the uterine smooth muscle.

Ergotamine tartrate

Ergotamine tartrate is used almost exclusively in the treatment of migraine and other vascular headaches, and its effects can be best illustrated by describing its actions when administered to a patient suffering from such headaches.

Migraine is a severe periodic headache often associated with nausea and vomiting, a so-called sick headache. Little is known about the basic pathogenesis of this condition except that vascular phenomena must play an important role in its causation. The attacks are usually preceded by certain prodromal symptoms and some visual disturbances. At the height of the headache such extracranial vessels as the temporal arteries are highly pulsatile and may even be edematous on the affected side.

It is believed by workers in this field that during the early stages of the attack there is constriction of blood vessels, followed by their marked dilatation.[19] The early visual disturbances are attributed to constriction of retinal vessels, whereas the headache itself may be related to dilatation and edema of the extracranial vessels.

Ergotamine tartrate is the drug of choice in the treatment of migraine and is believed to act by vasoconstriction. The drug may be given orally or injected subcutaneously or intramuscularly. Its effectiveness in relieving a headache is considered to be of diagnostic value.

Although the drug is very effective it is not suitable for long-continued or prophylactic use because of serious adverse effects such as severe vasoconstriction and gangrene of the extremities. For prophylaxis of migraine, methysergide (discussed previously) is commonly used, but it also has many untoward effects and contraindications.

Adverse effects caused by ergotamine tartrate include nausea, vomiting, diarrhea, vasoconstriction, and gangrene of the extremities. Because of its adverse effects the drug is contraindicated in pregnancy and all vascular diseases.

Preparations of ergotamine tartrate (Gynergen) include 1 mg. tablets and solution for injection, 0.5 mg./ml. Ergotamine tartrate is also available in sublingual tablets, 2 mg., and for inhalation in Medihalers, which dispense 0.36 mg. of the drug in each inhalation.

Ergonovine maleate

Ergonovine maleate (Ergotrate maleate) and its derivative, methylergonovine (Methergine), are used exclusively in obstetrics. They are less effective than ergotamine in migraine.

Ergonovine and methylergonovine are powerful oxytocics and have significant vasoconstrictor effects, but they lack the adrenergic blocking action of ergotamine. They are well absorbed from the gastrointestinal tract, whereas the larger amino acid alkaloids are only partially absorbed. They may produce hypertension.

Ergonovine and methylergonovine are used in obstetrics in the third stage of labor, principally to decrease postpartum bleeding through their powerful effect on direct contraction of the uterine smooth muscle.

Although ergonovine and methylergonovine have powerful effects on the uterus they do not promote normal uterine contractions as does oxytocin. For this reason they should not be employed for initiation of labor.

Adverse effects to ergonovine and methylergonovine include nausea, vomiting, and elevations of blood pressure.

Ergonovine maleate (Ergotrate maleate) is available in tablets containing 0.2 mg. and in solution for injection, 0.2 mg./ml. Methylergonovine maleate (Methergine) is available in tablets, 0.2 mg., and solution for injection, 0.2 mg./ml.

Dihydroergotoxine mesylate

The dihydrogenated alkaloids of the ergotoxine group are available in the preparation known as dihydroergotoxine mesylate (Hydergine), which contains 0.1 mg. of each of the three alkaloids in the injectable solution. This preparation has both adrenergic blocking actions and an inhibitory effect on sympathetic tone through depression of central autonomic regulations. It can cause bradycardia and considerable lowering of blood pressure. The drug produces side effects of nausea, vomiting, headache, and nasal stuffiness. It has some uses in the treatment of peripheral vascular diseases, being administered intravenously or intramuscularly in doses of 0.3 to 1 mg.

Ergot poisoning

Poisoning with ergot alkaloids occasionally follows ingestion of bread prepared from ergot-contaminated rye. There were large epidemics in the past, and occasional outbreaks still occur in some parts of the world. Poisoning may also be produced when patients take ergot alkaloids in fairly large doses over a long period of time for migraine or for the purpose of inducing abortion.

The symptoms and signs of ergot poisoning depend upon whether the poisoning is acute or chronic. In chronic poisoning the clinical picture is dominated by gangrene. In acute poisoning there may be vomiting, diarrhea, headache, vertigo, paresthesia, convulsions, and gangrene of the fingers, toes, nose, or ears. The skin may be cold and cyanotic. The pulse may be slow, but more frequently it is rapid and weak. Treatment with vasodilators such as papaverine and sympathetic nerve block has been tried, but there is no consensus on its effectiveness. The most important preventive measure is avoidance of long-continued use of ergotamine tartrate for vascular headaches.

References

1 Axelrod, J.: Discussion of paper by Uden-friend, S.: Amine metabolism and its pharmacological implications. In Neuropharmacology, Transactions of the Fifth Conference, New York, 1960, Josiah Macy, Jr., Foundation.

2 Brodie, B. B., Olin, J. S., Kuntzman, R. G., and Shore, P. A.: Possible interrelationship between release of brain norepinephrine and serotonin by reserpine, Science 125:1293, 1957.

3 Brodie, B. B., Spector, S., Kuntzman, R. G., and Shore, P. A.: Rapid biosynthesis of brain serotonin before and after reserpine administration, Naturwissenschaften 45:343, 1958.

4 Dahlstrom, A., and Fuxe, K.: Evidence for the existence of monoamine-containing neurons in the central nervous system. I. Demonstration of monoamines in the cell bodies of brain stem neurons, Acta Physiol. Scand. (supp. 232) 62:1, 1965.

5 Dudley, H. W., and Moir, C.: Substance responsible for traditional clinical effect of ergot, Brit. Med. J. 1:520, 1935.

6 Engelman, K., Lovenberg, W., and Sjoerdsma, A.: Inhibition of serotonin synthesis by para-chlorophenylalanine in patients with the carcinoid syndrome, New Eng. J. Med. 277:1103, 1967.

7 Erspamer, V.: Pharmacology of indolealkyl-amines, Pharmacol. Rev. 6:425, 1954.

8 Feldberg, W., and Sherwood, S. L.: Injections of drugs into the lateral ventricles of the cat, J. Physiol. (London) 123:148, 1954.

9 Haverback, B. J., Dutcher, T. F., Shore, P. A., Tomich, E. G., Terry, L. L., and Brodie, B. B.: Serotonin changes in platelets and brain induced by small daily doses of reserpine, New Eng. J. Med. 256:343, 1957.

10 Kety, S. S.: Biochemical theories of schizophrenia, Science 129:1528, 1590, 1959.

11 Lauer, J. W., Inskip, W. M., Bernsohn, J., and Zeller, E. A.: Observations on schizophrenic patients after iproniazid and tryptophan, Arch. Neurol. Psychiat. 80:122, 1958.

12 Marrazzi, A. S.: The effects of certain drugs on cerebral synapses, Ann. N. Y. Acad. Sci. 66:496, 1957.

13 Moncy, E.: Evaluation of topical methysergide on experimental cerebral vasospasm, Texas Med. 65:74, 1969.

14 Oates, J. A., Melmon, K., Sjoerdsma, A., Gillespie, L., and Mason, D.: Release of a kinin peptide in the carcinoid syndrome, Lancet 1:514, 1964.

15 Page, I. H.: Serotonin (5-hydroxytryptamine), Physiol. Rev. 34:563, 1954.

16 Purpura, D. P., Girado, M., Smith, T. G., Callan, D. A., and Grundfest, H.: Structure-activity determinants of pharmacological effects of amino acids and related compounds on central synapses, J. Neurochem. 3:238, 1959.

17 Rapport, M. M., Green, A. A., and Page, I. H.: Serum vasoconstrictor (serotonin): isolation and characterization, J. Biol. Chem. 176:1243, 1948.

18 Udenfriend, S.: Amine metabolism and its pharmacological implications. In Neuropharmacology, Transactions of the Fifth Conference, New York, 1960, Josiah Macy, Jr., Foundation.

19 de Whurst, W. G.: New theory of cerebral amine function and its clinical application, Nature 218:1130, 1968.

20 Wolff, H. G.: Headache and other pains, London, 1948, Oxford University Press.

Recent reviews

21 Erspamer, V., subeditor: Handbook of experimental pharmacology. 5-Hydroxytryptamine and related indolealkylamines, vol. 19, New York, 1966, Springer-Verlag New York.

22 Salmoiraghi, G. C., Costa, E., and Bloom, F. E.: Pharmacology of central synapses, Ann. Rev. Pharmacol. 5:213, 1965.

23 Sandler, M.: The role of 5-hydroxyindoles in the carcinoid syndrome, Advances Pharmacol. 6B:127, 1968.

24 Toman, J. E. P.: Some aspects of central nervous pharmacology, Ann. Rev. Pharmacol. 3:153, 1963.

18 Kinins and prostaglandins

In addition to various amines that act as neurotransmitters, there are numerous polypeptides and acidic lipids that exert powerful effects on various smooth muscles and glands. Since these compounds occur normally in the body, they probably perform important regulatory functions. The *kinins* are vasodilator polypeptides; among them the plasma kinins *bradykinin* and *kallidin* are of greatest interest. The *prostaglandins* are acidic lipids widely distributed in the body and having great pharmacologic activity.

KININS
GENERAL CONCEPT

A variety of polypeptides have effects somewhat similar to those of histamine on vascular smooth muscle, capillary permeability, and bronchial and intestinal smooth muscle.

Bradykinin is a biologically active nonapeptide, a product of the enzyme *kallikrein* on its alpha$_2$ globulin substrate. It is a potent agent to which many functions have been attributed, such as the regulation of the microcirculation of exocrine glands, circulatory changes occurring after birth, and mediation of inflammatory processes.

Numerous related kinins occur widely distributed in nature, such as in wasp venom and in the salivary gland of the octopus. What makes bradykinin of special interest, however, is the ease with which it may be made and destroyed in the body. It could have great importance in physiologic and pathologic processes, but its exact role is not likely to be defined until specific antagonists become available.

HISTORY AND NOMENCLATURE

The early studies on the kinins were carried out by two groups of investigators, one in Germany (Werle and co-workers[11]) and the other in Brazil (Rocha e Silva and co-workers[20]). Until recently the nomenclature on kinins was quite confusing because of the conflicting terms used by the various groups. The German group named their polypeptide *kallidin* and its plasma precursor *kallidinogen;* the enzyme that acted on kallidinogen was named *kallikrein.* The hypotensive substance was found in the urine and also in the pancreas, whose Greek name is *kallikreas* (although some Greeks disagree).

Independently the Brazilian group found that when snake venoms or trypsin acted on plasma globulin, a substance was produced that caused a slow contraction of the guinea pig ileum. The term *bradykinin* (from the Greek word *bradys,* meaning "slow") was coined to designate this substance.

Now that the structure of these peptides has been established and confirmed by synthesis, the terminology has become standard. Bradykinin is a polypeptide composed of a chain of nine amino acids (arginine-proline-proline-glycine-phenylalanine-serine-proline-phenylalanine-arginine). Kallidin is a decapeptide that contains an additional N-terminal lysine residue. The precursor of the kinins is called *kininogen*, sometimes referred to as bradykininogen or kallidinogen. The precursor of active *kallikrein* is *prekallikrein*. Enzymes that release kinins in general should be called kininogenases. Thus kallikrein and trypsin are kininogenases. The relationships between these factors are shown below:

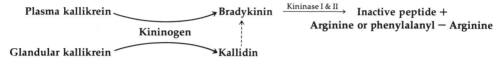

Hageman factor ⤳ Activated Hageman factor ⤳ Hageman factor fragment (prekallikrein activator)[10]

Plasma prekallikrein ⤳ Kallikrein

Plasma kallikrein ⟶ Bradykinin $\xrightarrow{\text{Kininase I \& II}}$ Inactive peptide + Arginine or phenylalanyl — Arginine

Kininogen

Glandular kallikrein ⟶ Kallidin

Bradykinin is split by at least two enzymes. Kininase I[29] is also known as carboxypeptidase N. Kininase II[28] appears to be identical with the angiotensin I converting enzyme. Kininase I inactivates other biologically active peptides,[28,29] for example, an anaphylatoxin derived from the activation of the complement system.[2]

The actual events are much more complex than indicated in the schema. Kininogen may be acted upon by trypsinlike proteases. There are activators in tissues whose nature is not understood. The subcutaneous injection of human plasma causes it to acquire kininlike properties.[16] Glandular tissues, such as in the salivary glands or pancreas, and urine are among the richest sources of kallikrein. There are also kallikrein inhibitors in tissues.

Kallikrein inhibitor: aprotinin

Aprotinin (Trasylol) is a peptide extracted from bovine salivary glands. It inhibits kallikrein and many other proteases. It is being tried clinically, particularly in Germany, in various types of shock, acute pancreatitis, and fibrinolytic states. Its therapeutic value is impossible to evaluate at this time.

Roles of bradykinin

Some interesting relationships may exist between bradykinin and angiotensin (p. 168). Both are polypeptides split from plasma proteins. Angiotensin is a potent vasoconstrictor, whereas bradykinin has the opposite effect on vascular smooth muscle. The converting enzyme in the angiotensin system is a powerful inactivator of bradykinin. Further work is necessary, however, for establishing the physiologic significance of these interrelationships.

A converting enzyme inhibitor is being tested at present both in hypertension and for its effect on the destruction of bradykinin. This nonapeptide (Pyr-Trp-Pro-Arg-Pro-Gln-Ile-Pro-Pro) blocks the conversion of angiotensin I to angiotensin II. It was found effective in the early phases of experimental renal hypertension in the dog.[28]

The plasma kinins very likely play a role in inflammatory processes. They can reproduce the cardinal signs of inflammation such as vasodilatation, increased capillary permeability, and pain. Furthermore, they can be produced rather easily in the tissues following injury.

It is attractive to think of some types of inflammation as having two phases. In an early phase histamine and other mediators are released rather explosively. In a secondary phase kinins may be constantly produced and destroyed to perpetuate the inflammatory process. Interestingly, many of the kinins in fairly high concentration can cause histamine release from mast cells,[9] although their primary action in the body is probably not a consequence of histamine release.

PHARMACOLOGIC EFFECTS

On a molar basis the plasma kinins are the most potent vasodilators known. They also cause increased capillary permeability and pain when applied to a denuded surface such as the base of a blister or after intraperitoneal injection. Pain produced by bradykinin is antagonized by aspirin, and some investigators believe that this antagonism is at the peripheral nerve endings.[12]

Bradykinin also constricts the bronchial smooth muscle. Much has been made of the observation that aspirin in very high doses antagonizes the action of the peptide on the guinea pig bronchi.[4] It is likely that the significance of this observation has been overestimated.

Other smooth muscle effects

Bradykinin constricts the uterine smooth muscle and most gastrointestinal smooth muscles. The anomalous relaxing effect on the rat duodenum may be a consequence of catecholamine release. Bradykinin can cause the release of catecholamines from the adrenal medulla.[7]

CLINICAL SIGNIFICANCE OF PLASMA KININS

In view of the ease with which plasma and tissue prekallikreins are activated and the availability of kininogen in the plasma, it is not surprising that numerous roles are being attributed to the kinins in health and disease. Plasma prekallikrein may be activated by the prior activation of the Hageman factor, antigen-antibody reactions, inflammation, trauma, trypsin, snake venoms, acid milieu, endotoxins, and heat. Similarly, tissue kallikreins may be activated and released by trauma, inflammation, toxins, and heat.

Some of the clinical conditions in which the kinins are believed to play a pathogenetic role are endotoxin shock, carcinoid syndrome (p. 206), hereditary angioneurotic edema[5,34] with its deficiency of a kallikrein inhibitor, anaphylaxis, arthritis (particularly gout where urate crystals activate the Hageman factor), and acute pancreatitis. In addition, bradykinin may play a role in constricting the umbilical artery and the ductus arteriosus and in the transformation of the fetal to the neonatal circulation.[14] An orthostatic syndrome, hyperbradykininemia, has recently been described.[25]

OTHER HYPOTENSIVE PEPTIDES

In addition to bradykinin and kallidin, there are other peptides with somewhat similar properties. *Substance P* is present in the brain and in larger amounts in the intestine.[29] *Eledoisin* is a powerful hypotensive peptide obtained from the salivary gland of the octopus.[29]

PROSTAGLANDINS

The prostaglandins, so named because they were first isolated from seminal fluid, represent a series of acidic lipids having powerful pharmacologic activity. Their widespread occurrence in tissues (including those of the nervous system) suggests for these acidic compounds a regulatory function that may be exerted as a very basic control system related to adenyl cyclase. Great efforts are being made to develop this new class of agents into medically useful drugs. Preliminary indications are that they may find applications in the induction of labor, as abortifacients, and as nasal vasoconstrictors. All these uses and the many others that are being investigated must be considered as strictly experimental at present.

HISTORY AND NOMENCLATURE

In 1930 two New York gynecologists reported that fresh human semen could cause contraction or relaxation of strips of human uterus. A few years later, Goldblatt in England[8] and von Euler in Sweden[6] studied the pharmacologic effects of lipid extracts of seminal fluid. The name *prostaglandin* was coined by von Euler in 1935, and the structures of two were established by Sune Bergström at the Karolinska Institute. Work on the pharmacology of prostaglandins has accelerated greatly since synthetic compounds have become available.

Prostaglandins are present in greatest amounts in human and sheep seminal plasma. In various species they occur also in the uterus, lung, brain, iris, thymus, pancreas, kidney, and in human menstrual blood. It is quite likely that the numerous acidic lipids with pharmacologic activity isolated over the years from various tissues are actually prostaglandins.

As shown in the schema below, the prostaglandins are derivatives of *prostanoic acid,* a C_{20} acid that contains a five-membered ring. Biosynthetically it originates from arachidonic acid. The four major groups of prostaglandins are designated as E, F, A, and B on the basis of their ring structure. The numeral in the subscript position indicates the degree of unsaturation in the side chains.

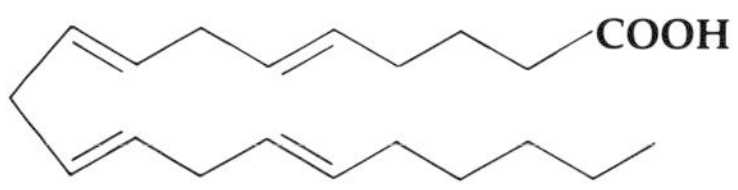

Arachidonic acid

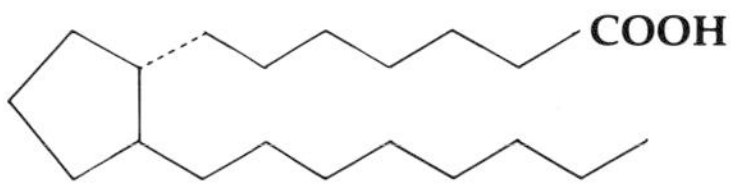

Prostanoic acid

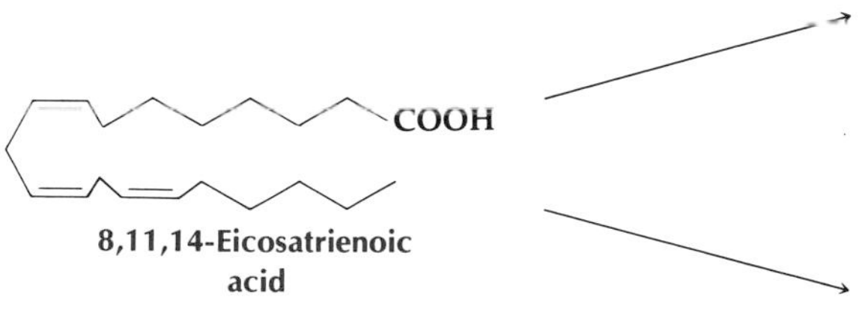

8,11,14-Eicosatrienoic acid

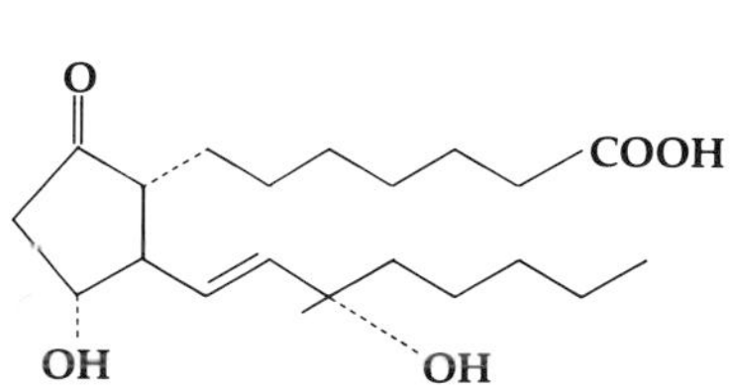

Prostaglandin E_1 (PGE$_1$)

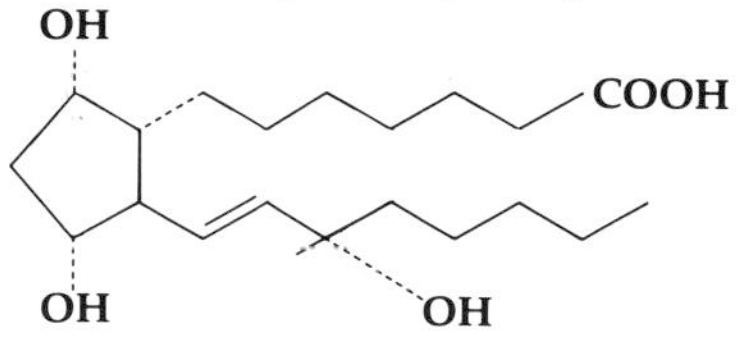

Prostaglandin $F_{1\alpha}$ (PGF$_{1\alpha}$)

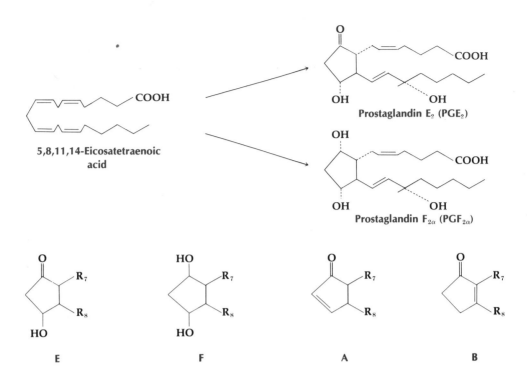

5,8,11,14-Eicosatetraenoic
acid

Prostaglandin E$_2$ (PGE$_2$)

Prostaglandin F$_{2\alpha}$ (PGF$_{2\alpha}$)

E   F   A   B

PHARMACOLOGIC EFFECTS

Interest in the prostaglandins stems from the fact that these potent endogenous hormones may play a role not only in reproductive physiology but also in a variety of clinical conditions. Their most prominent investigational use is in the area of induction of abortion.

The major pharmacologic activity of the prostaglandins is exerted on the uterus, cardiovascular system, bronchi, gastrointestinal tract, platelets, nervous system, and inflammatory and immune mechanisms.[18,35] Such widespread pharmacologic activity suggests an action on some basic control mechanism, and a positive effect of the prostaglandins on cyclic AMP formation has indeed been demonstrated. The widespread pharamacologic activity of these compounds makes their systemic use impractical. They are more likely to find therapeutic applications in clinical situations where the drugs may be administered in close proximity to the intended site of action. Thus prostaglandins given by the intravaginal, intrauterine, or intra-amniotic route were found effective in terminating first- and second-trimester pregnancy with minor side effects.[33]

PGE$_1$ and PGE$_2$ are powerful vasodilators having a short duration of action. The potency of these compounds is such that an intravenous injection of 1 μg/kg. in man will cause a considerable lowering of the blood pressure. When injected into the skin, these same prostaglandins produce a wheal-and-flare response[26] but no pain.

The prostaglandins PGE$_1$ and PGE$_2$ dilate bronchioles (although PGF$_{2\alpha}$ is a bronchoconstrictor) and are being tried in the treatment of asthma where they may be administered by aerosols. They increase intestinal motility and may cause diarrhea. PGE$_1$ inhibits platelet aggregation. Injected into the cerebral ventricles, it causes fever,[15] which is not prevented by the administration of antipyretics.

The possible role of the prostaglandins in inflammation and immune phenomena is of great interest. The intracutaneous injection of various prostaglandins has histamine-like effects.[76] In addition, it has been shown[27] that aspirin blocks the synthesis of prostaglandins by human platelets, guinea pig lungs, and some other tissues. On the basis of these findings it has been suggested[26] that the action of aspirin and perhaps other nonsteroidal anti-inflammatory drugs may be attributed to inhibition of prostaglandin synthesis.[26] A flaw in this provocative idea is the failure of the known prostaglandins to cause pain by intracutaneous injection in man, although aspirin is a potent analgesic against pain caused by inflammation.

POSSIBLE THERAPEUTIC APPLICATIONS

The prostaglandins are being tried as possible abortifacients.[33] Their usefulness in asthma, hypertension, and peptic ulcer is far from proved. As knowledge concerning the physiologic roles of the prostaglandins increases, inhibitors of their synthesis may find interesting applications.

References

1 Bergström, S., and Samuelsson, B.: Prostaglandins. Ann. Rev. Biochem. 34:101, 1965.

2 Bokisch, V. A., and Muller-Eberhard, H. J.: Anaphylatoxin inactivator of human plasma: its isolation and characterization as a carboxypeptidase, J. Clin. Invest. 49:2427, 1970.

3 Coffman, J. D.: The effect of aspirin on pain and hand blood flow responses to intraarterial injection of bradykinin in man, Clin. Pharmacol. Ther. 7:26, 1966.

4 Collier, H. O. J.: The action and antagonism of kinins on bronchioles, Ann. N. Y. Acad. Sci. 104:290, 1963.

5 Donaldson, V. H.: Serum inhibitor of C'1-esterase in health and disease, J. Lab. Clin. Med. 68:369, 1966.

6 von Euler, U. S.: Zur Kenntnis der pharmakologischen Wirkungen von Nativsekreten und Extrackten männlicher accessorischer Geschechtdrüsen, Arch. Exp. Path. Pharmakol. 175:78, 1934.

7 Feldberg, W., and Lewis, G. P.: The action of peptides on the adrenal medulla release of adrenaline by bradykinin and angiotensin, J. Physiol. (London) 171:98, 1964.

8 Goldblatt, M. W.: A depressor substance in seminal fluid, J. Soc. Chem. Ind. 52:1056, 1933.

9 Johnson, A. R., and Erdös, E. G.: Release of histamine from mast cells by vasoactive peptides, Proc. Soc. Exp. Biol. Med. 142:1252, 1973.

10 Kaplan, A. P., and Austen, K. F.: A pre-albumin activator of prekallikrein, J. Immunol. 105:802, 1970.

11 Kraut, F., Frey, E. K., and Werle, E.: Der Nachweis eines Kreislaufhormons in der Pankreasdrüse, Z. Physiol. Chem. 189:97, 1930.

12 Lim, R. K. S., Guzman, F., Rodgers, D. W., Goto, K., Braun, C., Dickerson, G. D., and Engle, R. J.: Site of action of narcotic and non-narcotic analgesics determined by blocking bradykinin-evoked visceral pain, Arch. Int. Pharmacodyn, 152:28, 1964.

13 Mason, D. T., and Melmon, K. L.: Abnormal forearm vascular responses in the carcinoid syndrome, J. Clin. Invest. 45:1685, 1966.

14 Melmon, K. L., Cline, M. J., Hughes, T., and Nies, A. S.: Kinins: possible mediators of neonatal circulatory changes in man, J. Clin. Invest. 47:1295, 1968.

15 Milton, A. S., and Wendlandt, S.: Effects on body temperature of prostaglandins of the A, E and F series on injection into the third ventricle of unanaesthetized cats and rabbits, J. Physiol. 218:325, 1971.

16 Oates, J. A., Pettinger, W. A., and Doctor, R. B.: Evidence for the release of bradykinin in carcinoid syndrome, J. Clin. Invest. 45:173, 1966.

17 Orloff, J., Handler, J. S., and Bergström, S.: Effect of prostaglandin (PGE₁) on the permeability response of toad bladder to vasopressin, theophylline and adenosine 3′,5′-monophosphate, Nature 205:397, 1965.

18 Ramwell, P. W., Shaw, J. E., Corey, E. J., and Andersen, N.: Biological activity of synthetic prostaglandins, Nature, 221:1251, 1969.

19 Ratnoff, D. D., and Miles, A. A.: Induction of permeability-increasing activity in human plasma by activated Hageman factor, Brit. J. Exp. Path. 45:328, 1964.

20 Rocha e Silva, M., Beraldo, W. T., and Rosenfeld, G.: Bradykinin, a hypotensive and smooth muscle stimulating factor released from plasma globulin by snake venoms and by trypsin, Amer. J. Physiol. **156**:261, 1949.

21 Rowley, D. A.: Venous constriction as the cause of increased vascular permeability produced by 5-hydroxytryptamine, histamine, bradykinin, and compound 48/80 in the rat, Brit. J. Exp. Path. **45**:56, 1964.

22 Schachter, M.: Kinins — a group of active peptides, Ann. Rev. Pharmacol. **4**:281, 1964.

23 Smith, J. B., and Willis, A. L.: Aspirin selectively inhibits prostaglandin production in human platelets, Nature **231**:235, 1971.

24 Steinberg, D., Vaughan, M., Nestel, P. J., and Bergstrom, S.: Effects of prostaglandin E opposing those of catecholamines on blood pressure and on triglyceride breakdown in adipose tissue, Biochem. Pharmacol. **12**:764, 1963.

25 Streeten, D. H. P., Kerr, C. B., Kerr, L. P., Prior, J. C., and Dalakos, T. G.: Hyperbradykininism: a new orthostatic syndrome, Lancet **2**:1048, 1972.

26 Vane, J. R.: Inhibition of prostaglandin synthesis as a mechanism of action for aspirin-like drugs, Nature **231**:232, 1971.

Recent reviews

27 Bergstrom, S., Carlson, L. A., and Weeks, J. R.: The prostaglandins: a family of biologically active lipids, Pharmacol. Rev. **20**:1, 1968.

28 Erdös, E. G., editor: Handbook of experimental pharmacology: bradykinin, kallidin, and kallikrein, Berlin, 1970, Springer-Verlag.

29 Erdös, E. G., editor: Structure and function of biologically active peptides: bradykinin, kallidin, and congeners, Ann. N. Y. Acad. Sci. **104**:1, 1963.

30 von Euler, U. S.: Prostaglandins, Clin. Pharmacol. Ther. **9**:228, 1968.

31 Frey, E. K., Kraut, H., and Werle, E.: Das Kallikrein-kinin Systemand seine Inhibitoren, Stuttgart, 1968, Ferdinand Enke Verlag.

32 Horton, E. W.: Hypotheses on physiological roles of prostaglandins, Physiol. Rev. **49**:122, 1969.

33 Karim, S. M. M.: Prostaglandins as abortifacients, New Eng. J. Med. **285**:1534, 1971.

34 Kellermeyer, R. W., and Graham, R. C.: Kinins — possible physiologic and pathologic roles in man, New Eng. J. Med. **279**:754, 802, 859, 1968.

35 Ramwell, P. W., and Shaw, J. E., editors: Prostaglandins, Ann. N. Y. Acad. Sci. **180**:1971.

SECTION THREE

PSYCHOPHARMACOLOGY

19 Antipsychotic and antianxiety drugs

GENERAL CONCEPT

Antipsychotic and antianxiety drugs are the newer terms for major and minor tranquilizers, respectively. The antipsychotic drugs, represented by the *phenothiazines, thioxanthenes,* and *butyrophenones,* produce a specific improvement in the mood and behavior of psychotic patients without excessive sedation and without causing addiction.

The antianxiety drugs include the *benzodiazepines, meprobamate,* and related drugs. The antianxiety drugs may not be basically different from the sedative-hypnotics except for some characteristics of the benzodiazepines that probably account for their great popularity and overuse. They are less likely to produce tolerance and physical dependence, and they are much safer than the sedative-hypnotics when taken in suicidal overdoses.

BRAIN AMINES AND MENTAL DISEASE

Several lines of evidence implicate brain amines and in particular the catecholamines (dopamine and norepinephrine) in severe mental illness such as schizophrenia. First, amphetamine, a drug related to the catecholamines, produces a toxic psychosis that is difficult to distinguish from some manifestations of schizophrenia. Second, the phenothiazines and butyrophenones can block adrenergic and dopaminergic receptors. Additional evidence indicates that inhibition of the synthesis of catecholamines by the administration of α-methyltyrosine potentiates the effects of phenothiazines[4] in schizophrenics. Although it is premature to formulate a general theory of the chemical basis of mental illness, there is evidence to implicate some imbalance between dopamine and norepinephrine as a part of "the biologic vulnerability in schizophrenia."[27]

DEVELOPMENT

The field of tranquilizing agents was opened up by the almost simultaneous introduction of two powerful drugs, chlorpromazine and reserpine. Chlorpromazine originated in France as a result of studies on those antihistaminics having a phenothiazine structure, such as promethazine. Preparations of *Rauwolfia serpentina* have been used in India for centuries for the treatment of various illnesses. Reserpine, one of its alkaloids, was isolated in 1952.

It was soon found that even at subhypnotic levels these drugs exert striking calming effects on the behavior of wild animals and disturbed patients. The knowledge that these drugs could influence spontaneous and learned behavior in animals led to the development of extensive screening procedures for new drugs of a tranquilizing type. This activity produced not only a variety of phenothiazine derivatives and reserpine-like compounds but also many minor antianxiety drugs such as meprobamate, phenaglycodol, benactyzine, hydroxyzine, chlordiazepoxide, and others. The list of these drugs is still growing.

■ Antipsychotic drugs

The development of the antipsychotic drugs is an outgrowth of research on antihistamines. The prototype of the phenothiazine drugs, chlorpromazine, was developed as an antihistamine related to promethazine (Phenergan). Once the unusually beneficial effect of the drug in psychotic patients was recognized, a large number of related compounds were introduced. As a group, these drugs are characterized by their calming effect on psychotics without excessive sedation, their extrapyramidal effects, and their unusual property of not inducing dependence. Most of these drugs have indications also as antiemetics, and some are used as antipruritics.

From a chemical standpoint the antipsychotic drugs comprise the *phenothiazines, thioxanthenes,* and *butyrophenones.* The properties of these drugs are so similar that emphasis in this discussion will be placed primarily on the phenothiazines. Reserpine was at one time used as a "major tranquilizer" but has been essentially abandoned in psychiatric practice. Its use as an antihypertensive is discussed in Chapter 14.

PHENOTHIAZINE DERIVATIVES

Numerous phenothiazine derivatives are in current use. They resemble chlorpromazine in action but differ from it in potency, clinical indications, and toxicity.

Chemistry

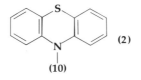

Phenothiazine nucleus

	Substitution in (2)	Substitution in (10)	Average oral dose (mg.)
		Aliphatic	
Chlorpromazine (Thorazine)	Cl	$CH_2-CH_2-CH_2-N-(CH_3)_2$	25-50
Promazine (Sparine)	—	$CH_2-CH_2-CH_2-N-(CH_3)_2$	25-50
Triflupromazine (Vesprin)	CF_3	$CH_2-CH_2-CH_2-N-(CH_3)_2$	10-25

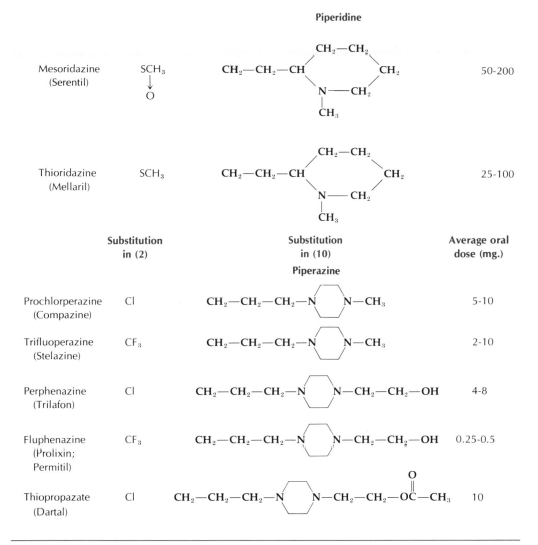

Piperidine

	Substitution in (2)	Substitution in (10)	Average oral dose (mg.)
Mesoridazine (Serentil)	$SCH_3 \downarrow O$	(Piperidine)	50-200
Thioridazine (Mellaril)	SCH_3	(Piperidine)	25-100
		Piperazine	
Prochlorperazine (Compazine)	Cl	$CH_2-CH_2-CH_2-N \quad N-CH_3$	5-10
Trifluoperazine (Stelazine)	CF_3	$CH_2-CH_2-CH_2-N \quad N-CH_3$	2-10
Perphenazine (Trilafon)	Cl	$CH_2-CH_2-CH_2-N \quad N-CH_2-CH_2-OH$	4-8
Fluphenazine (Prolixin; Permitil)	CF_3	$CH_2-CH_2-CH_2-N \quad N-CH_2-CH_2-OH$	0.25-0.5
Thiopropazate (Dartal)	Cl	$CH_2-CH_2-CH_2-N \quad N-CH_2-CH_2-OC-CH_3$ (O)	10

PHENOTHIAZINE DERIVATIVES AS ANTIPSYCHOTIC DRUGS

The first widely used phenothiazine tranquilizer, chlorpromazine, was synthesized in France in 1950. The compound is closely related chemically to promethazine, a potent antihistaminic drug. The drug was used by Laborit in France for production of artificial hibernation and as part of the so-called lytic cocktail, which consisted of promethazine, meperidine, and chlorpromazine. The purpose of this unusual mixture was to cause profound inhibition of the autonomic nervous system.

The potent tranquilizing and antiemetic actions of chlorpromazine led to widespread use of the drug in various fields of medicine. Subsequently, many other phenothiazine tranquilizers were synthesized. At present there are at least twelve of these in clinical use.

The pharmacologic effects of the phenothiazine tranquilizers are quite complex. In addition to their behavioral effects, these drugs are potent antiemetics and have important actions on the autonomic nervous system at various levels. In large doses they also produce significant toxic side effects such as parkinsonism.

The phenothiazines are classified on the basis of their chemistry and pharmacology into three groups (p. 222). The differences result from substitutions on the nitrogen in the phenothiazine ring. The *aliphatic* or *dimethylaminopropyl* compounds include chlorpromazine (Thorazine), promazine (Sparine), and triflupromazine (Vesprin). The *piperidine* derivatives are represented by thioridazine (Mellaril) and mesoridazine (Serentil). Among the numerous *piperazine* compounds, some of the most widely used are prochlorperazine (Compazine), trifluoperazine (Stelazine), perphenazine (Trilafon), fluphenazine (Prolixin; Permitil) and thiopropazate (Dartal).

The *thioxanthene* group of antipsychotic drugs resembles in all respects the phenothiazines, particularly the *aliphatic* or *dimethylaminopropyl* derivatives such as chlorpromazine. The thioxanthenes include chlorprothixene (Taractan) and thiothixene (Navane). The *butyrophenone* haloperidol (Haldol) is also very similar pharmacologically to the phenothiazines.

Major differences among the phenothiazine derivatives

The aliphatic or dimethylaminopropyl compounds have greater sedative action and are more useful in agitated schizophrenics. The piperazine group may be more useful in depressed or withdrawn schizophrenics. The piperidyl group resembles the aliphatic compounds in most respects.

The various groups of phenothiazines differ in the likelihood of causing certain adverse effects. In addition to causing drowsiness, the aliphatic group also tends to cause parkinsonism, whereas thioridazine (Mellaril) of the piperidyl group is less likely to do so. The piperazine compounds also produce extrapyramidal symptoms and dyskinesia.

Chlorpromazine will be discussed as the prototype of the phenothiazine tranquilizers.

CHLORPROMAZINE

Chlorpromazine (Thorazine), an aliphatic or dimethylaminopropyl phenothiazine, is a sedative antipsychotic drug. In addition to its usefulness in agitated psychotics, the drug has other medical applications such as prevention of nausea and vomiting. It is used also for its ability to potentiate the actions of other drugs such as anesthetics.

The structural formulas of chlorpromazine (Thorazine) and the antihistaminic drug promethazine (Phenergan) are as follows:

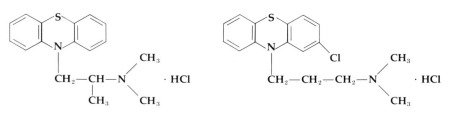

Promethazine hydrochloride   Chlorpromazine hydrochloride

Effects in man

When a person takes 25 to 50 mg. of chlorpromazine, he becomes drowsy and calm in about 1 hour and remains in this state for about 5 hours. If he takes an even larger dose, he may become quite sleepy and ataxic. His face acquires an expression characteristic of Parkinson's disease. Even when he becomes quite sleepy, he responds easily to painful stimuli. He definitely does not resemble someone who has swallowed a large dose of "sleeping pills."

His blood pressure tends to fall, more so if the drug has been given by intramuscular or intravenous injection, and he may have tachycardia. If he is in a cool environment, his temperature will be lower than normal. If he has also taken a barbiturate, he will sleep much longer than he would without the chlorpromazine.

If the person has schizophrenia, chlorpromazine will improve his thought disorder, change his blunted affect, alter his withdrawal and autistic behavior, and relieve his hallucinations, hostility, and resistiveness.[27]

Mode of action

Chlorpromazine exerts important effects on the central nervous system. In addition, it has some adrenergic blocking effects, together with weak antihistaminic, anticholinergic, and antispasmodic actions. It potentiates the hypnotics and blocks the emetic action of apomorphine.

The actions on the central nervous system are still not well understood although they have been studied extensively, using psychological and neurophysiologic techniques. The drug tends to inhibit conditioned reflexes in animals, decreasing hostility and spontaneous motor activity. It tends to oppose the psychomotor stimulant actions of caffeine and amphetamine but will not block the convulsant actions of strychnine.

The difference between chlorpromazine and a barbiturate is illustrated nicely in an experiment proposed by Lasagna.[14] This experiment is based on the previous observation that the toxicity of amphetamine in mice is markedly influenced by the environment. The LD_{50} of amphetamine for isolated mice was found to be 111 mg./kg. when injected intraperitoneally. When three mice were placed in a small cage, a much smaller dose of amphetamine, about 15 mg./kg., produced death. Apparently the anxiety induced by the hyperactive neighbors added to the central stimulant actions of amphetamine.

When either phenobarbital or chlorpromazine was injected in addition to amphetamine, the results in the grouped mice were similar to those obtained with the isolated mice. In other words, the LD_{50} of amphetamine in the grouped mice now went up to about 110 mg./kg., essentially the same as for isolated mice. This may be interpreted as a reduction of the damaging influence of crowded conditions on amphetamine toxicity. There was a great difference, however, between phenobarbital and chlorpromazine in this respect. Phenobarbital had to be raised to anesthetic levels in order to obtain protection, whereas chlorpromazine prevented the lethal actions of amphetamine even at dose levels that did not produce unconsciousness. This is a remarkable example of a tranquilizing drug reducing the adverse effects of the environment. It should be emphasized that these results cannot be explained on the basis of pharmacologic antagonism to amphetamine, since in single mice neither phenobarbital nor chlorpromazine produced an important increase in the LD_{50} of amphetamine.

It is quite likely that chlorpromazine acts on many different portions of the brain. Its ability to block vomiting induced by apomorphine suggests that it has an effect on the chemoreceptor trigger area.[11] The drug may also interfere with vasomotor reflexes mediated through the hypothalamus.[5]

Among the peripheral actions of chlorpromazine, perhaps the most important is its adrenergic blocking effect. Of less importance is its ability to antagonize to a slight extent the actions of histamine, serotonin, and acetylcholine.

Mechanism of antipsychotic effect

Although the exact mechanism of the antipsychotic effect of chlorpromazine and other phenothiazines is not known, the blocking action of these drugs on central catecholamine receptors is currently being emphasized. This is in line with some current thinking that attributes schizophrenic disorders to a possible overactivity of dopamine, an insufficiency of norepinephrine at appropriate synapses, or an imbalance between the two.[27]

Problem 19-1. Assuming that the antipsychotic effect of the phenothiazines is related to blockade of central catecholamine receptors, what would be the effect of inhibition of catecholamine synthesis on the efficacy of phenothiazines? This problem was put to a test.[4] The antipsychotic action of thioridazine or chlorpromazine was markedly potentiated by the tyrosine hydroxylase inhibitor, α-methyltyrosine. The dosage of the phenothiazine could be greatly lowered under these conditions. Although this study was performed only in five schizophrenic patients, its implications are great.

Metabolism

Chlorpromazine is well absorbed from the gastrointestinal tract, and its administration by the intramuscular or intravenous route is seldom justified. The peak effect occurs in about an hour, and the duration of action is about 4 or 5 hours following oral administration. One of the metabolic products of chlorpromazine has been identified as the sulfoxide. About 10% of an administered dose is excreted in the urine in this form. Very little of the unchanged chlorpromazine appears in the urine, and the liver appears to be the chief site of detoxication. Since the drug is used in treatment of vomiting in uremia, it is of some importance to know that as much as 100 mg. daily for 10 days has been tolerated by uremic patients in the absence of urinary excretion.[10] This, of course, would be a toxic dose in the absence of metabolic degradation.

It has been suggested that chlorpromazine has a more potent sedative action in patients with liver disease.[16] This is compatible with the proposed role of the liver in the metabolic degradation of the drug.

Comparison of chlorpromazine and reserpine

Superficially the central actions of these two drugs are similar. Both can have a potent tranquilizing effect in man and animals, and both promote the action of hypnotics and inhibit certain central autonomic regulations. There are certain important differences, however.

Chlorpromazine does not influence the binding and release of serotonin and norepinephrine and has many peripheral actions exemplified by its adrenergic blocking action. Finally, if the administration of reserpine is preceded by iproniazid, an MAO inhibitor, excitement may result. Iproniazid does not reverse the sedative action of chlorpromazine.

It has been postulated that chlorpromazine may block the actions of catecholamines in the brain, just as it does in the periphery. This interesting idea may contribute to the understanding of the similarities between the central actions of chlorpromazine and reserpine.

Adverse effects

Chlorpromazine is a potentially dangerous drug, and it has caused adverse effects of many different types. These include extrapyramidal symptoms, orthostatic hypotension, dryness of mouth, photosensitivity, cholestatic hepatitis, and blood dyscrasias. By its potentiation of other central nervous system depressants it can cause adverse effects in patients who are taking drugs such as barbiturates or alcohol. Because of its atropine-like action, chlopromazine is contraindicated in patients with glaucoma or prostatic hypertrophy.

Hypotension. Hypotension can be marked, particularly when the drug is given parenterally. The orthostatic nature of the hypotensive response is suggested by the observation that it is particularly likely to occur in ambulatory patients. Marked hypotension has occurred in patients who received general anesthesia following chlorpromazine administration.

Jaundice. Jaundice has been observed in approximately 2% of the patients taking the drug. Surprisingly, liver function studies have shown that this jaundice resembles the obstructive rather than the hepatocellular type. Apparently the bile canaliculi become edematous and inflamed in these patients, a condition leading to obstructive jaundice. It is believed that this is a peculiar allergic response to the drug, similar to what has been observed following use of arsphenamine and methyltestosterone. The jaundice usually disappears when the drug is discontinued. It has persisted, however, in some cases, and a few patients have died as a consequence of liver failure. Such an outcome is more likely in the presence of preexisting liver damage.

Drug hypersensitivity. Hypersensitivity to chlorpromazine may occur. Dermatitis and light sensitization have been reported. Agranulocytosis is fortunately rare.

Other toxic effects. The potentiation of the action of hypnotics and anesthetics can lead to toxic complications. Gastrointestinal disturbances may develop. In rare cases, gynecomastia in males and lactation in females have been reported as complications of chlorpromazine therapy.

Clinical uses

The drug is used for many purposes, but the most common uses are based on the tranquilizing and antiemetic properties.

Agitated psychotic and psychoneurotic patients may be calmed and made more receptive to psychotherapy. The drug is also useful in toxic psychosis. The agitation of alcoholics may be controlled with this medication.

As an antiemetic, chlorpromazine is particularly effective against nausea and vomiting induced by certain drugs and by certain disease states. It is not particularly effective in motion sickness; antihistaminics and scopolamine are distinctly superior.

The drug is effective against vomiting caused by narcotics and anesthetics but not against nausea induced by veratrum alkaloids and digitalis. It has been used successfully as an antiemetic in uremia and hyperemesis gravidarum.

The dose of chlorpromazine is usually 25 mg. three or four times a day by mouth. Similar doses may be given parenterally, but precautions must be taken to avoid orthostatic hypotension.

In psychiatric practice, markedly larger doses of chlorpromazine have been used, even several grams a day. This application of the tranquilizers has done much to decrease the patient load on mental hospitals.

PHENOTHIAZINE DERIVATIVES AS ANTIEMETICS

The phenothiazines are highly effective in blocking the action of drugs on the chemoreceptor trigger zone but are generally ineffective in the prevention of motion sickness. For this reason, the antihistaminic and anticholinergic drugs are most widely used for the prevention of motion sickness (p. 199). Phenothiazines are among the most useful antiemetics for preventing not only drug-induced nausea but also that which follows surgical operations, radiation sickness, and some disease states. The antihistaminic phenothiazine, promethazine (Phenergan), is effective in motion sickness also.

The phenothiazine antiemetics include chlorpromazine (Thorazine), fluphenazine dihydrochloride (Prolixin; Permitil), perphenazine (Trilafon), prochlorperazine (Compazine), thiethylperazine (Torecan), and triflupromazine hydrochloride (Vesprin).

PHENOTHIAZINE DERIVATIVES AS ANTIPRURITICS

Some of the phenothiazines with powerful antihistaminic activity are widely used and are effective in the relief of itching of various skin diseases. Promethazine hydrochloride is a powerful antihistaminic having a phenothiazine structure. Trimeprazine tartrate (Temaril) is related structurally to promazine. Methdilazine (Tacaryl) is another antihistaminic phenothiazine commonly used as an antipruritic. In general, these antihistaminic phenothiazines can cause drowsiness and all the toxic effects described previously. All precautions applicable to the other phenothiazines should be observed in their use.

THIOXANTHENE DERIVATIVES

The thioxanthene derivatives chlorprothixene (Taractan) and thiothixene (Navane) are very similar chemically and pharmacologically to the phenothiazine derivatives. In the thioxanthene drugs a carbon is substituted for the nitrogen that is present in the central ring of the phenothiazines.

Chlorprothixene (Taractan) is effective in psychotic conditions in which agitation and anxiety are prominent symptoms. The drug is available in tablets of 10, 25, 50, and 100 mg. and in solutions for injection containing 12.5 mg./ml.

Thiothixene (Navane) is useful in the treatment of chronic schizophrenics who are apathetic. The drug is available in capsules containing 1, 2, 5, and 10 mg.

SUBSTITUTED BUTYROPHENONES

A series of substituted butyrophenones synthesized in Belgium since 1956 have been used increasingly as major tranquilizers, particularly in psychiatry and anesthesiology.[26] Haloperidol (Haldol), the prototype of this series, has the following structure:

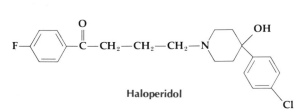

Haloperidol

Haloperidol is a potent antiemetic. It blocks apomorphine-induced vomiting, acting probably on the chemoreceptor trigger zone. From a pharmacologic standpoint, in this and other respects the butyrophenones resemble the phenothiazines. Haloperidol improves psychotic behavior, but extrapyramidal reactions to the drug are frequent. The drug is usually administered to adults in doses of 1 to 2 mg. two or three times daily.

The tranquilizing (so-called neuroleptic) butyrophenones are used also in anesthesiology in combination with some potent narcotic analgesic. The substituted butyrophenone droperidol, in combination with a meperidine-like analgesic (fentanyl), has been introduced recently for so-called neuroleptanalgesia. The combination is available under the trade name Innovar.

LITHIUM CARBONATE IN MANIC PSYCHOSIS

Lithium carbonate, a simple inorganic compound, shows some effectiveness in the treatment of the manic phases of manic-depressive psychosis. In 1949 Cade[3] of Australia instituted the study of its effect on psychotic behavior following the observation that lithium carbonate caused lethargy in guinea pigs.

Patients in acute manic phases usually require doses as high as 600 mg. three times a day, which should produce a serum lithium level of 0.5 to 1.5 mEq./L. As soon as a good response is achieved, the dosage should be reduced to 300 mg. three times a day. Serum lithium levels should be monitored and should not be allowed to exceed 2 mEq./L. Diarrhea, vomiting, drowsiness, and ataxia are among the early signs of lithium intoxication. Thyroid involvement may occur. Lithium is distributed in the total body water. Its renal clearance is proportional to its concentration in plasma. By interfering with sodium reabsorption, lithium may promote sodium depletion.[32,33]

The dose-related adverse effects of lithium carbonate administration may progress from *mild* symptoms such as nausea, vomiting, diarrhea, and muscle fasciculations to *moderately severe* symptoms that include hyperactive reflexes, epileptiform convulsions, and somnolence, leading finally to peripheral circulatory collapse, generalized convulsions, coma, and death. The very severe reactions are associated with serum lithium levels of 2.5 mEq./L. or more.

The mechanism of action of lithium carbonate in manic psychosis is not understood. Since there are many similarities in the biologic actions of sodium and lithium and since sodium is required for catecholamine uptake by the amine pump, current research is focusing on the possible effect of lithium on catecholamine uptake. Lithium appears to accelerate the uptake of norepinephrine by isolated nerve-ending particles (synaptosomes).[20]

Lithium carbonate is available in capsules (Eskalith; Lithonate) and in tablets (Lithane), all containing 300 mg. of the drug.

■ Antianxiety drugs

In contrast with the antipsychotic drugs, a group of compounds termed antianxiety agents are commonly prescribed, sometimes unnecessarily, for nervousness and tension in normal or neurotic individuals. These drugs are sometimes referred to as "minor tranquilizers," a term that should be abandoned because it implies a similarity to the antipsychotic drugs, or "major tranquilizers." The majority of the antianxiety drugs have sedative and even hypnotic effects and are centrally acting skeletal muscle relaxants; they do not produce extrapyramidal side effects or interfere with autonomic nervous system functions. On the other hand, and in contrast to the phenothiazines, they produce physical dependence.

The major group of antianxiety drugs, benzodiazepines and drugs related to meprobamate, includes chlordiazepoxide hydrochloride (Librium), diazepam (Valium), oxazepam (Serax), meprobamate (Equanil; Miltown), oxanamide (Quiactin), phenaglycodol (Ultran), mephenoxalone (Trepidone), hydroxyphenamate (Listica), and tybamate (Solacen; Tybatran).

A miscellaneous group of drugs includes certain antihistaminic and anticholinergic drugs and others that are difficult to classify. Hydroxyzine (Atarax; Vistaril) and buclizine (Softran) are antihistaminic and anticholinergic agents, and benactyzine (Suavitil) is an anticholinergic drug.

BENZODIAZEPINE DRUGS

The benzodiazepines, chlordiazepoxide hydrochloride (Librium), diazepam (Valium), and oxazepam (Serax), are widely used antianxiety drugs having central skeletal muscle–relaxing properties. The related drug flurazepam (Dalmane) is promoted as a hypnotic. The pharmacology of the benzodiazepines is basically similar to that of the barbiturate hypnotics except that in some tests they can achieve effects without excessive sedation or ataxia. Thus they have a taming effect on monkeys and other animals in doses that are not incapacitating, and behavioral studies in animals indicate that these drugs have a greater margin between the dosage needed for altering behavior and the ones that are generally depressant. The benzodiazepines prevent convulsions caused by strychnine or pentylenetetrazole. In this respect they are similar to the barbiturates and are quite different from the phenothiazines or reserpine, which are not anticonvulsants. The benzodiazepines have no extrapyramidal or autonomic side effects of significance.

The great popularity of the benzodiazepines is probably dependent on two differences between them and the barbiturates.[36] They are not as likely to produce tolerance and physical dependence, and they are remarkably safe when taken in large suicidal doses.[24]

Adverse effects produced by the benzodiazepines include drowsiness, ataxia, syncope, paradoxical excitement, rash, nausea, and altered libido.[9] Parenteral benzodiazepines such as diazepam should be used with caution in patients who are taking concomitantly such drugs as barbiturates, alcohol, antihypertensive drugs, anticonvulsants, opiates, or other drugs that depress the central nervous system.[6]

The half-life of chlordiazepoxide in the body is of the order of 24 hours. Diazepam is also a long-acting drug, and one of its major metabolic products is oxazepam.

Chlordiazepoxide (Libritabs) is available in tablets containing 5, 10, and 25 mg. Preparations of chlordiazepoxide hydrochloride (Librium) include capsules of 5, 10, and 25 mg. and powder for injection, 100 mg. Preparations of diazepam (Valium) include tablets containing 2, 5, and 10 mg. and solution for injection, 5 mg./ml. Oxazepam (Serax) is available in capsules containing 10, 15, and 30 mg. and in tablets containing 15 mg.

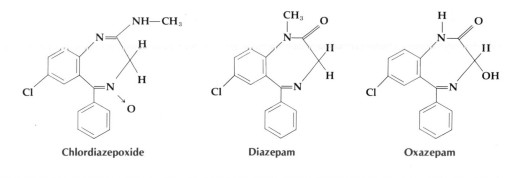

Chlordiazepoxide   Diazepam   Oxazepam

MEPROBAMATE

Meprobamate (Miltown; Equanil) was developed as a result of studies on mephenesin-like drugs. Clinical trials of this central muscle relaxant indicated that the drug has sedative and tranquilizing properties.

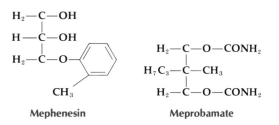

Mephenesin   Meprobamate

Meprobamate is available in 400 mg. tablets. The oral administration of one of these tablets has very slight effects, causing only very mild sedation. Larger doses tend to produce some drowsiness and reduction of muscle spasm without interference with normal proprioceptive tone. In sufficiently large doses the drug causes ataxia.

The behavioral effects of meprobamate can be shown in wild animals such as monkeys. These animals become less aggressive and hostile after its administration, although they may become somewhat ataxic. This drug decreases anxiety in patients without causing significant side effects.

The central muscle relaxant effect of meprobamate is illustrated by its reduction of experimental tremors induced by strychnine. The drug is also a fairly potent anticonvulsant and can protect mice against convulsions and death produced by pentylenetetrazol.

Mode of action

It is believed that meprobamate has a blocking action on interneurons, since it has been shown that the drug has no effects on knee jerk whereas flexor and crossed extensor reflexes are diminished by it. There are no interneurons interposed between the afferent and efferent reflex arcs in knee jerk. Thus the drug produces muscle relaxation without directly influencing transmission from motor nerve to skeletal muscle.

It is the opinion of many clinical pharmacologists that the muscle relaxant sedatives, although offered as tranquilizers, should be regarded simply as nonspecific sedatives similar in action to the barbiturates.[7] Not only do they cause somnolence and ataxia when used in large enough doses but also addiction, generally similar to barbiturate addiction, develops in patients who take large doses for a long time. Serious withdrawal symptoms characterized by muscle twitching and even convulsions may result when these drugs are discontinued abruptly.

Despite their lack of specificity, the muscle relaxants are used widely, perhaps too widely. Their mild sedative effect and lack of autonomic and extrapyramidal actions make them very attractive to physicians and patients alike.

Metabolism

Studies so far indicate that meprobamate is largely metabolized in the body. Only about 10% of the drug is excreted unchanged in the urine. Conjugation with glucuronic acid appears to be important in the metabolism of meprobamate, although it is first changed to hydroxymeprobamate.

Side effects and toxicity

Drowsiness occurs when fairly large doses of meprobamate are used. Skin rash, gastrointestinal disturbances, and purpura may rarely be caused by the drug.

Habituation and addiction to the drug may occur when large doses of meprobamate are taken for long periods of time. Sudden withdrawal may result in muscular twitching and even convulsions. It is very unlikely for these withdrawal symptoms to occur if the patient takes only two or three tablets a day. The drug should be withdrawn slowly and gradually.

PHENAGLYCODOL

Phenaglycodol (Ultran) has pharmacologic effects quite similar to those of meprobamate.

The indications for phenaglycodol are essentially the same as for meprobamate. It is administered orally in capsules (300 mg.) and tablets (200 mg.), usually three times a day.

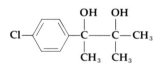

Phenaglycodol

MISCELLANEOUS SEDATIVES
ANTIHISTAMINIC SEDATIVES — HYDROXYZINE

The chemical structure of hydroxyzine (Atarax; Vistaril) as shown below is closely related to some of the antihistaminic drugs.

The drug produces drowsiness and has been introduced into therapeutics as an antianxiety drug with antihistaminic and antiemetic properties. In addition to its antihistaminic actions,[15] the drug has a slight atropine-like action and also a slight adrenergic blocking action. It has not achieved as widespread use as many of the other tranquilizing drugs, and its exact position in psychopharmacology is difficult to state.

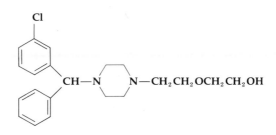

Hydroxyzine

Hydroxyzine is being tried experimentally for certain cardiac arrhythmias. It may have a weak quinidine-like effect, which is not unusual among the antihistaminic drugs. Hydroxyzine hydrochloride (Atarax) is available in tablets of 10, 25, 50, and 100 mg. and also as a solution for injection (Atarax; Vistaril hydrochloride) containing 25 or 50 mg./ml.

ANTICHOLINERGIC DRUG — BENACTYZINE

Benactyzine (Suavitil) is basically an anticholinergic drug with many central nervous system actions. It is closely related to adiphenine (Trasentine), which has been employed as a mild antispasmodic for many years. The structural formulas of benactyzine and adiphenine are shown below.

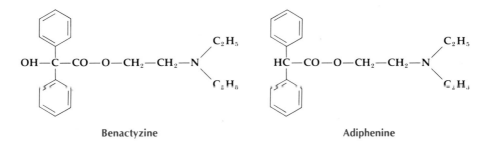

Benactyzine   Adiphenine

Just as do other atropine-like drugs, benactyzine produces mydriasis and inhibition of salivation and is an antispasmodic. It has relatively more potent effects on behavior than have equipotent anticholinergic doses of atropine. Its effects in man are characterized by drowsiness and inability to concentrate. It has not achieved widespread usefulness in the treatment of psychoneuroses.

References

1 Berger, F. M.: The similarities and differences between meprobamate and barbiturates, Clin. Pharmacol. Ther. 4:209, 1963.

2 Brodie, B. B.: Biochemical sites of action of psychotropic drugs. In Neuropharmacology, Transactions of the Fifth Conference, New York, 1960, Josiah Macy, Jr., Foundation.

3 Cade, J. F. J.: Lithium salts in the treatment of psychotic excitement, Med. J. Aust. 36:349, 1949.

4 Carlsson, A., Persson, T., Roos, B.-E., and Walinder, J.: Potentiation of phenothiazines by α-methyltyrosine in treatment of chronic schizophrenia, J. Neural Transmission 33:83, 1972.

5 Dasgupta, S. R., and Werner, G.: Inhibition of hypothalamic, medullary and reflex vasomotor responses by chlorpromazine, Brit. J. Pharmacol. 9:389, 1954.

6 Diazepam as a muscle relaxant, The Medical Letter 15:1, 1973.

7 Domino, E. F.: Sites of action of some central nervous system depressants, Ann. Rev. Pharmacol. **2**:215, 1962.

8 Erspamer, V.: The biological significance of 5-hydroxytryptamine: present status of the problem, Proceedings of the 21st International Congress of Physiological Sciences, Symposia and Special Lectures, 1959.

9 Friend, D. G.: Current concepts of therapy, tranquilizers. III. Meprobamate, phenaglycodol and chlordiazepoxide, New Eng. J. Med. **264**: 870, 1961.

10 Friend, D. G., and Cummins, J. F.: Use of chlorpromazine in the treatment of nausea and vomiting of uremia, New Eng. J. Med. **250**:997, 1954.

11 Glaviano, V. V., and Wang, S. C.: Dual mechanism of the antiemetic action of chlorpromazine, Fed. Proc. **13**:358, 1954.

12 Hendley, C. D., Lynes, T. E., and Berger, F. M.: Effect of 2-methyl, 2-n-propyl-1,3-propanediol dicarbamate (Miltown) on central nervous system, Proc. Soc. Exp. Biol. Med. **87**:608, 1954.

13 Killam, K. F., and Killam, E. K.: Central action of chlorpromazine and reserpine. In Neuropharmacology, Transactions of the Fifth Conference, New York, 1960, Josiah Macy, Jr., Foundation.

14 Lasagna, L., and McCann, W.: Effect of tranquilizing drugs on amphetamine toxicity in aggregated mice, Science **125**:1241, 1957.

15 Levis, S., Preat, S., Beersaerts, J., Dauby, J., Beelen, L., and Baugniet, V.: Pharmacological study on hydroxyzine, U. C. B. 492, a disubstituted piperazine derivative, Arch. Int. Pharmacodyn. **109**:127, 1957.

16 Moyer, J. H., Kinross-Wright, V., and Finney, R. M.: Chlorpromazine as a therapeutic agent in clinical medicine, Arch. Intern. Med. **95**:202, 1955.

17 Prensky, A. L., Raff, M. C., Moore, M. J., and Schwab, R. S.: Intravenous diazepam in the treatment of prolonged seizure activity, New Eng. J. Med. **276**:779, 1967.

Recent reviews

18 Cerletti, A., and Bove, F. J.: The present status of psychotropic drugs, Amsterdam, 1969, Excerpta Medica Foundation.

19 Cook, L., and Kelleher, R. T.: Effects of drugs on behavior, Clin. Pharmacol. Ther. **3**:599, 1962.

20 Davis, J. M., and Fann, W. E.: Lithium, Ann. Rev. Pharmacol. **11**:285, 1971.

21 Domino, E. F.: Human pharmacology of tranquilizing drugs, Clin. Pharmacol. Ther. **3**:599, 1962.

22 Essig, C. F.: Newer sedative drugs that can cause states of intoxication and dependence of barbiturate type, J. A. M. A. **196**:714, 1966.

23 Hollister, L. E.: Complications from psychotherapeutic drugs—1964, Clin. Pharmacol. Ther. **5**:322, 1964.

24 Hollister, L. E.: Mental disorders—antianxiety and antidepressant drugs, New Eng. J. Med. **286**:1195, 1972.

25 Itil, T. M.: Electroencephalography and pharmacopsychiatry. In Freyhan, F. A., Petrilowitsch, N., and Pichot, P., editors: Modern problems of pharmacopsychiatry, vol. 1, Clinical psychopharmacology, Basel, 1968, S. Karger, A. G.

26 Jansen, P. A. J.: The pharmacology of haloperidol, Int. J. Neuropsychiat. (supp.) **3**:10, 1967.

27 Kety, S. S.: Toward hypotheses for a biochemical component in the vulnerability to schizophrenia, Seminars in Psych. **4**:233, 1972.

28 Murphy, D. L., Goodwin, F. K., and Bunney, W. E.: A reevaluation of biogenic amines in manic and depressive states, Hosp. Practice, p. 85, Dec. 1972.

29 National Institute of Mental Health Psychopharmacology Service Center (collaborative study group): Phenothiazine treatment in acute schizophrenia, Arch. Gen. Psychiat. **10**:246, 1964.

30 Randall, L. O., Scheckel, C. L., and Pool, W.: Pharmacology of medazepam and metabolites, Arch. Internat. Pharmacodyn. **185**:135, 1970.

31 Scheckel, C. L.: Pharmacology and chemistry of thioxanthenes with special reference to chlorprothixene. In Freyhan, F. A., Petrilowitsch, N., and Pichot, P., editors: Modern problems of pharmacopsychiatry, vol. 2, The thioxanthenes, New York, 1969, S. Karger, A. G.

32 Schildkraut, J. J.: Neuropsychopharmacology and the affective disorders, New Eng. J. Med. **281**:197, 248, 302, 1969.

33 Schou, M.: Lithium in psychiatric therapy and prophylaxis, J. Psychiat. Res. **6**:67, 1968.

34 Shepherd, M., and Wing, L.: Pharmacological aspects of psychiatry, Advances Pharmacol. **1**:229, 1962.

35 Symposium on anxiety and a decade of tranquilizer therapy, J. Neuropsychiat. **5**:1, 1964.

36 Zbinden, G., and Randall, L. O.: Pharmacology of benzodiazepines: laboratory and clinical correlations, Advances Pharmacol. **5**:213, 1967.

20 Antidepressant and psychotomimetic drugs

GENERAL CONCEPT

The treatment of depression with drugs is a somewhat controversial area.[29] The *monoamine oxidase inhibitors* were introduced as the first antidepressants. *Iproniazid* was soon replaced by somewhat less toxic MAO inhibitors such as phenelzine (Nardil), isocarboxazid (Marplan), nialamide (Niamid), and tranylcypromine (Parnate).

The *tricyclic antidepressant* imipramine (Tofranil) was discovered accidentally during clinical testing for antipsychotic drugs. It was followed soon by related drugs such as amitriptyline (Elavil) and protriptyline (Vivactil) and their demethylated metabolites, such as desipramine (Pertofrane) and nortriptyline (Aventyl).

In addition to these groups of antidepressants, sympathomimetic drugs, such as dextroamphetamine (Dexedrine) and methylphenidate (Ritalin) are still used occasionally in depressed patients.

The *mechanism of action* of all of these drugs is attributed to the catecholamine hypothesis.[23] The various antidepressants increase the catecholamine stores or the effective level of catecholamines in the central nervous system. Thus the MAO inhibitors increase the concentration of catecholamines in the brain, whereas the tricyclic antidepressants interfere with the catecholamine reuptake after its release from nerve endings. Finally, the sympathomimetic amines such as dextroamphetamine release catecholamines and may act directly on central catecholamine receptors.

ANTIDEPRESSANTS—HYDRAZINE MAO INHIBITORS

Among the many disadvantages of the hydrazine MAO inhibitors, the following may be listed: slow action, hepatotoxicity, overstimulation, postural hypotension, insomnia, constipation, weight gain, and paradoxical behavior. Because of these disadvantages, they are being replaced by nonhydrazine MAO inhibitors and newer drugs.

The pharmacology of iproniazid is discussed because of its theoretical interest. The drug is no longer available, having been withdrawn because of hepatotoxicity.

DEVELOPMENT OF MAO INHIBITORS—IPRONIAZID

Iproniazid (Marsilid) was synthesized in 1951 as a chemotherapeutic agent for tuberculosis. It is the isopropyl derivative of isoniazid (Rimifon), which was previously shown to be a highly potent inhibitor of the growth of the tubercle bacillus. The structural formulas of iproniazid and isoniazid follow.

235

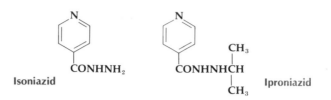

Isoniazid   Iproniazid

The pharmacology of iproniazid will be discussed first, and only the major differences between it and the newer MAO inhibitors will be mentioned.

EFFECTS OF IPRONIAZID IN MAN AND ANIMALS

When the drug is given orally in doses of 2 to 4 mg./kg., there may be a delay of days or weeks before many of the symptoms attributable to the medication develop. Among the effects that may be noted are central nervous system stimulation, characterized by elevation of mood, euphoria, and increase in appetite, and also dizziness, tinnitus, paresthesias, and even toxic psychosis. Additional central nervous system effects may result in hyperreflexia, tremors, jitteriness, and clonus.

Autonomic nervous system actions of iproniazid are indicated by hypotension, dryness of the mouth, and constipation. Toxic effects and idiosyncrasies are evidenced by skin rashes as well as by jaundice on the basis of hepatic involvement.

MODE OF ACTION OF MAO INHIBITORS

The enzyme MAO is widely distributed in the body. Histochemical studies show its presence in practically all tissues. Its function may be the oxidative deamination of such compounds as serotonin, tyramine, and dopamine, since the potency of these amines is greater in animals pretreated with the inhibitors of MAO.

There are several points in favor of the idea that the MAO inhibitors exert their pharmacologic effects as a consequence of enzyme inhibition and the accumulation of various amines. (See Table 20-1.) First of all, the onset of action of these compounds is slow. It may take from 4 to 20 days for their antidepressant action to become manifest. With some of the more potent compounds, the onset of action may be only 12 to 24 hours. In animal experiments it has been shown that the effect of these drugs is better correlated with the degree of enzyme inhibition than with the presence of the drugs in the body.[9] It is important also that when administration of the MAO inhibitors is discontinued, their antidepressant effects may persist for several days.

Table 20-1. Effect of iproniazid on concentration of serotonin in brains of normal and reserpine-treated rabbits*†

Drug	Brain serotonin (μg/gram, average)	Effect
None	0.55	—
Reserpine	0.10	Sedation
Iproniazid	0.63	None
Iproniazid followed by reserpine	0.42	Excitement
Reserpine followed by iproniazid	0.10	Sedation

*From Brodie, B. B., and Shore, P. A.: Ann. N. Y. Acad. Sci. **66**:631, 1957.
†Rabbits were given reserpine intravenously, 5 mg./kg. Iproniazid (100 mg./kg.) was given intravenously 2 hours before or after reserpine. Animals were killed 1 hour after the last drug administration.

NONHYDRAZINE MAO INHIBITORS — TRANYLCYPROMINE

Tranylcypromine (Parnate) is a potent nonhydrazine MAO inhibitor that also has a direct amphetamine-like stimulant action. Thus it is a *bimodal antidepressant*.

The drug is closely related to amphetamine.

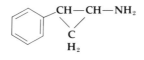

Tranylcypromine

Tranylcypromine provides fast, direct stimulation similar to that of amphetamine, but its action is sustained, probably as a consequence of its MAO inhibitory action. Its fast action is an advantage over the hydrazine drugs, but it shares with the latter the ability to cause postural hypotension. It is a remarkable fact that all MAO inhibitors cause postural hypotension. Tranylcypromine may cause overstimulation, and its use may be combined with a phenothiazine to combat the overstimulation.

Severe hypertensive reactions have occurred in patients treated with tranylcypromine following the ingestion of aged cheese.[4,31] These reactions may be attributed to the presence of tyramine and other monoamines that would normally be detoxified by MAO.

For the treatment of depressive reactions, tranylcypromine is administered orally, 10 mg. twice a day for several weeks.

• • •

Pargyline is discussed with the antihypertensive drugs on p. 173.

TRICYCLIC ANTIDEPRESSANTS

The tricyclic antidepressants such as imipramine (Tofranil) and amitriptyline (Elavil) and their desmethyl derivatives are chemically similar to the phenothiazines. Their pharmacologic properties are also similar, but empirically they have been found useful as antidepressants.

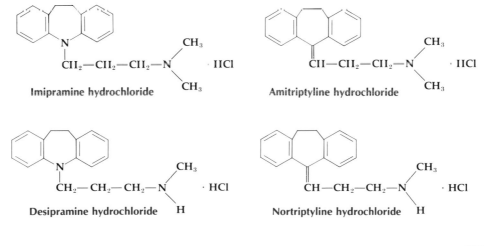

Imipramine hydrochloride

Amitriptyline hydrochloride

Desipramine hydrochloride

Nortriptyline hydrochloride

The basic pharmacology of imipramine and amitriptyline is quite complex. These drugs do not inhibit MAO, but they do have anticholinergic, antiserotonin, and antihistaminic actions. In fact, amitriptyline is a potent antihistaminic. The basic mechanism of their antidepressant action may be related to the fact that imipramine can block the uptake of norepinephrine by the brain and other organs.[5,7,12]

Imipramine and related drugs have a cocainelike effect on uptake and binding of injected norepinephrine in vivo. One could speculate that the common denominator between the actions of the MAO inhibitors and imipramine is the presence of elevated free norepinephrine levels in the brain.

Imipramine and amitriptyline are metabolized in the body to *N*-desmethyl derivatives, which are pharmacologically active. These derivatives have been introduced into therapeutics under the names of desipramine hydrochloride (Pertofrane) and nortriptyline hydrochloride (Aventyl). A closely related antidepressant is available under the name protriptyline hydrochloride (Vivactil).

Desipramine is chemically a tricyclic antidepressant and is pharmacologically related to imipramine. In fact, it is a metabolic product of the latter. The adverse reactions are also similar but may occur less frequently. The adverse reactions are in part atropine-like—dryness of the mouth, blurred vision, and constipation. But in addition, other adverse reactions to both imipramine and desipramine may occur, including ataxia, orthostatic hypotension, parkinsonism-like symptoms, agitation, and anxiety.

ADVERSE EFFECTS OF TRICYCLIC ANTIDEPRESSANTS

Common adverse effects after the use of tricyclic antidepressants are related to autonomic nervous system dysfunction and include dryness of the mouth, constipation, urinary retention in men, and hypotension. Cholestatic jaundice has been reported as a result of the use of these drugs. First-degree atrioventricular block indicates that these drugs can slow atrioventricular conduction.

DIBENZOXEPINES

Just as the tricyclic antidepressants resulted from modifications of the central ring of the phenothiazines, an additional modification has led to a new family of psychotherapeutic agents—the dibenzoxepines. **Doxepin** (Sinequan) is claimed to have a mixture of antipsychotic and antidepressant properties. The drug is administered in a daily dosage range of 25 to 300 mg. in three divided doses. Its exact position in relation to the phenothiazines and the other tricyclic antidepressants is impossible to assess at the present.

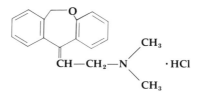

Doxepin hydrochloride

TOXICITY OF COMBINATION OF ANTIDEPRESSANTS

It is unwise and dangerous to combine some of the antidepressant medications. The simultaneous administration of MAO inhibitors and amitriptyline or imipramine may produce severe *atropine-like reactions, with tremors, hyperpyrexia, convulsions, delirium, and death.*[10, 15] A 1-week interval is recommended between the time an MAO inhibitor is discontinued and a suppressant antidepressant is administered. (For a contrary view see reference 21.)

PSYCHOMOTOR STIMULANTS

Amphetamine has been used for years as a mood elevator in depressed patients. Its disadvantages are its cardiovascular effects and the letdown that follows the short period of stimulation. Some mild stimulants, probably related in action and chemistry to amphetamine, are sometimes used in depressive states. These are pipradrol (Meratran) and methylphenidate (Ritalin).

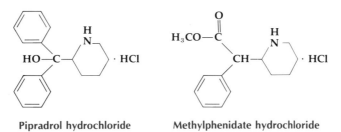

Pipradrol hydrochloride Methylphenidate hydrochloride

Pipradrol has been used as an antidepressant in depressive states, but its effectiveness is questionable. The related drug, methylphenidate hydrochloride is more widely used and abused.

Methylphenidate resembles dextroamphetamine in its pharmacology except for its lower potency. The drug is used widely as a mild stimulant in depressive states but is not basically superior to dextroamphetamine. Its use in hyperkinetic children may be justified and is quite effective. It is often used in the treatment of narcolepsy and is one of the favorites of medical students just before examinations.

Although methylphenidate in the usual adult dosage of 10 mg. taken orally does not elevate the blood pressure, it should not be used in hypertensives or any patients in whom sympathetic stimulation may be hazardous.

Preparations of methylphenidate hydrochloride (Ritalin hydrochloride) include tablets containing 5, 10, and 20 mg. and powder for injection, 100 mg.

PSYCHOTOMIMETIC DRUGS

Certain drugs can produce toxic psychosis in small doses. Interest in these compounds has been great, partly because they have some usefulness in experimental psychiatry and partly because their actions suggest that perhaps there may be a chemical basis for mental illness. The various chemical theories of mental illness have been critically reviewed by Kety.[13] The conclusion is that they are not convincing.

Some of the most interesting psychotomimetic agents are lysergic acid diethylamide, mescaline, and psilocybin.

Lysergic acid diethylamide (LSD; Delysid) is closely related to the ergot alkaloids. Its structural formula and that of mescaline are as follows:

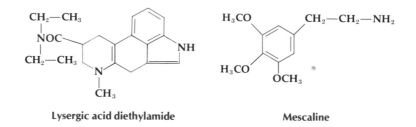

Lysergic acid diethylamide   **Mescaline**

The discovery of its hallucinogenic properties was made by the chemist who synthesized the drug and noted these reactions on himself. Subjects who take a few micrograms of LSD develop auditory and visual hallucinations. The body may feel distorted, the arms, for example, appearing to be at a great distance. The subject may become fearful and irrational.

In animal experiments, LSD may cause excitement and hyperthermia. Upon repeated administration, considerable tolerance to the drug develops.

LSD is a potent antagonist of the action of serotonin on smooth muscles. The association of this antiserotonin activity and the psychic effects suggested many interesting speculations concerning the role of serotonin in behavior. It should be remembered, however, that there is no evidence to indicate that the central actions of LSD are due to its antagonistic effect on serotonin. These actions may simply be a direct effect of an unusual amine. Brom-lysergic acid diethylamide has antiserotonin effects on smooth muscles similar to those of LSD, but the drug has no hallucinogenic properties. There is also no evidence for the normal occurrence of an LSD-like substance in mammals.

Mescaline is obtained from the cactus known as peyote or mescal (*Lophophora williamsii*) found in the southwestern region of the United States. This cactus is used by some Indians in religious ceremonies. Persons who have ingested dried peyote buttons report that they cause a stuporous state with unusual visual hallucinations. Colored lights, which are reported to be extremely beautiful, are the most striking feature of these hallucinations. Interestingly, some volunteers report that they have seen colors they did not know existed.

Mescaline, the active principle of peyote, is 3,4,5-trimethoxyphenethylamine, a structure resembling the sympathomimetic amines. The compound has some interest in experimental psychiatry. It is used experimentally in doses of 300 to 500 mg.

Psilocybin (*O*-phosphoryl-4-hydroxy-*N*,*N*-dimethyltryptamine) has been isolated from Mexican mushrooms that have hallucinogenic effects. Chemically it is closely related to serotonin.

It is of great interest that compounds related to the endogenously occurring amines have hallucinogenic properties. Further research is needed to explain why this should be so.

The abuse of psychotomimetic drugs is discussed in detail in Chapter 25.

References

1 Brodie, B. B., Prockop, D. J., and Shore, P. A.: An interpretation of the action of psychotropic drugs, Postgrad. Med. 24:296, 1958.

2 Carlsson, A., Corrodi, H., Fuxe, K., and Hokfelt, T.: Effect of antidepressant drugs on the depletion of intraneuronal brain 5-hydroxytryptamine stores caused by 4-methyl-α-ethyl-meta-tyramine, Europ. J. Pharmacol. 5:357, 1969.

3 Corrodi, H., and Fuxe, K.: Decreased turnover in central 5-HT nerve terminals induced by antidepressant drugs of the imipramine type, Europ. J. Pharmacol. 7:56, 1969.

4 Davies, E. B.: Tranylcypromine and cheese, Lancet 2:691, 1963.

5 Dengler, H. J., Michaelson, I. A., Spiegel, H. E., and Titus, E. O.: The uptake of labeled norepinephrine by isolated brain and other tissues of the cat, Int. J. Neuropharmacol. 1:23, 1962.

6 De Ritter, E., Drekter, L., Scheiner, J., and Rubin, S. H.: Urinary excretion of hydrazine derivatives of isonicotinic acid in normal humans, Proc. Soc. Exp. Biol. Med. 79:654, 1952.

7 Glowinski, J., and Axelrod, J.: Inhibition of uptake of tritiated-noradrenaline in the intact rat brain by imipramine and structurally related compounds, Nature 204:1318, 1964.

8 Harthorne, J. W., Marcus, A. M., and Kaye, M.: Management of massive imipramine overdosage with mannitol and artificial dialysis, New Eng. J. Med. 268:33, 1963.

9 Hess, S., Weissbach, H., Redfield, B. G., and Udenfriend, S.: The relationship between iproniazid metabolism and the duration of its effect on monoamine oxidase, J. Pharmacol. Exp. Ther. 124:189, 1958.

10 Himwich, W. A., and Petersen, J. C.: Effect of combined administration of imipramine and monoamine oxidase inhibitor, Amer. J. Psychiat. 117:928, 1961.

11 Hudgens, R. W., Tanna, V. L., Harley, J. D., and Leary, D. J.: Visual hallucinations with iminodibenzyl antidepressants, J.A.M.A. 198:81, 1966.

12 Iversen, L. L.: Inhibition of norepinephrine uptake by drugs, J. Pharm. Pharmacol. 17:62, 1965.

13 Kety, S. S.: Biochemical theories of schizophrenia, Science 129:1528, 1590, 1959.

14 Lehmann, H. E.: Tranquilizers and other psychotropic drugs in clinical practice, Canad. Med. Ass. J. 79:701, 1958.

15 Luby, E. D., and Domino, E. F.: Toxicity from large doses of imipramine and MAO inhibitor in suicidal intent, J.A.M.A. 177:68, 1961.

16 Pfeiffer, C. C., Goldstein, L., Munoz, C., Murphree, H. B., and Jenney, E. H.: Quantitative comparisons of the electroencephalographic stimulant effects of deanol, choline, and amphetamine, Clin. Pharmacol. Ther. 4:461, 1963.

17 Rickels, K., Raab, E., DeSilverio, R., and Etemad, B.: Drug treatment of depression, J.A.M.A. 201:675, 1967.

18 Rowe, G. G., Afonso, S., Castillo, C. A., Kyle, J. C., Leicht, T. R., and Crumpton, C. W.: Systemic and coronary hemodynamic effects of an amine oxidase inhibitor and of serotonin, Clin. Pharmacol. Ther. 4:467, 1963.

19 Scherbel, A. L.: Clinical experience in treatment of over 2000 cases with amine oxidase inhibitors, Dis. Nerv. Sys. (supp.) 21:67, 1960.

20 Schiele, B. C.: Newer drugs for mental illness, J.A.M.A. 181:126, 1962.

21 Schuckit, M., Robins, E., and Feighner, J.: Tricyclic antidepressants and monoamine oxidase inhibitors, Arch. Gen. Psychiat. 24:509, 1971.

22 Zeller, E. A., and Barsky, J.: In vivo inhibition of liver and brain monoamine oxidase by 1-isonicotinyl-2-isopropylhydrazine, Proc. Soc. Exp. Biol. Med. 81:459, 1952.

Recent reviews

23 Axelrod, J.: Biogenic amines and their impact in psychiatry, Seminars in Psychiat. 4:199, 1972.

24 Cohen, S.: Psychotomimetic agents, Ann. Rev. Pharmacol. 7:301, 1967.

25 Friend, D.: Antidepressant drug therapy, Clin. Pharmacol. Ther. 6:805, 1965.

26 Himwich, H. E., and Alpers, H.: Psychopharmacology, Ann. Rev. Pharmacol. 10:313, 1970.

27 Hollister, L. E.: Chemical psychoses, Ann. Rev. Med. 15:203, 1964.

28 Hollister, L. E.: Overdoses of psychotherapeutic drugs, Clin. Pharmacol. Ther. 7:142, 1966.

29 Hollister, L. E.: Mental disorders — antianxiety and antidepressant drugs, New Eng. J. Med. 286:1195, 1972.

30 Jacobsen, E.: The clinical pharmacology of the hallucinogens, Clin. Pharmacol. Ther. 4:480, 1963.

31 Kline, N. S.: The practical management of depression, J.A.M.A. 190:732, 1964.

32 Lennard, H. L., Epstein, L. J., Bernstein, A., and Ransom, D. C.: Hazards implicit in prescribing psychoactive drugs, Science 169:438, 1970.

33 Sulser, F., and Sanders-Bush, E.: Effect of drugs on amines in the CNS, Ann. Rev. Pharmacol. 11:209, 1971.

SECTION FOUR

DEPRESSANTS AND STIMULANTS OF THE CENTRAL NERVOUS SYSTEM

21 Hypnotic drugs

GENERAL CONSIDERATIONS

A variety of drugs can produce a state of depression of the central nervous system resembling normal sleep. These drugs are referred to as *hypnotics*. In smaller doses many of these drugs can produce a state of drowsiness, and when used in this manner, they are referred to as *sedatives*. When used in larger doses, hypnotics may produce anesthesia, poisoning, and death. These progressive dose-related effects may be indicated as follows:

$$\text{Sedation} \rightleftarrows \text{Hypnosis} \rightleftarrows \text{Anesthesia} \rightleftarrows \text{Coma} \rightarrow \text{Death}$$

Hypnotics have many important uses in medicine. Sleeping pills are used properly and improperly by many people. In addition, hypnotics are helpful in combination with analgesics in painful states, are antidotes for stimulant and convulsant drugs, and are useful in convulsive disorders and as adjuncts to anesthesia.

The most important hypnotics are the barbiturates, which were introduced as early as 1903 by Fischer and von Mering. When properly used, they are highly effective and safe medications. While the barbiturates are habit-forming and may even lead to addiction, the newer sedative-hypnotics, offered with the implication of being safer, are not truly superior. The piperidinediones such as glutethimide and methyprylon, introduced as "nonbarbiturate hypnotics," are actually chemically related to the barbiturates and offer no special advantages.

In addition to the barbiturates and the piperidinediones, there are many other classes of drugs that properly belong to the sedative-hypnotic group. Carbamates such as urethan and related drugs, bromides, alcohols, and paraldehyde are also classified as sedative-hypnotics.

A new benzodiazepine, flurazepam (Dalmane), has been introduced as a hypnotic agent for all types of insomnia.

BARBITURATES
Chemistry

The combination of urea with organic acids results in monoureides and diureides that have hypnotic properties. The combination of urea and malonic acid is malonylurea, or barbituric acid, the parent compound of the barbiturate series. The structural formulas of urea, malonic acid, and barbituric acid follow.

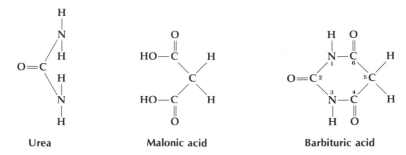

| Urea | Malonic acid | Barbituric acid |

The majority of the clinically useful barbiturates are obtained by making appropriate substitutions in position 5 of the molecule. Thus phenobarbital is ethylphenylbarbituric acid. In some cases an additional substitution is made by replacing a hydrogen in the ring. Thus mephobarbital (Mebaral) differs from phenobarbital in having a CH_3 group attached to a nitrogen atom. Finally, if thiourea instead of urea is combined with malonic acid, the resulting thiobarbituric acid is the parent compound of the ultrashort-acting barbiturate intravenous anesthetics such as thiopental (Pentothal).

Classification

The therapeutically useful barbiturates have traditionally been classified according to their duration of action, based on animal experiments.[84] Thus the pharmacologic literature describes ultrashort-, short-, intermediate-, and long-acting barbiturates, as indicated in Table 21-1.

Clinical experience indicates, however, that this classification is misleading.[46,84] In particular, the distinction between short- and long-acting barbiturates is not borne out by controlled clinical trials. Thus 100 mg. doses of secobarbital, pentobarbital, and phenobarbital were equally effective in inducing sleep in patients with chronic

Table 21-1. Classification, structure, and dosage of commonly used barbiturates

Names	Substituents in position 5	Hypnotic dose	Duration of action
Thiopental* (Pentothal)	Ethyl, 1-methylbutyl		Ultrashort
Thiamylal* (Surital)	Allyl, 1-methylbutyl		(intravenous
Hexobarbital† (Evipal)	Methyl, cyclohexenyl		anesthetics)
Secobarbital (Seconal)	Allyl, 1-methylbutyl	0.1-0.2 Gm.	Short
Pentobarbital (Nembutal)	Ethyl, 1-methylbutyl	0.1 Gm.	
Butabarbital (Butisol)	Ethyl, sec-butyl	0.1-0.2 Gm.	Intermediate
Amobarbital (Amytal)	Ethyl, isoamyl	0.05-0.2 Gm.	
Vinbarbital (Delvinal)	Ethyl, 1-methyl-1-butenyl	0.1-0.2 Gm.	
Phenobarbital (Luminal)	Ethyl, phenyl	0.1-0.2 Gm.	Long
Mephobarbital† (Mebaral)	Ethyl, phenyl	0.1-0.2 Gm.	
Barbital (Veronal)	Ethyl, ethyl	0.3-0.5 Gm.	

*Thiobarbiturate.
†A CH_3 group is attached to the nitrogen atom.

diseases.[38] In the same study, hangover was not greater with the long-acting pheno-barbital than with secobarbital or pentobarbital.

It is a reasonable suggestion that barbiturates be simply classified according to their therapeutic indications as "sedative-hypnotic barbiturates" and "anesthetic barbiturates."[84] Within the former group the physician may find that phenobarbital may be more slowly absorbed and metabolized and is thus more suitable for maintained sedation than secobarbital or pentobarbital. Nevertheless, for their most common usage, the promotion of sleep, duration of action has been overemphasized.

Physicochemical factors and pharmacokinetic behavior in the barbiturate series

Barbiturates are weak acids that cross biologic membranes in their undissociated form as a function of their *lipid solubility*. The variations in absorption, distribution, protein binding, speed of metabolic degradation, tissue localization, duration of action, and renal excretion are well correlated with the lipid solubility of the undissociated barbituric acid derivative.

The relationship between lipid solubility of a series of barbiturates and their therapeutic classification is shown in Table 21-2. Clearly, the ultrashort-acting intravenous anesthetics are highly lipid soluble, the short- and intermediate-acting sedative-hypnotics are much less so, and the long-acting drugs such as phenobarbital and barbital are even less lipid soluble.

Table 21-3 shows the pharmacokinetic characteristics of three representative barbiturates in relation to their lipid solubilities. Phenobarbital, having a low lipid solubility compared with secobarbital or thiopental, is generally classified as a "long-acting" sedative-hypnotic. This is a consequence of its slow absorption from the gastrointestinal tract and its slower rate of metabolism. The renal excretion of 30% of the administered

Table 21-2. Lipid solubility of a series of barbiturates as determined by their partition coefficients between methylene chloride and water*

Drug	Partition coefficient†	Classification
Methohexital	1,000	Intravenous anesthetic
Thiopental	580	Intravenous anesthetic
Secobarbital	52	Sedative-hypnotic, short acting
Amobarbital	42	Sedative-hypnotic, short or intermediate acting
Pentobarbital	39	Sedative-hypnotic, short or intermediate acting
Phenobarbital	3	Sedative-hypnotic, long acting
Barbital	1	Sedative-hypnotic, long acting

* Based on data from Bush, M. T.: In Root, W. S., and Hofmann, F. G., editors: Physiological pharmacology, vol. 1, New York, 1963, Academic Press, Inc.

† Partition coefficient between methylene chloride and water at approximately 25° C. of the un-ionized form. The partition coefficient is defined as the ratio: (concentration in organic solvent)/(concentration in aqueous phase) at equilibrium. Methylene chloride is a typical lipid solvent.

Table 21-3. Pharmacokinetic behavior of three representative barbiturates in relation to their lipid solubility

Characteristics	Phenobarbital	Secobarbital	Thiopental
Partition coefficient*	3	52	580
Absorption from stomach†	Slow	Rapid	Rapid (not used orally)
Plasma protein binding†	2%	44%	65%
Rate of entry into CNS	Slow	Rapid	Very rapid
Renal excretion of unchanged drug	30%	Negligible	Negligible

* Between methylene chloride and water.
†Data from Bush.[72]

phenobarbital is a consequence of several factors—slower rate of metabolism, less protein binding, and less tubular reabsorption. In the case of barbital, which is even less lipid soluble, as much as 65 to 90% of the administered dose is excreted unchanged.

The rate of entry into the central nervous system is strongly influenced by lipid solubility. When thiopental is injected intravenously, it produces anesthesia almost instantaneously. On the other hand, when sodium phenobarbital was injected intravenously into mice, there was a delay of 12 minutes before anesthesia occurred.[7]

In addition to lipid solubility, ionization of barbiturates plays a role in their distribution and excretion. For practical purposes this is important only when the pK_a of the drug is about the same as the physiologic pH. The pK_a of phenobarbital is 7.3. As a consequence, relatively slight changes in the pH of the body fluids will exert a significant effect on the degree of ionization of phenobarbital. It has been demonstrated that alkalinization with sodium bicarbonate infusions or hyperventilation will favor a movement of phenobarbital from the tissues to the plasma.[64] For the same reasons administration of sodium bicarbonate, with its alkalinizing effect on the urine, will favor the excretion of phenobarbital.[64]

Pharmacologic effects

The primary action of the barbiturates is on nervous tissue. The consequences of this primary action are manifested as (1) hypnosis and anesthesia, (2) anticonvulsant effects, and (3) miscellaneous effects such as analgesia, autonomic nervous system actions, respiratory effects, and others.

Hypnosis and anesthesia. Following the administration of a hypnotic dose of a barbiturate, the only significant effect consists of sleep from which the individual can be awakened by various stimuli. When larger amounts are administered, a state of anesthesia ensues from which the person or animal cannot be awakened until the drug is metabolized or, in the case of the ultrashort-acting compounds, until the blood level of the drug falls as a consequence of its distribution in the body. The same barbiturate may be a sedative, a hypnotic, or an anesthetic or may be lethal as increasing doses are administered. This relationship between dosage and effect is illustrated in Fig. 21-1.

It may be seen from the data that the therapeutic index, expressed as LD_{50}/hypnotic dose$_{50}$, is quite favorable. On the other hand, the anesthetic dose is dangerously close

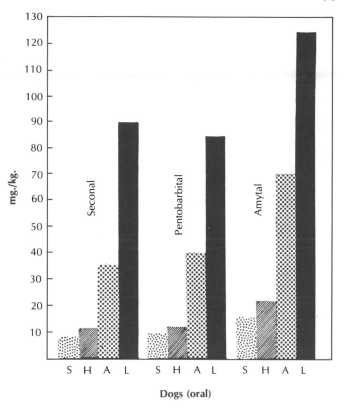

Fig. 21-1. Activity of three barbiturates in dogs. A comparison of three barbiturates with regard to sedative, hypnotic, anesthetic, and lethal doses. **S,** Sedative dose$_{50}$; **H,** hypnotic dose$_{50}$; **A,** anesthetic dose$_{50}$; **L,** lethal dose$_{50}$. Note that SD$_{50}$ is approximately one fourth of AD$_{50}$, HD$_{50}$ is about one third of AD$_{50}$, and AD$_{50}$ is about one half of LD$_{50}$. (From Chen, K. K.: In Symposium on sedative and hypnotic drugs, Baltimore, 1954, The Williams & Wilkins Co.)

to the lethal dose. This is an important reason why the ordinary sedative-hypnotic barbiturates are not suitable for general anesthesia in patients, although they are commonly used in experimental animals. The ultrashort-acting barbiturates are used in anesthesia for induction and supplementation of inhalation agents because their rapid redistribution in the body allows a minute-to-minute adjustment of the intensity of their effect. The cause of death following administration of large doses is respiratory failure as a consequence of depression of the respiratory center.

Very little is known about the mechanism of the hypnotic effect, just as there is little understanding of the mechanism of normal sleep. Recent pharmacologic and neurophysiologic studies that suggest a relationship between brain serotonin and sleep have been summarized and discussed by Jouvet.[30]

Of great current interest is the effect of barbiturates and other drugs on the various sleep states. It is now recognized that sleep consists of two main functional states. One is called "slow wave," nondreaming, or non-rapid eye movement (NREM) sleep. The other is referred to as "paradoxical," dreaming, or rapid eye movement (REM) sleep. Dream deprivation or suppression of REM sleep causes adverse effects in normal subjects. Since sedative-hypnotic drugs tend to suppress REM sleep, evaluation of the long-range consequences of their chronic use is an important research problem.[74, 87] Certain newer sedative-hypnotics that are being promoted are claimed to have less effect on REM sleep, but any such conclusion would seem premature. The recently introduced drug flurazepam hydrochloride (Dalmane), for example, is said not to decrease dream time as reflected by REM. The significance of this finding remains to be demonstrated.

The studies of Magoun[43] indicate that barbiturates have a selective effect on the reticular activating system and are capable of blocking ascending conduction in this area. It has also been shown that the barbiturates increase the recovery time and raise the threshold for neurons in general.[62] The selective effect on the ascending reticular formation may be related to the extensive chain of synaptic connections in this area or to a lower factor of safety at the individual synapses.

Anticonvulsant effects. The barbiturates are potent antidotes of the convulsant drugs, and they can also abolish convulsions that arise in disease states such as tetanus and eclampsia. Some of the barbiturates are effective also as antiepileptic drugs, but not all are useful in this respect.

The antidotal action of the barbiturates against convulsant drugs is of great practical importance. It is possible to protect experimental animals against as many as ten lethal doses of strychnine and pentylenetetrazol and also against the convulsant and lethal action of local anesthetics such as procaine and cocaine. It is important to point out, however, that whereas the barbiturates are very potent antidotes against the convulsant drugs, the mutual antagonism works much better in this sequence than in the reverse direction; that is, convulsant drugs are only moderately effective against barbiturate depression and can protect experimental animals against only *very few* lethal doses of barbiturates.

The barbiturates are often employed for preventing or abolishing convulsions in disease states. For this purpose the drugs are usually injected intravenously or intramuscularly.

When a barbiturate is used as an anticonvulsant, it is important to realize that if the duration of action of the barbiturate outlasts the duration of action of the convulsant, serious depression of respiration may result. For this reason the ultrashort-acting or short-acting barbiturates are much preferred in the management of convulsive emergencies.

In addition to this general usefulness of the barbiturates as anticonvulsants, some members of the series are also antiepileptic drugs. Phenobarbital, mephobarbital, and metharbital have special anticonvulsant and antiepileptic properties. Clinically these drugs are potent in the management of grand mal epilepsy, and experimental studies indicate also that these three barbiturates have anticonvulsant actions in situations in which other members of the series are ineffective.

Miscellaneous effects. Miscellaneous effects include analgesia, autonomic nervous system actions, respiratory effects, and others.

Analgesia. It is generally believed that barbiturates are not primarily analgesic, or at least they do not elevate the pain threshold significantly. A patient still perceives painful stimuli when subanesthetic doses of barbiturates are given. Also, a patient experiencing severe pain may become agitated and delirious if barbiturates are administered without analgesics. On the other hand, barbiturates may modify the reaction to pain. It has been shown that intravenous hypnotic doses of pentobarbital produced relief from postoperative pain in 50% of the patients in one series, whereas a placebo relieved only 20%.[32] Morphine produced relief in 80% of these patients.

It appears likely, then, that although the barbiturates are not primarily analgesics, they may modify the reaction of patients to pain and may be useful in combinations with analgesics.

Autonomic nervous system actions. Ordinary hypnotic doses of the barbiturates have no important actions on the autonomic nervous system. On the other hand, anesthetic doses can produce many effects on autonomic function.

Central autonomic regulations are influenced by these drugs. The body temperature tends to fall in barbiturate anesthesia, partly as a result of central interference with temperature regulation. Direct hypothalamic stimulation produces a lessened blood pressure rise in barbiturate-anesthetized animals. Intravenously injected barbiturates can markedly lower the blood pressure by a depression of the vasomotor centers.

Peripheral autonomic mechanisms may be influenced by the barbiturates. Ganglionic transmission is depressed by amobarbital and to a lesser extent by other barbiturates.[12] Serum cholinesterase activity can be inhibited by various barbiturates, but this has questionable importance in their therapeutic uses in man.[57]

Respiratory effects. While hypnotic doses of barbiturates cause only minor depression of respiration, larger doses depress the respiratory center and diminish its responsiveness to CO_2. The cause of death in acute barbiturate poisoning is respiratory depression.

It is generally believed that in severe barbiturate depression the respiratory center is still responsive to anoxia through the carotid chemoreceptor mechanism. There is experimental evidence to indicate that oxygen may further depress respiration in profound barbiturate anesthesia by eliminating the anoxic drive.[2]

Other respiratory effects consist of hiccoughing, coughing, and laryngospasm, which may follow the intravenous administration of the ultrashort-acting and short-acting barbiturates. Although this is referred to as a vagal action, the mechanism is not clear.

Other effects. Hypnotic doses of the barbiturates exert no effects on the heart. In heart-lung preparations, large experimental doses of the barbiturates can produce failure, which responds to digitalis glycosides. However, concentrations used in these experiments are much higher than those that can be obtained in patients. The low blood pressure in barbiturate poisoning is probably a consequence of both impaired gaseous exchange secondary to respiratory depression and actions on central and peripheral components of the autonomic nervous system.

The gastrointestinal tract is not influenced by hypnotic doses of the barbiturates. The clinical uses of barbiturates in diseases of the gastrointestinal tract are based on the central nervous system actions of these hypnotics.

The barbiturates in anesthetic doses have some effects on renal function. Urine volume tends to decrease, partly as a result of hemodynamic changes and partly due to the release of antidiuretic hormone.

Metabolism

The barbiturates are absorbed rapidly from the stomach, intestine, rectum, subcutaneous tissue, and muscle. Their sodium salts are employed when given by injection.

Following absorption, the barbiturates are bound to a varying extent to plasma proteins. Thiopental is bound up to 60 or 70%, pentobarbital about 50%, and the long-acting phenobarbital only to a very slight extent.

Just as plasma binding varies with the different barbiturates, their binding by tissues also shows important differences. The concentration of thiopental or pentobarbital in the brain is not very different from their concentration in plasma. On the other hand, thiopental may be six times more concentrated in body fat than in plasma, whereas pentobarbital is not concentrated in fatty tissue.[3,4]

Some of the barbiturates penetrate into the brain more slowly than others, even following intravenous injection. Barbital shows an "anesthetic lag," which has been correlated with its slow equilibration with brain tissue.[5] This in turn correlates well with the low fat solubility of the nonionized barbital, as contrasted with that of pentobarbital.

The metabolic degradation of the various barbiturates follows four general paths: (1) oxidation of radicals in the 5 position, (2) removal of N-alkyl radicals, (3) conversion of thiobarbiturates to their oxygen analogs, and (4) cleavage of the ring. The first mechanism is important for pentobarbital, phenobarbital, and many others, including the thiobarbiturates. The second mechanism has been demonstrated for mephobarbital,[8] whereas the importance of mechanisms 3 and 4 in man is not known.

The long-acting barbiturate phenobarbital is metabolized quite slowly to p-hydroxyphenobarbital. As a consequence, as much as 30% of a dose of phenobarbital in man may be recovered in the urine. Renal handling of the various barbiturates appears to be glomerular filtration with partial tubular reabsorption. In the case of phenobarbital, excretion of the drug is markedly influenced by the urinary pH. Excretion of the drug is promoted by an alkaline pH. This has been explained on the basis of the principle that alkalinity increases the percentage of ionized phenobarbital. The ionic form, being less lipid soluble, is not reabsorbed effectively through the tubules, and thus increased excretion results.[64] This principle has practical applications in the management of phenobarbital poisoning.

Factors that influence action

Many factors have been described that either oppose or potentiate the action of the barbiturates, but only a few of these have practical significance.

The various central nervous system stimulants such as caffeine, strychnine, picrotoxin, pentylenetetrazol, and bemegride (β,β-methylethylglutarimide; Megimide) tend to oppose the action of the barbiturates, particularly when they are administered at about the same time. This antagonism does not have the same specificity as the well-known antagonism of nalorphine and morphine. In severe, prolonged barbiturate anesthesia the antidotal action of the central nervous system stimulants is weak.

With the exception of the stimulants, the only procedures that may shorten the action of the barbiturates are those that promote the removal of the drug from the body. Alkalinization of the urine promotes excretion of phenobarbital but cannot be expected to be effective in the case of the short-acting and intermediate-acting compounds, since their pK' is higher.[64]

The action of the barbiturates is intensified by several factors. These can be divided into two categories: factors that interfere with the metabolism or excretion of the barbiturates and drugs that exert synergistic effects with the barbiturates on the central nervous system.

Factors that interfere with metabolism or excretion of barbiturates. Liver and kidney diseases may intensify the action of the barbiturates by interfering with their metabolism or excretion. The side chain oxidation of the barbiturates is carried out in the liver microsomes. The factor of safety must be great, however, since degradation of the barbiturates proceeds quite adequately even in patients with cirrhosis. Kidney disease is expected to prolong the half-life of those barbiturates normally excreted in the urine. In uremia the toxicity of the barbiturates is increased out of proportion to the deficient clearance of the drugs by the kidney; the mechanisms are not clear.

Drugs that inhibit the hepatic microsomal enzymes interfere with the metabolism of barbiturates. An experimental preparation, SKF-525 A, the propyl derivative of adiphenine (Trasentine), is a powerful inhibitor of microsomal enzymes. Some MAO inhibitors have an additional effect on microsomal enzymes and prolong the action of barbiturates.

Drugs that intensify the action of barbiturates. Alcohol, reserpine, the phenothiazine tranquilizers, other sedative-hypnotics, and many other drugs may intensify the actions of the barbiturates. For this reason it is inadvisable to administer drugs in combination with barbiturates without considering possible drug interactions. Another reason is the capacity of some barbiturates (phenobarbital, for example) to accelerate the metabolism of a variety of drugs by enzyme induction in the hepatic microsomes (p. 33).

Toxicity

The barbiturates are safe and effective drugs when administered in hypnotic doses to normal persons. Untoward effects may arise in an occasional person as unexplained idiosyncrasies or in all persons as a result of acute or chronic overdosage. Barbiturates are strictly contraindicated in porphyria, since they may produce severe toxic effects, even paralysis.[66]

A few persons, particularly elderly persons, may exhibit idiosyncratic excitement instead of depression following the use of the barbiturates. A few may also show skin reactions, vague pains and aches, and gastrointestinal symptoms. The incidence of these unusual responses is extraordinarily low.

Acute barbiturate poisoning

Barbiturate poisoning is one of the most common problems in toxicology. The intake of large doses of barbiturates may be intentional in suicide or it may be accidental.

The cause of death in acute, overwhelming barbiturate poisoning is undoubtedly cessation of respiration as a consequence of depression of the respiratory center. If the ingested dose is not quite lethal or absorption from the gastrointestinal tract is delayed, the individual may survive for many hours or days. Under these conditions he will often be comatose, his respiration slow, his skin and mucous membranes cyanotic, and various reflexes will be diminished or absent. Body temperature will be low, blood pressure may be diminished, and the pupils may be somewhat constricted and may or may not respond to light.

Although respiratory depression is the primary cause of death in acute, overwhelming barbiturate poisoning, other factors may contribute to lethality if the patient does not succumb in the first few hours. Impairment of circulation, hypostatic pneumonia, and perhaps unknown mechanisms may still cause death even if adequate oxygenation is ensured.

Treatment. Maintenance of adequate respiration and circulation should be the most important objectives in the treatment of acute poisoning. In addition, efforts at eliminating the drug may contribute to recovery. Such efforts include the administration of osmotic diuretics such as mannitol or hemodialysis and in phenobarbital poisoning the administration of sodium bicarbonate to produce an alkaline urine.

Alkalinization of the urine in the case of phenobarbital is based on a sound principle that has been confirmed by animal experiments.[64] The pK_a of phenobarbital is 7.3. At a urinary pH of 8, achievable with bicarbonate administration, 86% of the phenobarbital in the renal tubular fluid becomes ionized and 14% nonionized. It will be recalled (p. 22) that it is the ionized fraction which escapes tubular reabsorption. The reason for the ineffectiveness of alkalinization in promoting the urinary excretion of other commonly used barbiturates becomes obvious by examining their acid dissociation constants. The pK_a of pentobarbital is 8.1. Even if the urinary pH is brought to 8 with bicarbonate, as much as 44% of the drug would still be un-ionized and thus reabsorbable by the tubules.

The experimental administration of central nervous system stimulants in the early stages of poisoning can protect animals against an otherwise lethal dose of barbiturates. Artificial respiration will do the same by reversing the adverse effects of hypoxia and hypercapnia. Although central nervous system stimulants were widely used at one time in the treatment of barbiturate poisoning, they have fallen into disfavor as compared with the physiologic approach first promoted by a Danish group of investigators.[49] Excessive use of central nervous system stimulants can lead to secondary depression of respiration and aggravation of the clinical state of the poisoned individual. There are no specific pharmacologic antagonists for sedative-hypnotic drugs.

According to the best current evidence, supportive therapy with early gastric aspiration and efforts at elimination of the drug from the body are more rewarding than "desperate efforts at arousal."[85]

Psychic and physiologic dependence

The barbiturates are unquestionably habit-forming. Some individuals who perhaps unnecessarily become accustomed to taking one of these drugs at bedtime may find it difficult to give up the habit and may develop some craving for the drug. For many years it was assumed that chronic habituation to the barbiturates was an unimportant problem when compared with the chronic use of the morphine type of narcotics. It is now generally accepted that chronic administration of large doses of barbiturates results in serious withdrawal symptoms in both men and animals.[27] The manifestations of withdrawal consist of anxiety, tremors, occasional convulsive phenomena, and craving for the barbiturate.

The most important principle in the medical management of the barbiturate addict is gradual withdrawal of the drug. Sudden withdrawal can produce marked excitement and even convulsions.

The tolerance to the barbiturates that develops with their chronic use is not nearly so great as the tolerance to morphine and similar narcotics. Most barbiturate addicts ingest about ten to fifteen hypnotic doses, or 1 to 1.5 Gm. of the drug in 24 hours, whereas the morphine addict may take a hundred times the usual therapeutic dose of morphine. Tolerance to the lethal effect of the barbiturates is probably not very great in the addict, whereas the morphine addict is resistant to many lethal doses of the narcotic.

NONBARBITURATE SEDATIVE-HYPNOTICS

Although the barbiturates are quite satisfactory as sedative-hypnotics, a large variety of other drugs are available for essentially the same indications. Some (chloral hydrate, for example) are old but still quite useful medications. Others, introduced more recently for competitive reasons, have few, if any, advantages over the barbiturates.

Bromides and ethanol also belong to the sedative-hypnotic group of drugs. Both are obsolete as therapeutic agents but are of interest because of their toxicology, basic mechanisms of action, and (at least in the case of ethanol) widespread abuse. A classification of sedative-hypnotic drugs follows:

Classification of nonbarbiturate sedative-hypnotics

Alcohols
    Tertiary alcohols
        Ethchlorvynal (Placidyl)
        Methylparafynol (Dormison)
    Other alcohols
        Ethanol
        Tricholoethanol
        Phenaglycodol (Ultran)
Piperidinediones
    Methyprylon (Noludar)
    Glutethimide (Doriden)
    Thalidomide

Carbamates
    Urethan
    Ethinamate (Valmid)
Chloral hydrate and related drugs
    Chloral hydrate
    Petrichloral (Periehlor)
    Chloral betaine (Beta-Chlor)
Cylic ether
    Paraldehyde
Bromides
Miscellaneous sedative-hypnotics
    Methaqualone (Quaalude)
    Flurazepam (Dalmane)

ALCOHOLS

Tertiary alcohols

The structural formulas of **ethchlorvynol** (Placidyl) and **methylparafynol** (Dormison) are as follows:

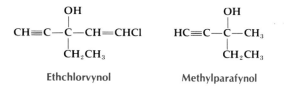

Ethchlorvynol   Methylparafynol

Ethchlorvynol induces sleep rapidly when administered in doses of 0.3 to 0.5 Gm. Its duration of action is similar to that of secobarbital, although its has considerably less potency. In insomnia as much as 1 Gm. may have to be administered for a satisfactory result.

Methylparafynol is so weak that it seldom deserves consideration as a hypnotic.

Other alcohols

Ethanol is undoubtedly the most widely used sedative, although it is not commonly prescribed by physicians. Its pharmacology will be discussed at the end of this chapter.

Trichloroethanol is a metabolic product of chloral hydrate and will be discussed in relation to the action of that hypnotic (p. 257).

Phenaglycodol (Ultran) is a sedative related structurally and in its pharmacology to meprobamate. Phenaglycodol is a derivative of butanediol, while meprobamate and its congeners are derivatives of propanediol. The drug is used as a sedative in the form of capsules (300 mg.) and tablets (200 mg.), which may be administered to an adult three times a day.

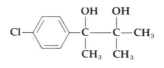

Phenaglycodol

PIPERIDINEDIONES

The two widely used piperidinedione hypnotics, **methyprylon** (Noludar) and **glute-thimide** (Doriden), are structurally related to the barbiturates, with few if any advantages over the older drugs. Methyprylon is used much the same way as pentobarbital or secobarbital. The usual adult dose is one capsule (300 mg.) or one to two tablets (200 mg. per tablet).

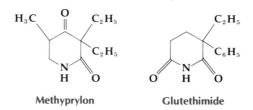

Methyprylon   Glutethimide

Glutethimide is similar in its clinical uses to a moderately long-acting barbiturate. In its toxicology it has some unusual features. In glutethimide intoxication the pupils may be widely dilated; the patient may go into coma many hours after return to consciousness and may die unexpectedly. It has been suggested that very slow absorption from the intestine may be responsible for the irregular course of glutethimide intoxication. Laryngospasm and convulsions are other unusual features. In addition to these disadvantages, hemodialysis is of only limited usefulness in the treatment of glutethimide poisoning. Glutethimide is just as addictive as the barbiturates, and sudden withdrawal may lead to convulsions. It is difficult to see what advantages this non-barbiturate hypnotic could have over the barbiturates. Glutethimide is available in the form of tablets and capsules, and the usual adult dose for insomnia is 0.5 Gm.

The piperidinedione hypnotic **thalidomide** was responsible for thousands of children's being born with disastrous defects such as absence of limbs, especially in Germany. Pregnant women ingesting a single hypnotic dose of the drug between the twenty-fourth and thirty-sixth day of their pregnancy have delivered severely deformed babies. Although the potent teratogenic action of the drug precludes its clinical use, its pharmacology is quite remarkable. Despite its hypnotic potency, which is similar to that of the barbiturates, its acute toxicity is so low that it would be almost impossible to commit suicide by taking the drug. Except for its teratogenic action, thalidomide is almost an ideal hypnotic. Elucidation of its basic mechanism of action would probably contribute to the understanding of the chemical basis of sleep.

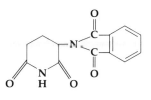

Thalidomide

It is believed that the teratogenic action of thalidomide is mediated by some of its metabolites, among which phthalylglutamic acid and its decarboxylated derivative may play an important role.[33] Interference with glutamic acid metabolism is an interesting possibility.

The thalidomide disaster stimulated the adoption of strict regulations in the testing of new drugs in the United States. It also called attention to the teratogenic potential of other drugs when used during pregnancy. The common antiemetic antihistaminic drugs such as cyclizine must now carry a warning of their possible teratogenicity as demonstrated in rat experiments. Also, physicians are becoming cautious in the use of almost any drug during the first trimester of pregnancy.

CARBAMATES

Carbamic acid esters of various alcohols have sedative and hypnotic properties. Ethyl carbamate, or **urethan**, is a weak hypnotic used as an injectable anesthetic in animals only. While it is obsolete as a hypnotic in medicine, it exerts some antineoplastic effect (p. 588 in the fifth edition).

Several of the carbamates are used as mild sedatives, hypnotics, and muscle relaxants. **Ethinamate** (Valmid) is a short-acting sedative hypnotic. Available in 0.5 Gm. tablets, the drug is administered in doses of one to two tablets.

A number of dicarbamates such as meprobamate (Miltown; Equanil) and related drugs are looked upon by the medical profession as "minor tranquilizers" or antianxiety drugs rather than ordinary mild sedatives. These drugs were discussed in Chapter 19.

CHLORAL HYDRATE AND RELATED DRUGS

Chloral hydrate is an old but still useful hypnotic. It is often prescribed for elderly patients who may show idiosyncratic reactions to the barbiturates. It is metabolically altered in the tissues to trichloroethanol.[6] Since this compound is also effective as a hypnotic, it is quite likely that much of the hypnotic action of chloral hydrate may be mediated by this metabolic product.[6] Some of the drug is oxidized also to trichloroacetic acid. Trichloroethanol is excreted as the glucuronide. It gives a false positive reaction for glucose in the urine by reducing Fehling's solution or similar alkaline copper reagents.

$$Cl_3C-CHOH$$
$$|$$
$$OH$$

Chloral hydrate

Chloral hydrate is administered to adults in the usual dosage of 1 Gm. It causes some gastric irritation in the concentrated form. When diluted in some flavored solution, it is less irritating but still not as convenient to take as the barbiturates. The drug produces refreshing sleep, usually for 4 to 8 hours.

The toxicity of chloral hydrate is low but is increased by the simultaneous administration of alcohol. This is the basis of "knockout drops." The lethal dose of the drug is quite variable but probably lies between 3 and 30 Gm. It is likely that heart disease or impaired detoxication may account for the wide variation in the lethal dose of chloral hydrate. Although ordinary hypnotic doses have no demonstrable adverse effect on the heart, overdosage may affect the cardiac muscle and should be avoided in patients suffering from heart disease.

The main disadvantage of chloral hydrate as compared with the barbiturates is gastric irritation and its characteristic odor. To avoid these disadvantages, preparations have been created that can be administered in tablet form, chloral hydrate being released from these tablets in the gastric juice.

Petrichloral (Perichlor) is a combination of chloral and pentaerythritol, from which the hypnotic is released slowly in the stomach. It is claimed that the combination causes less gastric irritation than does chloral hydrate. The hypnotic dose of petrichloral is 0.3 to 0.6 Gm. for adults.

Chloral betaine (Beta-Chlor) is a combination of chloral and betaine. It is available in stable, tasteless tablets. In the tablet form, 870 mg. of the complex is equivalent to 500 mg. of chloral hydrate. The complex is absorbed as such from the gastrointestinal tract and is hydrolyzed in the tissues. The hypnotic dose of chloral betaine is one to two tablets for adults, which is equivalent to 0.5 to 1 Gm. of chloral hydrate. It is claimed that the betaine complex causes less gastric irritation than chloral hydrate alone.

CYCLIC ETHER

Paraldehyde, a cyclic ether obtained through the polymerization of acetaldehyde, is an effective hypnotic with limited usefulness because of its offensive odor. It is unique among the hypnotics in that a significant fraction of the administered dose is excreted through the lungs. The remainder is metabolized through the stage of acetaldehyde. Drugs that block the oxidation of acetaldehyde, such as disulfiram, elicit severe reactions when paraldehyde is ingested.

Paraldehyde is administered orally, usually in a cold beverage to disguise its taste. A dose of 4 to 8 ml. is sufficient to facilitate sleep. Its use is restricted almost entirely to the management of hospitalized patients undergoing alcohol withdrawal and convulsive states such as eclampsia or tetanus. It is sometimes employed in patients with renal shutdown, since as much as 28% of the drug administered may be eliminated through the pulmonary route and the remainder is metabolized to carbon dioxide and water.

Paraldehyde may be injected by the intramuscular route, although it is quite damaging to tissues at the site of injection. Intravenous use of the drug has resulted in fatalities and should be avoided. Paraldehyde is well absorbed following rectal administration. When administered rectally, the drug is often dissolved in two or three parts of olive oil.

The lethal dose of paraldehyde is quite variable, depending on the route of administration and other factors. As little as 12 to 24 ml. of the drug administered rectally has caused death, whereas doses as high as 100 ml. have been given to some patients with ultimate recovery. Liver damage increases the toxicity of paraldehyde, probably because of delayed metabolic transformation. For the same reason the drug should not be prescribed for any patient who is taking disulfiram.

BROMIDES

The bromide ion exerts a sedative and antiepileptic effect. Until recently it has been widely utilized in medicine and by the laity. With recognition of the dangers of chronic bromide intoxication and the cumulative action of the drug and with the development of much more effective sedatives and antiepileptic drugs, the modern physician finds few uses for bromides. The pharmacology of the bromides remains important, however, because of the problem of bromide intoxication.

Pharmacologic effects

The administration of 2 to 5 Gm. of sodium bromide or other bromide salts produces sedation, drowsiness, and sleep. The mechanism whereby this halide influences the central nervous system is mysterious. Since the body does not easily distinguish the bromide from the chloride ion, it is suspected that the replacement of brain chloride by bromide may alter the functions of nerve cells. Chronic administration of several grams of bromide tends to produce mental depression, confusion, and lethargy.

Bromide is the oldest antiepileptic drug, having been introduced for this purpose in 1857 by Charles Locock.

Metabolism

When a bromide is ingested, it becomes distributed in the body in a manner very similar to that of chloride. Bromide remains largely extracellular, with the exception of the red cell, which normally contains a high concentration of chloride. The ratio of bromide to chloride will be very similar in most tissues, indicating that bromide is essentially distributed in the chloride space. The brain and spinal fluid may contain relatively less bromide than chloride. The kidney does not readily distinguish between bromide and chloride either, although the tubules may reabsorb bromide somewhat more readily than chloride.

If administration of bromide is stopped, considerable time is required to rid the body of the drug. Large amounts of chloride given to such a patient will accelerate the elimination of bromide because the total daily halide excretion will be increased.

Toxicity

Mental and neurologic symptoms are most prominent, and it is important for the physician to consider the possibility of chronic bromide intoxication in the differential diagnosis of confused and lethargic patients.

In addition, various skin lesions, gastrointestinal disturbances, and involvement of the mucous membranes of the eyes and respiratory passages are not uncommon in bromide intoxication.

MISCELLANEOUS SEDATIVE-HYPNOTICS

Many of the "minor tranquilizers" and "antianxiety agents" are difficult to distinguish from the sedative-hypnotic class of drugs from the standpoint of clinical pharmacology, although sophisticated neurophysiologic and behavioral experiments performed in animals do reveal some differences. There is an increasing tendency on the part of clinical pharmacologists to view the antianxiety drugs as members of the sedative-hypnotic class, quite different from the true tranquilizers or antipsychotic drugs such as the phenothiazines. This last group of drugs does not present the characteristic sequence of sedation-hypnosis-anesthesia-coma-death when increasing doses are administered. Furthermore, in contrast with the sedative-hypnotics, abrupt withdrawal of an antipsychotic drug following chronic administration does not lead to convulsive manifestations.

Some of the antihistaminic drugs exert considerable sedative-hypnotic effects and they are promoted as sleep-inducing medications in over-the-counter products. One such antihistaminic, doxylamine, has proved effective as a hypnotic in a controlled clinical trial.[58] In doses of 25 and 50 mg. the drug performed better than a 100 mg. dose of secobarbital but was somewhat inferior to a dose of 200 mg. secobarbital. The pharmacology of the antihistaminics was discussed in Chapter 16.

Methaqualone (Quaalude), a relatively new hypnotic, is similar in action to the barbiturates. It has no proven advantages except in patients who show idiosyncratic reactions to the barbiturates. Chemically, methaqualone is 2-methyl-3-*o*-tolyl-4(3H)-quinazolone. It is available in 150 mg. tablets, and the dose for adults is 150 to 300 mg. given at bedtime.

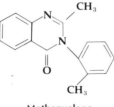

Methaqualone

Flurazepam (Dalmane), a recently introduced benzodiazepine, is said to be a hypnotic useful in all types of insomnia. It is supplied in 15 and 30 mg. capsules. It is claimed that the drug does not decrease dream time as measured by REM.[31] It is too early to evaluate the advantage this may have.

CLINICAL PHARMACOLOGY OF HYPNOTICS

The safe and effective use of hypnotics requires the application of certain simple pharmacologic principles.[82]

1. Hypnotics should be used only if obvious causes of insomnia such as painful conditions or too much coffee have been eliminated. The drugs should be used only when necessary and in doses as low as possible.

2. Inability to go to sleep is somewhat different from difficulty in staying asleep, the latter being the more common problem. A few minutes' delay in going to sleep should not require sleep medications, all of which are habit-forming.

3. While there are differences in the onset of action of the various hypnotics, these differences are of little practical significance. Liquid preparations of chloral hydrate, paraldehyde, or elixirs of the barbiturates act rapidly but are inconvenient to use. Capsules of secobarbital, pentobarbital, and chloral hydrate act quite rapidly, while phenobarbital may have a somewhat delayed effect.

4. The duration of action of the various hypnotics has received much attention in

pharmacology and in drug promotion, but the rigid classifications of "short acting," "medium acting," and "long acting" are not very important in actual practice (p. 246). It should be remembered that duration of action is greatly influenced by dose. Nevertheless, it is traditional to look upon secobarbital, pentobarbital, chloral hydrate, paraldehyde, and methyprylon as short-acting, amobarbital and glutethimide as intermediate-acting, and phenobarbital as long-acting hypnotics. The antianxiety agents are also employed as hypnotics, with the meprobamate-type drug being intermediate-acting and the benzodiazepines such as chlordiazepoxide behaving as long-acting sedative-hypnotics.

5. The hypnotic dose of a drug varies greatly in different individuals and should be adjusted carefully. On the other hand, liver disease and moderate impairment of renal function do not greatly influence the duration of action of hypnotics. Other sedative-hypnotics, tranquilizers, or alcohol do modify the dose and duration of action of sleep-producing medications. Sudden withdrawal of all such drugs is dangerous.

6. Habituation, addiction, and the dangers of sudden withdrawal are greater hazards than direct toxic effects when sedative-hypnotics are properly used in therapeutics.

ETHYL ALCOHOL

As a therapeutic agent, ethyl alcohol is only of moderate importance. It has great toxicologic interest, however, and chronic alcoholism is one of the great social problems of mankind.

Pharmacologic effects

The main action of ethyl alcohol is exerted on the central nervous system. It may be looked upon as an unusual hypnotic and anesthetic. There is general agreement that the apparent stimulant action of the drug is a consequence of primary depression of the higher centers, resulting in uninhibited behavior.

In addition to its action on behavior and consciousness, alcohol influences cardiovascular, gastrointestinal, and renal functions.

Cutaneous vasodilatation and a feeling of warmth are generally observed following the ingestion of an alcoholic beverage. This vasodilatation is not a direct effect of the drug on blood vessels but is a consequence of its central nervous system actions. There is a popular impression that alcohol dilates the coronary vessels, but it has been shown that alcohol does not prevent the electrocardiographic evidences of coronary insufficiency following exercise tolerance.[55] Alcohol may lessen precordial pain, but this action is likely to be exerted on the brain rather than on the coronary vessels. Adverse myocardial responses to alcohol have been demonstrated in animal experiments.[88]

The ingestion of alcohol promotes the secretion of acid gastric juice. It has been postulated that this action may be mediated through the release of histamine or gastrin in the stomach wall.[11, 69]

The diuresis observed in drinkers of alcoholic beverages is partly due to the ingestion of water. Inhibition of the release of antidiuretic hormone from the posterior pituitary lobe by alcohol has also been demonstrated.[63]

Metabolism

Ingested alcohol is absorbed rapidly from the stomach and the small intestine. The rate of absorption is influenced by the concentration of the alcohol ingested and most

Table 21-4. Relative concentration of alcohol in various body fluids, tissues, and alveolar air (concentration in blood is 1.0)

Serum	1.15
Urine	1.3
Saliva	1.3
Spinal fluid	1.15
Brain or liver	0.85 to 0.90
Kidney	0.83
Alveolar air	1/2,100 of blood concentration

importantly by the presence of food in the stomach. On an empty stomach the drinking of an alcoholic beverage produces peak blood levels in less than 1 hour. There may be considerable delay if the stomach is filled with food.

Once absorbed, alcohol is distributed in total body water. The concentration of alcohol in different tissues and body fluids correlates well with the concentration of water at these sites. If the concentration of alcohol in blood is assigned the value of 1.0, the relative values given in Table 21-4 may be expected in the various body fluids, tissues, and alveolar air.

The concentration of alcohol in the blood has great medicolegal importance since it is generally accepted that a blood level of alcohol of 150 mg./100 ml. may be taken as evidence that the person is drunk. It is of some importance to know also the relationship between the quantities of alcohol ingested and the blood levels that may be expected. The concentration of alcohol in the blood will depend on the following factors: (1) quantity of alcohol ingested and rate at which it is drunk, (2) speed of absorption, (3) body weight and the percentage of total body water, and (4) rate of metabolism of alcohol.

The blood levels of alcohol that may be expected following the ingestion of various alcoholic beverages may be calculated.[21] Since intoxication occurs when a blood level of 150 mg. of alcohol/100 ml. of blood is reached (0.15%), it can be calculated that this will occur if approximately 8 fluid ounces of a distilled spirit containing 45% alcohol is drunk rapidly. If a distilled spirit is drunk over a period of several hours, the number of ounces required for producing a blood level of 0.15% may be calculated by the following formula: $8 + H =$ number of ounces of distilled spirits required to cause intoxication, where H is the number of hours during which the beverage is drunk.

The corresponding formula for fortified wine (containing 20% alcohol) is $18 + 2H$; for ordinary wine (containing 10% alcohol) it is $36 + 4H$; for beer (containing 4.5% alcohol) the figure would be $80 + 10H$.

The relationships between the ingestion of various beverages, blood levels of alcohol, and prognosis in terms of ability in driving an automobile are shown in Fig. 21-2.

Elimination

The quantity of alcohol excreted in the urine, exhaled through the lungs, or lost in the perspiration ordinarily represents less than 10% of the total ingested. The remainder is metabolized; the end products are carbon dioxide and water.

The steps in the metabolism of alcohol appear to be as follows[29]:

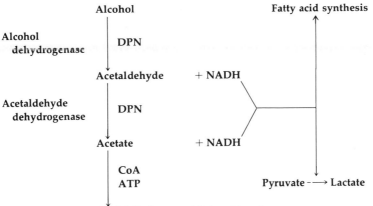

The liver plays an important role in the metabolic transformation of alcohol. The first step occurs almost entirely in the liver.

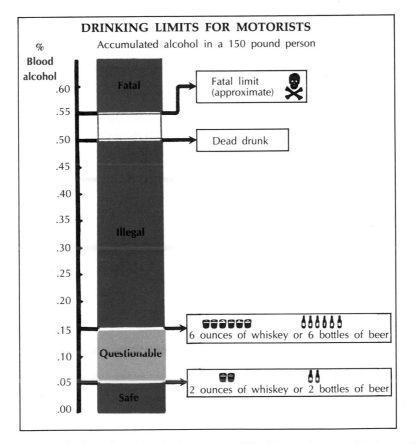

Fig. 21-2. Level of alcohol in blood of an automobile driver relative to his being "under the influence." (From Harger, R. N. In Economos, J. P., and Kreml, F. M., editors: Judge and prosecutor in traffic court, Chicago, 1951, American Bar Association and The Traffic Institute, Northwestern University.)

The average person metabolizes 6 to 8 Gm. (7.5 to 10 ml.) of alcohol per hour. This figure is fairly constant for a given individual and is independent of the quantity present in the body. Habitual drinkers may metabolize alcohol slightly more rapidly than abstainers.[16]

It has been claimed that the administration of glucose and insulin, various vitamins, dinitrophenol, and muscular exercise accelerate the metabolism. However, most of these claims have been denied.

The metabolism of 1 Gm. of alcohol yields 7 calories. Since the maximal amount that can be metabolized in 24 hours is approximately 170 Gm., it may be calculated that alcohol can contribute up to 1,200 calories per day to the metabolic requirements of an individual.

Metabolic effects

The influence of alcohol on carbohydrate and lipid metabolism has received much attention in recent years. Hypoglycemia can be induced in human beings by the ingestion of 35 to 50 ml. of ethanol after a 2-day fast. Such individuals must have low liver glycogen because they do not respond to glucagon with the characteristic increase in blood glucose.[13] Animal studies indicate that alcohol can inhibit glycogen synthesis, probably by interfering with glyconeogenesis from amino acids.

It is quite likely that acute hyperlipemia following alcohol ingestion and the hyperlipemia of the chronic alcoholic have different mechanisms. The acute hyperlipemia is probably mediated through sympathetic activation, norepinephrine release, and lipolysis from fat depots. This effect of norepinephrine can be prevented by beta adrenergic blocking agents. On the other hand, hyperlipemia in the chronic alcoholic may depend to a large extent on deficient removal of lipid from the blood. Evidence for decreased lipoprotein lipase activity in alcoholic patients has been presented.[42]

Fatty livers are commonly observed in alcoholic patients. The most likely explanations would appear to be (1) increased mobilization from fat depots, (2) increased esterification to triglycerides rather than to phospholipids and cholesterol esters, and (3) decreased triglyceride release from the liver.

Tolerance and addiction

It is commonly known that the experienced drinker shows fewer and less marked effects from moderate amounts of alcohol than does the abstainer. This moderate tolerance cannot be explained on the basis of what is known about absorption, distribution, and metabolism in the chronic alcoholic. It is concluded, therefore, that the experienced drinker has learned to behave and to perform habitual tasks at blood alcohol levels that would seriously disturb the unaccustomed individual. This apparent tolerance probably does not extend to the lethal effect of alcohol, and blood levels exceeding 550 mg./100 ml. may produce death in the chronic alcoholic.

Treatment of the acute hallucinosis of alcohol withdrawal is controversial. Alcohol and paraldehyde are the "time-honored" medications, but chlordiazepoxide also has its advocates.[17]

Acute intoxication

There is no specific treatment for acute alcoholic intoxication. The most important measures consist of supportive therapy, including correction of fluid and electrolyte disturbances, good caloric intake, and vitamin supplements. Alcoholics may have hypokalemia and serum potassium levels must be monitored, particularly when glucose-containing fluids are administered. There may also be hypomagnesemia, which may be corrected with the parenteral administration of magnesium sulfate if renal function is normal.[70] As regards drug treatment, there is no consensus, but recent studies tend to favor chlordiazepoxide and diazepam over the barbiturates or paraldehyde for the prevention of hallucinations and seizures.[70]

The blood alcohol levels that may be lethal are usually in excess of 0.5% or 500 mg./100 ml. If the person has taken some other central nervous system depressant such as a barbiturate, even lower blood alcohol levels may result in a lethal outcome.

Chronic alcoholism

It has been estimated that there are several million persons in the United States who drink to excess. More than one million of these may be classified as chronic alcoholics on the basis of a compulsive and unmanageable desire to drink.

A variety of pathologic changes occur in the alcoholic with much greater frequency than in the general population. Chronic gastritis, cirrhosis of the liver, and the neuropsychiatric condition known as the Korsakoff syndrome have received considerable attention. The mechanism of production of these abnormalities is difficult to state because the chronic alcoholic often suffers from nutritional deficiencies also. When benefited by psychiatric treatment or the organization known as Alcoholics Anonymous, about 50% of chronic alcoholics may be able to abstain from drinking.

Another approach to the problem has been the administration of drugs that will make the effects of alcohol extremely unpleasant or even dangerous. The best known of these is disulfiram.

Disulfiram. The development of the disulfiram approach (Antabuse) to chronic alcoholism was the consequence of a chance observation.[24] While testing certain new drugs as potential anthelmintics, it was observed that following ingestion of tetraethylthiuram disulfide even a few bottles of beer caused very unpleasant side effects. Careful study of this unusual occurrence led to the discovery of the probable mechanism involved and to the eventual introduction of disulfiram into therapeutics.

From a chemical standpoint, disulfiram is tetraethylthiuram disulfide. Certain other disulfides have similar properties with respect to alcohol intolerance.

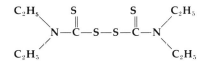

Disulfiram

If alcohol is ingested several hours after taking disulfiram in doses of 1 to 2 Gm., the individual develops the typical reaction characterized by nausea, vomiting, flushing, palpitation, and headache. There may be lowering of the blood pressure, even to shock levels. These symptoms are so unpleasant that the patient simply cannot drink alcohol while he is on a maintenance dose of 0.25 to 0.5 Gm. of disulfiram. Even when the drug administration is stopped, it may take a week before the alcohol intolerance disappears.

Disulfiram by itself can cause some effects. Dizziness, metallic taste, reduced sexual potency, electroencephalographic changes, and skin reactions have occurred following its use.

It seemed reasonable to assume that disulfiram interfered with the metabolism of alcohol, resulting in the accumulation of some toxic intermediate. Indeed, it has been demonstrated that acetaldehyde accumulates in the blood when the patient ingests alcohol while taking disulfiram.[29] Blood acetaldehyde levels under these conditions may be of the order of 1 mg./100 ml. It has also been demonstrated that the intravenous infusion of acetaldehyde, which would produce comparable blood levels, reproduces the manifestations of the "Antabuse reaction." It has also been demonstrated in experimental animals that the administration of disulfiram delays the metabolism of administered acetaldehyde.

On the basis of these facts it may be concluded that disulfiram inhibits the second step in alcohol metabolism: the further utilization of acetaldehyde. This intermediate is a very potent pharmacologic agent with vasopressor and vasodepressor properties.

Acetaldehyde apparently can cause the release of catecholamines from the tissues and thus behaves as an indirect-acting sympathomimetic drug.[65] It is quite likely that it releases other amines also, which may account for the symptoms of the "Antabuse reaction."

Disulfiram is usually administered in a dosage of 1 to 2 Gm. the first day, the quantity administered being gradually decreased in 4 days to about 0.5 Gm., but it may be even further reduced to 0.25 Gm. as a maintenance dose.

Other drugs that create intolerance to alcohol and may elicit an "Antabuse reaction" are calcium carbimide (Temposil), metronidazole (Flagyl), and rarely the antidiabetic sulfonylureas such as tolbutamide (Orinase).

OTHER ALCOHOLS

The aliphatic alcohols other than ethyl alcohol are of interest in medicine largely because they are sometimes involved in cases of poisoning.

METHANOL

Generally the toxicity of the alcohols increases with the chain length. An exception to this statement is methyl alcohol, which is unique in producing marked acidosis and blindness in primates but not in lower animals. As little as 30 ml. of methanol has caused serious poisoning, and even death has been attributed to this quantity or even less. In addition to the acidosis, methanol intoxication involves the central nervous system, with the production of headache, dizziness, delirium, and coma. Blindness, which is a common accompaniment of these effects, may be total or partial.

Although methanol is metabolized in part to formaldehyde and formic acid, the amount of the latter is not sufficient to explain the profound metabolic acidosis that may result from ingestion of relatively small quantities of the alcohol. Blindness is probably a consequence of the toxic effects of formaldehyde on the retina. Interference with adenosine triphosphate generation by uncoupling of oxidative phosphorylation has been postulated.[73]

Metabolism of methyl alcohol in the body is very much slower than that of ethyl alcohol, a fact that further complicates the management of methanol poisoning. The treatment of methanol poisoning is based largely on the correction of the acidotic state with appropriate intravenous fluids. Another approach is based on the observation that ethanol delays the metabolic transformation of methanol.[53] Although some investigators favor the use of ethanol in treating methanol poisoning, it must be kept in mind that correction of the acidotic state with sodium bicarbonate given orally or intravenously (500 ml. of a 5% solution) is the most important therapeutic procedure.

ISOPROPYL ALCOHOL

Isopropyl alcohol has some toxicologic interest also. It is metabolized to acetone in the body. Severe renal damage is found in patients who have recovered from ingestion of a few ounces of isopropyl alcohol. The fatal dose is estimated as 120 to 240 ml.

References

1 Anton, A. H.: Ethanol and urinary catecholamines in man, Clin. Pharmacol. Ther. **6**:462, 1965.

2 Beecher, H. K., and Moyer, C. A.: Mechanisms of respiratory failure under barbiturate anesthesia (Evipal, Pentothal), J. Clin. Invest. **20**:549, 1952.

3 Brodie, B. B., Bernstein, E., and Mark, L. C.: The role of body fat in limiting the duration of action of thiopental, J. Pharmacol. Exp. Ther. **105**:421, 1952.

4 Brodie, B. B., Burns, J. J., Mark, L. C., Lief, P. A., Bernstein, E., and Papper, E. M.: The fate of pentobarbital in man and dog and a method for its estimation in biological material, J. Pharmacol. Exp. Ther. **109**:26, 1953.

5 Burstein, C. L., and Rovenstine, E. A.: Respiratory parasympathetic action of some shorter acting barbituric acid derivatives, J. Pharmacol. Exp. Ther. **63**:42, 1938.

6 Butler, T. C.: The metabolic fate of chloral hydrate, J. Pharmacol. Exp. Ther. **92**:49, 1948.

7 Butler, T. C.: The rate of penetration of barbituric acid derivatives into the brain, J. Pharmacol. Exp. Ther. **100**:219, 1950.

8 Butler, T. C.: Quantitative studies of the metabolic fate of mephobarbital (N-methyl phenobarbital), J. Pharmacol, Exp. Ther. **106**:235, 1952.

9 Cares, R. M., Newman, B., and Mauceri, J. C.: Poisoning by methylparafynol (Dormison), Amer. J. Clin. Path. **23**:129, 1953.

10 Clemmesen, C., and Nilsson, E.: Therapeutic trends in the treatment of barbiturate poisoning. The Scandinavian method, Clin. Pharmacol. Ther. **2**:220, 1961.

11 Dragstedt, C. A., Gray, J. S., Lawton, A. H., and de Arellano, M. R.: Does alcohol stimulate gastric secretion by liberating histamine? Proc. Soc. Exp. Biol. Med. **43**:26, 1940.

12 Exley, K.: Autonomic ganglion depressant properties of barbiturates, Nature **170**:242, 1952.

13 Field, J. B., Williams, H. E., and Mortimore, G. E.: Studies on the mechanism of ethanol-induced hypoglycemia, J. Clin. Invest. **42**:497, 1963.

14 Frew, J. L., and Rosenheim, M. L.: The labile neurogenic component of hypertension: comparison of the effects of tetraethyl-ammonium bromide and a rapidly acting barbiturate (Seconal), Clin. Sci. **7**:217, 1949.

15 Friend, D. G.: Sedative hynotics, Clin. Pharmacol. Ther. **1**:5, 1960.

16 Goldberg, L.: Quantitative studies on alcohol tolerance in man, Acta Physiol. Scand. (supp. 16) **5**:1, 1943.

17 Golbert, T. M., Sanz, C. J., Rose, H. D., and Leitschuh, H.: Comparative evaluation of treatments of alcohol withdrawal syndromes, J.A.M.A. **201**:99, 1967.

18 Goldstein, A., and Aranow, L.: The duration of action of thiopental and pentobarbital, J. Pharmacol. Exp. Ther. **128**:1, 1960.

19 Goldstein, A., and Judson, B. A.: Alcohol dependence and opiate dependence: lack of relationship in mice, Science **172**:290, 1971.

20 Goldstein, D. B., and Pal, N.: Alcohol dependence produced in mice by inhalation of ethanol: grading the withdrawal reaction, Science **172**:288, 1971.

21 Greenberg, L. A.: The definition of an intoxicating beverage, Quart. J. Stud. Alcohol **16**:316, 1955.

22 Gruber, C. M., Jr., Kohlstaedt, K. G., Moore, R. B., and Peck, F. B., Jr.: A study of the effects of Valmid, a non-barbiturate central nervous system depressant, in humans, J. Pharmacol. Exp. Ther. **112**:480, 1954.

23 Hadden, J., Johnson, K., Smith, S., Price, L., and Giardina, E.: Acute barbiturate intoxication, J.A.M.A. **209**:893, 1969.

24 Hald, M., Jacobsen, E., and Larsen, V.: The sensitizing effect of tetraethyl-thiuram disulfide (Antabuse) to ethyl alcohol, Acta Pharmacol. 4:285, 1948.

25 Hiatt, E. P.: Replacement of chlorides in tissues and body fluids of dogs by nitrates, Amer. J. Physiol. 126:533, 1939.

26 Hughes, F. W., and Forney, R. B.: Comparative effect of three antihistaminics and ethanol on mental and motor performance, Clin. Pharmacol. Ther. 5:414, 1964.

27 Isbell, H., and Fraser, H. F.: Addiction to analgesics and barbiturates, Pharmacol. Rev. 2:355, 1950.

28 Israel, Y., Kalant, H., LeBlanc, E., Bernstein, J. C., and Salazar, I.: Changes in cation transport and (Na + K)-activated adenosine triphosphatase produced by chronic administration of ethanol, J. Pharmacol. Exp. Ther. 174:330, 1970.

29 Jacobsen, E.: The metabolism of ethyl alcohol, Pharmacol. Rev. 4:107, 1952.

30 Jouvet, M.: Neurophysiology of the states of sleep, Physiol. Rev. 47:117, 1967.

31 Kales, A.: Psychophysiological and biochemical changes following use and withdrawal of hypnotics. In Kales, A., editor: Sleep: physiology and pathology, Philadelphia, 1967, J. B. Lippincott Co.

32 Keats, A. S., and Beecher, H. K.: Pain relief with hypnotic doses of barbiturates and a hypothesis, J. Pharmacol. Exp. Ther. 100:1, 1950.

33 Keberle, H., Loustalot, R. K., Maller, J. W., and Schmid, K.: Biochemical effects of drugs on the mammalian conceptus, Ann. N. Y. Acad. Sci. 123:252, 1965.

34 Keller, A. D., and Fulton, J. F.: The action of anesthetic drugs on the motor cortex of monkeys, Amer. J. Physiol. 97:537, 1931.

35 Keplinger, M. L., and Wells, J. A.: The effect of disulfiram on the action and metabolism of paraldehyde, J. Pharmacol. Exp. Ther. 119:19, 1957.

36 Landauer, A. A., Milner, G., and Patman, J.: Alcohol and amitryptiline effects on skills related to driving behavior, Science 163:1467, 1969.

37 Larrabee, M. G., and Holaday, D. A.: Depression of transmission through sympathetic ganglia during general anesthesia, J. Pharmacol. Exp. Ther. 105:400, 1952.

38 Lasagna, L.: A study of hypnotic drugs in patients with chronic diseases; comparative efficacy of placebo, methyprylon, (Noludar), meprobamate (Miltown, Equanil), pentobarbital, phenobarbital, secobarbital, J. Chronic Dis. 3:122, 1956.

39 Lasagna, L.: The newer hypnotics, Med. Clin. N. Amer. 41:359, 1957.

40 Lasagna, L.: The effect of pharmacological agents on the nervous system, Baltimore, 1959, The Williams & Wilkins Co.

41 Levine, H. A., Gilbert, A. J., and Bodansky, M.: The pulmonary and urinary excretion of paraldehyde in normal dogs and in dogs with liver damage, J. Pharmacol. Exp. Ther. 69:316, 1940.

42 Losowsky, M. S., Jones, D. P., Davidson, C. S., and Lieber, C. S.: Studies of alcoholic hyperlipemia and its mechanism, Amer. J. Med. 35:794, 1963.

43 Magoun, H. W.: A neural basis for the anesthetic state. In Symposium on sedative and hypnotic drugs, Baltimore, 1954, The Williams & Wilkins Co.

44 Magoun, H. W.: The waking brain, Springfield, Ill., 1958, Charles C Thomas, Publisher.

45 Maher, J. F., Schreiner, G. E., and Westervelt, F. B.: Acute glutethimide intoxication. I. Clinical experience (twenty-two patients) compared to barbiturate intoxication (sixty-three patients), Amer. J. Med. 33:70, 1962.

46 Mark, L. C.: Metabolism of barbiturates in man, Clin. Pharmacol. Ther. 4:504, 1963.

47 Marshall, E. K., Jr., and Owens, A. H., Jr.: Absorption, excretion and metabolic fate of chloral hydrate and trichloroethanol, Bull. Hopkins Hosp. 95:1, 1954.

48 Maxwell, J. M., Cook, L., Davis, G. J., Toner, J. J., and Fellows, E. J.: Effects of β-diethylaminoethyldiphenylpropylacetate hydrochloride (SKF No. 525-A) on a series of hypnotics, Fed. Proc. 12:349, 1953.

49 Nilsson, E.: On treatment of barbiturate poisoning; a modified clinical aspect, Acta Med. Scand. (supp. 253) 139:1, 1951.

50 Owens, A. H., Jr., Marshall, E. K., Jr., Broun, G. O., Jr., Zubrod, C. G., and Lasagna, L.: A comparative evaluation of the hypnotic potency of chloral hydrate and trichloroethanol, Bull. Hopkins Hosp. 96:71, 1955.

51 Perlman, P. L., Sutter, D., and Johnson, C. B.: Further studies on the metabolic disposition of Dormison (3-methyl-pentyne-ol-3) in dogs and man, J. Amer. Pharm. Ass. 42:750, 1953.

52 Riegelman, S., Rowland, M., and Epstein, W. L.: Griseofulvin-phenobarbital interaction in man, J.A.M.A. 213:426, 1970.

53 Roe, O.: The metabolism and toxicity of methanol, Pharmacol. Rev. 7:399, 1955.

54 Rubin, E., and Lieber, C. S.: Alcohol-induced hepatic injury in nonalcoholic volunteers, New Eng. J. Med. 278:869, 1968.

55 Russek, H. I., Urbach, K. F., and Doerner,

A. A.: Choice of a coronary vasodilator in clinical practice, J.A.M.A. **153**:207, 1953.

56 Schallek, W., Kuehn, A., and Seppelin, D. K.: Central depressant effects of methyprylon, J. Pharmacol. Exp. Ther. **118**:139, 1956.

57 Schutz, F.: An effect of barbiturates on serum cholinesterase, J. Physiol. **102**:259, 1943.

58 Sessions, J. T., Jr., Minkel, H. P., Bullard, J. C., and Ingelfinger, F. J.: The effect of barbiturates in patients with liver disease, J. Clin. Invest. **33**:1116, 1954.

59 Shideman, F. E.: Clinical pharmacology of hypnotics and sedatives, Clin. Pharmacol. Ther. **2**:313, 1961.

60 Sjoquist, F., and Lasagna, L.: The hypnotic efficacy of doxylamine, Clin. Pharmacol. Ther. **8**:48, 1967.

61 Straw, R. N., and Mitchell, C. L.: A comparison of the effects of phenobarbital and pentobarbital on motor cortical threshold and righting reflex response in the cat, J. Pharmacol. Exp. Ther. **156**:598, 1967.

62 Toman, J. E. P., and Davis, J. P.: The effects of drugs upon the electrical activity of the brain, Pharmacol. Rev. **1**:425, 1949.

63 Van Dyke, H. B., and Ames, R. G.: Alcohol diuresis, Acta Endocr. **7**:110, 1951.

64 Waddell, W. J., and Butler, T. C.: The distribution and excretion of phenobarbital, J. Clin. Invest. **36**:1217, 1957.

65 Walsh, M. J., Hollander, P. B., and Truitt, E. B., Jr.: Sympathomimetic effects of acetaldehyde on the electrical and contractile characteristics of isolated left atria of guinea pigs, J. Pharmacol. Exp. Ther. **167**:173, 1969.

66 Weatherall, M.: Drugs and porphyrin metabolism, Pharmacol. Rev. **6**:133, 1954.

67 Webb, W. R., and Degerli, I. U.: Ethyl alcohol and the cardiovascular system, J.A.M.A. **191**:1055, 1965.

68 Widmark, E. M. P.: Die theoretischen Grundlagen und die praktische Verwendbarkeit der gerichtlich-medizinischen Alkoholbestimmung, Berlin, 1932, Urban & Schwarzenberg.

69 Woodward, E. R., Slotten, D. S., and Tillmans, V. C.: Mechanism of alcoholic stimulation of gastric secretion, Proc. Soc. Exp. Biol. Med. **89**:428, 1955.

Recent reviews

70 Becker, C. E., and Scott, R.: The treatment of alcoholism, Rational Drug Ther. **6**:1, Oct., 1972.

71 Burns, J. J.: Implications of enzyme induction for drug therapy, Amer. J. Med. **37**:329, 1964.

72 Bush, M. T.: Sedatives and hypnotics. In Root, W. S., and Hofmann. F. G., editors: Physiological pharmacology, vol. 1, New York, 1963, Academic Press, Inc.

73 Cooper, J. R., and Kini, M. M.: Biochemical aspects of methanol poisoning, Biochem. Pharmacol. **2**:405, 1962.

74 Dement, W. C.: The effect of dream deprivation, Science **131**:1705, 1960.

75 Essig, C. F.: Addiction to nonbarbiturate sedative and tranquilizing drugs, Clin. Pharmacol. Ther. **5**:334, 1964.

76 Forney, R. B., and Hughes, F. W.: Combined effects of alcohol and other drugs, Springfield, Ill., 1968, Charles C Thomas, Publisher.

77 Israel, Y.: Cellular effects of alcohol, Quart. J. Stud. Alcohol **31**(2):293, 1970.

78 Isselbacher, K. J., and Greenberger, N. J.: Metabolic effects of alcohol on the liver, New Eng. J. Med. **270**:351, 1964.

79 Johns, M. W.: Methods for assessing human sleep, Arch. Intern. Med. **127**:484, 1971.

80 Kales, A., and Kales, J. D.: Evaluation, diagnosis, and treatment of clinical conditions related to sleep, J.A.M.A. **213**:2229, 1970.

81 Kales, A., and Kales, J. D.: Sleep laboratory evaluation of psychoactive drugs, Pharmacol. Physicians **4**(9):1, 1970.

82 Lasagna, L.: The pharmacological basis for the effective use of hypnotics, Pharmacol. Physicians **1**(2):1, 1967.

83 Mardones, J.: The alcohols. In Root, W. S., and Hofmann, F. G., editors: Physiological pharmacology, vol. 1, New York, 1963, Academic Press, Inc.

84 Mark, L. C.: Archaic classification of barbiturates; commentary, Clin. Pharmacol. Ther. **10**:287, 1969.

85 Mark, L. C., and Papper, E. M.: Changing therapeutic goals in barbiturate poisoning, Pharmacol. Physicians **1**(3):1, 1967.

86 Mendelson, J. H.: Biologic concomitants of alcoholism, New Eng. J. Med. **283**:24, 71, 1970.

87 Oswald, I.: Drugs and sleep, Pharmacol Rev. **20**:273, 1968.

88 Regan, T. J., Koroxenidis, G., Moschos, C. B., Oldewurtel, H. A., Lehan, P. H., and Hellems, H. K.: The acute metabolic and hemodynamic responses of the left ventricle to ethanol, J. Clin. Invest. **45**:270, 1966.

89 Strickler, J. C.: Forced diuresis in the management of barbiturate intoxication, Clin. Pharmacol. Ther. **6**:693, 1965.

90 Wallgren, H., and Barry, H.: Actions of alcohol, New York, 1970, American Elsevier Publishing Co., Inc.

22 Central nervous system stimulants of the convulsant type

GENERAL CONCEPT

A variety of drugs exert widespread stimulant action on the central nervous system and produce convulsions when given in sufficient doses. They tend to stimulate respiration and oppose the depressant action of moderate doses of barbiturates. Because of their awakening effect, they are often referred to as *analeptics*.

It has been traditional to classify the central nervous system stimulants on the basis of their predominant site of action. The majority of the analeptics — such as pentylenetetrazol, picrotoxin, nikethamide, and bemegride — act predominantly on the brainstem. Strychnine has some selective stimulant action on the spinal cord. Caffeine, amphetamine, ephedrine, cocaine, atropine, pipradrol (Meratran), and methylphenidate (Ritalin) are generally considered to have a predominant cerebral site of action. Many of the latter group of drugs are potent psychomotor stimulants rather than convulsant analeptics.

The importance of the convulsant group of analeptics has been decreasing in medical practice. The only therapeutic indication for the use of these drugs is for respiratory stimulation. Even this indication is somewhat debatable at present, and many competent investigators feel that some mechanical method of artificial respiration may be just as effective without the danger of inducing convulsions.

MECHANISMS OF CONVULSANT ACTION

The overall effect of the convulsant drugs is to lower the threshold of excitability of the central nervous system. They produce cerebral dysrhythmia by directly or indirectly reducing synaptic resistance.

The finer mechanisms by which these drugs act are not known, but some advance has been made toward understanding the convulsant action in the case of strychnine and the experimental convulsant thiosemicarbazide.

With strychnine, the stimulant effect on motor function may be due to removal of inhibitory influences on motoneurons.[2] The Renshaw cells in the spinal cord exert such inhibitory actions on motoneurons, and strychnine reduces this inhibitory influence. The chemical nature of the transmitter released from the axon of the Renshaw cell is not known, and consequently the mode of action of strychnine on this particular synaptic transmission cannot be stated. It is also believed by the Australian investigators that tetanus toxin may exert a similar opposing action on inhibitory mechanisms.[3] This is an interesting hypothesis in view of the similarities between strychnine poisoning and tetanus. It is possible that these interesting effects of strychnine on inhibitory mechanisms may be only a part of the explanation of its convulsant action. Significantly, pentylenetetrazol and picrotoxin do not share with strychnine the property of blocking the inhibitory action of the Renshaw cell. Picrotoxin may act by depression of presynaptic inhibition.[3]

The antagonism between strychnine and glycine on spinal motoneurons is discussed on p. 72.

The convulsant action of thiosemicarbazide and semicarbazide is interesting because it suggests a biochemical mechanism for at least one type of convulsant drug. These aldehyde reagents are known to block enzymatic reactions that require pyridoxal as a cofactor, as is the case with many decarboxylations. Interestingly, convulsions produced in animals or man by thiosemicarbazide can be stopped by the injection of pyridoxine. It has been suggested that the aldehyde reagents may reduce the brain concentration of γ-aminobutyric acid (GABA), and the latter may exert an inhibitory or modulating activity on brain function.[5,6] Although the semicarbazides reduce the brain γ-aminobutyric acid concentration, as does pyridoxine deficiency, there is no certainty about a cause-and-effect relationship, since many other enzymatic reactions are probably inhibited as well in these deficiency states. In any case, these studies represent an interesting example of attempts to correlate metabolism and pharmacologic action.

CENTRAL NERVOUS SYSTEM STIMULANTS

Only the essential features of the pharmacology of the various central nervous system stimulants will be considered.

PENTYLENETETRAZOL

The structural formula of pentylenetetrazol (Metrazol) is as follows:

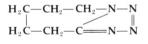

Pentylenetetrazol

There is much experience with the convulsant action of pentylenetetrazol in man because the drug has been used extensively in shock treatment for mental disease. When approximately 5 ml. of a 10% solution of pentylenetetrazol is injected rapidly by the intravenous route, the individual becomes apprehensive and in a few seconds goes into convulsions and becomes unconscious. The major convulsive movements are tonic at first but rapidly become clonic. The convulsive phase may last only a minute but is followed by exhaustion and sleep.

Muscular contractions may be so powerful that fractures of vertebrae and other bones may occur. For this reason muscle relaxants such as succinylcholine may be administered along with the convulsant.

Pentylenetetrazol is now largely obsolete both as an analeptic and for convulsive therapy.

PICROTOXIN

Picrotoxin is a nonnitrogenous compound obtained from an East Indian shrub. It is available in injectable solution containing 3 mg./ml.

The drug is a typical convulsant of the pentylenetetrazol rather than the strychnine type. In normal animals it stimulates respiration only in doses close to the convulsant dose. Barbiturate-anesthetized animals may show significant respiratory stimulation without a convulsant action because the barbiturates antagonize the convulsive tendency.

Picrotoxin, once widely used as an analeptic in barbiturate poisoning, is seldom used today and is largely obsolete.

NIKETHAMIDE

Nikethamide (Coramine) is closely related to nicotinamide and is converted to the vitamin in the body. The structural relationships are as follows:

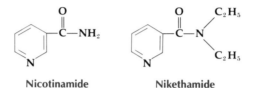

Nicotinamide   Nikethamide

Nikethamide is a respiratory stimulant and analeptic of low potency. In large doses the drug can produce clonic convulsions. The site of its respiratory stimulant action has been debated. It was believed for some time that nikethamide stimulates the carotid body, but subsequent work indicated that medullary stimulation may be more important.[4]

Nikethamide is available in ampules containing 0.4 Gm./1.5 ml. or 1.25 Gm./5 ml. The drug is not a cardiac stimulant, and as an analeptic it is seldom used today.

BEMEGRIDE

Bemegride (Megimide), a central nervous system stimulant, has been claimed to be an antagonist of the barbiturates. Its structural formula shows some relationship to the barbiturate structure, and it was believed by some investigators that it might be a competitive inhibitor of the action of the barbiturate hypnotics.

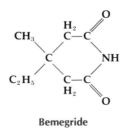

Bemegride

Present evidence indicates, however, that it stimulates respiration and other neural functions by mechanisms similar to those of the other analeptics.[7,10]

ETHAMIVAN

Ethamivan (Emivan) is claimed to be a respiratory stimulant useful in hypoventilatory states.[9] It is used as an adjunct to the management of chronic pulmonary disease with depressed respiration, particularly when aggravated by sleep or oxygen therapy.

Ethamivan may be injected intravenously in a dose of 100 mg. It may also be given by slow intravenous infusion. The oral administration of 20 mg. doses may not cause effective respiratory stimulation, but much larger doses have been effective in some cases.

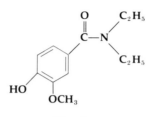

Ethamivan

DOXAPRAM

Doxapram (Dopram) is an analeptic that is claimed to have outstanding respiratory stimulant effects.[12] Its therapeutic index, expressed as convulsant dose$_{50}$/respiratory stimulant dose$_{50}$, is higher than that of the older analeptics, as determined in animals. This ratio may be as high as 25. The drug is administered intravenously in doses of 1 to 1.5 mg./kg. of body weight.

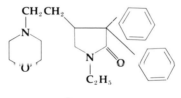

Doxapram

STRYCHNINE

Strychnine is a complex alkaloid obtained from the seeds of the plant *Strychnos nuxvomica.*

Strychnine exerts a predominant effect on the spinal cord, in which it lowers the threshold of excitability of various neurons.[1] More recent studies[2] indicate that it opposes the inhibitory influence of Renshaw cells on the motoneurons. Strychnine convulsions differ from pentylenetetrazol seizures in man by the predominance of the tonic extensor phase, opisthotonos being characteristic of both this type of poisoning

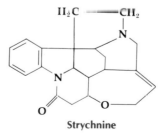

Strychnine

and of tetanus. The individual becomes highly susceptible to various stimuli, so that any sudden stimulation such as noise precipitates a tonic extensor seizure.

Death in strychnine poisoning is probably due to asphyxia or to exhaustion after a prolonged series of seizures. Barbiturates are effective antagonists against the convulsant and lethal actions of strychnine. The muscle relaxants such as mephenesin (Tolserol) are also capable of protecting animals against strychnine poisoning.

Treatment of strychnine poisoning is based on the prompt use of intravenous barbiturates. The stomach may be lavaged with a dilute potassium permanganate solution in order to remove and alter the poison at the early stages of intoxication.

CAFFEINE

Caffeine (1,3,7-trimethylxanthine) is one of the most widely used stimulants by the lay public and it also has some medical uses. Coffee contains approximately 1.3% caffeine, and a cup of coffee may contain from 100 to 150 mg. of the alkaloid. It has been estimated that the annual consumption of caffeine in the United States in the form of coffee is about 7,000,000 kg.

The structural formula of caffeine, a methylated xanthine, is as follows:

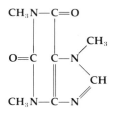

Caffeine

This drug is closely related to theophylline but has greater central nervous system stimulant action.

The main pharmacologic actions of caffeine are exerted on the central nervous system and the cardiovascular system. In addition, the drug is a diuretic and stimulates gastric secretion. In large experimental doses the drug can cause unusual contracture of skeletal muscle, but this has no clinical importance.

Caffeine stimulates the cerebral cortex and medullary centers. In ordinary doses it causes wakefulness, restlessness, and mental alertness. These actions of caffeine are considered pleasant by most persons, and it is not surprising that wherever a caffeine-containing plant grows, the inhabitants of the area have usually learned to utilize the drug. Some habituation to the use of caffeine occurs, but the drug is not truly addictive.

In larger doses, caffeine can stimulate respiration and can also precipitate clonic convulsions in experimental animals.

Caffeine has some stimulant action on the myocardium and can cause an increase in cardiac output. Increased coronary blood flow is probably a consequence of the increased myocardial work. Systemic blood pressure is not changed by ordinary doses of caffeine, although the drug directly dilates some blood vessels. The cerebral vessels are constricted by caffeine. These effects are similar to those of aminophylline.[9]

The end product of caffeine metabolism in the body appears to be 1-methyluric acid and other methyl derivatives of uric acid. It is quite certain that caffeine does not increase the miscible pool or urinary excretion of uric acid itself and is not contraindicated in gout.

For therapeutic use, caffeine is available as caffeine sodium benzoate in ampules of 0.25 and 0.5 Gm. in 2 ml. for intramuscular injection. For oral administration, citrated caffeine is available in 60 and 120 mg. tablets. In addition, caffeine is often added to headache remedies containing salicylates and acetophenetidin and to ergotamine (Cafergot) for the treatment of migraine.

Although the basic mechanism of action of caffeine and other methylxanthines is not known, it is of great interest that some relationship may exist between these drugs and the tissue levels of cyclic adenylic acid. It has been shown that methylxanthines inhibit the enzyme phosphodiesterase,[11] which inactivates cyclic adenosine-3',5'-phosphate. Since catecholamines promote the formation of the cyclic nucleotide whereas the methylxanthines inhibit its destruction, a very interesting hypothesis could be constructed for explaining similarities of pharmacologic action at many sites such as the heart and the bronchial smooth muscle. The action of methylxanthines and epinephrine on cyclic adenylic acid metabolism is discussed further on p. 99.

References

1 Dusser de Barenne, J. G.: The mode and site of action of strychnine in the nervous system, Physiol. Rev. **13**:325, 1933.

2 Eccles, J. C.: The physiology of nerve cells, Baltimore, 1957, The Johns Hopkins Press.

3 Eccles, J. C., Schmidt, R., and Willis, W. D.: Pharmacological studies on presynaptic inhibition, J. Physiol. **168**:500, 1963.

4 Eckenhoff, J. E.: A status report on analeptics, J.A.M.A. **139**:780, 1949.

5 Killam, K. F.: Possible role of gamma-aminobutyric acid as an inhibitory transmitter, Fed. Proc. **17**:1018, 1958.

6 Killam, K. F., and Bain, J. A.: Convulsant hydrazides: in vitro and in vivo inhibition of vitamin B_6 enzymes by convulsant hydrazides, J. Pharmacol. Exp. Ther. **119**:255, 1957.

7 Kimura, E. T., and Richards, R. K.: A comparative study of bemegride (β,β-methylethylglutarimide; NP-13; Megimide) as an analeptic in mice, Arch. Int. Pharmacodyn. **110**:29, 1957.

8 Miller, W. F., Archer, R. K., Taylor, H. F., and Ossenfort, W. F.: Severe respiratory depression. Role of a respiratory stimulant, ethamivan, in the treatment, J.A.M.A. **180**:905, 1962.

9 Moyer, J. H., Miller, S. I., Tashnek, A. B., and Bowman, R.: The effect of theophylline with ethylene diamine (aminophylline) on cerebral hemodynamics in the presence of cardiac failure with and without Cheyne-Stokes respiration, J. Clin. Invest. **31**:267, 1952.

10 Plum, F., and Swanson, A. G.: Barbiturate poisoning treated by physiological methods with observations on effects of beta, beta-methylethylglutarimide and electrical stimulation, J.A.M.A. **163**:827, 1957.

11 Sutherland, E. W., and Rall, T. W.: The relation of adenosine-3'5'-phosphate to the action of catecholamines. In Adrenergic mechanisms, Ciba Foundation and Committee for Symposium on Drug Action, Boston, 1960, Little, Brown & Co.

12 Wasserman, A. J., and Richardson, D. W.: Human cardiopulmonary effects of doxapram, a respiratory stimulant, Clin. Pharmacol. Ther. **4**:321, 1963.

Recent reviews

13 Adriani, J., Drake, P., and Arens, J.: Use of antagonists in drug-induced coma, J.A.M.A. **179**:752, 1962.

14 Bader, M. E., and Bader, R. A.: Respiratory stimulants in obstructive lung disease, New York, 1964, Academic Press, Inc.

15 Eccles, J. C.: The physiology of synapses, Amer. J. Med. **38**:165, 1965.

23 Antiepileptic drugs

GENERAL CONCEPT

Epilepsy is a manifestation of paroxysmal cerebral dysrhythmia. The overt clinical picture may vary from frank convulsions to momentary losses of consciousness. There may be as many as 500,000 epileptics in the United States, and the state of well-being of these patients depends almost entirely upon adequate drug therapy.

The antiepileptic drugs are central nervous system depressants whose selectivity is such that they can prevent epileptic seizures in doses that do not cause excessive drowsiness. Although all antiepileptic drugs have some undesirable features and the perfect medication has not been discovered, the fact that some measure of protection can be offered against attacks in at least 80% of epileptics may be considered an outstanding success in the pharmacologic approach to disease.

The several convulsive disorders encountered in clinical practice may be classified as (1) grand mal, including generalized, focal, and jacksonian seizures, (2) petit mal, including pure petit mal and myoclonic and akinetic epilepsy, (3) psychomotor epilepsy, and (4) autonomic or visceral epilepsy.

Bromides were the earliest antiepileptic drugs. They were gradually abandoned after the introduction of phenobarbital in 1912 and the later development of diphenylhydantoin. Although many new antiepileptic drugs of high potency and fair selectivity have subsequently been discovered, most of them have considerable toxicity.

ANTIEPILEPTIC DRUGS
Methods of testing

Although clinical trial is the only certain method for determining the usefulness of antiepileptic drugs, preliminary estimates can be made by screening procedures in animals. These screening procedures are usually carried out in mice, and convulsions are produced either by application of an electric current or by injection of pentylenetetrazol (Metrazol).

In the electroconvulsive method, electrodes are placed in the ears or eyes of these animals, and alternating or interrupted direct current is applied for a short period of time. The convulsions that are produced are characterized by a short tonic extensor period followed by clonic convulsions. When premedication is used, the effect of the drug on the threshold and on the characteristics of the convulsions can be determined.

The ability of a potential antiepileptic drug to elevate the threshold to pentylenetetrazol-induced convulsions is also determined. Finally, the relationship between the dosage elevating the convulsive threshold and the dosage producing sedation gives some preliminary indication of the therapeutic index.

Experience indicates that the drugs which can modify maximal electroshock seizure in animals are usually effective in grand mal epilepsy. On the other hand, some of these drugs (for example, diphenylhydantoin) may be quite ineffective against seizures induced by pentylenetetrazol. Some drugs that are very effective against the drug-induced convulsions, such as trimethadione, turned out to be effective in the management of petit mal.

Mode of action

The mechanism whereby the anticonvulsant drugs protect patients against attacks in the various types of epilepsy is not known with certainty.[14]

It is believed that seizures are produced by discharges of abnormal foci in the brain. The spread of these discharges creates long-chain reverberating circuits. The antiepileptic drugs could either suppress the abnormally discharging foci or prevent spread of the discharges by reducing the excitability of the otherwise normal neurons involved in the reverberating circuits.

It has been observed that anticonvulsant drugs can protect patients against grand mal epileptic convulsions without preventing the electroencephalographic evidences of the disease. This finding suggests that the abnormal focus is not suppressed but that the spread of the discharges may be prevented.

In the petit mal type of epilepsy the effective drugs are capable of affecting both the clinical and the electroencephalographic evidences of the disease.

Although carbonic anhydrase inhibitors have anticonvulsant activity, it is unlikely that the major antiepileptic drugs act by a similar mechanism. Phenobarbital, diphenylhydantoin, and trimethadione, in anticonvulsant doses, have no effect on brain carbonic anhydrase in animals.[12] Similarly, alterations in acid-base and electrolyte balance as well as in the hormones of the adrenal cortex have important influences on seizure threshold,[15] but there is no reason to believe that the antiepileptic drugs act through such mechanisms.

Classes of antiepileptic drugs

From a chemical standpoint the various drugs used in epilepsy may be listed in the following categories:

Barbiturates and related drugs
Phenobarbital (Luminal)
Mephobarbital (Mebaral)
Metharbital (Gemonil)
Primidone (Mysoline)
Hydantoins
Phenylethylhydantoin (Nirvanol)
Mephenytoin (Mesantoin)
Diphenylhydantoin (Dilantin)
Oxazolidones
Trimethadione (Tridione)
Paramethadione (Paradione)

Succinimides
Phensuximide (Milontin)
Methsuximide (Celontin)
Ethosuximide (Zarontin)
Miscellaneous anticonvulsants
Phenacemide (Phenurone)
Bromides
Acetazolamide (Diamox)
Aminoglutethimide (Elipten)
Diazepam
Meprobamate

An examination of the basic structural formulas of the barbiturates, hydantoins, oxazolidines, and succinimides reveals certain obvious similarities.

Whereas barbituric acid is malonylurea, hydantoin has a five-membered ring that

277

may be considered to be a combination of acetic acid and urea. In the oxazolidine derivatives the nitrogen in the hydantoin ring is replaced by oxygen. The succinimides obviously resemble the oxazolidines.

Main areas of usefulness

The major areas of usefulness of the various groups of drugs may be listed as follows, although some overlap does occur:

Barbiturates and primidone
  Grand mal epilepsy
  Psychomotor epilepsy
Hydantoins
  Grand mal epilepsy
  Psychomotor epilepsy
Oxazolidones
  Petit mal epilepsy
Succinimides
  Petit mal epilepsy

Phenacemide
  Psychomotor epilepsy
Acetazolamide
  Grand mal epilepsy
  Petit mal epilepsy
Diazepam
  Petit mal epilepsy
  Status epilepticus
Meprobamate
  Petit mal epilepsy

BARBITURATES AND RELATED DRUGS

Phenobarbital (Luminal) is one of the oldest antiepileptic drugs. It is administered in a total daily dose of 0.1 to 0.2 Gm. Phenobarbital differs from most of the other barbiturate hypnotics in possessing a significant antiepileptic effect at dose levels that do not cause excessive sedation or sleep. When phenobarbital is used, care must be taken never to withdraw it suddenly because this procedure can precipitate a grand mal attack.

The major usefulness of phenobarbital is in the management of grand mal epilepsy. It has little effect on petit mal but may be advantageous in combination with trimethadione in patients who have both types of epilepsy.

Mephobarbital (Mebaral) is N-methylphenobarbital. Its indications and uses are very similar to those of phenobarbital. In fact, it has been shown that the compound is demethylated to a significant extent to phenobarbital in the body.[4] As a consequence, the antiepileptic effects of mephobarbital may be due, at least in part, to phenobarbital. The dosage of mephobarbital is 300 to 600 mg./day.

Metharbital (Gemonil) is N-methylbarbital and is probably demethylated in the body to barbital. Its dosage is 100 mg. two or three times a day.

Primidone (Mysoline), although not a true barbituric acid, shows considerable similarity in structure to phenobarbital. It may produce considerable drowsiness and vertigo. Because of this, it should be started in small doses, about 50 mg., with a gradual increase to as much as 250 mg. three times a day. Primidone is converted, at least in part, to phenobarbital in the body.[3]

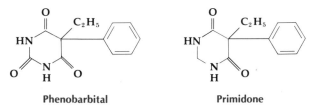

Phenobarbital   Primidone

HYDANTOINS

The structural formulas for phenylethylhydantoin, mephenytoin, and diphenyl-hydantoin follow:

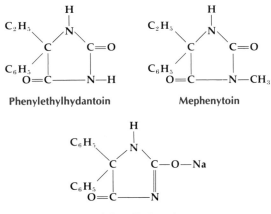

Phenylethylhydantoin   Mephenytoin

Diphenylhydantoin

Phenylethylhydantoin (Nirvanol) was used as a sedative as early as 1916. The drug was abandoned because it tended to produce an extraordinarily high incidence of drug fever, skin sensitization, and eosinophilia. Interestingly, the replacement of the ethyl radical by a phenyl group yielded the highly useful drug diphenylhydantoin.

On the other hand, **mephenytoin** (3-methyl-5-ethyl-5-phenylhydantoin; Mesantoin), which is the N-methyl derivative of phenylethylhydantoin, is demethylated in the body to this highly toxic and sensitizing drug. It is not surprising, therefore, that a high incidence of drug reactions has been reported following the use of mephenytoin. Some of these are skin rashes and fever, granulocytopenia, and aplastic anemia. Clearly the drug should be used only if other compounds are ineffective.

Diphenylhydantoin (Dilantin), introduced in 1938, is still one of the most valuable antiepileptic drugs. It is administered in capsules containing 0.1 Gm. of the drug as its sodium salt. The daily dose in adults varies from 0.2 to 0.6 Gm.

The main advantage of diphenylhydantoin in the management of grand mal and psychomotor epilepsy is that it exerts little sedative action at effective dose levels. However, in large doses it can cause ataxia, tremors, and nausea.

Adverse effects of diphenylhydantoin. The unwanted effects of diphenylhydantoin are of three categories.[18] It has *toxic effects,* true *side effects,* and *idiosyncratic reactions.* Intoxication is characterized by sedation, ataxia, and nystagmus. These manifestations are dose-related and appear at plasma levels of 20 to 40 μg per milliliter.

Side effects include osteomalacia and hypocalcemia caused probably by an interference with vitamin D metabolism. Long-term use of diphenylhydantoin may lead to lowered serum folic acid levels resulting in megaloblastic anemia.

An unusual side effect caused by diphenylhydantoin is the hypertrophy of the gums. It occurs in 20% of patients and is generally attributed to a disorder of fibroblastic activity.

Drugs of the hydantoin group may produce blood dyscrasias and rarely a clinical picture resembling malignant lymphoma. Diphenylhydantoin has antiarrhythmic effects.[16] Its use as an antiarrhythmic drug is discussed on p. 399.

OXAZOLIDONES

The structural formulas of the oxazolidine derivatives **trimethadione** (Tridione) and **paramethadione** (Paradione) are as follows:

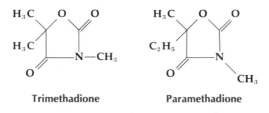

Trimethadione   Paramethadione

Trimethadione and paramethadione are useful in the mangement of petit mal. They are available in capsules containing 0.3 Gm., and the daily dose varies from 1 to 2 Gm.

In clinical use of the oxazolidine derivatives,[1, 9] the following toxic effects have been reported: drowsiness and ataxia, photophobia, and a strange visual disturbance consisting of a white halo around various objects. Bone marrow depression and kidney damage have also been reported following prolonged use of the oxazolidines. Skin rashes and alopecia also have been reported.

SUCCINIMIDES

Succinimides such as **phensuximide** (Milontin), **methsuximide** (Celontin), and **ethosuximide** (Zarontin) are useful in the management of petit mal. They may be less toxic than the oxazolidones, although dizziness or skin rashes may occur following their use. Rare cases of neutropenia and other blood dyscrasias have also been reported.

Usual dosages of these drugs are phensuximide, 0.5 to 1 Gm. three times a day; methsuximide, 0.3 to 0.6 Gm. three times a day; and ethosuximide, 0.5 Gm. two to four times a day. Ethosuximide is now considered the drug of choice in the treatment of petit mal.

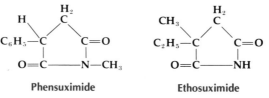

Phensuximide   Ethosuximide

MISCELLANEOUS ANTICONVULSANTS

Phenacemide (Phenurone), a very potent but quite toxic anticonvulsant, should be used rarely, if at all, only after all other measures fail. When used in doses of 0.5 Gm. three times a day, it may cause severe bone marrow depression, hepatocellular damage, and toxic psychoses.

Bromides were used extensively at one time but are now obsolete. Their use is associated with mental depression, toxic psychoses, and skin rashes.

Acetazolamide (Diamox), a carbonic anhydrase inhibitor, is used occasionally. Mild metabolic acidosis induced by a ketogenic diet was at one time used in epilepsy. The carbonic anhydrase inhibitors, which produce metabolic acidosis, have been found useful in all types of epilepsy. There is a possibility that their effectiveness is not due to systemic acidosis but to inhibition of carbonic anhydrase in the central nervous system. Acetazolamide is given in doses of 250 to 500 mg. two or three times a day.

Aminoglutethimide (Elipten) is a drug chemically related to the hypnotic glutethimide (Doriden). Although it is claimed to be effective in all types of epilepsy, it was withdrawn because of its toxicity.

Diazepam (Valium) and **meprobamate** (Miltown; Equanil) are antianxiety drugs that have some usefulness as antiepileptic drugs. Both have some effectiveness in the treatment of petit mal, and diazepam given by injection is quite useful in terminating an attack of status epilepticus. Childhood epilepsy responds remarkably well to diazepam treatment.[6]

CLINICAL PHARMACOLOGY OF ANTIEPILEPTIC DRUGS

The various groups of anticonvulsants may be listed according to the clinical form of the disease in which they are most useful:

Grand mal or focal seizures
  Barbiturates and primidone
  Hydantoins
  Carbonic anhydrase inhibitors
Petit mal seizures
  Oxazolidones
  Succinimides
  Carbonic anhydrase inhibitors
Psychomotor seizures
  Hydantoins
  Primidone and barbiturates
  Phenacemide

In *status epilepticus*, diphenylhydantoin may be injected parenterally. It is best to administer the drug by slow intravenous infusion, although intramuscular injection of 500 mg. of the drug may be useful for terminating an attack. Phenobarbital sodium may also be used for this purpose, although respiration may be seriously depressed by the drug. Paraldehyde has been administered for status epilepticus in doses of 6 mg. by intramuscular injection. Diazepam is considered by some as the drug of choice for status epilepticus. It is given by slow intravenous injection or intramuscularly, 5 to 10 mg. in adults or 2 to 5 mg. in children.

In patients who have both grand mal and petit mal epilepsy, it has been reported that the oxazolidones may precipitate grand mal attacks, whereas diphenylhydantoin may aggravate petit mal. To avoid these paradoxical effects, skillful selection of the various drugs is mandatory.

The toxic potentiality of the antiepileptic drugs should be kept in mind by both the physician and patient so that their adverse effects may be recognized at an early stage. Skin rash, blood dyscrasias, lymphadenopathy, lupus erythematosus, disturbances in hair growth, gingival hyperplasia, bleeding tendency, and fever are some of the complications that should be looked for in patients on anticonvulsant therapy.

Drug interactions

Numerous drug interactions of clinical significance may be seen in the treatment of epilepsy. Phenobarbital speeds up the metabolism of diphenylhydantoin and thereby decreases its effectiveness. This interaction is not readily recognized and is of no great importance, since the two drugs are additive in their antiepileptic effect.

The barbiturates speed up the metabolism of coumarin anticoagulants, and this interaction becomes dangerous when the barbiturate is suddenly discontinued, since bleeding may develop. The coumarins inhibit the metabolism of diphenylhydantoin, an interaction that could lead to intoxication with the antiepileptic drug.

The metabolism of diphenylhydantoin is also inhibited by isoniazid, aminosalicylic acid, and disulfiram (Antabuse). Barbiturates may become more toxic when certain MAO inhibitors are used because of inhibition of drug metabolism. Finally, reserpine tends to lower convulsive thresholds and may antagonize the actions of diphenyl-hydantoin. For further detail on drug interactions and references Chapter 58 should be consulted.

References

1 Abbott, J. A., and Schwab, R. S.: Medical progress: the serious side effects of the newer antiepileptic drugs; their control and prevention, New Eng. J. Med. **242**:947, 1950.

2 Benton, J. W., Tynes, B., Register, H. B., Jr., Alford, C., and Halley, H. L.: Systemic lupus erythematosus occurring during anticonvulsive drug therapy, J.A.M.A. **115**:115, 1962.

3 Bogan, J., and Smith, H.: Relation between primidone and phenobarbital blood levels, J. Pharm. Pharmacol. **20**:64, 1968.

4 Butler, T. C.: Quantitative studies of the metabolic fate of mephobarbital (N-methyl phenobarbital), J. Pharmacol. Exp. Ther. **106**: 235, 1952.

5 Camerman, A., and Camerman N.: Diphenyl-hydantoin and diazepam; molecular structure similarities and steric basis of anticonvulsant activity, Science **168**:1458, 1970.

6 Geller, M., and Christoff, N.: Diazepam in the treatment of childhood epilepsy, J.A.M.A. **215**: 2087, 1971.

7 Gunn, C. G., Gogerty, J., and Wolf, S.: Clinical pharmacology of anticonvulsant compounds, Clin. Pharmacol. Ther. **2**:733, 1961.

8 Lennox, W. G.: The treatment of epilepsy, Med. Clin. N. Amer. **29**:1114, 1945.

9 Lennox, W. G.: Tridione in the treatment of epilepsy, J.A.M.A. **134**:138, 1947.

10 Lennox, W. G.: Convulsive states. In Cecil, R. L., and Loeb, R. F., editors: Textbook of medicine, ed. 9, Philadelphia, 1955, W. B. Saunders Co.

11 Livingston, S., Pauli, L., and Najmabadi, A.: Ethosuximid in the treatment of epilepsy, J.A.M.A. **180**:822, 1962.

12 Merritt, H. H., and Putnam, T. J.: Sodium diphenylhydantoinate in the treatment of convulsive disorders, J.A.M.A. **111**:1068, 1938.

13 Millichap, J. G., Woodbury, D. M., and Goodman, L. S.: Mechanism of the anticonvulsant action of acetazolamide, a carbonic anhydrase inhibitor, J. Pharmacol. Exp. Ther. **115**:251, 1955.

14 Putnam, T. J., and Merritt, H. H.: Experimental determination of anticonvulsant properties of some phenyl derivatives, Science **85**:525, 1937.

15 Toman, J. E. P., and Goodman, L. S.: Anticonvulsants, Physiol. Rev. **28**:409, 1948.

16 Unger, A. H., and Sklaroff, H. J.: Fatalities following the intravenous use of sodium diphenylhydantoin for cardiac arrhythmias, J.A.M.A. **200**:335, 1967.

17 Woodbury, D. M.: Relation between the adrenal cortex and the central nervous system, Pharmacol. Rev. **10**:275, 1958.

Recent reviews

18 Kutt, H., and Louis, S.: Untoward effects of anticonvulsants, New Eng. J. Med. **286**:1316, 1972.

19 Livingston, S.: Drug therapy for epilepsy, Springfield, Ill., 1966, Charles C Thomas, Publisher.

20 Rose, S. W., Smith, L. D., and Penry, J. K.: Blood level determinations of antiepileptic drugs, Bethesda, Md., 1971, National Institutes of Neurological Diseases and Stroke; National Institutes of Health.

21 Scholl, M. L.: Treatment of seizure disorders (epilepsy), New Eng. J. Med. **269**:1304, 1421, 1963.

24 Narcotic analgesic drugs

Relief of pain is one of the great objectives in medicine. Drugs with a predominant pain-relieving action are called *analgesics* and are commonly classified as *narcotic* and *nonnarcotic*. The narcotic analgesics include the alkaloids of opium and many related synthetic drugs. Their use in most instances is regulated by the Federal Controlled Substances Act of 1970.

The classification of analgesics as narcotic and nonnarcotic is based on legal considerations. From a medical standpoint it would be more useful to classify them as *strong* and *mild*, since what the physician is interested in is the capability of a drug to relieve *severe* or only *moderate* pain. However, most of the narcotic analgesics are strong and most of the nonnarcotics are mild, and the traditional classification will be followed in this discussion.

Opium has been used by man throughout recorded history. The chemist has succeeded in modifying the structures of the opium alkaloids and in creating related drugs. Although morphine is still a very important narcotic analgesic, some of the synthetic drugs are welcome additions to therapeutics. The great incentive for the development of new analgesics has been the possible dissociation of the analgesic from the euphoriant effects of these drugs and the elimination of addiction liability. Some success has been achieved in these efforts and in the synthesis of opiate antagonists.

THE OPIATE RECEPTOR

Recent evidence indicates that there is a specific receptor for opiates in nervous tissue.[25] The existence of such a receptor has been suspected from the basic structural similarity of all active opioid drugs, their stereospecificity, and the availability of specific opiate antagonists. One of these, naloxone (tritiated) was found to bind to certain portions of mammalian brain. Competition could be demonstrated between various opiates and their antagonists, which parallelled their pharmacologic potency. The opiate receptor could also be demonstrated in the innervated but not in the denervated intestine. This and other evidence indicates that the opiate receptor is confined to nervous tissue.

METHODS OF STUDY OF ANALGESIC ACTION

Quantitative studies on analgesics are very difficult because the pain experience in man depends not only on the perception of the painful stimulus but also on psychological factors.

Two types of experimental approaches are commonly used for evaluation of analgesic action. In one, the threshold for pain is determined in man or animals by the application of painful stimuli of graded intensity. In the other method, analgesics are administered to postoperative patients, and their pain-relieving potency is compared with that of a placebo,[4] which has a distinct analgesic effect.

CHEMISTRY AND CLASSIFICATION OF NARCOTIC ANALGESICS

Narcotic analgesics can be divided into five categories as follows:

Natural opium alkaloids
  Morphine
  Codeine
Synthetic derivatives of opiates
  Dihydromorphinone (Dilaudid)
  Heroin
  Methyldihydromorphinone (metopon)
  Hydrocodone (Hycodan)
Synthetic opiate-like drugs
  Phenazocine (Prinadol)
  Meperidine (Demerol)
  Alphaprodine (Nisentil)
  Anileridine (Leritine)
  Piminodine (Alvodine)
  Diphenoxylate (with atropine, as Lomotil)
  Methadone (Dolophine)
  Levorphanol (Levo-Dromoran)
Synthetic opiate-like drugs of low addiction liability and potency
  Propoxyphene (Darvon)
  Ethoheptazine (Zactane)
  Pentazocine (Talwin)
Narcotic antagonists
  Nalorphine (Nalline)
  Levallorphan (Lorfan)
  Naloxone hydrochloride (Narcan)

Pharmacologic studies indicate a basic similarity among the various addictive analgesics. They are all potent against severe pain, all can be substituted for each other in the addict (although great tolerance develops to all of them), and all are antagonized by such drugs as nalorphine or levallorphan. It could be anticipated from these facts that some basic chemical similarity must exist in this series; and, in fact, examination of the formulas of all of these drugs reveals the presence of a common moiety, γ-phenyl-N-methyl-piperidine.

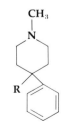

γ-**Phenyl-N-methylpiperidine**

NATURAL OPIATES AND SYNTHETIC DERIVATIVES
MORPHINE

Morphine, which has been used extensively for many years, remains the most important narcotic analgesic. Its pharmacology will be discussed in some detail, and it will serve as a standard of comparison with the other narcotics.

Chemistry

Morphine is an alkaloid obtained from opium, which is the dried juice of the poppy plant *Papaver somniferum*. The many different alkaloids found in opium fall into two categories: the phenanthrene alkaloids and the benzylisoquinoline compounds. Of the latter group, only papaverine has achieved any medical importance as an antispasmodic and vasodilator. It is not an analgesic and is now excluded from the opiates covered by the Harrison Narcotic Act.

Morphine and codeine are the only important narcotics obtainable from the phenanthrene group of opium alkaloids. Opium contains 10% morphine and 0.5% codeine.

Morphine, the chief alkaloid of opium, was isolated as early as 1803 by Sertürner but was not totally synthesized until 1952.[19] The synthesis confirmed the structure proposed by Gulland and Robinson in 1925.

The two hydroxyl groups, one phenolic and the other alcoholic, are of great importance, since some of the natural morphine derivatives are obtained by simple modifications of one or both of these groups. For example, codeine is methylmorphine, the substitution being in the phenolic hydroxyl. Heroin is diacetylmorphine. In dihydromorphinone the alcoholic hydroxyl is replaced by a ketonic oxygen and the double bond adjacent to it is removed. While most of the useful semisynthetic alkaloids are prepared by substitutions in the hydroxyl groups, the antidotal compound nalorphine is prepared by replacement of the CH_3 group on the nitrogen by the allyl radical $-CH_2CH=CH_2$.

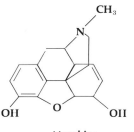

Morphine

Morphine sulfate is the most commonly employed salt. It is available in ampules of 1 ml. or in tablets of various sizes for preparing the injectable solution. It is also available in ampules of larger sizes. An ampule is not a dose. The subcutaneous dosage range is 8 to 15 mg.

Analgesic and other central nervous system effects

When morphine is administered by the subcutaneous route to a normal person in the amount of 10 to 15 mg., it produces drowsiness and euphoria in some but anxiety and nausea in others. The individual may go to sleep, his respiration slow, and his pupils constrict.

Practically all forms of pain can be relieved by morphine, but it is more effective against dull, constant pain than against sharp painful episodes. In its analgesic action, morphine differs significantly from the nonnarcotic analgesics such as the salicylates. The latter group of drugs is ineffective against visceral pain, whereas morphine is a potent analgesic against all modalities of pain.

There are at least two factors involved in the pain relief afforded by morphine. The drug elevates the pain threshold and alters the reaction of the individual to the painful experience.

There are differences of opinion concerning the relative importance of elevated pain threshold and altered reaction to pain in the effectiveness of morphine. Some investigators have been impressed with the similarity of the action of morphine and frontal lobotomy with regard to painful experiences; both are capable of bringing about separation of the painful experience from associated suffering. It has even been suggested that morphine may interrupt impulses between the frontal lobes and the diencephalon.[35] The effect of morphine on the psychic reaction to painful experience is probably the essential feature of the analgesic action.

The optimal dose of morphine for the average adult is 8 to 15 mg. This dose may elevate the threshold for pain perception by 60 to 70%. It has also been shown that 10 mg. of morphine gave relief of moderate postoperative pain to at least 90% of the patients.[5] This percentage is reduced to 70 in severe postoperative pain. A dose of 15 mg. may raise this percentage to 80. Interestingly, placebo administration provided relief to 30% of the patients and morphine by the oral route to only 40%.

The exact site of the analgesic action of morphine has not been elucidated. It is generally recognized, however, that morphine is far more selective with regard to analgesia than could be expected from a nonspecific depressant of the central nervous system. It has been shown that subjective depression and maximal analgesic action in man are not parallel.[29] For example, when morphine is injected intravenously, the maximal subjective depression occurs in about 5 minutes, whereas maximal analgesia occurs some 15 minutes later. Although some specific mechanism may be operative in the analgesic action of morphine, there is little doubt that the drug exerts widespread effects within the central nervous system.

Respiration

The respiratory center is markedly depressed by morphine, and stoppage of respiration is the cause of death in morphine poisoning. Therapeutic doses of morphine cause some lowering of respiratory minute volume and lessened response to carbon dioxide inhalation without much change in respiratory rate.[24] Larger doses also depress the rate of respiration, and carbon dioxide retention becomes severe. The onset of respiratory depression following injection of morphine is dependent on the method of administration.[15] Maximal depression of respiration occurs within about 5 minutes following intravenous injection, whereas it may be delayed for 60 minutes or longer if the drug is injected by the intramuscular route. As tolerance develops to the analgesic and euphoric actions of morphine, the respiratory center becomes tolerant also. This is the reason the addict may exhibit resistance to otherwise lethal doses of morphine.

Carbon dioxide retention is the probable cause of the cerebral vasodilatation and increased intracranial pressure that follow the administration of morphine.

Morphine is not a uniform depressant of neural structures. It does not oppose the action of stimulants such as strychnine or picrotoxin. Indeed, it may be synergistic with such drugs. Also, morphine may enhance monosynaptic reflexes, whereas it depresses multineuronal reflexes. Thus it has been shown by Wikler[34] that the knee and ankle jerks in the cat with spinal cord section were enhanced or not affected, whereas the flexor and crossed extensor reflexes were depressed.

Excitation

Morphine may actually be excitatory in certain persons and in several species of animals. Some patients may become nauseated and vomit following a morphine injection and may even become delirious. Similarly, cats and horses are stimulated by morphine. The violent excitement of cats caused by morphine is still present in decortication, requiring experimental lesions in the hypothalamus for its prevention.

Emesis

The emetic effect of morphine may be exerted on the chemoreceptor trigger zone in the medulla.[33] Interestingly, apomorphine, which is obtained from morphine through a major chemical modification, is a most potent stimulant of the chemoreceptor trigger zone.

Miscellaneous effects

Other effects of morphine include pupillary, gastrointestinal, biliary, cardiovascular, bronchial, antidiuretic, and metabolic.

Effect on pupils. The pupils are constricted by morphine, and this action is antagonized by atropine. Pupillary constriction is a consequence of the central nervous system action of the drug. Addicts do not develop tolerance to the pupillary constrictor action of morphine, and during withdrawal their pupils become widely dilated. Animals excited by morphine show pupillary dilatation.

Gastrointestinal effects. Morphine has a marked constipating effect, and opiates are time-honored remedies in the management of diarrhea.

In general, morphine tends to increase the tone of intestinal smooth muscle and decrease propulsive movements. Morphine delays gastric emptying through decreased gastric motility and contraction of the pylorus and perhaps of the duodenum as well. Atropine tends to partially oppose this spasmogenic action of morphine.

The constipating effect of morphine may be due to several factors. The most important ones are (1) increased tone and decreased propulsive activity throughout the gastrointestinal tract and (2) failure to perceive sensory stimuli that would otherwise elicit the defecation reflex.

The intestinal hypermotility that contributes to the constipating action of morphine appears to be mediated by the release of serotonin,[11] at least in the perfused dog's small intestine.

Problem 24-1. If the intestinal effect of morphine is mediated by serotonin, what would be the effect of reserpine pretreatment on this action of morphine? Experimental studies show[10] that reserpine pretreatment, which is known to deplete serotonin in tissues, reduced the response of the intestine to morphine.

Effect on biliary tract. Morphine increases intrabiliary pressure as a consequence of constricting the smooth muscles of the biliary tract. Pain relief under these conditions must be due to its central analgesic action. Atropine may not be effective in relieving severe spasm of the biliary tract induced by morphine.

Cardiovascular effects. The cardiovascular effects of morphine are generally unimportant when the drug is given in therapeutic doses. This is fortunate because the drug is often used in cardiac patients to relieve the pain of myocardial infarction and in the management of acute pulmonary edema of cardiac origin.

After the administration of large doses, morphine may cause central vasomotor depression. Hypoxia may play an important role in the fall of blood pressure, but more complex mechanisms are involved in the sharp hypotensive action that follows the intravenous injection of the drug. Under these circumstances morphine may produce its effects reflexly by initiating afferent activity in the vagus nerve.[18] The depressor response to intravenous morphine can be abolished by vagal section or hexamethonium. It is reduced but not abolished by atropine. In addition, histamine release in some species and a direct depressant action on the heart may contribute to the hypotension caused by morphine administered intravenously.

Effect on bronchial smooth muscle. The bronchial smooth muscle is contracted by morphine. Since death has occurred in asthmatic patients following morphine injection, many investigators attribute this adverse effect to the bronchoconstrictor action of morphine. It is quite possible, however, that this reaction of the asthmatic patient may be related to the depressant action of morphine on the responses of the respiratory center to carbon dioxide. According to this view, carbon dioxide narcosis, rather than bronchial constriction, may be the cause of death; however, the question is not settled.

Effect on genitourinary tract. The smooth muscle of the urinary tract is affected by morphine. The narcotic tends to contract the ureter and the detrusor muscle of the bladder and to cause an increase in the tone of the vesical sphincter. Atropine tends to relieve the ureteral spasm induced by morphine. Despite its smooth muscle effect, morphine is often used in the relief of ureteral colic, where its effectiveness must be due to its analgesic action.

The urinary retention that may follow administration of morphine is due to difficulty in micturition and decreased perception of the stimulus for micturition. Morphine is also an antidiuretic. It causes release of the antidiuretic hormone, and its hemodynamic actions also contribute to this antidiuretic effect.

Uterine contractions during labor are not significantly affected by a therapeutic dose of morphine, although they may be slowed somewhat.

Metabolic effects. One metabolic effect of morphine is some lowering of total oxygen consumption, probably due to decreased activity and muscle tone. Hyperglycemia of varying intensity has been observed after the injection of morphine. It is generally believed that this is a consequence of increased sympathetic activity, since total sympathectomy will prevent the rise in blood sugar.[7]

Metabolism

Morphine is readily absorbed following subcutaneous or intramuscular injection. It is estimated that about 60% of subcutaneously injected morphine is absorbed in the first 30 minutes. Absorption is strongly influenced by cutaneous circulation. Its absorption from the gastrointestinal tract is slow, however, and the drug is not given by this route.

About 90% of an administered dose can be recovered from the urine in a conjugated form, and a small percentage can be recovered from the feces. Biliary excretion may account for the presence of morphine in the feces. It has been shown that a microsomal enzyme in the liver can convert morphine to its glucuronide.[31]

A small amount of morphine is demethylated in the body to normorphine. Interesting studies have been carried out on the increase of demethylating enzyme activity in animals on chronic administration of morphine.[1,2]

Tolerance

A striking feature of the pharmacology of morphine and related drugs is the gradual tolerance that develops to some of its effects.

If a patient in chronic pain is given 10 to 15 mg. of morphine sulfate by the subcutaneous route twice a day, it is often observed that after a week or so he will not receive as much pain relief as he did at the beginning. The dose must be gradually increased. This tolerance extends not only to the analgesic but also to the respiratory depressant actions of morphine. On the other hand, no tolerance develops to the gastrointestinal or pupillary constrictor actions of morphine nor to the excitatory effects of the drug.

If the administration of morphine is prolonged, both a normal person and an addict will require progressively larger doses of morphine in order to obtain the same subjective effects. The tolerance may reach almost incredible proportions. Addicts have been known to take as much as 4 Gm. of the drug in 24 hours. This quantity is far greater than the lethal dose in a nontolerant person. The duration of tolerance is 1 to 2 weeks, and following this period of abstinence the individual again responds to a small dose of the drug. Addicts may die as a consequence of taking their usual large dose of morphine after a period of abstinence during which they have lost their tolerance.

Problem 24-2. Could tolerance to morphine be a consequence of altered absorption, increased rate of metabolism, and excretion? Obviously not, because the tolerant addict can administer doses of morphine intravenously that would depress the respiratory center of a nonaddict permanently. There must be a true cellular tolerance of some nervous elements. In agreement with this view, experimental studies[13] failed to show a difference in the metabolism of morphine in tolerant and nontolerant dogs.

Many factors influence the development of tolerance. Regular frequent administration of the drug is more likely to produce tolerance than widely spaced, irregular modes of administration. The administration of the narcotic antagonists nalorphine or naloxone produces acute withdrawal symptoms in individuals who are tolerant to large doses of morphine.

The mechanism of tolerance to the opiates is not well understood, but there are some interesting hypotheses that attempt to explain the relationships between tolerance and addiction. For example, according to the hypothesis of Goldstein and Goldstein,[20] morphine could inhibit an enzyme whose synthesis is repressed by its product. The immediate drug effect could be due to the enzyme inhibition. Tolerance would result from increased enzyme synthesis, which would be a consequence of low concentrations of the product. Withdrawal of the drug would lead to symptoms that are generally the opposite of the drug effect. The addict would have an excess of the enzyme that is constantly repressed by his drug intake. He would be in a steady state until the drug was withdrawn or an opiate antagonist was administered.

Morphine poisoning

In *acute* morphine poisoning the individual is comatose and cyanotic, his respirations are slow, and the pupils are of pinpoint size.

The management of a patient in acute morphine poisoning is quite different from that of the barbiturate-poisoned patient. First, central stimulant drugs such as picrotoxin or pentylenetetrazol (Metrazol) should not be used, since there is experimental evidence for lack of antidotal value. Morphine, in contrast to the barbiturates, has many excitatory actions and may be synergistic with the convulsants.

The major development in the treatment of acute morphine poisoning has been the discovery of the antidotal action of nalorphine. Intravenous injection of 5 to 10 mg. of this drug produces striking improvement in respiration and circulation of the acutely poisoned individual. The dosage may be repeated but should not exceed a total of 40 mg. This action of nalorphine does not extend to the barbiturates or general anesthetics but is so specific for morphine and related narcotics that it can be of diagnostic significance.

Naloxone hydrochloride (Narcan) is a new narcotic antagonist of great importance discussed on p. 295.

CODEINE

Codeine, or methylmorphine, is a very important analgesic and antitussive drug. In therapeutic doses it is less sedative and analgesic than morphine, but tolerance to the drug develops more slowly, and codeine is less addictive than morphine. It has less effect also on the gastrointestinal and urinary tracts and on the pupil and causes less nausea and constipation than morphine.

Codeine administered orally is not as effective an analgesic as when it is injected subcutaneously. In one study performed on postoperative patients, 60 mg. of codeine administered by mouth produced relief in 40% of the patients, whereas a placebo was effective in 33%.[5] On the other hand, administered subcutaneously, the drug was effective in 60% of the patients, whereas 10 mg. of morphine provided relief in 71%. Although effective, codeine is not quite as effective an analgesic as morphine, even when its dosage is six times higher.

Codeine phosphate is widely used in oral doses of 15 to 64 mg. for moderately severe pain when the nonaddictive analgesics prove to be ineffective. It is given by subcutaneous injection for severe pain.

Codeine is partly demethylated to morphine in the body and is partly changed to norcodeine. The conjugated forms of these compounds are excreted in the urine.

SYNTHETIC DERIVATIVES

Heroin, or diacetylmorphine, is a highly euphoriant and analgesic drug. It is much preferred by the addict, who may take it by the intravenous route in order to obtain a peculiar orgastic sensation. Because of its great addictive liability, heroin may not be legally manufactured in or imported into the United States.

Hydrocodone (Hycodan) resembles codeine but may be a more effective antitussive compound and is also more addictive. The recommended oral dose for adults is 5 to 15 mg., which may be given three to four times a day.

Dihydromorphinone (Dilaudid) is up to ten times as potent an analgesic as is morphine. Its respiratory depressant effect is correspondingly greater, although it may be less nauseating and constipating. Doses for hypodermic injection are about one tenth of the morphine dose, or 1 to 2 mg.

Methyldihydromorphinone, or metopon, is more potent than morphine, but it has no significant advantages over the latter, except that it is effective by oral administration.

Pantopium (Pantopon) contains the alkaloids of opium in the same proportion as they exist naturally. Since it contains about 50% morphine, its dosage is correspondingly higher. It has no significant advantages over morphine.

SYNTHETIC OPIATE-LIKE DRUGS

Phenazocine (Prinadol) is a synthetic addictive analgesic that is about four times as active as morphine but is without other significant advantages.

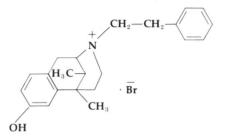

Phenazocine bromide

Meperidine (pethidine; isonipecaine; Demerol; Dolantin) was introduced originally as an antispasmodic of the atropine type.[16]

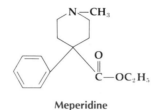

Meperidine

The analgesic potency of meperidine is such that 50 mg. is equivalent to 8 mg. of morphine and 100 mg. is equivalent to 12 mg. of morphine.

Despite early claims, it appears that meperidine is just as depressant to respiration as morphine when the two drugs are compared in equianalgesic doses. The drug may be slightly less sedative than morphine, but there is no basis for the belief that it has a significantly different action on the gastrointestinal or biliary tract or on the bronchial smooth muscle. Intravenous injection of meperidine may be followed by severe hypotension, caused at least in part by histamine release. Meperidine is definitely addictive.

The liver plays an important role in the metabolism of meperidine, which may be toxic in persons with liver disease.

Alphaprodine (Nisentil) is a piperidine derivative resembling meperidine. Its analgesic action is prompt and of short duration, but its superiority to meperidine remains to be demonstrated.

Anileridine (Leritine) is related to meperidine but is slightly more potent. The oral dose in adults is 25 to 50 mg. It may be given intramuscularly in 40 mg. dosage for severe pain.

Piminodine (Alvodine) and **diphenoxylate** (with atropine, as Lomotil) are related chemically to meperidine. Piminodine is used primarily as an analgesic orally or by injection. Diphenoxylate has been recommended for the control of diarrhea in doses of 5 mg. three times a day by mouth. It may cause addiction.

Methadone (Amidone; dolophine) was discovered in Germany during World War II. Although the structural formula of methadone does not obviously resemble that of morphine, its analgesic potency and some other effects, including the antagonistic action of nalorphine, are quite similar.

The analgesic potency of *dl*-methadone is largely due to the levo isomer. Isomethadone differs from methadone only in the position of the methyl group in the side chain.

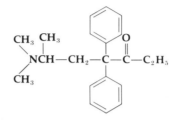

Methadone

The analgesic potency of methadone is about as great as that of morphine but is of longer duration. As a consequence, it is administered in doses of 10 mg. and is quite effective following oral administration. It causes considerable respiratory depression, but its emetic and constipating actions are less than those of morphine. Development of tolerance and addiction to methadone are known to occur.

Methadone is widely employed as an analgesic. Sedation and euphoria are slight. A unique application of methadone is in the treatment of morphine addiction.[14] If the drug can be substituted for morphine, subsequent withdrawal will be less severe, but it may be more prolonged. The use of methadone in addicts is discussed in Chapter 25.

The **morphinan series** of drugs includes levorphanol, dextrorphan, and dextromethorphan.

Levorphanol (Levo-Dromoran) is a synthetic drug that is closely related chemically to morphine.

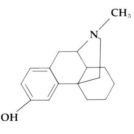

Levorphanol

The levo isomer is about five times as analgesic as morphine and consequently is administered in dosages of 2 mg. Its duration of action is somewhat longer than that of morphine. Respiratory depression and addiction liability are marked, but emetic and constipating actions are only moderate.

The dextro isomer, **dextrorphan**, has little analgesic action but possesses some antitussive properties.

Dextromethorphan (Romilar) the methyl ether of dextrorphan, has about the same antitussive potency as codeine, with no analgesic, euphoric, or respiratory-depressant properties. It is widely used as a cough suppressant, an action that is clearly unrelated to any narcotic analgesic property. It is a fairly harmless drug.[12]

SYNTHETIC OPIATE-LIKE DRUGS OF LOW ADDICTION LIABILITY AND POTENCY

Propoxyphene and ethoheptazine are related to methadone and meperidine, respectively, but have much lower potency and addiction liability. Pentazocine is one of the narcotic antagonists with some analgesic potency and low addiction liability.

Propoxyphene (Darvon) is widely used, often in combination with aspirin, phenacetin, and caffeine, the so-called Darvon Compound. It is commonly stated that its analgesic potency is similar to that of codeine, but this is doubtful. For many of its uses, aspirin contributes an anti-inflammatory analgesic effect to the Darvon Compound, which then may be more potent than codeine for specific applications. Pure propoxyphene is a weaker analgesic than codeine.

When its widespread use is considered, the number of individuals who have become addicted to propoxyphene is very low, although tolerance and addiction to the drug are possible. Doses of 32 or 64 mg. of propoxyphene should suffice for most of its indications, but some individuals take the larger dose six or more times a day. In chronic painful conditions it is often difficult to know if one is dealing with iatrogenic addiction.

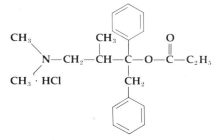

Propoxyphene hydrochloride

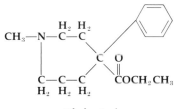

Ethoheptazine

Problem 24-3. How does propoxyphene compare in analgesic efficacy with aspirin? In a recent double-blind crossover study,[23] propoxyphene (65 mg.) gave no significant evidence of therapeutic activity and aspirin was clearly superior. It should be kept in mind, however, that these studies involved single administration to patients who had definite pain problems caused by cancer. It is conceivable that on continued administration the results would have been different.

Acute propoxyphene intoxication resembles morphine poisoning. The respiratory depression responds to the administration of a narcotic antagonist such as nalorphine.

Ethoheptazine (Zactane) is related to meperidine and, like propoxyphene, is of low potency and addiction liability. It is not nearly as popular as the latter.

Pentazocine (Talwin) is a synthetic analgesic structurally related to phenazocine.

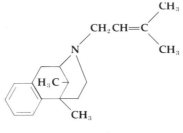

Pentazocine

Pentazocine is actually a weak narcotic antagonist with a significant analgesic effect of its own. Its potency is moderate and of short duration, but its low addiction liability makes it useful in chronic illnesses in which the more addictive drugs would constitute a hazard. Administered in 20 to 40 mg. doses by the subcutaneous or intramuscular route,[3] pentazocine may be as effective as 10 mg. of morphine. Larger doses do not increase its analgesic power. Pentazocine is also available in tablet form (50 mg.) for oral administration. It is difficult to evaluate its analgesic potency compared with that of other drugs by the oral route.

NARCOTIC ANTAGONISTS

Competitive antagonism of the narcotic analgesics, particularly their respiratory depressant actions, results from certain substitutions on the nitrogen atom of morphine or levorphanol. Nalorphine and levallorphan are important narcotic antagonists. Pentazocine is a weak antagonist and is much more useful as an analgesic of low addiction liability.

Nalorphine (Nalline) is N-allylnormorphine. Although there was evidence in the literature for many years that N-allyl derivatives of certain opiate drugs might antagonize the respiratory depressant effects of the various narcotics,[32] it was not until 1950 that nalorphine received clinical recognition.

Nalorphine is capable of antagonizing practically all the effects of morphine and other narcotics, including meperidine and methadone. It is a most important antidote in cases of poisoning from these drugs and can also precipitate acute withdrawal symptoms in an addicted person.

Interestingly, in the normal person, nalorphine behaves only as weak morphine. It has been suggested that the antidotal action of the drug may be due to competitive inhibition with replacement of potent drugs by a weak compound having higher affinity for the receptors. The drug itself is not a respiratory stimulant in normal persons, and it should not be employed in poisoning due to barbiturates or other hypnotics or anesthetics.

Nalorphine is administered in doses of 5 to 10 mg., usually by the intravenous route in cases of poisoning. The dosage should not exceed 40 mg.

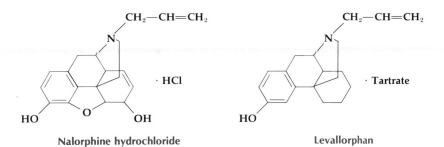

Nalorphine hydrochloride   Levallorphan

Levallorphan (Lorfan) is a morphine antagonist that is very similar in indications to nalorphine. From the chemical and pharmacologic standpoints, it has the same relationship to levorphanol as nalorphine has to morphine. Levallorphan is used in doses of 0.3 to 1.2 mg. by injection.

Naloxone hydrochloride (Narcan) is an important new narcotic antagonist, which is the *N*-allyl derivative of oxymorphone hydrochloride (Numorphan). It is available for intravenous, intramuscular, or subcutaneous administration in ampules and vials containing 0.4 mg./ml.

Naloxone reverses the respiratory-depressant action of the narcotics related to morphine, meperidine, and methadone. It differs from the other narcotic analgesics in several important respects. By itself, naloxone does not cause respiratory depression, pupillary constriction, sedation, or analgesia. It antagonizes the actions of pentazocine. Although naloxone does not antagonize the respiratory-depressant effects of barbiturates and other hypnotics, it does not aggravate their depressant effects on respiration. Just like the other narcotic antagonists, naloxone precipitates an abstinence syndrome when administered to patients addicted to opiate-like drugs.

CONTRAINDICATIONS TO THE USE OF MORPHINE AND RELATED AGENTS

The following medical conditions are generally considered to be contraindications to the use of morphine and related drugs:

Head injuries and following craniotomy
Bronchial asthma
Acute alcoholism
Convulsive disorders

PHYSICAL DEPENDENCE

The important problem of physical dependence to narcotics will be discussed in detail in Chapter 25.

CLINICAL PHARMACOLOGY OF ANTITUSSIVE DRUGS

From a pharmacologic standpoint, cough may be suppressed by action on the neural component of the reflex or by procedures that influence the quantity or viscosity of respiratory tract fluid. Drugs that act on the neural component may act on the central nervous system or on sensory endings in the mucous membranes of the respiratory tract. The specific effectiveness of antitussives is difficult to determine because non-specific sedation and placebos can be of benefit. Furthermore, in many of the cough mixtures the demulcent action of vehicles may play a significant part in the effects claimed.

In an attempt at quantitation, experiments have been designed in both animals and man in which the action of various drugs is determined through inducing coughing by the inhalation of irritant substances.[6,39] It is believed by clinical pharmacologists, however, that these experimental studies may not correlate well with the effectiveness of drugs in pathologic coughing.

There is little doubt that morphine and the synthetic opiate-like drugs are potent cough suppressants. However, because of their addiction liability, they are seldom used for this purpose. Codeine is the traditional cough suppressant, and all nonaddictive antitussives should be compared with codeine in controlled clinical trials. Claims for their effectiveness are often based on uncontrolled clinical trials and on experimental studies that may not be relevant.

Codeine is the standard narcotic antitussive. It is highly effective, and its addiction liability is not nearly as great as that of the strong narcotics. Nausea, constipation, and drowsiness are among the common side effects of codeine. In contrast with morphine, excessive doses of codeine may cause convulsions, especially in children. These convulsions are attributed to an effect of codeine on the spinal cord. The usual adult dosage of codeine phosphate USP is 8 to 15 mg. three or four times daily.

Hydrocodone bitartrate (Dicodid) is a somewhat more potent antitussive than codeine, but its addiction liability is greater. It is available in 5 mg. tablets.

Dextromethorphan (Romilar) is a substituted dextro isomer of the narcotic levorphan (Dromoran). It is not analgesic and is not addictive. It is claimed that it approaches codeine in antitussive potency. The usual dose is 10 to 20 mg. by mouth.

Noscapine (Nectadon) is the isoquinoline alkaloid narcotine found in opium. The drug is not addictive and has little analgesic action but is claimed to be antitussive. The dose is 15 to 30 mg. by mouth three times a day.

Benzonatate (Tessalon) is a local anesthetic related to tetracaine. It is claimed to be an effective antitussive when used in doses of 100 mg. It is believed to influence the cough reflex both at the stretch receptors in the lungs and within the central nervous system. It does not depress respiration.

Antihistaminics are also claimed to be of benefit as antitussives. Although there may be some reason for this action in asthmatic bronchitis of allergic etiology, their mode of action in other types of cough is not understood and according to some investigators is not well documented. Drugs of this type include carbetapentane (Toclase), dimethoxanate (Cothera), a phenothiazine, and other antihistaminic drugs.

Levopropoxyphene (Novrad), in contrast to its dextro form (Darvon), is claimed to have antitussive properties without being an analgesic. It may be too early to evaluate these claims on the basis of the evidence presented so far, although the drug is claimed to be as potent as codeine.

In addition to the antitussives that depress the cough reflex, drugs may be beneficial in the treatment of respiratory illnesses associated with coughing because they may reduce the viscosity of thick mucus.

Glyceryl guaiacolate (Guaianesin) apparently increases the volume and decreases the viscosity of bronchial secretions. Its dose is 100 to 200 mg. by mouth, which may be repeated in 2 to 4 hours. The formula appears on p. 297. Its efficacy is in doubt.

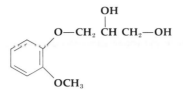

Glyceryl guaiacolate

Iodides are sometimes employed in bronchial asthma. The mode of action of these drugs is not known with certainty, but they may decrease the viscosity of bronchial mucus.

Ipecac and **ammonium chloride** are believed to cause thinning of bronchial mucus, perhaps by some reflex mechanism.

As a general statement, the antitussive drugs may be valuable in reducing a useless cough. They are purely symptomatic medications, and their use should not obviate the necessity of determining the cause of the cough. Claims made for the many non-addictive antitussives should be examined critically.

References

1 Axelrod, J.: The enzymatic demethylation of narcotic drugs, J. Pharmacol. Exp. Ther. **117**: 322, 1956.

2 Axelrod, J.: Possible mechanism of tolerance to narcotic drugs, Science **124**:263, 1956.

3 Beaver, W. T., Wallenstein, S. L., Houde, R. W., and Rogers, A.: A comparison of the analgesic effects of pentazocine and morphine in patients with cancer, Clin. Pharmacol. Ther. **7**:740, 1966.

4 Beecher, H. K.: Appraisal of drugs intended to alter subjective responses, symptoms. Report to Council on Pharmacy and Chemistry, J.A.M.A. **158**:399, 1955.

5 Beecher, H. K.: Measurement of subjective responses, New York, 1959, Oxford University Press.

6 Bickerman, H. A., Cohen, B. M., and German, E.: Cough response of healthy human subjects stimulated by critic acid aerosol. XI. Evaluation of antitussive agents, Amer. J. Med. Sci. **234**:191, 1957.

7 Bodo, R. C., Cotui, F. W., and Benaglia, A. E.: Studies on the mechanism of morphine hyperglycemia: role of the sympathetic nervous system, with special reference to the sympathetic supply to the liver, J. Pharmacol. Exp. Ther. **62**:88, 1938.

8 Bonica, J. J.: The management of pain, Philadelphia, 1953, Lea & Febiger.

9 Bucher, K.: Pathophysiology and pharmacology of cough, Pharmacol. Rev. **10**:43, 1958.

10 Burks, T. F.: Mediation by 5-hydroxytryptamine of morphine stimulant actions in dog intestine, J. Pharmacol. Exp. Ther. **185**:530, 1973.

11 Burks, T. F., and Long, J. P.: Release of intestinal 5-hydroxytryptamine by morphine and related agents, J. Pharmacol. Exp. Ther. **156**:267, 1967.

12 Cass, L. J., Frederik, W. S., and Andosca, J. B.: Quantitative comparison of dextromethorphan hydrobromide and codeine, Amer. J. Med. Sci. **227**:291, 1954.

13 Cochin, J., Haggart, J., Woods, L. A., and Seevers, M. H.: Plasma levels, urinary and fecal excretion of morphine in non-tolerant and tolerant dogs, J. Pharmacol. Exp. Ther. **111**:74, 1954.

14 Dole, V. P., and Nyswander, M.: A medical treatment for diacetylmorphine (heroin) addiction: a clinical trial with methadone hydrochloride, J.A.M.A. **193**:646, 1965.

15 Dripps, R. D., and Comroe, J. H., Jr.: Clinical studies on morphine: immediate effect of morphine administered intravenously and intramuscularly upon the respiration of normal man, Anesthesiology **6**:464, 1945.

16 Eisleb, O., and Schaumann, O.: Dolantin, ein neuartiges Spasmolytikum und Analgetikum (chemisches und pharmakologisches), Deutsch. Med. Wschr. **65**:967, 1939.

17 Evans, A. G. J., Nasmyth, P. A., and Stewart, H. C.: The fall of blood pressure caused by intravenous morphine in the rat and cat, Brit. J. Pharmacol. **7**:542, 1952.

18 Fennessy, M. R., and Rattray, J. F.: Cardiovascular effects of intravenous morphine in the anaesthetized rat, Europ. J. Pharmacol. **14**:1, 1971.

19 Gates, M., and Tschudi, G.: Synthesis of morphine, J. Amer. Chem. Soc. **78**:1380, 1956.

20 Goldstein, D. B., and Goldstein, A.: Possible

role of enzyme inhibition in repression in drug tolerance and addiction, Biochem. Pharmacol. **8**:48, 1961.

21 Gross, E. G.: Effect of liver damage on urinary morphine excretion, Proc. Soc. Exp. Biol. Med. **51**:61, 1942.

22 Kay, D. C., Gorodetzky, C. W., and Martin, W. R.: Comparative effects of codeine and morphine in man, J. Pharmacol. Exp. Ther. **156**:101, 1967.

23 Moertel, C. G., Ahmann, D. L., Taylor, W. F., and Schwartau, N.: A comparative evaluation of marketed analgesic drugs, New Eng. J. Med. **286**:813, 1972.

24 Papadopoulos, C. N., and Keats, A. S.: Studies of analgesic drugs. VI. Comparative respiratory depressant activity of phenazocine and morphine, Clin. Pharmacol. Ther. **2**:8, 1961.

25 Pert, C. B., and Snyder, S. H.: Opiate receptor: demonstration in nervous tissue, Science **179**: 1011, 1973.

26 Ralph, N.: Evaluation of new cough suppressant, Amer. J. Med. Sci. **227**:297, 1954.

27 Reynolds, A. K., and Randall, L. O.: Morphine and allied drugs, Toronto, 1957, University of Toronto Press.

28 Sadove, M., Balagot, R. C., and Pecora, F. N.: Pentazocine—a new nonaddicting analgesic, J.A.M.A. **189**:199, 1964.

29 Seevers, M. H., and Pfeiffer, C. C.: A study of the analgesia, subjective depression, and euphoria produced by morphine, heroin, dilaudid, and codeine in the normal human subject, J. Pharmacol. Exp. Ther. **56**:166, 1936.

30 Seevers, M. H., and Woods, L. A.: The phenomena of tolerance, Amer. J. Med. **14**:546, 1953.

31 Strominger, J. L., Kalkar, H. M., Axelrod, J., and Maxwell, E. S.: Enzymatic oxidation of uridine diphosphate glucose to uridine diphosphate glucuronic acid, J. Amer. Chem. Soc. **76**:6411, 1954.

32 Unna, K.: Antagonistic effect of N-allylnormorphine upon morphine, J. Pharmacol. Exp. Ther. **79**:27, 1943.

33 Wang, S. C., and Glaviano, V. V.: Locus of

emetic action of morphine and hydergine in dogs, J. Pharmacol. Exp. Ther. **111**:329, 1954.

34 Wikler, A.: Studies on the action of morphine on the central nervous system of the cat, J. Pharmacol. Exp. Ther. **80**:176, 1944.

35 Wikler, A.: Sites and mechanisms of action of morphine and related drugs in the central nervous system, Pharmacol. Rev. **2**:435, 1950.

36 Winter, C. A., and Flataker, L.: Antitussive compounds: testing methods and results, J. Pharmacol. Exp. Ther. **112**:99, 1954.

37 Wolff, B. B., Kantor, T. G., Jarvik, M. E., and Laska, E.: Response of experimental pain to analgesic drugs. I. Morphine, aspirin and placebo, Clin. Pharmacol. Ther. **7**:224, 1966.

38 Wolff, H. G., Hardy, J. D., and Goodell, H.: Studies on pain: measurement of the effect of morphine, codeine, and other opiates on the pain threshold and an analysis of their relation to the pain experience, J. Clin. Invest. **19**:659, 1940.

Recent reviews

39 Bickerman, H. A.: Clinical pharmacology of antitussive agents, Clin. Pharmacol. Ther. **3**:353, 1962.

40 Cohen, M., Keats, A. S., Krivoy, W., and Ungar, G.: Effect of actinomycin D on morphine tolerance, Proc. Soc. Exp. Biol. Med. **119**:381, 1965.

41 Fraser, H. F., and Harris, L. S.: Narcotic and narcotic antagonist analgesics, Ann. Rev. Pharmacol. **7**:277, 1967.

42 Lasagna, L.: The clinical evaluation of morphine and its substitutes as analgesics, Pharmacol. Rev. **16**:47, 1964.

43 Lewis, J. W., Bentley, K. W., and Cowan, A.: Narcotic analgesics and antagonists, Ann. Rev. Pharmacol. **11**:241, 1971.

44 Murphree, H. B.: Clinical pharmacology of potent analgesics, Clin. Pharmacol. Ther. **3**:473, 1962.

45 Vandam, L. D.: Clinical pharmacology of the narcotic analgesics, Clin. Pharmacol. Ther. **3**:827, 1962.

25 Contemporary drug abuse

Gregory G. Dimijian, M.D.

Contemporary drug abuse encompasses an extraordinary variety of drugs, techniques of administration, and sought-after effects. It is not only the layman who feels bewildered by the complexity of the "drug scene"; many physicians feel unequipped to help the drug user. Much remains unknown of the risk inherent in the various patterns of drug abuse, and on what is known, even the "experts" often disagree. The present survey is an attempt to provide, for the medical student and physician, a fundamental orientation to the current modes of drug abuse, with the understanding that many issues are unresolved and new issues are arising daily.

The term *abuse* implies that a particular application of a drug is more destructive than constructive for society or the individual. Needless to say, it is sometimes difficult to decide whether an application is preponderantly destructive or constructive. Are the Inca Indians abusing cocaine when they chew coca leaves for optimal endurance? Is a student abusing dextroamphetamine if he takes it to study all night before an exam? Does social drinking represent abuse of ethyl alcohol? Some observers[77] assert that the connotation of "drug abuse" represents solely a cultural value judgment, a biased accusation; it is nevertheless obvious that some drug usage would be considered abusive from almost any cultural frame of reference. Prolonged dependence on amphetamines in high doses, for example, invariably invokes a progressive organic brain syndrome; it is conceivable that in some cultures self-destruction would not be considered abusive, but this would seem to be stretching the point.

It is important to distinguish between *drug abuse* and *drug dependence;* the two concepts are not synonymous. Drug abuse may exist without drug dependence, drug dependence without drug abuse, or both may coexist. A single administration of a hazardous drug may represent abuse without dependence, whereas the maintenance of a diabetic on insulin represents dependence without abuse. The concept of abuse also depends in part on cultural values, unlike the concept of dependence.

Most abused drugs are drugs with a primary action on the central nervous system. The reason is obvious: the drug user wishes to modify his mental state. Abuse of drugs without primary central nervous system activity is mostly a matter of misuse by medical or paramedical personnel, such as the indiscriminate prescription of penicillin and the "treatment" of obesity with digitalis, thyroid hormone, and diuretics.[43]

Drug dependence has traditionally been conceptualized in terms of a rigid duality: psychologic dependence and physical dependence. This duality probably originates in the ancient distinction between mind and body.[93] The dual concepts are still used today, and are incorporated into the discussions of individual drugs in this chapter. If a physiologically disruptive withdrawal illness follows the abrupt discontinuation of a drug taken over a prolonged period of time, the drug is said to be physically addicting. Physically addicting drugs include the opiates, barbiturates, antianxiety agents,

299

ethanol, and some nonbarbiturate sedatives. Psychologic drug dependence, on the other hand, has been described as a craving for a drug producing a desired effect and to which one has become accustomed by habit; the habit has become a crutch and may assume enormous importance to the individual. It is said that psychologic dependence, not physical dependence, drives an opiate addict back to his drug after months or years of successful abstinence.

Bridging the gap between psychologic and physical dependence would now seem feasible. Studies of central neurotransmitter action have led to the theory of noradrenergic reward, in which pleasurable drug effects appear to occur in association with potentiation of catecholamine action at central synapses, although the mechanism of potentiation may differ with different drugs. If the theory is correct, it partially bridges the gap between psychologic and physical dependence in that psychologic dependence on a drug occurs in association with a physicochemical change at central synapses.[93] The gap is not fully bridged by this theory, however, as psychologic dependence also embodies the concept of dependence on established habit patterns; thus one may become dependent on a drug or on any oft-repeated behavior, such as eating a hearty breakfast each morning.

The concept of intrinsic activity of drugs, considered in Chapter 2, is helpful in understanding adverse drug effects. Although it is true in some cases that a drug of low potency will produce the same effect in very high doses as another more potent drug of the same type, this is not always the case. Some drugs have a higher intrinsic activity than others and produce effects of a magnitude that cannot be achieved by the weaker drug at any dose. It is doubtful, for example, that mescaline or psilocybin at any dose could produce the psychotomimetic effect of a substantial dose of LSD.

The major categories of commonly abused drugs will be considered separately.

OPIATES AND OPIATE-LIKE DRUGS

In some state statutes the legal category "narcotics" embraces the opiates, opiate-like drugs, marihuana, and cocaine. Medically defined, however, the term *narcotic* refers only to drugs having both a sedative and an analgesic action and is essentially restricted to the opiates and opiate-like drugs. These drugs are classified on p. 284.

Physical dependence and tolerance

Marked physical dependence develops rapidly during continued administration of any of the narcotic drugs. A striking tolerance also develops to all but the miotic action; the addict continues to have constricted pupils, even after low doses. A high degree of cross-tolerance exists among all the opiates and opiate-like drugs in spite of chemical dissimilarities.

Characteristics of abuse

Of all the narcotic drugs, heroin is generally the one most preferred by the drug user because of its slightly greater euphorogenic properties. In regions of the United States where good-quality heroin is hard to obtain, however, the addict may prefer "drugstore dope" (usually morphine or hydromorphone stolen from drugstores). Until recently narcotic addiction in this country has been mostly confined to the lower socio-

Table 25-1. Comparison of commonly abused centrally acting drugs

Drug category	Physical dependence*	Tolerance	Psychotogenic in high doses
Opiates	X	X	
Marihuana			X
Ethanol	X	X	
Barbiturates	X	X	
Amphetamines		X	X
Cocaine			X
Psychotomimetics		X	X
Phenothiazines			
Antianxiety agents	X		
Inhalants†		?	X

*An abstinence syndrome results from abrupt discontinuation of any drug producing physical dependence.
†See text for details.

economic classes of the larger cities and to members of the medical profession; it is now spreading alarmingly into the ranks of the newer drug "subculture."

The veteran heroin addict seeks two principal desired effects from his drug: avoidance of the withdrawal illness and a feeling described most commonly as "relief." These effects are usually more important to the addict than the transitory "kick" or "rush" felt immediately after intravenous injection. The opiates tend to leave the user in a state of drive satiation; everything is "as it should be." Accordingly, sexual drive is usually diminished.

There is no evidence that the opiates produce organic central nervous system damage or other organ pathology, even after years of continuous use. An 84-year-old physician morphine addict was found to exhibit no evidence of mental or physical deterioration after continuous use for 62 years.[14,36] Complications of parenteral administration, however, are legion and include viral hepatitis, bacterial and fungal endocarditis, systemic and pulmonary mycoses, lung abscess, pulmonary fibrosis or granulomatosis, pneumonia, chronic liver disease (of obscure type), transverse myelitis, osteomyelitis (frequently pseudomonas), acute and chronic polyneuropathy, acute and chronic myopathy, acute rhabdomyolysis with myoglobinuria, tetanus, malaria (now rare in the United States), thrombophlebitis, cellulitis, local abscesses, and sclerosis and occlusion of veins.[60,107,117,135] In addition, there is a constant risk of overdose and death from an unexpectedly concentrated sample of heroin; the triad of coma (or stupor), respiratory depression, and pinpoint pupils strongly suggests opiate overdose. Death from overdose may be a result of respiratory depression or acute pulmonary edema[138] or both; the mechanism of production of pulmonary edema is obscure. Still another ever-present hazard is the masking of pain, which may delay awareness of a serious medical condition; cigarette burns between the fingers of opiate addicts are a common finding.

Additional dangers arise from foreign substances intentionally added to the sample by the supplier. Heroin is commonly "cut" with lactose or quinine; other adulterants include barbiturates, procaine, mannitol, aminopyrine, methapyrilene, and baking soda.[60]

301

Social consequences of narcotic addiction include crime, interruption of employment, and personal and family neglect. Criminal activity is usually restricted to property offenses and peddling, which may become necessary in the absence of employment in order to support the habit. Some addicts become functionally disabled, spending much of the 24-hour period "nodding" (remaining inactive in a semistuporous state) or suffering withdrawal symptoms; other addicts who have an uninterrupted drug supply and are careful with dosage may lead a seemingly normal life at work and at home. The concept of the opiate addict as a dangerous "dope fiend" is not justified; in contrast to alcohol, the opiates tend to quell aggressive drives. When an addict's supply of drugs is exhausted, however, he may resort to violence to obtain a continuing supply. Another incentive for assaultive behavior may be fear of police detection. A fellow addict suspected of collaborating with the police may be silenced permanently by an overdose of drug, either arranged through a supplier who provides an unusually concentrated sample of heroin to the victim or accomplished more directly by assault and enforced injection. The apparent cause of death in either case is accidental overdose.

Abstinence syndromes

Morphine or heroin. Symptoms first appear about 8 hours after the last dose, reaching peak intensity between 36 and 72 hours. Lacrimation, rhinorrhea, yawning, and diaphoresis appear between 8 and 12 hours. Shortly thereafter, at about 13 hours, a restless sleep (the "yen") may intervene. At about 20 hours, gooseflesh, dilated pupils, agitation, and tremors may appear. During the second and third day, when the illness is at its peak, symptoms and signs include weakness, insomnia, chills, intestinal cramps, nausea, vomiting, diarrhea, violent yawning, muscle aches in the legs, severe low back pain, elevation of blood pressure and pulse rate, diaphoresis, and waves of gooseflesh. The skin may have the appearance of a cold plucked turkey, hence the expression "cold turkey," denoting abrupt withdrawal. Fluid depletion during the withdrawal period has at times resulted in cardiovascular collapse and death. At any point during the course of withdrawal, administration of an opiate in adequate dosage will dramatically eliminate the symptoms and restore a state of apparent normalcy. The duration of the syndrome is roughly 7 to 10 days.

Other narcotic drugs. Most narcotic abstinence syndromes are similar to that of morphine or heroin. Narcotics with a shorter duration of action tend to produce a shorter and more severe abstinence syndrome; those with a longer duration of action or slower rate of elimination, such as methadone, usually produce a milder and more prolonged syndrome.

Withdrawal by methadone substitution

Withdrawal from an opiate may be accomplished simply by administering smaller and smaller doses of the same opiate over a period of days. A method preferred by many treatment centers, however, involves immediate discontinuation of the opiate and substitution of methadone in equivalent dosage; the methadone is then tapered slowly in the same manner. This method appears to have several advantages. Methadone, a synthetic opiate-like drug, substitutes well for most other opiates and is well absorbed from the gastrointestinal tract, unlike morphine or heroin; parenteral administration is thereby avoided during the withdrawal period, and the addict is weaned from the needle at an earlier time. In addition, methadone has a longer duration of action than other opiates, permitting administration only once or twice in a 24-hour period. Finally, the total period of drug administration is shortened, as methadone remains in the body for 36 to 72 hours after the last dose.

Methadone maintenance

In 1964 Dole and Nyswander introduced a method of treatment in which the ambulatory addict is maintained on oral methadone for an indefinite period of time. A single daily maintenance dose of 80 to 120 mg. is common. Addicts on this regimen no longer have a craving for heroin and no longer derive euphoria from a "fix." This method of treatment is currently being evaluated on a wide scale.[66,99] Opponents of the method argue that the long-term substitution of one opiate for another is not "treatment" and is medically unethical.[4,5] The appeal of methadone maintenance derives from the relative ineffectiveness of other large-scale treatment approaches to the narcotic addict and from the substitution of a legitimate, orally administered drug for a parenterally administered black-market drug.

A synthetic congener of methadone, l-α-acetylmethadol hydrochloride (l-methadyl acetate), can prevent withdrawal symptoms for more than 72 hours. Because of this relative advantage, acetylmethadol is currently being evaluated as a substitute for methadone.[110,111]

Narcotic antagonists

An intensive search is now under way for the "ideal" narcotic antagonist, namely, a pharmacologic agent that blocks the effects of opiates, has few or no "side effects" of its own, requires relatively infrequent administration, and is not prohibitively expensive to produce. No drug has yet met these criteria, but some have come close. Naloxone, for example, abolishes the euphoria, respiratory depression, nausea, and gastrointestinal disturbances produced by opiates, and produces virtually no side effects, it is expensive, however, and its limited duration of action requires more than one dose per day for the treatment or prevention of addiction.[145] A number of new agents are being tested.[121]

The earliest known narcotic antagonists were nalorphine (Nalline) and levallorphan (Lorfan). Administration of a narcotic antagonist precipitates a telltale abstinence syndrome if physical dependence on an opiate has become established. The use of antagonists is not without hazard, however. A severe abstinence syndrome may be precipitated that cannot be suppressed during the period of action of the antagonist, and the antagonist itself, except for naloxone, may further embarrass respiration that has been compromised by alcohol, barbiturates, or other nonnarcotic depressants.

ETHYL ALCOHOL

It is often forgotten that alcoholism is still the most serious form of drug abuse in western society. It is estimated that over 9 million Americans are alcoholics, and that over 50% of crimes and over 50% of highway accidents in the United States are alcohol-related.

Physical dependence and tolerance

A marked degree of physical dependence and a moderate degree of tolerance develop to ethanol when ingested regularly and in large amounts. Tolerance may be explained in part by induced hypertrophy of hepatic smooth endoplasmic reticulum with stimulation of ethanol metabolism.[136]

Characteristics of abuse

Ethyl alcohol is a primary and continuous depressant of the central nervous system. Even a small amount decreases mental acuity and impairs motor coordination; at times, however, this deficit may be more than compensated for by the improved performance accompanying the induced state of euphoria and release from inhibitory attitudes.

In chronic alcoholism one may observe organ pathology and clinical syndromes not usually associated with other types of drug abuse, including fatty metamorphosis and cirrhosis of the liver, peripheral polyneuropathy, alcoholic gastritis, Korsakoff's psychosis, Wernicke's encephalopathy, and the complications of portal hypertension. Some of these changes are thought to be the result of nutritional deficiency rather than the direct action of ethanol; unlike other commonly abused drugs, ethanol supplies calories, depressing the appetite and encouraging a dietary deficit in the face of a deceptive maintenance of body weight. It is believed that ethanol is directly incriminated, however, in the pathogenesis of alcoholic fatty liver.[118]

Chronic ethanol consumption leads to hypertrophy of hepatic smooth endoplasmic reticulum, with consequent stimulation of drug metabolism. This finding may explain in part the tolerance of alcoholics, *when sober,* to drugs such as barbiturates. *When inebriated,* alcoholics display a *heightened* sensitivity to barbiturates, not only because of the synergistic action of the two drugs but perhaps also because hepatic metabolism of other drugs is temporarily slowed during the active metabolism of ethanol.[136]

In the history of many opiate addicts there occurs a turning from alcohol to opiates. The addict recalls that he was frequently "getting into fights" while under the influence of alcohol, and that such poorly controlled behavior diminished or disappeared entirely "behind heroin."

Abstinence syndrome

After prolonged, heavy intake of alcohol, withdrawal symptoms may appear within a few hours after the last dose; these include tremulousness, weakness, anxiety, intestinal cramps, and hyperreflexia. Between 12 and 24 hours the stage of "acute alcoholic hallucinosis" may appear, in which visual hallucinations are reported, at first only with the eyes closed. By 48 hours an acute brain syndrome may become apparent, with confusion, disorientation, and delusional thinking. When this syndrome is accompanied by gross tremulousness, it is called "delirium tremens." Major convulsive seizures ("rum fits") may occur but are less common than in barbiturate withdrawal. The chronic alcoholic may be in too poor a condition to withstand the stress of withdrawal; if death is not the price, recovery occurs by the fifth to the seventh day.

MARIHUANA

Slang equivalents: grass, weed, pot, dope, hemp; marihuana cigarette = joint, "j," number, reefer, root; cigarette butt = roach, snipe

Although marihuana is not medically a narcotic, it is classified legally as a narcotic in some states for purposes of control. It is inadequately described by any one drug category, since it possesses properties of a sedative, euphoriant, and hallucinogen.

The source of marihuana is the Indian hemp plant *Cannabis sativa,* an herbaceous annual growing wild in temperate climates all over the world. The plant is dioecious; that is, male and female flowers are borne on separate plants. The active compounds are most concentrated in the resinous exudate of the female flower clusters.

In the United States the term *marihuana* refers to any part or extract of the plant. The smoking mixture termed "bhang" consists only of the cut tops of uncultivated female plants. The most concentrated natural supply of cannabinols is found in the preparations called "hashish" and "charas," which consist largely of the actual resin from the flower clusters of cultivated female plants. The potency of any marihuana preparation varies with the plant strain and the growth conditions.

The principal psychoactive compound in marihuana appears to be *l*-Δ^9-trans-tetrahydrocannabinol (hereafter referred to as Δ^9THC; Δ^1THC and Δ^9THC represent different systems of nomenclature for the same compound). A varying, usually small, amount of $\Delta^{8(9)}$THC may also be present.[116, 123, 124]

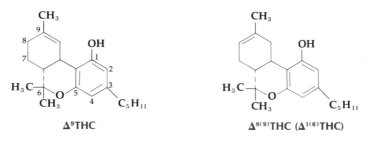

Δ^9THC $\Delta^{8(9)}$THC ($\Delta^{1(6)}$THC)

Physical dependence and tolerance

Neither physical dependence nor tolerance is known to develop. In one study,[100] tolerance failed to develop to THC administered to chimpanzees for 63 consecutive days. Two studies have failed to demonstrate cross-tolerance between Δ^9THC and LSD in man[39] or between Δ^9THC and mescaline in rats.[137] On the other hand, one study has demonstrated a dose-related cross-tolerance between Δ^9THC and ethanol,[130] and the cross-tolerance is symmetrical (i.e., either drug induces cross-tolerance to the other).

Characteristics of intoxication

Anecdotal reports. Most users report that marihuana induces a dreamy, euphoric state of altered consciousness, with feelings of detachment, gaiety, and jocularity and preoccupation with simple and familiar things. Cognitive abilities are said to remain keen unless drowsiness and sleep intervene, as may occur if the smoker is alone. In the company of others there is a tendency toward laughter and loquaciousness. Perceptual distortion of space and time is regularly reported; distances may be judged inaccurately, and things may seem to be happening very slowly or very rapidly.

Dissociative phenomena such as partial amnesia or a feeling of being outside of oneself looking on are frequently reported. Libido is variably affected; since sexual desire may be enhanced, marihuana has gained a reputation as an aphrodisiac. There may be an unusually vivid remembrance or reliving of experiences or mood states of the past. The continuity of a story or movie may be lost, to be replaced by an intense experiencing of individual segments or scenes. Users are sometimes recognized by the characteristic hilarity of their mutual laughter, which may become prolonged and uncontrolled. Appetite and appreciation of the flavor of food are usually enhanced, and weight gain may accompany regular smoking.

A paranoid state is sometimes reported, in which the smoker is keenly sensitive of others watching him; some forsake marihuana for this reason. Antisocial behavior under the influence of marihuana appears to be rare; the user ordinarily withdraws from company that he finds unpleasant.

Adverse reactions to unadulterated preparations of marihuana are relatively rare, but they may be serious when they do occur. Such reactions include acute paranoid states, dissociative states, and less commonly, acute psychotic reactions. Adverse reactions to marihuana appear to be dose-related (they are more frequent with hashish) and highly individualized (some users regularly have adverse reactions and some never do). The evaluation of reports of adverse reactions is complicated by the fact that marihuana is frequently adulterated with other drugs; some reports have failed to take this possibility into consideration.[49, 69]

Regular use of marihuana may result in a pervasive feeling of apathy, the so-called "amotivational syndrome." The user discovers that "things just don't seem important to me any more." This development may be especially damaging to the psychologic maturation of the adolescent. Such a syndrome is undoubtedly multi-determined, but in many adolescents undergoing psychotherapy, its development has been observed to coincide temporally with regular use of marihuana.

Clinical studies. An early study by Isbell and co-workers[38] demonstrated that Δ^9THC produces effects similar to those of crude marihuana preparations, and that the psychotomimetic effects are dose-related. Isbell subsequently compared the effects of Δ^9THC and LSD and showed that (1) pupillodilatation and hyperreflexia occurred with LSD but not with THC; (2) heart rate was increased markedly by THC; (3) conjunctival injection and pseudoptosis were produced by THC but not LSD; (4) differences in the subjective states induced by the two drugs were difficult to determine; and (5) no cross-tolerance between the two drugs could be demonstrated.[39]

Hollister[106] has found that perceptual and psychologic changes in man to measured doses of synthetic THC include euphoria, sleepiness (deep sleep followed higher doses), alteration in time sense, visual perceptual distortion, depersonalization, difficulty in concentrating, dreamlike states, and decreased aggressiveness with increasing dose. Psychometric tests demonstrated reduced accuracy in some cases and slowing of performance in other cases to a mild degree. Physiologic effects were limited to regular and constant increase in pulse rate, no change or slight decrease in blood pressure, two instances of orthostatic hypotension, regular conjunctival injection (no smoke was present), and muscle weakness (measured in the fingers). For comparison, the synthetic THC homolog, synhexyl, was also administered orally to human subjects; effects were similar to Δ^9THC, but synhexyl was approximately one third as potent.

Marihuana smoking was shown to produce an increase in pulse rate and limb blood flow with a slight rise in both systolic and diastolic pressure.[90] The fact that an increase in limb flow was unaccompanied by a fall in systemic pressure suggests that circulatory adjustments occur in other vascular beds. Propranolol, a beta adrenergic blocker, prevented both the tachycardia and the increased limb flow; atropine increased the pulse rate but not limb flow. Cooling the hand with ice failed to evoke the normal reduction in blood flow to the hand. It is apparent from this study that marihuana smoking may impair vascular reflex responses and render the individual more vulnerable both to blood loss in the event of peripheral injury and to hypotension in the event of blood loss. The risk of aggravating or prolonging marihuana-induced tachycardia by administration of atropine is also revealed by the study.

The question of partial pyrolytic inactivation of THC in the burning cigarette was investigated by Mikes and Waser,[127] who found that smoke from a cigarette impregnated with Δ^9THC and cannabidiol contained 21 to 23% of the starting amount, with apparent partial cyclization of the cannabidiol to THC. No new pyrolyzed products were found.

A study of marihuana-induced temporal disintegration was conducted at the Stanford University School of Medicine,[125,126] using doses of 20, 40, and 60 mg. of THC (the higher two doses were admittedly larger than the dose to be expected from ordinary social smoking). All three doses significantly impaired serial operations in performing a task requiring sequential cognitive functions. Progressively more errors were made with increasing dose. The subjects reported a feeling of timelessness and uncertainty of how much time had elapsed; the time line extending from past to future seemed discontinuous, and past and future seemed unrelated to the present. One subject stated, ". . . I can't stay on the same subject. . . . I can't remember what I just said or what I want to say . . . because there are just so many thoughts that are broken in time, one chunk there and one chunk here." Impairment of immediate memory with emergence of loose associations was noted, and the latter was considered to have its probable origin in the former. The serious implications of such an effect over a prolonged period of time are clear.

Apparent overestimation of the passage of time was also reported in chimpanzees to whom Δ^9THC was administered by the oral route.[94] Temporally spaced responses of the chimps came to be made closer and closer together as the dose of THC was increased, suggesting that the chimps perceived shorter and shorter intervals of time as being of the original familiar duration.

A study of driving skills and marihuana[13] suggests that marihuana may have little effect on driving safety. The question remains unanswered, however, of how the subjects might have performed behind the wheel had they not been taking a test.

A report of 31 American soldiers who were heavy hashish smokers suggests that respiratory tract irritation may be a prominent feature of hashish smoking.[143] Bronchitis, asthma, rhinopharyngitis, and sinusitis were common findings, with a mild obstructive pulmonary dysfunction in five who underwent pulmonary function studies. It was noted that the uvula becomes swollen and edematous while hashish is smoked and remains so for 12 to 24 hours afterward.

A three-year study of 720 hashish smokers in an American Army population[142] revealed a marked difference in the effects of light vs. heavy hashish smoking. Occasional smoking in small, intermittent doses caused only minor respiratory ailments with no adverse mental effects. Heavier smoking, several times a day, resulted in a chronic intoxicated state with frequent acute adverse effects, such as disorientation, panic reaction, or acute psychotic reaction. Many chronic users became psychotic for long periods of time and were unresponsive to treatment with antipsychotic agents. Symptoms of chronic intoxication were similar to those of long-term dependence on depressant-hypnotic drugs, and included apathy, dullness, and lethargy with mild to severe impairment of judgment, concentration, and memory. The heavy user, dubbed a "hashaholic" in Army jargon, appeared dull and maintained poor hygiene. He rarely resorted to violence or overt criminal behavior. His consumption of hashish reached 500 to 600 Gm. per month, the equivalent of several thousand American marihuana cigarettes. The frequent practice of abusing ethanol and hashish simultaneously was reported to greatly increase the likelihood of adverse reaction and long-term morbidity.

A study of the acute pulmonary physiologic effects of marihuana in healthy young men suggests that both smoked marihuana and orally administered Δ^9THC produce significant bronchodilatation of relatively long duration (6 hours for the 20 mg. dose).[138a]

Administered to rats, [^{14}C]Δ^9THC was shown to accumulate in tenfold greater concentrations in fat than in other tissues[112]; 11-hydroxy THC, an active metabolite of Δ^9THC, showed a similar distribution, with highest concentration in body fat. The importance of fat localization of drugs in prolonging pharmacologic activity is well known; it is conceivable that slow release from fat stores may help explain the phenomenon of "reverse tolerance," in which regular users of marihuana achieve a "high" more quickly and easily than sporadic users.

The psychologic effects, disposition, and excretion of [^{14}C]Δ^9THC in man were compared in a recent study.[115] High plasma levels of unchanged [^{14}C]Δ^9THC were rapidly achieved after intravenous administration and inhalation, whereas after oral administration plasma levels remained low, requiring several hours to peak. It was found that 90 to 95% of an oral dose of THC is absorbed from the gastrointestinal tract; the low plasma levels are explained by the slower absorption. Psychologic effects were maximal in all subjects at the times of maximal plasma levels of metabolites, lending support to the growing suspicion that a metabolite of Δ^9THC is indeed the active compound responsible for the psychologic effects of marihuana.

Further evidence in support of this belief was provided by a study in which 11-hydroxy-Δ^9THC was administered intravenously to man.[113] The metabolite produced tachycardia and a "high" that was difficult to evaluate but was somewhat comparable to a marihuana "high." The disposition and metabolism of 11-hydroxy-Δ^9THC were similar to the disposition and metabolism of THC, as indicated by rate of disappearance from plasma, rate of excretion, and metabolic profile in urine and feces.

Further considerations

Marihuana is sometimes said to "lead to other drugs." Many drug users experiment first with marihuana, and in this sense marihuana may serve as a "stepping stone" to the more potent agents. Most drug users feel strongly, however, that they would have eventually tried other drugs whether or not they had first smoked marihuana.

Marihuana is often compared to alcohol. Unlike alcohol, marihuana is not known to be physically addicting and tolerance does not develop to the effects of ordinary marihuana preparations. When inebriated, the alcoholic usually suffers a greater temporary loss of judgment and control than the marihuana user, whose "highs" are usually characterized by mild alterations in perception and mood without marked loss of behavioral control. Hostility and aggression are commonly released by alcohol but rarely by marihuana. The appetite is stimulated by marihuana, whereas calories are provided by alcohol; nutritional deficiency commonly complicates the syndrome of chronic alcoholism. The hangover of the alcoholic is unknown to the "pothead," who awakens the next morning feeling refreshed. Psychologic dependence on either drug may develop, and both drugs may impair the physical performance essential to safe automobile driving. Acute paranoid states, dissociative reactions, and near-psychotic reactions are occasionally seen with marihuana use; moderate drinking rarely if ever induces such reactions. There is strong suggestive evidence that chronic marihuana use interferes with motivational and goal-directed thinking; chronic alcoholism may do the same and ultimately result in brain damage and general physical deterioration.

In summary, in the light of our present incomplete knowledge, the principal medical risks in the use of marihuana appear to be (1) the occasional adverse reaction, relatively uncommon with the milder preparations but far more likely with hashish or THC; (2) alteration of time and space perception, with loosening of associations and impairment of driving skills; (3) loss of motivation and drive, associated with regular and frequent use; and (4) probable impairment of vascular reflex responses.

BARBITURATES

Slang equivalents:
Barbiturates in general = goofballs, fool pills
Short-acting: secobarbital (Seconal) = red birds, red devils, reds; pentobarbital (Nembutal) = yellow jackets
Intermediate-acting: amobarbital (Amytal) = blue heavens
Long-acting: phenobarbital (Luminal) = purple hearts
Combinations: secobarbital + amobarbital (Tuinal) = tooies, Christmas trees, rainbows

Physical dependence and tolerance

A marked degree of both physical dependence and tolerance develops to all the barbiturates. There is a sharp upper border to the tolerance, so that a slight increase in dosage may precipitate toxic symptoms.

Characteristics of abuse

The effects of ordinary doses of barbiturates include sedation (without analgesia), decreased mental acuity, slowed speech, and emotional lability. Toxic symptoms resulting from overdose include ataxia, diplopia, nystagmus, difficulty in accommodation, vertigo, and a positive Romberg sign. There is risk of overdose as a result of the delayed onset of action of the longer-acting barbiturates and also as a result of perceptual time distortion, which induces the user to ingest more than he intended in a short period of time. Death from overdose, as with the opiates, results from respiratory depression; the respiratory depression of barbiturate overdose, however, is not antagonized by nalorphine or levallorphan.

In contrast to opiate addiction, the direct harm to the individual and society stems more from the toxic effects of the drug than from the difficulty of maintaining a continuing supply.

Abstinence syndrome

The barbiturate abstinence syndrome is one of the most dangerous drug withdrawal syndromes. Symptoms progress from weakness, restlessness, tremulousness, and insomnia to abdominal cramps, nausea, vomiting, hyperthermia, blepharoclonus (clonic blink reflex), orthostatic hypotension, confusion, disorientation, and eventually major convulsive seizures. The syndrome is sometimes mistaken for the "delirium tremens" of alcohol withdrawal. The seizures may become prolonged, as in status epilepticus. Agitation and hyperthermia may lead to exhaustion and cardiovascular collapse. With the short-acting barbiturates, convulsions are most likely to appear during the second or third day of abstinence; with the longer-acting barbiturates, convulsions are less likely to occur and usually appear between the third and the eighth day.

The barbiturate type of abstinence syndrome is occasionally observed in an addict being withdrawn from heroin who insists that he has used no other drug. In such cases one should suspect that the lot of heroin last used by the patient had been "cut" (diluted) with barbiturates, a practice that is known to exist. A barbiturate withdrawal regimen is then instituted immediately.

Withdrawal from barbiturates

Hospitalization is advisable for the duration of the withdrawal period. Instead of accepting the addict's word for the level of barbiturate to which he has become addicted, an objective test is made to determine the level of tolerance to barbiturates.[97] An ordinary therapeutic dose of pentobarbital is administered, and the patient is observed for clinical signs of drug effect. If the sedative action of the drug is not soon apparent, it is concluded that the patient's level of tolerance is higher and that he has become accustomed to higher individual doses. Additional increments of pentobarbital are administered until drug effect is evident; at this point the total dose of drug administered is considered the base line from which subsequent doses are tapered over the ensuing 7 to 14 days. The long withdrawal period is advisable to minimize the likelihood of convulsions.

NONBARBITURATE SEDATIVES

Glutethimide (Doriden). Marked physical dependence develops, resulting in a severe abstinence syndrome characterized by nausea, vomiting, abdominal cramps, tachycardia, pyrexia, hyperesthesia, dysphagia, and major convulsive seizures.[45,58]

Methaqualone (Quaalude; Sopor; Parest). Nicknamed "quaas" and "sopors," methaqualone has become a popular "downer" with the young. Overdose, in contrast to barbiturate overdose, may result in restlessness, hypertonia, and convulsive seizures. Pulmonary edema has been reported with large overdoses. Death may occur from respiratory arrest, pulmonary edema, or other causes. It appears that physical dependence may develop after prolonged use in high doses.

Chloral hydrate (Noctec; Somnos). Moderate physical dependence develops, as manifest by the occurrence of a "chloral delirium" upon abrupt withdrawal, characterized by agitation, confusion, disorientation, and hallucinations.[73] Slight to moderate tolerance develops; a "break in tolerance" may result from abrupt impairment of the mechanism of hepatic detoxification, with resulting overdose and death.[31]

Methyprylon (Noludar). Abrupt withdrawal has resulted in confusion, agitation, hallucinations, and generalized convulsions.[7,44]

Paraldehyde. Moderate physical dependence develops, as evidenced by withdrawal symptoms that include tremulousness, visual and auditory hallucinations, and a state of agitation and disorientation similar to delirium tremens.[31]

Bromides. Physical dependence has not been demonstrated.[31] In low doses, bromides act as sedatives; in toxic doses, they produce a so-called bromide psychosis characterized by confusion, disorientation, vivid hallucinations, and eventually coma. The slow elimination of bromide from the body may lead to chronic accumulation when it is administered over a period of time, with the subtle onset of the toxic syndrome.

AMPHETAMINES

Slang equivalents:

Dextroamphetamine (Dexedrine) = dexies, co-pilots, oranges
Amphetamine (Benzedrine) = bennies, splash, peaches
Methamphetamine (Methedrine; Desoxyn) = meth, speed, crystal, crank, white cross (tablets)
Dextroamphetamine + amphetamine (Diphetamine; Biphetamine) = footballs

Proprietary combinations with other drugs:

Daprisal = dextroamphetamine + amobarbital + aspirin + phenacetin
Desbutal = methamphetamine + pentobarbital
Dexamyl = dextroamphetamine + amobarbital
Esidral = amphetamine + aspirin + phenacetin
Eskatrol = dextroamphetamine + prochlorperazine (Compazine)
Obedrin-LA = methamphetamine + pentobarbital + vitamins

Physical dependence and tolerance

It appears that little if any physical dependence develops to the amphetamines. A change in sleep pattern upon abrupt withdrawal has been reported in association with minimal EEG changes,[67] but there is no physiologically disruptive abstinence syndrome. Abrupt withdrawal is physiologically safe and is characterized by the onset of lethargy, somnolence, and often a precipitous depressive reaction; the possibility of suicide should be kept in mind. Some consider the period of lethargy and somnolence an abstinence syndrome in itself.[53]

Proprietary formulas combining an amphetamine with another drug are often used out of expediency or preference. Withdrawal is complicated, of course, by the other drug, which may be a barbiturate.

Tolerance to amphetamines develops slowly and becomes marked. At any level of tolerance the margin between euphoria and toxic psychosis remains narrow.

Characteristics of abuse

The amphetamines are direct central nervous system stimulants and in ordinary therapeutic doses produce the following effects: euphoria, with increased sense of well-being; heightened mental acuity, until fatigue sets in from lack of sleep; nervousness, with insomnia; and anorexia. Amphetamines are useful in circumstances demanding optimal endurance and mental acuity; they have been prescribed for airmen in the military and for astronauts during difficult maneuvers. They are commonly abused by students, housewives, truck drivers, and all-night workers who self-administer the drugs for extended periods of time. Liberal dispensing by physicians of amphetamines for dietary management has contributed significantly to the abuse of these agents. Perhaps the most serious current form of abuse is the "mainlining" of methamphetamine.

Undesirable and potentially hazardous effects accompany the prolonged use of amphetamines. As many a student has learned the hard way, fatigue eventually sets in and blocks coherent thought at inopportune times, such as during an examination. In addition, brief lapses of alertness, with sudden drooping of the head ("nodding"), may occur without warning as fatigue "breaks though"; this phenomenon, like the seizure of the epileptic, may result in a catastrophic loss of control in dangerous circumstances.

High doses of amphetamines reduce mental acuity and impair performance of complex acts, even in the absence of fatigue. Behavior may become irrational. A peculiar phenomenon observed among amphetamine users is a condition described as being "hung up." The user may get stuck in a repetitious behavioral sequence, repeating an act ritually for hours; the perseverative behavior may become progressively more irrational.

The "amphetamine psychosis" [6] may develop during long-term or short-term abuse of amphetamines and is characterized by visual and auditory hallucinations and paranoid delusions in the setting of a clear sensorium and full orientation. The psychosis clears within a few days after the drug is discontinued.

In a recent study, [105] the psychosis was compared to a severe paranoid state that closely resembled paranoid schizophrenia, with fixed, systematized delusions that were aggravated by attempts at intervention.

The expressions "meth is death" and "speed kills" reflect the belief, widespread among drug users, that brain damage may result from administration of methamphetamine in large doses. In most cases a prolonged acute brain syndrome follows withdrawal.

Tolerance develops to such a degree that the habitual user may come to inject several hundred milligrams of an amphetamine every few hours. A total 24-hour dose of methamphetamine estimated at over 10 Gm. has been reported. [53] Some users report that the subjective effects of intravenous amphetamines are similar to the effects of intravenous cocaine except for the longer duration of action of the amphetamines.

Physiologic effects of high doses of amphetamines include mydriasis, elevation of blood pressure, and hyperreflexia. Hypertensive crisis with intracerebral hemorrhage has been reported following oral and intravenous administration of methamphetamine. [48, 103]

Other sympathomimetic agents that are chemically related to the amphetamines and commonly abused include ephedrine, phenmetrazine (Preludin), mephentermine (Wyamine and Dristan inhalers), and methylphenidate (Ritalin). These drugs all produce central stimulation much like the amphetamines, but generally less marked. As with the amphetamines, physical dependence is not known to develop.

COCAINE

Slang equivalents: coke, snow, candy, girl, Charlie, big C

Legally classified with the narcotic drugs, cocaine is not medically a narcotic, but a topical anesthetic and powerful central nervous system stimulant. It occurs naturally in the leaves of the coca plant *Erythroxylon coca* and in other species of *Erythroxylon*, which are indigenous to Peru and Bolivia. The leaves have been chewed by the Inca

Indians for centuries to increase endurance and make possible arduous ascents into the Andes while carrying heavy loads.

Physical dependence and tolerance

Neither physical dependence nor tolerance is known to develop to the prolonged use of cocaine. It is possible that heightened responsiveness actually develops in some cases.[40]

Characteristics of abuse

Euphoric excitement, often of orgastic proportions, is rapidly produced even when cocaine is sniffed nasally ("snorted" or "horned"). Grandiose feelings of great mental and physical prowess may cause the user to overestimate his capabilities. Strong sexual desire is often aroused, and the drug is sometimes used expressly for this effect. After intravenous injection, spontaneous ejaculation in the absence of genital stimulation has been reported; some users joke about letting the drug "replace" a sexual partner (as suggested by the slang names "girl" and "Charlie").

The effect of each injection is fleeting, and to recapture it the user injects repeated doses at 5- to 15-minute intervals, often leaving the needle in place. Users have been known to lock themselves in a room and enjoy 3 days and nights of uninterrupted cocaine euphoria, sharing a large supply of cocaine until it is exhausted.

If dosage is not watched carefully, signs of toxicity may appear, such as rapid heart rate with palpitations, hallucinations (visual, auditory, and tactile), and paranoid delusions. At times delusions have been so compelling that the user has assaulted an innocent party without provocation. When the user perceives that he has exceeded a safe dose, he often chooses to "come down" comfortably by injecting an opiate and delaying his next dose of cocaine.

A complication that is not uncommon among cocaine sniffers is perforation of the nasal septum, occurring as a result of ischemic necrosis in the wake of the intense and prolonged vasoconstriction induced by the drug.

In spite of its vasoconstrictor action, cocaine is absorbed topically from mucous membranes. A common topical application is to the glans penis and vaginal mucosa; some users report that this enhances the pleasure of sexual relations and promotes a prolonged erection.

Physiologic disturbances from high doses of cocaine include pyrexia, dilated pupils, tachycardia, irregular respiration, abdominal pain, vomiting, and major convulsive seizures. Central stimulation is followed by depression; the higher centers are the first to become depressed, making this transition while the lower centers are still excited. Death results from medullary paralysis and respiratory failure. Acute poisoning may pursue a rapid course.

TRANQUILIZERS
PHENOTHIAZINES (ANTIPSYCHOTIC DRUGS)

The phenothiazines, sometimes called the "major tranquilizers" because of their potent antipsychotic effect, include chlorpromazine (Thorazine), thioridazine (Mellaril), trifluoperazine (Stelazine), prochlorperazine (Compazine), perphenazine (Trilafon), promazine (Sparine), and others. It is remarkable that no significant physical dependence develops during long-term administration of these drugs in high doses. One author has described a syndrome characterized by anxiety, insomnia, and gastrointestinal disturbances following the abrupt discontinuation of phenothiazines,[9] but, as in the case of amphetamine withdrawal, there is no gross physiologic disturbance. The issue of whether or not to call this an "abstinence syndrome" is largely a matter of semantics.

Moderate tolerance develops to the sedative effects of the phenothiazines; it is not known whether a true tolerance develops to the antipsychotic effects.

ANTIANXIETY DRUGS ("MINOR TRANQUILIZERS")

Drugs in this category, unlike the phenothiazines, characteristically produce a marked physical dependence of the barbiturate type, as evidenced by the common occurrence of major convulsive seizures after abrupt withdrawal. Barbiturates may, in fact, be substituted for any of the following drugs for purposes of controlled withdrawal.

Meprobamate (Equanil; Miltown; Meprospan). Withdrawal symptoms may progress from insomnia, tremors, ataxia, and vomiting to an acute psychotic reaction, major convulsive seizures, coma, and death.[25,79] Seizures occur between 24 and 48 hours after the last dose.

Chlordiazepoxide (Librium). Withdrawal symptoms are reported to progress from agitation and insomnia to major convulsive seizures.[34] Because of slow elimination of the drug, seizures may be delayed as long as a week after the last dose.

Ethchlorvynol (Placidyl). Abrupt withdrawal may result in agitation, hallucinations, and generalized convulsions.[10]

Diazepam (Valium). Major convulsive seizures have been reported during the withdrawal illness.[3,33]

Ethinamate (Valmid). Abrupt withdrawal has resulted in agitation, confusion, hallucinations, and generalized convulsions.[23]

PSYCHOTOMIMETIC (HALLUCINOGENIC, PSYCHOTOGENIC, PSYCHEDELIC, AND DYSLEPTIC) DRUGS

Considered in this category are drugs taken primarily for their psychotomimetic effects. Many other drugs such as the amphetamines and cocaine are also psychotogenic in high doses.

LSD

Slang equivalent: acid; many different local names. The term "mikes" refers to micrograms; "clinical mikes" refers to actual micrograms, "street mikes" to a fictional microgram one third to one fourth as potent.

LSD (LSD-25; D-lysergic acid diethylamide tartrate) was first synthesized from the alkaloids of ergot (*Claviceps purpurea*), a fungus that parasitizes rye and other grains in Europe and North America. The ergot alkaloids, which include ergotamine and ergonovine, are active oxytocics and vasoconstrictors. The chance synthesis of LSD was accomplished in 1938 by a research chemist working for Sandoz, Ltd., who attached a diethylamide radical to lysergic acid, the skeletal structure common to all the ergot alkaloids. The sample was set aside until 1943, when it was first tested by the researcher and found to have strange and potent central effects.

Physical dependence and tolerance

Physical dependence is not known to develop. Tolerance, however, develops rapidly and is lost as rapidly after discontinuance of LSD. The usual initial dose of 200 to 400 μg is often raised to several thousand micrograms after a few days of continuous use. Cross-tolerance between LSD, mescaline, and psilocybin has been shown[96]; it appears that cross-tolerance between LSD and DMT (dimethyltryptamine) and between LSD and Δ^9THC does not develop.[22, 39]

Characteristics of abuse

The nature of the "trip" taken with LSD is not predictable in advance but is influenced to some degree by the state of mind, mood, and expectations at the time the drug is taken. This is also true of one's response to marihuana, which may act as a stimulant, aphrodisiac, or sedative, depending largely on the environment and the state of mind. The usual trip with LSD is characterized by exhilarating feelings of strangeness and newness of experience, vividly colored and changing hallucinations, reveries, "free thinking," and "new insight." Colors become alive and may seem to glow; the space between objects may take on greater subjective importance as a thing in itself; and there is dazed wonderment at the beauty in common things. The introspective experience may be intense and sobering; it has been described as an intellectual earthquake in which conditioned attitudes and feelings are reevaluated and values are reshuffled. To some degree there appears to be a regression to primary process thinking.

Unpleasant experiences with LSD are relatively frequent and may involve an uncontrollable drift into confusion, dissociative reactions, acute panic reactions, a reliving of earlier traumatic experiences, or an acute psychotic reaction. Some of these effects may become prolonged and require psychiatric hospitalization.[59, 72] Prolonged nonpsychotic reactions have included dissociative reactions, time and space distortion, body image changes, and a residue of fear or depression stemming from morbid or terrifying experiences under the drug.

Catastrophic reactions to LSD are better understood when one conceptualizes the disruption by the drug of psychologic defense mechanisms such as repression and denial in an individual precariously defended against confrontation of conflict material. With the failure of the usual defenses, the onslaught of repressed material overwhelms the integrative capacity of the ego, and a psychotic reaction results. It appears that this disruption of long-established patterns of adapting may be a lasting or semipermanent effect of the drug.

It also appears that LSD removes the usual intrinsic restraints on the intensity of affective response. It is well known to LSD users that a specific emotional response, whether it be fear, dread, delight, or sadness, may become rapidly more intense under the influence of the drug until it reaches overwhelming proportions. The user is then virtually in the grip of the reaction; he may indeed derive insight from the introspective experience, as most users report, but he may become so disturbed as to engage in behavior that endangers his own life. Deaths while under the influence of LSD have occurred by drowning, falling from a window,[51] and walking into the path of a car. The meaningless question has been asked, "Was it accident or suicide?" An instance of homicide by a 22-year-old student during an LSD-induced psychotic reaction has been reported[134]; the student, not previously psychotic except for one other experience with LSD, killed a stranger with a knife in response to persecutory delusions. During four years of observation after the episode, the student was not again psychotic.

Disturbing implications are inherent in the finding by many "acid heads" that after twenty-five or fifty trips the frequency of taking LSD may be reduced progressively without sacrificing the desired state of mind. The user may discover that between trips he begins to feel as he did while under the influence of the drug, until he eventually finds himself on a continuous trip with no further ingestion of the drug. He states that his thinking has become different, and he no longer "needs" the drug. Indeed, his changed behavior is apparent to others; with no further drug ingestion, he remains preoccupied with any trivial thing at hand, feels "at one" with all living things, and acts as he often did while under the influence of the drug. The ultimate duration of these changes as well as their significance remains unknown.

Symptoms occurring during an LSD trip may recur unpredictably days, weeks, or months after a single dose. Strangest of drug effects, these "flashback" reactions may occur at intervals following the administration of many drugs with central nervous system activity, but most commonly follow an LSD reaction. Flashback symptoms vary from gentle mood states to severely disruptive changes in thought and feeling and may occur with or without further administration of the drug. The reaction may be initiated voluntarily in some cases. The mechanism remains unknown, but the existence of the phenomenon suggests a residual impairment of psychologic defense mechanisms, with periodic emergence of repressed feelings. Flashback reactions may also be "triggered" by strong affective states or by administration of a drug with central nervous activity.

The physiologic effects of LSD are few and include mydriasis, hyperreflexia, and muscular incoordination.[32] Grand mal seizures have been observed following ingestion of LSD.[29]

It has been demonstrated that injections of LSD in rats decrease the turnover rate of serotonin (5-hydroxytryptamine).[57] Some investigators suggest that this may in part explain the psychotomimetic effects of LSD.

There is no evidence to date that LSD in moderate dosages induces mutation or produces significant chromosome damage in man.[98] In like manner, no evidence of teratogenic effect in man has appeared, although in one small sample of mothers exposed to LSD, an increase in the incidence of spontaneous abortion was found.[122] It must be admitted that the question of reproductive detriment still remains unanswered. Some recent studies suggest a role of LSD in fetal defects, but the studies are complicated by many other etiologic variables.[109]

Because it is water soluble, odorless, colorless, and tasteless and because by weight it is one of the most potent drugs known, LSD is easily administered to the unwary. At a party it will not be detected in the punch until its effects are evident.

LSD is usually taken by mouth. It is occasionally "mainlined,"[65] however, alone or in combination with other drugs. It is also absorbed through the lungs when marihuana, soaked in an LSD solution, is smoked.

It was once believed that a transient "model psychosis" resembling schizophrenia could be experimentally induced with LSD. It was soon recognized, however, that the psychotic reaction from LSD differs substantially from most types of schizophrenic reactions. In schizophrenia one usually finds a disordered thought pattern characterized by subtle or flagrant delusions that are systematized and integrated into the personality structure of the individual. The LSD psychosis, on the contrary, is characterized by a chaotic and unpredictable thought disturbance with little or no organization or integration. It resembles an acute brain syndrome more closely than it does most types of schizophrenic reaction, although it differs somewhat from a brain syndrome in the wide range of affective disturbance and in the complex nature of the hallucinatory experiences.

In the opinion of some investigators, LSD may become useful as a psychotherapeutic agent when administered under strictly controlled conditions in the course of psychotherapy.[54,82] Two studies, however, failed to demonstrate superiority of LSD in the treatment of alcoholism.[46,61]

Phenothiazines and barbiturates, singly or in combination, have sometimes been found effective in treating the acutely intoxicated state.[96] The regular LSD user knows this well and may keep a supply of chlorpromazine on hand.

PSYCHOTOMIMETIC AGENTS SIMILAR TO LSD

DMT (dimethyltryptamine), DET (diethyltryptamine), and DPT (dipropyltryptamine) are commonly abused for their psychotomimetic effects. All three tryptamine derivatives produce a syndrome resembling an LSD reaction but differing in the following ways: the onset is more rapid, increasing the likelihood of panic reaction; the duration of action is only 1 to 2 hours (the experience has been dubbed a "businessman's trip"); and the autonomic effects consisting of pupillodilatation and elevation of blood pressure are more marked than with LSD.[22] DMT is present in several South American snuffs, including cohoba snuff.

The labels "STP" and "DOM" have been given to the hallucinogenic drug 2,5-dimethoxy-4-methyl amphetamine.[77] It is said to induce an LSD-like reaction lasting 72 hours or longer. Many who have tried the drug dislike the long "come-down" period of 1 to 3 days; perhaps for this reason, among others, it is generally less popular than LSD.

Another psychotomimetic agent related to the amphetamines is "MDA," or the "love pill" (3-methoxy-4,5-methylenedioxy amphetamine),[76] which is said to induce a relatively mild LSD-like reaction lasting 6 to 10 hours. An amphetamine-like effect is also produced and tends to persist longer than the psychotomimetic effect, so that the period of "crashing" or "coming down" may be characterized by euphoria instead of the psychic depression that frequently concludes an LSD trip.

MORNING GLORY SEEDS

Varieties:
1. *Rivea corymbosa:* ololiuqui, Mexican morning glory, Heavenly Blue (used in ceremony by Aztec Indians of Mexico)
2. *Ipomoea versicolor* (alternate names: *I. violacea, I. tricolor*): Pearly Gates

Morning glory seeds, readily purchasable in stores, contain compounds similar to LSD—D-lysergic acid amide among others. Up to several hundred seeds are ingested at a time to produce effects; less commonly an extract is injected intravenously.

Symptoms include drowsiness, perceptual distortion, confusion, lability of affect, and hallucinations; giddiness and euphoria may alternate with intense anxiety.[28,35] Common side effects of oral ingestion include nausea, vomiting, and diarrhea.

An instance of suicide apparently related to a morning glory seed flashback reaction has been described.[11] A 24-year-old college student ingested 300 Heavenly Blue seeds and developed an acute psychotic reaction. Three weeks later the symptoms recurred for no apparent reason, and the student expressed a fear of losing his mind. The symptoms persisted and one morning he awoke, communicated his distress to others, and drove his car at an estimated 90 to 100 miles per hour down a hill to his death.

MESCALINE

The dumpling (peyote) cactus, *Lophophora williamsii*, is indigenous to the Rio Grande Valley. Protuberances atop the plant are cut off and dried in the sun to form the peyote or mescal buttons; these contain the active drug, mescaline (peyote; peyotl; 3,4,5,-trimethoxyphenethylamine). The buttons are prepared into cakes, tablets, or powder; the powder is water soluble and may be administered orally or parenterally. Peyote is used in ceremonies by the Indians of northern Mexico and by the Navahos,[1] Apaches, Comanches, and other tribes of the southwestern United States.

Mescaline produces effects similar to those of LSD, but it is less potent. Vivid and colorful hallucinations are reported. Flagrant psychotic reactions are far less common than with LSD.

Mescaline has been found in smaller quantities in another North American cactus, *Pelecyphora aselliformis*,[129] and is known also to occur in some species of South American cacti.

PSILOCYBIN AND PSILOCIN

The hallucinogenic agents psilocybin and psilocin, available in powder and liquid form, are extracted from the mushrooms *Stropharia* spp. and *Psilocybe* spp., which occur principally in Mexico.

A native religious cult in which these mushrooms are consumed as a sacrament has deep roots in Mexican tradition.[74] Psilocybin is now popular with drug users in the United States and produces an effect similar to mescaline.

ANTICHOLINERGICS

Commonly abused anticholinergic agents include atropine, scopolamine, synthetic atropine substitutes, and preparations or plants containing these agents (such as the over-the-counter preparation "Asthmador"[50] and the plant jimsonweed [*Datura stramonium*]).[27,104] In high doses these agents induce disorientation, confusion, hallucinations, and eventually coma. Other signs of anticholinergic intoxication are present, such as mydriasis, tachycardia, decreased salivary secretion, anhidrosis, urinary retention, and warm, flushed skin. Anticholinergic agents are abused for their psychotomimetic effects and are sometimes falsely marketed as LSD.

NUTMEG

Nutmeg (*Myristica*), a spice used throughout the world, is the powdered seed kernel of the East Indian tree *Myristica fragrans*. Unknown to many, it contains a hallucinogen thought to be myristicin. Ingestion of large amounts of nutmeg produces euphoria, hallucinations, and an acute psychotic reaction. Side effects, which may be confused with atropine poisoning, include flushing of the skin, tachycardia, and decreased salivary secretion. Unlike atropine, nutmeg may produce early pupillary constriction.[68,83]

INHALANTS

The term *inhalant,* as used here, includes gases and highly volatile organic compounds and excludes liquids sprayed into the nasopharynx (droplet transport required) and substances that must be ignited prior to inhalation (such as marihuana).

This category of drug abuse attracts the youngest customers. Not infrequently one learns of elementary schoolchildren who have experimented dangerously with inhalants for weeks or months before being discovered. The abuse of these agents is not limited, however, to children.

Among the more popular inhalants are model airplane glues, plastic cements, gasoline, brake and lighter fluids, paint and lacquer thinners, varnish remover, cleaning fluid (spot remover), and nail polish remover. These household agents contain a variety of volatile aliphatic and aromatic hydrocarbons, including benzene, toluene, xylene, carbon tetrachloride, chloroform, acetone, amyl acetate, trichloroethane, naphtha, ethyl alcohol, and isopropyl alcohol. Some of these compounds are depressants of the central nervous system and may produce anesthesia and death in high concentrations. Some have known toxic effects. Chloroform and carbon tetrachloride, for example, are toxic to the myocardium, liver, and kidney and may produce hepatic or renal failure or cardiac arrhythmias with severe hypotension; mild poisoning with either agent may produce a reversible oliguria of a few days' duration. Exposure to high concentrations of toluene may result in acute hepatic failure, bone marrow suppression, and permanent encephalopathy.[52] A case of fatal aplastic anemia secondary to glue sniffing has been reported.[70] A drug user habituated to one inhalant may resort to using another when the first inhalant is unavailable; a gasoline sniffer substituted carbon tetrachloride with near-fatal results.[20]

Symptoms produced by inhalation of the agents just listed are essentially similar for all. A sense of exhilaration and light-headedness are usually reported, progressing to hallucinations. Judgment and reality perception are impaired. Transient ataxia, slurred speech, diplopia, and vomiting have been reported in cases of glue sniffing. If inhalation is not interrupted, coma and death may result.[2,21,85]

The development of a definite tolerance has been reported.[67] Physical dependence is not known to develop.

Anesthetic agents such as nitrous oxide ("laughing gas"), diethyl ether, cyclopropane, trichloroethylene (Trilene), and halothane (Fluothane) are also subject to abuse. Nitrous oxide, currently a very popular inhalant, represents an exception to the general rule that inhalants are organic compounds.

One popular inhalant that is neither a household item nor an anesthetic agent is amyl nitrite, nicknamed "snappers," "poppers," and "whiffenpoppers." Amyl nitrite is a clear liquid with a pungent odor and is marketed in thin glass ampules called "vaporols" or "pearls." Each ampule is encased in an absorbent fabric envelope; when the ampule is crushed by light pressure between the fingers, the fabric provides the surface area for rapid volatilization. The effect of inhalation is almost instantaneous; light-headedness and dizziness are produced, with a feeling interpreted by some as euphoria. The experience has been dubbed a "60-second trip." The effects are enjoyed by some during sexual intercourse; one or both partners break an ampule at the moment of climax.

"Sudden sniffing death" is a new phenomenon associated with inhalant abuse.[89] In the usual reported case a young person inhales a volatile hydrocarbon deeply and gets the urge to run; after sprinting a short distance he falls to the ground, dead. The cause of death is assumed to be a cardiac arrhythmia induced by the inhaled agent and intensified by exercise and hypercapnia. Most reported cases have followed inhalation of fluoroalkane gases such as the pressurized propellants of many aerosol sprays. Once called "inert," fluoroalkane gases have been found to sensitize the hearts of mice to asphyxia-induced sinus bradycardia, atrioventricular block, and ventricular T-wave depression.[139] Inhalation of airplane glue or toluene has likewise been shown to sensitize the heart of mice to asphyxia-induced A-V block.[140] Fatal cardiac arrhythmias have been produced in dogs by inhalation of fluorinated hydrocarbons (trichloromonofluoromethane and dichlorodifluoromethane) in the absence of hypoxia, with careful maintenance of normal arterial oxygen tension, CO_2 tension, pH, serum CO_2 level, and base excess.[101]

MISCELLANEOUS DRUGS

Propoxyphene (Darvon). There is no evidence that significant physical dependence or tolerance develops when propoxyphene is administered in ordinary therapeutic doses. In very large doses, however, both physical dependence and tolerance have been observed to develop.[24,30,86] The withdrawal syndrome is characterized by chills, diaphoresis, rhinitis, yawning, muscle aches, irritability, abdominal cramping, and diarrhea.[24,86] Evidence suggesting that propoxyphene is pharmacologically related to the opiates is provided by the finding that it can suppress the morphine abstinence syndrome to a slight degree.[30,55] Perhaps the most convincing evidence of such a relationship is the finding that the toxic effects of an overdose of propoxyphene (muscular fasciculations, respiratory depression, and convulsive seizures) are antagonized by the narcotic antagonists nalorphine and levallorphan.

In a study at the Addiction Research Center in Lexington, Kentucky,[30] comparison of propoxyphene with codeine was made on the basis of the occurrence of an abstinence syndrome following abrupt withdrawal, suppression of morphine abstinence syndrome, and precipitation of an abstinence syndrome upon administration of nalorphine. It was concluded that propoxyphene induces considerably less physical dependence than codeine and has substantially less addiction liability than codeine. The same investigators also found that a toxic psychosis was induced by single doses of propoxyphene in excess of 900 mg. Propoxyphene overdosage may be rapidly fatal. Respiratory depression, convulsions, and pulmonary edema are common terminal events.[144]

A recent review of the literature on propoxyphene concludes that the potential for physical dependence on propoxyphene is low.[128] The actual *abuse* potential, however, seems to be fairly high. In some areas of the United States it appears to be one of the most commonly abused drugs.[131]

Nicotine. Nicotine is extracted from the tobacco plant *Nicotiana tabacum*, which has been cultivated from remote antiquity and in every country of the world where the climate has permitted. It has never been found as a wild plant and fails to survive outside of cultivation. Nicotine is one of the most toxic of all drugs; the dosage encountered in cigarettes is extremely small. Physiologic effects of nicotine include elevation of blood pressure, increased bowel activity, and an antidiuretic action. Apparently a moderate tolerance develops and a mild to moderate physical dependence.[31]

Caffeine. Caffeine occurs naturally in the coffee bean (seeds of *Coffea arabica* and related species), the leaves of the tea plant (*Thea sinensis*), and the seeds of the chocolate tree (*Theobroma cacao*). Caffeine is added to many soft beverages and over-the-counter medications. It stimulates the central nervous system at all levels, beginning with the cortex; a more rapid and clear flow of thought is produced and sense of fatigue is diminished. Physical dependence on caffeine has not been demonstrated. It appears that a mild degree of tolerance develops during continued use.

Cantharidin (Spanish fly). Spanish fly is erroneously reputed to have a specific aphrodisiac effect, presumably because priapism may result from irritation of the male urethra when the drug is excreted in the urine.[31] Ingestion of cantharidin is followed by stomatitis, abdominal cramps, vomiting, bloody diarrhea, urinary urgency, dysuria, hematuria, and priapism. Cantharidin is directly toxic to the kidneys; deaths from renal damage and cardiorespiratory collapse have been reported.[78,133]

Catnip *(Nepeta cataria).* The dried leaves of the catnip plant are smoked like marihuana or the extract is sprayed over ordinary tobacco. Effects are said to be euphoria and enhanced appreciation of sensory experiences.[41] No definite pharmacologic activity has yet been demonstrated. One wonders to what extent the alleged effects of catnip, like those of banana peels,[8] are the result of placebo effect and hyperventilation.

p-**Chlorophenylalanine.** *p*-Chlorophenylalanine ("PCPA") has been found to induce long-lasting sexual excitation in male rats.[80,102] Nicknamed "steam" by drug users, it has gained a reputation as a dangerous drug capable of inducing a prolonged psychotic reaction when taken in high doses. Drug users warn each other that "steam burns."

DRUG MIXING

Drug users are aware that the combination of two or more centrally active drugs may provide a novel dimension of feeling unobtainable with a single drug alone. A second drug may be taken to enhance the effects of the first drug, to prevent undesired effects of the first drug, or to reduce the discomfort of discontinuing the first drug. Unintentional mixing is virtually the rule with black-market drugs; users rejoice when they can obtain "good-quality acid" that has escaped adulteration with methamphetamine, STP, or strychnine.

CLINICAL EVALUATION OF THE DRUG USER

Unlike alcoholism and opiate addiction, the newer type of drug abuse is just over a decade old. Spreading relentlessly across socioeconomic and geographic barriers, it offers to youth the tempting illusion of asylum from conflicts and anxieties with promise of adventure in an uncharted inner world. The initial decision to experiment with drugs may be a response to normal curiosity or peer group pressure and may not involve serious risk. In contrast, the choice of making one or more drugs a "way of life" for extended periods of time is a response to unmet inner needs and is strongly correlated with the degree of emotional disturbance.

When drugs of abuse are classified as they are in this chapter and in Table C (p. 702), it is often forgotten that a large percentage of drugs taken by youngsters today are black-market samples and that three unknowns are thereby introduced: dose, actual identity, and purity. Any one of these three unknowns constitutes a serious danger in itself, and all three are present in any black-market sample.[91]

Fundamental to the diagnostic evaluation of the suspected drug user is an attempt to place the apparent drug-related symptoms into one or more of four categories: symptoms occurring during intoxication; symptoms of withdrawal; "flashback" symptoms; and the "masking" of symptoms of illness or injury by a drug.[97]

The lack of symptom specificity in cases of intoxication makes the evaluation tricky even for an experienced observer; manic excitement, panic reaction, dissociative reaction, paranoid reaction, and overt psychotic reactions may occur during a "bad trip" with most of the drugs discussed. An etiologic diagnosis is best reached through laboratory analysis of drug sample, gastric aspirate, blood, or urine; even laboratory identification may be difficult, however, because of introduction of new chemical agents in an evolving drug scene.[141] To make matters more complicated, a patient may be simultaneously in withdrawal from one drug and intoxicated with another.

Contrary to earlier thinking, it is now apparent that discontinuing almost any drug after heavy use is likely to result in serious abstinence symptoms. It may be unrealistic to describe the phenomenon of "crashing" (discontinuing a drug after heavy use or a large dose) in either physiologic or psychologic terms; it is clearly neither the one nor the other alone.

Symptoms of coincident illness or injury may not be reported by the intoxicated drug user because of the analgesic action of the drug or because of a mental state in which he is only vaguely aware of the symptoms (or lacks the incentive to report them). Heart attack or head injury may thereby escape detection. Systemic infection, metabolic disturbance (especially diabetic crisis), and head injury may contribute to the moribund state of patients who have taken a depressant drug.

It is important to remember that a patient under the influence of, or in withdrawal from, almost any drug may show no obvious symptoms or signs referable to recent drug use.

A syndrome of necrotizing angiitis associated with drug abuse has recently been described.[92] It appears to be pathologically indistinguishable from periarteritis nodosa and is manifest clinically by few or no symptoms in some patients and multiple-system involvement, with pulmonary edema, hypertension, pancreatitis, and renal failure, in others. Although the etiology is unclear, a frequent associated finding has been the intravenous injection of methamphetamine. The actual existence of this syndrome as a new drug-related phenomenon is challenged by some observers.[88]

Injection of oral drug preparations may be associated with deposition of tablet filler material in retina, lung, endocardium, liver, spleen, and kidney. Pulmonary angio-thrombotic granulomatosis has been reported, with consequent pulmonary hypertension and fatal cor pulmonale, as a result of deposition of talc (magnesium trisilicate) in the pulmonary vessels.[108] Ophthalmologic examination may reveal crystals of talc and cornstarch clustered in the macular region.[87] The list of tablet filler materials is endless, and includes lactose, colloidal silica, microcrystalline cellulose, magnesium stearate, and dibasic calcium phosphate. The list may be almost as long as that of contaminants added to black-market drugs.

Gangrene of an extremity is a common end result of inadvertent arterial injection of a drug. The mechanism of vascular injury is not known, but chemical damage to the intima by the concentrated drug may play an important role. Tissue ischemia after intra-arterial injection of *oral* drug preparations appears to be more severe than that after injection of parenteral preparations,[119] perhaps because of the presence of the many additives of the filler.

A drug habit carries a proportionately greater risk if (1) black-market drugs are used; (2) the higher-risk drugs such as LSD, amphetamines, or heroin are used; and (3) the route of administration is intravenous. The intravenous route introduces a number of risks of its own, including greater likelihood of adverse reaction or lethal overdose, viral hepatitis, bacterial endocarditis, serious sequelae of injecting filler from oral drug preparations, and development of a "needle habit" (craving for injection of anything by needle).

Drug abuse has reached the point of the ultimate flirtation with the unknown. Randomly selected chemicals and consumer products are "tested" for effect by the intravenous route. Rat poison containing strychnine is poured over marihuana and the preparation is smoked. An encapsulated mixture of LSD, strychnine, and arsenic is said to give that "special kick." With grim humor, a lapel button reads, "drop cyanide for the *ultimate* trip."

References

1 Aberle, D. F.: The peyote religion among the Navaho, Chicago, 1966, Aldine Publishing Co.

2 Ackerly, W. C., and Gibson, G.: Lighter fluid "sniffing," Amer. J. Psychiat. 120:1056, 1964.

3 Aivazian, G. H.: Clinical evaluation of diazepam Dis. Nerv. Syst. 25:491, 1964.

4 Ausubel, D. P.: The Dole-Nyswander treatment of heroin addiction, J.A.M.A. 195:949, 1966.

5 Bates, G. M.: Letter to the editor, J.A.M.A. 207:2439, 1969.

6 Bell, D. S.: Comparison of amphetamine psychosis and schizophrenia, Brit. J. Psychiat. 111:701, 1965.

7 Berger, H.: Addiction to methyprylon: report of a case of 24-year-old nurse with possible synergism with phenothiazine, J.A.M.A. 177:63, 1961.

8 Bozzetti, L., Jr., Goldsmith, S., and Ungerleider, J. T.: The great banana hoax, Amer. J. Psychiat. 124:678, 1967.

9 Brooks, G. W.: Withdrawal from neuroleptic drugs, Amer. J. Psychiat. 115:931, 1959.

10 Cahn, C. H.: Intoxication by ethclorvynol (Placidyl): report of four cases, Canad. Med. Ass. J. 81:733, 1959.

11 Cohen, S.: Suicide following morning glory seed ingestion, Amer. J. Psychiat. 120:1024, 1964.

12 Connell, P. H.: Clinical manifestations and treatment of amphetamine type of dependence, J.A.M.A. 196:718, 1966.

13 Crancer, A., Jr., Dille, J. M., Delay, J. C., Wallace, J. E., and Haykin, M. D.: Comparison of the effects of marihuana and alcohol on simulated driving performance, Science 164:851, 1969.

14 Cutting, W. C.: Morphine addiction for 62 years: a case report, Stanford Med. Bull. 1:39, 1942.

15 Deneau, G. A., and Seevers, M. H.: Pharmacological aspects of drug dependence, Advances Pharmacol. 3:267, 1964.

16 Dole, V. P., and Nyswander, M. E.: Medical treatment of diacetylmorphine (heroin) addiction, J.A.M.A. 193:646, 1965.

17 Dole, V. P., and Nyswander, M. E.: The treatment of heroin addiction (letter to the editor), J.A.M.A. 195:188, 1966.

18 Dole, V. P., and Nyswander, M. E.: Heroin addiction—a metabolic disease, Arch. Intern. Med. 120:19, 1967.

19 Dole, V. P., Nyswander, M. E., and Warner, A.: Successful treatment of 750 criminal addicts, J.A.M.A. 206:2708, 1968.

20 Durden, W. D., Jr., and Chipman, D. W.: Gasoline sniffing complicated by acute carbon tetrachloride poisoning, Arch. Intern. Med. 119:371, 1967.

21 Easson, W. M.: Gasoline addiction in children, Pediatrics 29:250, 1962.

22 Efron, D. H., editor-in-chief: Ethnopharmacologic search for psychoactive drugs, Public Health Service Publication No. 1645, Washington, D. C., 1967, U. S. Government Printing Office.

23 Ellinwood, E. H., Ewing, J. A., and Hoaken, P. C. S.: Habituation to ethinamate, New Eng. J. Med. **266**:185, 1962.

24 Elson, A., and Domino, E. F.: Dextro propoxyphene addiction: observations of a case, J. A. M. A. **183**:482, 1963.

25 Essig, C. F.: Newer sedative drugs that cause states of intoxication and dependence of barbiturate type, J.A.M.A. **196**:126, 1966.

26 Expert Committee on Addiction-Producing Drugs, Seventh Report, WHO Techn. Rep. Ser. 116, 1957.

27 Farnsworth, N. R.: Hallucinogenic plants, Science **162**:1086, 1968.

28 Fink, P. J., Goldman, M. J., and Lyons, I.: Recent trends in substance abuse: morning glory seed psychosis, Int. J. Addictions **2**:143, 1967.

29 Fisher, D. D., and Ungerleider, J. T.: Grand mal seizures following ingestion of LSD-25, Calif. Med. **106**:210, 1967.

30 Fraser, H. F., and Isbell, H.: Pharmacology and addiction liability of dl- and d-propoxyphene, Bull. Narcotics **12**:9, 1960.

31 Goodman, L. S., and Gilman, A., editors: The pharmacological basis of therapeutics, ed. 4, New York, 1970, The Macmillan Co.

32 Hollister, L. E.: Human pharmacology of lysergic acid diethylamide (LSD). In Efron, D. H., editor-in-chief: Psychopharmacology: a review of progress, 1957–1967, Public Health Service Publication No. 1836, Washington, D. C., 1968, U. S. Government Printing Office.

33 Hollister, L. E., Bennett, J. L., Kimbell, I., Savage, C., and Overall, J. E.: Diazepam in newly admitted schizophrenics, Dis. Nerv. Syst. **24**:746, 1963.

34 Hollister, L. E., Motzenbecker, F. P., and Degan, R. O.: Withdrawal reactions from chlordiazepoxide (Librium), Psychopharmacologia **2**:63, 1961.

35 Ingram, A. L., Jr.: Morning glory seed reaction, J.A.M.A. **190**:1133, 1964.

36 Isbell, H.: Medical aspects of opiate addiction, Bull. N. Y. Acad. Med. **33**:866, 1955.

37 Isbell, H., and Gorodetzky, C. W.: Effect of alkaloids of ololiuqui in man, Psychopharmacologia **8**:331, 1966.

38 Isbell, H., Gorodetzky, C. W., Jasinski, D., Claussen, U., Spulak, F. V., and Korte, F.: Effects of (—)-Δ⁹ trans-tetrahydrocannabinol in man, Psychopharmacologia **11**:184, 1967.

39 Isbell, H., and Jasinski, D. R.: A comparison of LSD-25 with (__)-Δ⁹-trans-tetrahydrocannabinol (THC) and attempted cross tolerance between LSD and THC, Psychopharmacologia **14**:115, 1969.

40 Isbell, H., and White, W. M.: Symposium on drug addiction: clinical characteristics of addictions, Amer. J. Med. **14**:558, 1953.

41 Jackson, B., and Reed, A.: Catnip and the alteration of consciousness, J.A.M.A. **207**:1349, 1969.

42 Jaffe, J. H.: Drug addiction and drug abuse. in Goodman, L. S., and Gilman, A., editors: The pharmacological basis of therapeutics, ed. 4, New York, 1970, The Macmillan Co.

43 Jelliffe, R. W., Hill, D., Tatter, D., and Lewis, E., Jr.: Death from weight-control pills, J.A.M.A. **208**:1843, 1969.

44 Jensen, G. R.: Addiction to Noludar: a report of two cases, New Zeal. Med. J. **59**:431, 1960.

45 Johnson, F. A., and Van Buren, H. C.: Abstinence syndrome following glutethimide intoxication, J.A.M.A. **180**:1024, 1962.

46 Johnson, F. G.: LSD in the treatment of alcoholism, Amer. J. Psychiat. **126**:481, 1969.

47 Judd, L. L., Brandkamp, W. W., and McGlothlin, W. H.: Comparison of the chromosomal patterns obtained from groups of continued users, former users, and nonusers of LSD-25, Amer J. Psychiat. **126**:626, 1969.

48 Kane, F. J., Jr., Keeler, M. H., and Reifler, C. B.: Letter to the editor, J. A. M. A. **210**:556, 1969.

49 Keeler, M. H.: Adverse reaction to marihuana, Amer. J. Psychiat. **124**:128, 1967.

50 Keeler, M. H., and Kane, F. J., Jr.: The use of hyoscyamine as a hallucinogen and intoxicant, Amer. J. Psychiat. **124**:852, 1967.

51 Keeler, M. H., and Reifler, C. B.: Suicide during an LSD reaction, Amer. J. Psychiat. **123**:884, 1967.

52 Knox, J. W., and Nelson, J. R.: Permanent encephalopathy from toluene inhalation, New Eng. J. Med. **275**:1494, 1966.

53 Kramer, J. C., Fischman, V. S., and Littlefield, D.C.: Amphetamine abuse: pattern and effects of high doses taken intravenously, J.A.M.A. **201**:305, 1967.

54 Kurland, A. A., Unger, S., Shaffer, J. W., and Savage, C.: Psychedelic therapy utilizing LSD in the treatment of the alcoholic patient: a preliminary report, Amer. J. Psychiat. **123**:1202, 1967.

55 Lasagna, L.: The clinical evaluation of morphine and its substitutes as analgesics, Pharmacol. Rev. **16**:47, 1964.

56 Lemere, F.: The danger of amphetamine dependency, Amer. J. Psychiat. **123**:569, 1966.

57 Lin, R. C., Ngai, S. H., and Costa, E.: Lysergic acid diethylamide: role in conversion of plasma tryptophan to brain serotonin (5-hydroxytryptamine), Science **166**:237, 1969.

58 Lloyd, E. A., and Clark, L. D.: Convulsions

and delirium incident to glutethimide (Doriden) withdrawal, Dis. Nerv. Syst. **20**:524, 1959.

59 Louria, D. B.: Lysergic acid diethylamide, New Eng. J. Med. **278**:435, 1968.

60 Louria, D. B., Hensle, T., and Rose, J.: The major medical complications of heroin addiction, Ann. Intern. Med. **67**:1, 1967.

61 Ludwig, A., Levine, J., Stark, L., and Lazar, R.: A clinical study of LSD treatment in alcoholism, Amer. J. Psychiat. **126**:59, 1969.

62 Malitz, S., and Hoch, P. H.: Drug therapy: neuroleptics and tranquilizers. In Arieti, S., editor: American handbook of psychiatry, vol. 3, New York, 1966, Basic Books, Inc., Publishers.

63 Martin, W. R., Gorodetzky, C. W., and McClane, T. K.: An experimental study in the treatment of narcotic addicts with cyclazocine, Clin. Pharmacol. Ther. **7**:455, 1966.

64 Massengale, O. N., Glaser, H. H., LeLievre, R. E., Dodds, J. B., and Klock, M. E.: Physical and psychologic factors in glue sniffing, New Eng. J. Med. **269**:1340, 1963.

65 Materson, B. J., and Barret-Conner, E.: LSD "mainlining": a new hazard to health, J.A.M.A. **200**:1126, 1967.

66 Methadone Maintenance Evaluation Committee, American Medical Association: Progress report of evaluation of Methadone Maintenance Treatment Program as of March 31, 1968, J.A.M.A. **206**:2712, 1968.

67 Oswald, I., and Thacore, V. R.: Amphetamine and phenmetrazine addiction, Brit. Med. J. **2**:427, 1963.

68 Payne, R. B.: Nutmeg intoxication, New Eng. J. Med. **269**:36, 1963.

69 Perna, D.: Psychotogenic effect of marihuana, J.A.M.A. **209**:1085, 1969.

70 Powars, D.: Aplastic anemia secondary to glue sniffing, New Eng. J. Med. **273**:700, 1965.

71 Press, E., and Done, A. K.: Solvent sniffing: physiologic effects and community control measures for intoxication from the intentional inhalation of organic solvents, Pediatrics **39**:451, 611, 1967.

72 Robbins, E., Frosch, W. A., and Stern, M.: Further observations on untoward reactions to LSD, Amer. J. Psychiat. **124**:393, 1967.

73 Robinson, J. T.: A case of chloral hydrate addiction, Int. J. Soc. Psychiat. **12**:66, 1966.

74 Schultes, R. E.: I. The plant kingdom and hallucinogens, Bull. Narcotics **21**:3, 1969.

75 Seevers, M. H.: Drug dependence and drug abuse: a world problem, The Pharmacologist **12**:172, 1970.

76 Shulgin, A. T.: 3-Methoxy-4, 5-methylenedioxy

77 Snyder, S. H., Faillace, L., and Hollister, L.: 2,5-Dimethoxy-4-methyl-amphetamine (STP): a new hallucinogenic drug, Science **158**:669, 1967.

78 Sollman, T.: A manual of pharmacology and its applications to therapeutics and toxicology, ed. 8, Philadelphia, 1957, W. B. Saunders Co.

79 Swanson, L. A., and Okada, T.: Death after withdrawal of meprobamate, J.A.M.A. **184**:780, 1963.

80 Tagliamonte, A., Tagliamonte, P., Gessa, G. L., and Brodie, B. B.: Compulsive sexual activity induced by p-chlorophenylalanine in normal and pinealectomized male rats, Science **166**: 1433, 1969.

81 Tatum, A. L., and Seevers, M. H.: Theories of drug addiction, Physiol. Rev. **11**:107, 1931.

82 Unger, M.: Mescaline, LSD, psilocybin, and personality change, Psychiatry **26**:111, 1963.

83 Weiss, G.: Hallucinogenic and narcoticlike effects of powdered Myristica (nutmeg), Psychiat. Quart. **34**:346, 1960.

84 Wickler, A.: Opiate addiction, Springfield, Ill., 1953, Charles C Thomas, Publisher.

85 Winek, C. L., Collom, W. D., and Wecht, C. H.: Fatal benzene exposure by glue-sniffing, Lancet **1**:683, 1967.

86 Wolfe, R. C., Reidenberg, M., and Vispo, R. H.: Propoxyphene (Darvon) addiction and withdrawal syndrome, Ann. Intern. Med. **70**:773, 1969.

Recent references

87 AtLee, W. E., Jr.: Talc and cornstarch emboli in eyes of drug abusers, J.A.M.A. **219**:49, 1972.

88 Baden, M. M.: Angiitis in drug abusers (letter to the editor), New Eng. J. Med. **284**:111, 1971.

89 Bass, M.: Sudden sniffing death, J.A.M.A. **212**: 2075, 1970.

90 Beaconsfield, P., Ginsburg, J., and Rainsbury, R.: Marihuana smoking: cardiovascular effects in man and possible mechanisms, New Eng. J. Med. **287**:209, 1972.

91 Cheek, F. E., Newell, S., and Joffe, M.: Deceptions in the illicit drug market, Science **167**: 1276, 1970.

92 Citron, B. P., Halpern, M., McCarron, M., et al.: Necrotizing angiitis associated with drug abuse, New Eng. J. Med. **283**:1003, 1970.

93 Collier, H. O. J.: The experimental analysis of drug dependence, Endeavour **31**:123, 1972.

94 Conrad, D. G., Elmore, T. F., and Sodetz, F. J.: Delta-9-tetrahydrocannabinol: dose-related effects on timing behavior in chimpanzee, Science **175**:547, 1972.

95 Council on Mental Health and Committee on Alcoholism and Drug Dependence: Dependence on Cannabis (marihuana), J.A.M.A. **201**:368, 1967.

96 Council on Mental Health and Committee on Alcoholism and Drug Dependence: Dependence on LSD and other hallucinogenic drugs, J.A.M.A. **202**:47, 1967.

97 Dimijian, G. G., and Radelat, F. A.: Evaluation and treatment of the suspected drug user in the emergency room, Arch. Intern. Med. **125**: 162, 1970.

98 Dishotsky, N. I., Loughman, W. D., Mogar, R. E., and Lipscomb, W. R.: LSD and genetic damage, Science **172**:431, 1971.

99 Dole, V. P.: Methadone maintenance treatment for 25,000 heroin addicts, J.A.M.A. **215**:1131, 1971.

100 Ferraro, D. P., and Grilly, D. M.: Lack of tolerance to delta-9-tetrahydrocannabinol in chimpanzees, Science **179**:490, 1973.

101 Flowers, N. C., and Horan, L. G.: Nonanoxic aerosol arrhythmias, J.A.M.A. **219**:33, 1972.

102 Gessa, G. L., Tagliamonte, A., and Tagliamonte, P.: Aphrodisiac effect of p-chlorophenylalanine, Science **171**:706, 1971.

103 Goodman, S. J., and Becker, D. P.: Intracranial hemorrhage associated with amphetamine abuse (letter to the editor), J.A.M.A. **212**:480 1970.

104 Gowdy, J. M.: Stramonium intoxication: review of symptomatology in 212 cases, J.A.M.A. **221**:585, 1972.

105 Griffith, J. D., Cavanaugh, J., Held, J., and Oates, J. A.: Dextroamphetamine: evaluation of psychomimetic properties in man, Arch. Gen. Psychiat. **26**:97, 1972.

106 Hollister, L. E.: Marihuana in man: three years later, Science **172**:21, 1971.

107 Holzman, R. S., and Bishko, F.: Osteomyelitis in heroin addicts, Arch. Intern. Med. **75**:693, 1971.

108 Hopkins, G. B.: Pulmonary angiothrombotic granulomatosis in drug offenders, J.A.M.A. **221**:909, 1972.

109 Jacobson, C. B., and Berlin, C. M.: Possible reproductive detriment in LSD users, J.A.M.A. **222**:1367, 1972.

110 Jaffe, J. H., and Senay, E. C.: Methadone and 1-methadyl acetate: use in management of narcotics addicts, J.A.M.A. **216**:1303, 1971.

111 Jaffe, J. H., Senay, E. C., Schuster, C. R., Renault, P. R., Smith, B., and DiMenza, S.: Methadyl acetate vs. methadone: a double-blind study in heroin users, J.A.M.A. **222**:437, 1972.

112 Kreuz, D. S., and Axelrod, J.: Delta-9-tetrahydrocannabinol: localization in body fat, Science **179**:391, 1973.

113 Lemberger, L., Crabtree, R. E., and Rowe, H. M.: 11-Hydroxy-delta-9-tetrahydrocannabinol: pharmacology, disposition, and metabolism of a major metabolite of marihuana in man, Science **177**:62, 1972.

114 Lemberger, L., Silberstein, S. D., Axelrod, J., and Kopin, I. J.: Marihuana, studies on the disposition and metabolism of delta-9-tetrahydrocannabinol in man, Science **170**:1320, 1970.

115 Lemberger, L., Weiss, J. L., Watanabe, A. M., Galantes, I. M., Wyatt, R. J., and Cardon, P. V.: Delta-9-tetrahydrocannabinol: temporal correlation of the psychologic effects and blood levels after various routes of administration, New Eng. J. Med. **286**:685, 1972.

116 Lerner, P.: The precise determination of tetrahydrocannabinol in marihuana and hashish, Bull. Narcotics **21**:39, 1969.

117 Lewis, R., Gorbach, S., and Altner, P.: Spinal pseudomonas chondro-osteomyelitis in heroin users, New Eng. J. Med. **286**:1303, 1972.

118 Lieber, C. S.: Liver adaptation and injury in alcoholism, New Eng. J. Med. **288**:356, 1973.

119 Lindell, T. D., Porter, J. M., and Langston, C.: Intra-arterial injections of oral medications, New Eng. J. Med. **287**:1132, 1972.

120 Louria, D. B.: Medical complications of pleasure-giving drugs, Arch. Intern. Med. **123**:82, 1969.

121 Maugh, T. H.: Narcotic antagonists: the search accelerates, Science **177**:249, 1972.

122 McGlothlin, W. H., Sparkes, R. S., and Arnold, D. O.: Effect of LSD on human pregnancy, J.A.M.A. **212**:1483, 1970.

123 Mechoulam, R.: Marihuana chemistry, Science **168**:1159, 1970.

124 Mechoulam, R., Shani, A., Edery, H., and Grunfeld, Y.: Chemical basis of hashish activity, Science **169**:611, 1970.

125 Melges, F. T., Tinklenberg, J. R., Hollister, L. E., and Gillespie, H. K.: Marihuana and temporal disintegration, Science **168**:1118, 1970.

126 Melges, F. T., Tinklenberg, J. R., Hollister, L. E., and Gillespie, H. K.: Marihuana and the temporal span of awareness, Arch. Gen. Psychiat. **24**:564, 1971.

127 Mikes, F., and Waser, P. G.: Marihuana components: effects of smoking on Δ^9 tetrahydrocannabinol and cannabidiol, Science **172**:1158, 1971.

128 Miller, R. R., Feingold, A., and Paxinos, J.:

Propoxyphene hydrochloride: a critical review, J.A.M.A. **213**:996, 1970.

129 Neal, J. M., Sato, P. T., and Howald, W. N.: Peyote alkaloids. identification in the Mexican cactus *Pelecyphora aselliformis* Ehrenberg, Science **176**:1131, 1972.

130 Newman, L. M., Lutz, M. P., Gould, M. H., and Domino, E. F.: Delta-9-tetrahydrocannabinol and ethyl alcohol: evidence for cross-tolerance in the rat, Science **175**:1022, 1972.

131 Owen, N. L.: Abuse of propoxyphene (letter to the editor), J.A.M.A. **216**:2016, 1971.

132 Pillard, R. C.: Medical progress: Marihuana, New Eng. J. Med. **283**:294, 1970.

133 Presto, A. J., and Muecke, E. C.: A dose of Spanish fly, J.A.M.A. **214**:591, 1970.

134 Reich, P., and Hepps, R. B.: Homicide during a psychosis induced by LSD, J.A.M.A. **219**:869, 1972.

135 Richter, R. W., Challinor, Y. B., Pearson, J. et al.: Acute myoglobinuria associated with heroin addiction, J.A.M.A. **216**:1172, 1971.

136 Rubin, E., and Lieber, C. S.: Alcoholism, alcohol, and drugs, Science **172**:1097, 1971.

137 Silva, M. T. A., Carlini, E. A., Claussen, U., and Korte, F.: Lack of cross-tolerance in rats among (−) Δ^9-*trans*-tetrahydrocannabinol (Δ^9THC), cannabis extract, mescaline and lysergic acid diethylamide (LSD-25), Psychopharmacologia **13**:332, 1968.

138 Steinberg, A. D., and Karliner, J. S.: The clinical spectrum of heroin pulmonary edema, Arch. Intern. Med. **122**:122, 1968.

138a Tashkin, D. P., Shapiro, B. J., and Frank, I. M.: Acute pulmonary physiologic effects of smoked marijuana and oral Δ^9 tetrahydrocannabinol in healthy young men, New Eng. J. Med. **289**:336, 1973.

139 Taylor, G. J., and Harris, W. S.: Cardiac toxicity of aerosol propellants, J.A.M.A. **214**:81, 1970.

140 Taylor, G. J., and Harris, W. S.: Glue sniffing causes heart block in mice, Science **170**:866, 1970.

141 Taylor, R. L., Maurer, J. I., and Tinklenberg, J. R.: Management of "bad trips" in an evolving drug scene, J.A.M.A. **213**:422, 1970.

142 Tennant, F. S., and Groesbeck, C. J.: Psychiatric effects of hashish, Arch. Gen. Psychiat. **27**:133, 1972.

143 Tennant, F. S., Preble, M., Prendergast, T. J., and Ventry, P.: Medical manifestations associated with hashish, J.A.M.A. **216**:1965, 1971.

144 Young, D. J.: Propoxyphene suicides, Arch. Intern. Med. **129**:62, 1972.

145 Zaks, A., Jones, T., Fink, M., and Freedman, A. M.: Naloxone treatment of opiate dependence, J.A.M.A. **215**:2108, 1971.

26 Nonnarcotic analgesics and anti-inflammatory drugs

GENERAL CONCEPT

In contrast to the narcotic analgesics, a group of widely used analgesic drugs exemplified by the salicylates are antipyretic, and most are anti-inflammatory as well. Salicylates, pyrazolones, aniline derivatives, and cinchophens belong to this group. Indomethacin and mefenamic acid are newer members of the series. All drugs in this group are *analgesic* and *antipyretic* and, with the exception of the aniline derivatives, are *anti-inflammatory* and *antirheumatic* as well.

The analgesics to be discussed in this chapter are *mild* in the sense that they are not potent enough to abolish severe pain. The mild group of analgesics should include not only the antipyretic and anti-inflammatory classes of drugs but also those newer drugs structurally related to the narcotics but having a lower potency, or power. Because of their chemical similarities to the narcotics, they are discussed in Chapter 24 dealing with that group of agents.

SALICYLATES

Salicylic acid, or *o*-hydroxybenzoic acid, is a simple organic compound that exerts remarkable analgesic, antipyretic, anti-inflammatory, antirheumatic, and uricosuric effects in man. Compounds closely related to this drug occur naturally in willow bark as the glycoside *salicin* and in oil of gaultheria (oil of wintergreen).

Since it is believed that compounds related to salicylic acid act either by conversion to this acid or by mechanisms similar to its mode of action, the various preparations related to salicylic acid are referred to as salicylates. Most commonly employed are sodium salicylate, acetylsalicylic acid, and salicylamide. The structural formulas of these drugs are shown below.

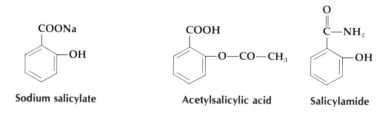

Sodium salicylate   Acetylsalicylic acid   Salicylamide

Although aspirin, sodium salicylate, and salicylamide are structurally very similar, some of their effects in the body may be quite diverse. Thus aspirin is more potent than sodium salicylate as an analgesic and antipyretic, and salicylamide is much less effective than either.

Pharmacologic effects

When as much as 600 mg. of sodium salicylate, acetylsalicylic acid, or salicylamide is taken orally by a normal adult, the effects are negligible. Some persons may notice slight drowsiness and may complain of gastric irritation, but generally no medically useful property could be anticipated from the effects on a normal person. In disease states or in certain painful conditions, however, the therapeutic actions of the salicylates become quite prominent.

Analgesic effect

It is well known that the pain of headache, arthralgia, and muscular ache responds remarkably well to acetylsalicylic acid. Opinions on the mechanism of pain relief by these drugs vary considerably.

Although the analgesic effect of the salicylates is generally assumed to result from an action on the central nervous system, the evidence for this is not impressive. There is increasing evidence, on the other hand, for some relationship between aspirin and the pain-producing polypeptide bradykinin. It has been known for years that aspirin blocks at least one action of bradykinin, bronchial constriction, in the guinea pig.[9]

Recent studies performed in man indicate that aspirin can block pain elicited by the intraperitoneal injection of bradykinin by a peripheral mechanism.[30] Intraperitoneally injected Na-aspirin was more effective than intravenous Na-aspirin in these experiments.

It is difficult to believe that antagonism to the action of bradykinin on sensory nerves completely explains the analgesia produced by aspirin and related drugs. Perhaps the anti-inflammatory action contributes also. In any case, aspirin is more analgesic than other salicylates, and according to some studies, aspirin blood levels correlate better with analgesia than do levels of the hydrolysis product—salicylate.

Inhibition of prostaglandin synthesis by aspirin may contribute to the understanding of its anti-inflammatory, but not its analgesic, effect.[48, 58]

There is an unfounded idea that mixtures of aspirin and acetophenetidin or various buffered preparations of aspirin are more effective analgesics than aspirin itself. A controlled study dispels this notion.[12] On the other hand, buffered preparations may have lesser gastric effects (p. 331).

Antipyretic effect

The salicylates decrease the temperature of patients who have fever but do not lower normal temperature. The same phenomenon can be demonstrated in experimental animals. Intravenous injections of bacterial suspensions such as typhoid vaccine can produce fever in rabbits. The salicylates oppose this experimental temperature elevation but do not lower normal body temperature.

Normal body temperature is maintained by the balance between heat production and heat dissipation. Central regulation of this process is accomplished in the hypothalamus. Under normal circumstances, increased heat production, such as is caused by muscular exercise, brings about increased heat dissipation through peripheral vasodilatation and sweating. Thus the constancy of body temperature is maintained within relatively narrow limits.

In fever there appears to be primarily a defect in heat dissipation. Although the production of heat may be increased, it is not followed by a corresponding increase in heat dissipation. The temperature-regulating centers behave under these conditions much as would a thermostat that has been set higher. The salicylates lower the temperature in fever by increasing heat loss through promotion of peripheral vasodilatation and sweating. Sweating is not essential for the antipyretic action, since temperature can be lowered by the salicylates even when sweating is prevented by atropine.

The possibility of prostaglandins' playing a role in temperature regulation is of great interest. Prostaglandins E_1 and E_2 produced hyperthermia when injected into the third ventricle of cats and rabbits.[33] This is especially interesting in view of the inhibitory action of several antipyretics on prostaglandin synthesis.[48,58]

Antirheumatic and anti-inflammatory effects

In rheumatic fever the administration of salicylates in large doses results in lowering of fever, relief of joint symptoms, and normalization of the elevated sedimentation rate. It is agreed by most investigators that whereas these drugs are highly effective against the joint manifestations of the disease, they have no effect on rheumatic carditis.

The antirheumatic effect of the salicylates is probably just a manifestation of their anti-inflammatory action. The latter action can be demonstrated experimentally in studies of inflammation following the injection of irritating compounds such as carrageenin, a sulfated polygalactose. The anti-inflammatory potency of a series of drugs correlates well with their antirheumatic usefulness in man.[61] The inhibitory action of aspirin on prostaglandin synthesis[48] is of great research interest.

Comparison of salicylates and cortisone

A number of similarities exist between the actions of the salicylates and those of cortisone. Both drugs are effective in rheumatic fever and rheumatoid arthritis and both have some anti-inflammatory actions, although those of cortisone are much more general and potent.

There was great interest when it was shown that large doses of salicylates administered to rats cause depletion of the ascorbic acid content of the adrenal gland,[21] an effect not seen in the hypophysectomized animals.

Somewhat prematurely the impression was gained that perhaps many of the actions of the salicylates are due to stimulant action on the pituitary-adrenal axis, with eventual production of anti-inflammatory steroids. Despite the attractiveness of this idea, overwhelming evidence indicates that this is not the case.

Compounds related to salicylic acid, such as *m*- and *p*-hydroxybenzoic acids, also cause adrenal ascorbic acid depletion, but these drugs have no antirheumatic effects.[44] The effects of the salicylates and those of cortisone on carbohydrate metabolism are also quite different. Cortisone administration increases the glycogen content of the liver, whereas the salicylates decrease it. Salicylates reduce glycosuria in diabetic rats, whereas cortisone increases it.[25] Furthermore, cortisone is effective against many experimental inflammations and in many human diseases such as bronchial asthma, in which the salicylates exert no effect at all.

Uricosuric action

Salicylates in large doses increase the excretion of uric acid in the urine, probably by preventing its tubular reabsorption. On the other hand, small doses such as used for analgesia not only are not uricosuric but actually prevent the effects of probenecid on uric acid excretion.[36]

Miscellaneous effects of salicylates

Salicylates also affect the gastrointestinal tract and respiration, exert an anti-inflammatory action, and have metabolic effects.

Gastrointestinal effects. Salicylates cause gastric irritation. Furthermore, gastric ulceration has been produced with salicylates in experimental animals, and occult blood can be demonstrated in the stools of patients who are taking salicylates.

Generally, salicylic acid in solid particles is more irritating to the gastric mucosa than is the sodium salt solution. Aspirin completely dissolved by the addition of sufficient alkali is less likely to cause gastric bleeding, although the ionized form is not as rapidly absorbed from the stomach as the nonionized form.

The gastric effects of aspirin create a very serious problem for those patients who must take the drug for long periods of time in high doses.

The mechanism of gastrointestinal bleeding induced by aspirin may be quite complex. Lesions of the gastric mucosa are more common after aspirin ingestion when intragastric pH is low. This finding suggests that hydrochloric acid plays an important role in causing the erosions and bleeding. It is likely also that bleeding is aggravated by the striking effect of aspirin on platelet aggregation and stickiness.[35]

Aspirin and platelet aggregation. It has been shown that aspirin, but not sodium salicylate, inhibits platelet aggregation induced by collagen in the test tube.[50] Ingestion of even small analgesic doses of aspirin prolongs the bleeding time in man, presumably by inhibiting platelet function. Such prolongation of bleeding time by aspirin ingestion has been noted also in a variety of diseases such as von Willebrand's disease, afibrinogenemia, and abnormalities of platelet aggregation.

The mode of action of aspirin in blocking platelet aggregation and its significance in the prevention of thrombosis are being investigated. Aspirin appears to block the release of ADP (adenosine diphosphate) induced by collagen, and this effect may explain its inhibitory action on platelet aggregation.[41]

Effect on respiration. Patients with salicylate poisoning show marked hyperpnea. Large oral doses in man or intravenous injections in animals result in marked stimulation of respiration. The immediacy of this response following intravenous injection of sodium salicylate suggests that it is a direct effect rather than a consequence of some metabolic alteration in the body. It has been shown experimentally that in cats and rabbits the respiratory stimulant action is due to a reflex mediated through vagal afferent nerve fibers not involving the carotid bodies.[17]

Metabolic effects. Salicylates affect intermediary metabolism, thyroid function, carbohydrate metabolism, and handling of water and electrolytes.

Salicylates uncouple oxidative phosphorylation.[5] This may be the reason for the increased heat production and oxygen consumption that can be demonstrated in isolated tissues or in whole animals. These drugs also inhibit biosynthesis of acid mucopolysaccharides.

Interference with thyroid function is more apparent than real. The salicylates interfere with binding of thyroxine by plasma proteins. As a consequence, certain tests of thyroid function, such as the protein-bound iodine test, are altered.

Salicylates lower blood sugar levels in diabetics, an effect not mediated by insulin. The drugs can deplete liver glycogen in experimental animals.

In toxic doses the salicylates cause disturbances in acid-base balance. As will be discussed in relation to salicylate poisoning, metabolic acidosis may be caused by these drugs in infants and young children, but respiratory alkalosis is more likely in older children and adults.

Metabolism

Both sodium salicylate and acetylsalicylic acid are rapidly absorbed from the stomach and small intestine. Salicylic acid is poorly ionized at the usual pH of the stomach contents, and its absorption is facilitated by this fact, the nonionized form being more diffusible through membranes.

The absorption of aspirin is greatly influenced by the dissolution characteristics of the tablets. Addition of sufficient alkali to dissolve aspirin would facilitate absorption but could have the disadvantage of inducing systemic alkalosis if large enough doses are administered.

Following their absorption the salicylates are unevenly distributed throughout the body. Salicylic acid is bound to plasma proteins, up to 80%. Acetylsalicylic acid is absorbed as such but is hydrolyzed fairly rapidly in the body to salicylic acid.

The half-life of salicylates in the body is about 6 hours following administration of a single dose. When aspirin is administered, the drug is hydrolyzed in an hour to salicylate. Toxic symptoms such as tinnitus generally develop in adults when the salicylate concentration reaches 30 mg./100 ml., although they may occur at much lower levels.

The salicylates are metabolically altered in the body. The various products of biotransformation, together with some unaltered salicylate, can be found in the urine. In man about 50% of sodium salicylate administered is excreted in 24 hours.[26] The urine contains a variable amount of free salicylate, glucuronides, salicyluric acid (conjugation product with glycine), and gentisic acid (2,5-dihydroxybenzoic acid). At one time it was suggested that the antirheumatic action of the salicylates might be due to their transformation to gentisic acid in the body. This is not believed at the present time because only a small percentage of the salicylate is converted to this product, and the antirheumatic action of sodium gentisate is about the same as that of the salicylates.

Plasma levels of salicylates are greatly influenced by the pH of the urine, since an acid urine favors tubular reabsorption but an alkaline urine is associated with increased salicylate excretion. The administration of sodium bicarbonate to a group of individuals taking 1 Gm. of aspirin four times a day changed the pH of the urine from 5.6–6.1 to 6.2–6.9. At the same time the mean salicylate plasma levels changed from 27 to 15 mg./100 ml.[29] It has been estimated that if an individual had plasma salicylate levels of 20 to 30 mg./100 ml. and a urine pH of 6.5, a change to pH 5.5 would more than double the plasma levels and could be quite hazardous.

Poisoning

Although the salicylates are remarkably safe drugs, they can cause adverse effects and even death when given in large doses. In addition, some individuals appear to have a true drug allergy to aspirin and other salicylates and may show anaphylactic reactions of the urticarial or asthmatic type following the administration of small doses of the drugs. Aspirin hypersensitivity can result in severe attacks of asthma, a fact not as widely known as it should be.

Salicylate intoxication may be mild or serious. The mild form is often called *salicylism* and is characterized by ringing of the ears, dizziness, headache, and mental confusion. The picture is similar to that seen after the administration of large doses of quinine. In the latter case the syndrome is called *cinchonism*.

Serious salicylate intoxication is characterized by hyperpnea, gastrointestinal symptoms, disturbances in acid-base balance, and petechial hemorrhage. The lethal dose of aspirin for adults is about 20 Gm.

Petechial hemorrhages in salicylate poisoning may be due to the ability of these drugs to depress the formation of prothrombin in a manner similar to that of the coumarin anticoagulants. Hemorrhages may reflect other mechanisms, and thrombocytopenic purpura has been reported to occur rarely after the use of the salicylates.

The disturbances in acid-base balance caused by toxic doses of salicylates are quite complex. Hyperventilation leads to respiratory alkalosis. Secondarily, and perhaps triggered by the lowered P_{CO_2}, lactic acid is released from the tissues. As a consequence, respiratory alkalosis may lead to metabolic acidosis, particularly in infants.

The treatment of salicylate poisoning is based on the correction of fluid and electrolyte disturbances. Hemodialysis may be useful for removing salicylates from the blood.

Salicylamide

Salicylamide is much less effective than aspirin as an analgesic and antipyretic. It has some central nervous system depressant actions, but there is serious question about its clinical usefulness.

Preparations

Aspirin USP is available in tablets containing 60, 75, 150, and 300 mg.; in enteric-coated tablets of 300 and 600 mg.; in capsules containing 300 mg.; and in rectal suppositories containing 60, 75, 120, 150, 200, 300, and 600 mg. and 1 Gm. Sodium salicylate USP is available in tablets and enteric-coated tablets, both containing 300, 500, and 600 mg. (Aluminum aspirin is poorly absorbed from the gastrointestinal tract; salicylamide is much less effective than aspirin.)

NONSALICYLATE ANALGESICS
PYRAZOLONE COMPOUNDS
Aminopyrine

Certain phenylpyrazolone derivatives such as aminopyrine and its predecessor antipyrine were widely used at one time as analgesics and antipyretic drugs. Antipyrine has been largely abandoned because the salicylates exert essentially the same beneficial effects without causing significant sensitization reactions. At present the only interest in antipyrine has to do with experimental investigations in which it or its derivative N-acetyl-4-aminoantipyrine may be used for measurement of total body water.

Although aminopyrine (Pyramidon) is an effective analgesic, antipyretic, and antirheumatic drug, its use has led to the development of agranulocytosis in a significant number of patients. As a result of this disadvantage and the greater safety of other analgesics, there is little reason for prescribing aminopyrine.

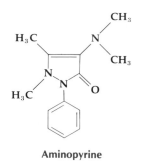

Aminopyrine

Dipyrone

The closely related drug dipyrone is also quite hazardous because of its capability of producing agranulocytosis.[23] The drug is popular in some circles because it is one of the few *injectable* nonnarcotic analgesics. There is some question, however, about its continued use since the drug has caused several deaths.

Because of its great tendency to cause blood dyscrasias, the use of dipyrone can rarely be justified. Nevertheless, when fever cannot be reduced by other drugs in malignant diseases or febrile convulsions in children, the intramuscular injection of dipyrone may be tried.

Preparations of dipyrone (Dimethone; Key-Pyone; Narone; Pyrilgin) include tablets of 300, 324, 600, and 648 mg.; liquid containing 500 mg./5 ml.; and solution for injection, 500 mg./ml.

Phenylbutazone and derivatives

Of much greater interest is another pyrazolone derivative, phenylbutazone (Butazolidin), as are the related drugs oxyphenbutazone (Tandearil) and sulfinpyrazone (Anturan).

The discovery of the therapeutic effectiveness of phenylbutazone has an interesting history. In order to increase the solubility of aminopyrine in an injectable preparation, phenylbutazone was added. Not only did this preparation prove very effective in the treatment of rheumatoid arthritis, but the duration of action also appeared much greater than what could be expected from aminopyrine alone. It was subsequently shown that the blood levels of phenylbutazone were higher and could be maintained for a much longer time than those of aminopyrine.

Pharmacologic actions. This drug is particularly effective in the treatment of rheumatoid arthritis, ankylosing spondylitis, osteoarthritis, and gout. The effectiveness of the drug is somewhere between that of the salicylates and that of the anti-inflammatory steroids.

In animals, phenylbutazone has been shown to inhibit inflammation caused by ultraviolet light or castor oil and to retard the inflammatory edema caused by egg albumin in the rat.[13]

Phenylbutazone has a uricosuric action and may cause sodium retention and edema.

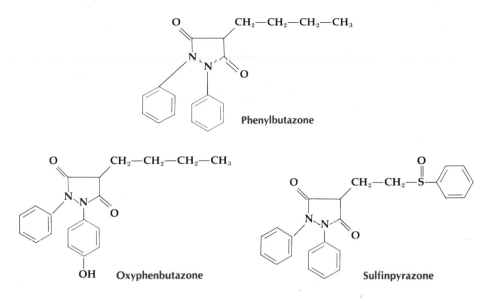

Phenylbutazone

Oxyphenbutazone

Sulfinpyrazone

Metabolism. The metabolism of phenylbutazone has been studied extensively.[6,7] The drug is absorbed much more readily from the gastrointestinal tract than from an intramuscular site. It is almost completely altered in the body, but its metabolism is so slow that its half-life in man may be 72 hours. The drug is bound to plasma proteins and is thus protected from metabolizing enzymes. When large doses are given, the plasma-binding capacity is exceeded and the free drug is metabolized rapidly.[7]

The metabolic alteration of phenylbutazone leads to two active compounds. Oxyphenbutazone, a drug produced by aromatic hydroxylation, has very similar activity and toxicity to those of the parent compound. Another metabolic product that results from alkyl chain oxidation is strongly uricosuric and is similar to sulfinpyrazone.

Toxic effects. It should be emphasized that phenylbutazone can produce many and varied toxic effects. As a consequence, it should be used only when safer medications do not suffice. It has been estimated that some toxic manifestations may appear in 25% of the patients on phenylbutazone treatment. Some of these manifestations are skin rash, gastrointestinal symptoms with activation of peptic ulcer, generalized hypersensitivity reactions similar to the sulfonamide-induced clinical picture, bone marrow depression, bleeding tendency, and jaundice. Thus phenylbutazone is another example of a potent drug that should not be used promiscuously because of the high incidence of adverse effects it may produce.

Dosage. The optimal blood level of phenylbutazone appears to be 10 mg./100 ml. This level may be obtained by administering an initial dose of 200 mg. daily. This dose may have to be increased gradually to 600 mg./day.[4]

Oxyphenbutazone is employed in oral doses of 100 mg. three times a day.

Both phenylbutazone (Butazolidin) and oxyphenbutazone (Tandearil) are available in tablets containing 100 mg.

ANILINE DERIVATIVES

Certain aniline derivatives such as acetanilid have been used as analgesic and antipyretic drugs for many years although they are quite toxic and tend to produce methemoglobinemia. A related compound, acetophenetidin (phenacetin), proved to be more satisfactory and is still in use, particularly in combination with the salicylates. The demonstration that acetophenetidin is converted in the body to N-acetyl-p-aminophenol suggested the possibility that the latter may be responsible for the therapeutic actions of acetophenetidin.[3] As a consequence, N-acetyl-p-aminophenol (acetaminophen) has been introduced as an analgesic and antipyretic.

Several generalizations can be made about the so-called *coal-tar antipyretics*. They are effective analgesics and antipyretics that differ from the salicylates in not having uricosuric or antirheumatic actions. Also, methemoglobinemia and hemolytic anemia may occur following the use of these drugs.

Of the many coal-tar antipyretics, only acetophenetidin and N-acetyl-p-aminophenol have widespread uses. The structural formulas of these two drugs are shown below.

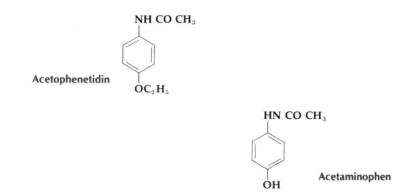

Although acetophenetidin is used widely in combination with the salicylates, there is an increasing tendency to question the necessity of such mixtures. The usefulness of acetophenetidin and caffeine in such mixtures is also questionable.[8]

In addition to hemolytic anemia and acidosis, acetophenetidin can cause methemoglobinemia, particularly in infants.[37] Kidney damage has also been reported following its use.[34] It must be admitted that serious toxic reactions occur very rarely, considering the enormous number of persons who take these headache remedies and the paucity of reports on serious toxic reactions.

Acetaminophen is an effective analgesic and antipyretic that has no anti-inflammatory actions. Although it is as effective as phenacetin, it causes essentially no methemoglobimemia or hemolytic anemia. It has the advantage over aspirin of not causing gastrointestinal bleeding or uric acid retention. The drug is available in tablets of 300 or 325 mg., in drops containing 60 mg./0.6 ml., and elixir or syrup, 120 mg./5 ml.

NEWER ANTI-INFLAMMATORY DRUGS

A number of potent new anti-inflammatory drugs were developed recently on the basis of screening procedures in experimental animals.

Indomethacin is comparable in effectiveness to phenylbutazone in rheumatoid arthritis. It is also used in the treatment of osteoarthritis, rheumatoid spondylitis, and gout.[20,59] Adverse effects caused by the drug include headache, gastrointestinal symptoms, blood dyscrasias, and peptic ulcer. Indomethacin (Indocin) is available in capsules containing 25 and 50 mg.

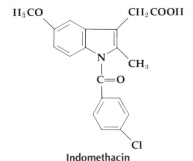

Indomethacin

Flufenamic acid is another potent new anti-inflammatory drug. Its exact position in therapeutics is impossible to state at the present time. It is used in doses of 300 mg. by mouth. The closely related mefenamic acid (Ponstel) appears to have no advantages over aspirin.

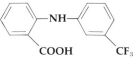

Flufenamic acid

Miscellaneous drugs used in rheumatic diseases

In addition to aspirin, phenylbutazone, oxyphenbutazone, and indomethacin, many other drugs may be useful in the treatment of rheumatic diseases. Some of these such as chloroquine and adrenal corticosteroids are discussed in Chapters 54 and 38, respectively. Gold salts such as aurothioglucose (Solganal) and gold sodium thiomalate (Myochrysine), available for intramuscular injection, have some limited usefulness also.

NONADDICTIVE PHENOTHIAZINE ANALGESIC

Methotrimeprazine (Levoprome), a phenothiazine closely related to chlorpromazine, has been introduced as a novel nonaddictive analgesic. In a carefully controlled clinical study, 20 mg. of methotrimeprazine was approximately equivalent to 10 mg. of morphine when both drugs were administered by the intramuscular route.[2] Special advantages claimed for this phenothiazine analgesic are a lack of respiratory depressant action and an antiemetic effect. On the other hand, marked sedation and possible orthostatic hypotension may limit its usefulness in some patients. The structural formula of methotrimeprazine as contrasted with that of chlorpromazine is shown below.

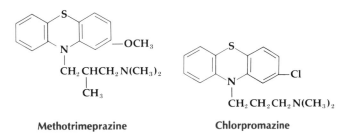

Methotrimeprazine   **Chlorpromazine**

References

1 Beaumont, J. L., and Willie, A.: Influence sur l'hémostase de l'hypertension artérielle, des antivitamines K, de l'héparine et de l'acide acétyl salicylique, Sang 26:880, 1955.

2 Beaver, W. T., Wallenstein, S. L., Houde, R. W., and Rogers, A.: A comparison of the analgesic effects of methotrimeprazine and morphine in patients with cancer, Clin. Pharmacol. Ther. 7:436, 1966.

3 Brodie, B. B., and Axelrod, J.: The fate of acetophenetidin (phenacetin) in man and methods for the estimation of acetophenetidin and its metabolites in biological material, J. Pharmacol. Exp. Ther. 97:58, 1949.

4 Brodie, B. B., Lowman, E. W., Burns, J. J., Lee, P. R., Chenkin, T., Goldman, A., Weiner, M., and Steele, J. M.: Observations on the antirheumatic and physiologic effects of phenylbutazone (Butazolidin) and some comparisons with cortisone, Amer. J. Med. 16:181, 1954.

5 Brody, T. M.: Action of sodium salicylate and related compounds on tissue metabolism in vitro, J. Pharmacol. Exp. Ther. 117:39, 1956.

6 Burns, J. J., Rose, R. K., Chenkin, T., Goldman, A., Schulert, A., and Brodie, B. B.: The physiological disposition of phenylbutazone (Butazolidin) in man and a method for its estimation in biological material, J. Pharmacol. Exp. Ther. 109:346, 1953.

7 Burns, J. J., Rose, R. K., Goodwin, S., Reichenthal, J., Horning, E. C., and Brodie, B. B.: The metabolic fate of phenylbutazone (Butazolidin) in man, J. Pharmacol. Exp. Ther. 113:481, 1955.

8 Cass, L. J., and Frederik, W. S.: The augmentation of analgesic effect of aspirin with phenacetin and caffeine, Curr. Ther. Res. 4:583, 1962.

9 Collier, H. O. J.: The action and antagonism of kinins on bronchioles, Ann. N. Y. Acad. Sci. 104:290, 1963.

10 Croft, D. N., and Wood, P. H. N.: Gastric mucosa and susceptibility to occult gastrointestinal bleeding caused by aspirin, Brit Med. J. 1:137, 1967.

11 Davison, C., Hertig, D. H., and DeVine, R.: Gastric hemorrhage induced by nonnarcotic analgetic agents in dogs, Clin. Pharmacol. Ther. 7:239, 1966.

12 DeKornfeld, T. J., Lasagna, L., and Frazier, T. M.: A comparative study of five proprietary analgesic compounds, J.A.M.A. 182:1315, 1962.

13 Domenjoz, R.: Some pharmacological aspects of phenylbutazone (Butazolidin), a new antirheumatic, Int. Rec. Med. 165:467, 1952.

14 Fraser, H. F., and Isbell, H.: Pharmacology and addiction liability of dl- and d-propoxyphene, Bull. Narcotics 12:9, 1960.

15 Gilman, A.: Analgesic nephrotoxicity. A pharmacological analysis, Amer. J. Med. 36:167, 1964.

16 Glander, G. W., Chaffee, J., and Goodale, F.: Studies on the antipyretic action of salicylates, Proc. Soc. Exp. Biol. Med. 126:205, 1967.

17 Graham, J. D. P., and Parker, W. A.: The toxic manifestations of sodium salicylate therapy, Quart. J. Med. 17:153, 1948.

18 Guerra, F.: Hyaluronidase inhibition by sodium salicylate in rheumatic fever, Science 103:686, 1946.

19 Guerra, F., and Barbour, H. G.: The mechanism of aspirin antipyresis in monkeys, J. Pharmacol. Exp. Ther. 79:55, 1943.

20 Hart, F. D., and Boardman, P. L.: Indomethacin: a new nonsteroid anti-inflammatory agent, Brit. Med. J. 2:965, 1963.

21 Hetzel, B. S., and Hine, D. C.: The effect of salicylates on the pituitary and suprarenal glands, Lancet 2:94, 1951.

22 Hollister, L. E., and Kanter, S. L.: Studies of delayed-action medication. IV. Salicylates, Clin. Pharmacol. Ther. 6:5, 1965.

23 Huguley, C. M.: Agranulocytosis induced by dipyrone, a hazardous antipyretic and analgesic, J.A.M.A. 189:938, 1964.

24 Hutchison, H. E., Jackson, J. M., and Cassidy, P.: Drug-induced hemolytic anemia, Lancet 2:1022, 1962.

25 Ingle, D. J.: Effects of aspirin aminopyrine, and HPC upon glycosuria in the diabetic rat. J. Amer. Pharm. Ass. 42:247, 1953.

26 Kapp, E. M., and Coburn, A. F.: Urinary metabolites of sodium salicylate, J. Biol. Chem. 145:549, 1942.

27 Katz, A. M., Pearson, C. M., and Kennedy, J. M.: A clinical trial of indomethacin in rheumatoid arthritis, Clin. Pharmacol. Ther. 6:25, 1965.

28 Leonards, J. R., and Levy, G.: Reduction of prevention of aspirin-induced occult gastrointestinal blood loss in man, Clin. Pharmacol. Ther. 10:571, 1969.

29 Levy, G., and Leonards, J. R.: Urine pH and salicylate therapy (letter to the editor), J.A.M.A. 217:81, 1971.

30 Lim, R. K., Miller, D. G., Guzman, F., Rodgers, D. W., Rogers, R. W., Wang, S. K., Chao, P. Y., and Shih, T. Y.: Pain and analgesia evaluated by the intraperitoneal bradykinin-evoked pain

method in man, Clin. Pharmacol. Ther. **8**:521, 1967.

31 Mandel, H. G., Rodwell, W. W., and Smith, P. K.: A study of the metabolism of C¹⁴ salicylamide in the human, J. Pharmacol. Exp. Ther. **106**:433, 1952.

32 Medical Research Council Report: Treatment of acute rheumatic fever in children; a cooperative clinical trial of A.C.T.H., cortisone, and aspirins, Brit. Med. J. **1**:555, 1955.

33 Milton, A. S., and Wendlandt, S.: Effects on body temperature of prostaglandins of the A, E and F series of injection into the third ventricle of unanaesthetized cats and rabbits, J. Physiol. (London) **218**:325, 1971.

34 Moolten, S. E., and Smith, I. B.: Fatal nephritis in chronic phenacetin poisoning, Amer. J. Med. **28**:127, 1960.

35 O'Brien, J. R.: Effects of salicylates on human platelets, Lancet **1**:779, 1968.

36 Pascale, L. R., Dubin, A., and Hoffman, W. S.: Therapeutic value of probenecid (Benemid) in gout, J.A.M.A. **149**:1188, 1952.

37 Ross, J. D., and Ciccarelli, R. F.: Acquired methemoglobinemia due to ingestion of acetophenetidin: report of a case in a small infant, New Eng. J. Med. **266**:1202, 1962.

38 Roth, J. L. A., Valdes-Dapena, A., Pieses, P., and Buchman, E.: Topical action of salicylates, Gastroenterology **44**:146, 1963.

39 Sahud, M. A., and Aggeler, P. M.: Platelet dysfunction—differentiation of a newly recognized primary type from that produced by aspirin, New Eng. J. Med. **280**:453, 1969.

40 Salassa, R. M., Bollman, J. L., and Dry, T. J.: The effect of para-aminobenzoic acid on the metabolism and excretion of salicylate, J. Lab. Clin. Med. **33**:1393, 1948.

41 Salzman, E. W., Harris, W. H., and DeSanctis, R. W.: Reduction in venous thromboembolism by agents affecting platelet function, New Eng. J. Med. **284**:1287, 1971.

42 Scott, D.: Aspirin: action on receptor in the tooth, Science **161**:180, 1968.

43 Smith, J. B., and Willis, A. L.: Aspirin selectively inhibits prostaglandin production in human platelets, Nature (New Biol.) **231**:235, 1971.

44 Smith, M. J. H.: Some recent advances in the pharmacology of salicylates, J. Pharm. Pharmacol. **5**:81, 1953.

45 Smith, P. K.: Certain aspects of the pharmacology of the salicylates, Pharmacol. Rev. **1**:353, 1949.

46 Stubble, L. T., Pietersen, J. H., and van Heulen, C.: Aspirin preparations and their noxious effect on the gastrointestinal tract, Brit. Med. J. **1**:675, 1962.

47 Ungar, G., Damgaard, E., and Hummel, F. P.: Action of salicylates and related drugs on inflammation, Amer. J. Physiol. **171**:545, 1952.

48 Vane, J. R.: Inhibition of prostaglandin synthesis as a mechanism of action of aspirin-like drugs, Nature **231**:232, 1971.

49 Vignec, A. J., and Gasparik, M.: Antipyretic effectiveness of salicylamide and acetylsalicylic acid in infants, J.A.M.A. **167**:1821, 1958.

50 Weiss, H. J., Aledort, L. M., and Kochwa, S.: The effects of salicylates on the hemostatic properties of platelets in man, J. Clin. Invest. **47**:2169, 1968.

51 Winter, C. A., Risley, E. A., and Nuss, G. W.: Carrageenin-induced edema in hind paw of the rat as an assay for antiinflammatory drugs, Proc. Soc. Exp. Biol. Med. **111**:544, 1962.

52 Wolff, H. G., Hardy, J. D., and Goodell, H.: Measurement of the effect on the pain threshold of acetylsalicylic acid, acetanilid, acetophenetidin, aminopyrine, ethyl alcohol, trichlorethylene, barbiturate, quinine, ergotamine tartrate and caffeine: an analysis of their relation to the pain experience, J. Clin. Invest. **20**:63, 1941.

53 Yu, T. F., and Gutman, A. B.: Study of the paradoxical effects of salicylate in low, intermediate, and high dosage on the renal mechanisms for excretion of urate in man, J. Clin. Invest. **38**:1298, 1959.

54 Atkins, E., and Bodel, P.: Fever, New Eng. J. Med. **286**:29, 1972.

Recent reviews

55 Cooperating Clinics Committee of the American Rheumatism Association: A three-month trial of indomethacin in rheumatoid arthritis, with special reference to analysis and inference, Clin. Pharmacol. Ther. **8**:11, 1967.

56 Davison, C.: Salicylate metabolism in man, Ann. N. Y. Acad. Sci. **179**:249, 1971.

57 Dixon, A. St. J., Martin, B. K., Smith, M. J. H., and Wood, P. H. N., editors: Symposium on salicylates, London, 1963, J. & A. Churchill, Ltd.

58 Krane, S. M.: Action of salicylates, New Eng. J. Med. **286**:317, 1972.

59 O'Brien, W. M.: Indomethacin: a survey of clinical trials, Clin. Pharmacol. Ther. **9**:94, 1968.

60 Vandam, L. D.: Analgesic drugs—the mild analgesics, New Eng. J. Med. **286**:20, 1972.

61 Winter, C. A.: Nonsteroid anti-inflammatory agents, Ann. Rev. Pharmacol. **6**:157, 1966.

SECTION FIVE

ANESTHETICS

27 Pharmacology of general anesthesia

GENERAL CONCEPT

The development of agents that allow the performance of surgical operations without pain is one of the great achievements in medicine. The objectives of general anesthesia are broader, however, than just abolition of pain. Anesthetic drugs should be capable of inducing sleep, eliminating noxious reflexes, and causing good muscular relaxation.

Any powerful depressant of the central nervous system that can accomplish all of these objectives is potentially dangerous because an extension of its effect to medullary centers can be lethal. It follows that the level of such a drug in the body should be subject to minute-to-minute control. Only drugs whose uptake and elimination are rapid can be adequately controlled.

The clinically useful general anesthetics are of two classes, the inhalation and the intravenous anesthetics. The inhalation agents not only provide (although to a varying degree) analgesia, loss of consciousness, areflexia, and muscular relaxation but also are highly controllable, since the lungs provide a large surface for the rapid diffusion of these agents in and out of the body. The intravenous anesthetics have many desirable features, but they are not as controllable as the inhalation anesthetics and lack significant analgesic and muscle-relaxing properties. Rectal anesthetics are now obsolete.

Among the inhalation anesthetics, *halothane* is favored by many anesthesiologists. It is potent and nonflammable, and induction with this agent is fast and smooth. *Ether, cyclopropane,* and *nitrous oxide* as well as newer halogenated agents are still employed. The intravenous agent *thiopental sodium* is widely employed for short operations and for induction. Combinations of narcotics and a butyrophenone such as the combination known as *Innovar* have their advocates. Similarly, "dissociative" agents such as *ketamine hydrochloride* are employed by some anesthesiologists. Muscle relaxants are commonly used also.

BRIEF HISTORY

While no attempt will be made to discuss the very interesting history of surgical anesthesia, a few important dates will indicate the first use or year of introduction of the various anesthetics.

Inhalation agents
- 1842 Ether
- 1845 Nitrous oxide
- 1846 Ether demonstration
- 1847 Chloroform
- 1923 Ethylene
- 1930 Vinyl ether
- 1934 Cyclopropane
- 1934 Trichloroethylene
- 1954 Fluroxene
- 1956 Halothane
- 1959 Methoxyflurane
- 1972 Enflurane

Intravenous agents
- 1935 Thiopental
- 1970 Ketamine

UPTAKE, DISTRIBUTION, AND ELIMINATION
OF INHALATION ANESTHETICS

The purpose in administering an inhalation anesthetic is to produce a certain partial pressure of the anesthetic gas in the brain. This partial pressure will depend on that of the blood, which in turn depends on the alveolar partial pressure and eventually on the concentration in the inhaled mixture. Henry's law states that the concentration of a gas in a liquid is directly related to the partial pressure of the gas. Once equilibrium is reached, the partial pressures of the gas in the liquid phase and the gaseous phase become equal. Their *concentrations*, however, can be quite different.

Equilibrium curve

The equilibrium curve depicts the rate at which equilibrium between alveolar and inhaled partial pressure is attained when an anesthetic is administered. The y axis represents the following ratio:

$$\frac{\text{Alveolar partial pressure (mm. Hg)}}{\text{Inhaled partial pressure (mm. Hg)}} \times 100$$

It may be seen in Fig. 27-1, right, that the curve has a steep *initial slope*, a "knee," and a *secondary slope*.

Factors that determine the rate of tension development in arterial blood and brain

The main factors that will determine the rate at which a certain partial pressure of the anesthetic is reached in the blood and brain are concentration in inspired gas mixture, alveolar concentration, uptake by blood, and uptake by tissues.

Concentration in inspired gas mixture. The inspired anesthetic concentration is regulated by metering devices or by controlled vaporization of volatile liquids. The dead space of the machine is also a factor that influences the final concentration of the gas in the inspired air.

Alveolar concentration. Alveolar concentration depends on the inspired anesthetic concentration, alveolar ventilation, residual volume of the lungs, and uptake by blood. The greater the alveolar ventilation, the faster the rate of equilibration of anesthetic partial pressure in the alveoli and arterial blood.

Uptake by blood. Blood uptake is determined largely by the following factors:

1. Passage across the alveolar membrane, which is usually unimpeded
2. The blood/air solubility of the anesthetic, which is similar in magnitude to the Ostwald solubility coefficients for a number of anesthetic gases
3. Cardiac output and pulmonary blood flow, which play a role in the rate of equilibration of the gas between alveolar air and blood (the higher the cardiac output, the more rapidly the pulmonary blood "drains" the alveoli of gases)

The Ostwald solubility coefficient is of great importance in determining the slope of the equilibrium curve. The higher the coefficient and the more soluble the anesthetic, the slower the "knee" of the equilibrium is reached. The lower the coefficient, the more rapidly the "knee" is reached (Fig. 27-1).

Uptake by tissues. The most important determinants of the tissue uptake of the anesthetic are as follows:

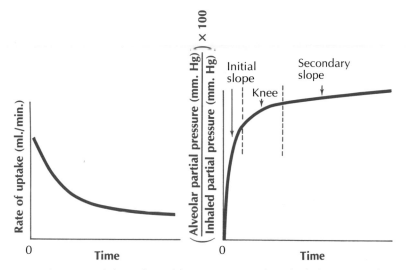

Fig. 27-1. Uptake curve (left) and equilibrium curve (right) of inhalation anesthetic agents. In the uptake curve the *y* axis represents the milliliters of anesthetic taken up by the subject per minute.

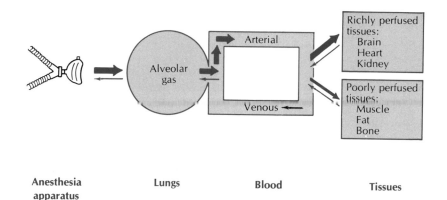

Fig. 27-2. Transfer of anesthetic agents from anesthesia apparatus to lungs, blood, and tissues. Arrows represent relative rates of transfer during induction stage.

1. Regional blood flow to the tissue
2. Tissue/blood solubility coefficient
3. Volume of the tissue compartment

Of these factors, the regional blood flow has the greatest practical importance (Fig. 27-2). The brain, which receives a large percentage of the cardiac output, will equilibrate much more rapidly with the arterial blood than skeletal muscle or fat, which per unit weight are not as well perfused. On the other hand, when the mask is removed from the patient, the brain will lose its anesthetic more rapidly than more poorly perfused tissue.

Table 27-1. Ostwald solubility coefficients of anesthetic gases at 37° C. and 760 mm. Hg*

	Water/gas	Blood/gas	Tissue/blood	
Cyclopropane	0.204	0.415	0.91	(muscle)
Nitrous oxide	0.435	0.468	1.13	(heart)
Halothane	0.74	2.3	2.6	(brain)
			3.5	(muscle)
			60.0	(fat)
Chloroform	3.8	10.3	1.0	(brain)
Diethyl ether	15.61	15.2	1.14	(brain)
Xenon	0.097		1.25	(brain, white matter)
			0.7	(brain, gray matter)

*Based on data from Papper, E. M., and Kitz, R. J., editors: Uptake and distribution of anesthetic agents, New York, 1963, McGraw-Hill Book Co.

Ostwald solubility coefficient and the speed of induction

As seen in Table 27-1, diethyl ether has a high Ostwald coefficient, while cyclopropane and halothane are relatively less soluble in water and blood. It is also well known that induction with ether is very slow but cyclopropane and halothane are fairly rapid-acting anesthetics. The usual explanation has to do with the rapidity with which the blood carries the anesthetic away from the alveoli. If the anesthetic is very soluble in blood, the alveolar concentration is constantly lowered by the pulmonary blood flow and it will take a long time before equilibrium is established between inspired air, alveolar air, and blood. The reverse happens with such anesthetics as cyclopropane, halothane, nitrous oxide, and ethylene, which are not very soluble in blood. Equilibration is rapid because the capacity of the pulmonary blood for the anesthetics is less.

It is quite likely that anesthetic drugs must reach a certain *relative saturation* of some brain lipid in order to be effective (p. 353). A high Ostwald coefficient and solubility in body fluids would prolong the time necessary for achieving such a relative saturation of a brain lipid. In addition to such purely physical factors, the irritating quality of some anesthetics such as ether makes it impossible to administer them in high concentrations in the inspired air. This factor contributes to the slowness of induction.

Miscellaneous factors that alter uptake and distribution of anesthetics

Metabolism of the anesthetic. Metabolism of the anesthetic is quantitatively small but may be of importance.

Diffusion through skin and into body cavities. Diffusion through skin and into the bowel is quantitatively unimportant.

Concentration effect.[12] When a weak anesthetic such as nitrous oxide is administered in high concentration (for example, 80% with 20% oxygen), the movement of gas from the inspired mixture is facilitated as pulmonary blood suddenly lowers gas pressure in the alveoli, thus adding what amounts to suction to ventilation.

Second gas effect.[15] The second gas effect is very similar in principle to the concentration effect. When a low concentration of an anesthetic such as halothane is administered with a high concentration of nitrous oxide, the rapid disappearance of a large volume of the gases from the alveoli to blood and tissues promotes the movement of the gas mixture and speeds the action or equilibration of halothane.

Diffusion hypoxia. The concept of diffusion hypoxia is related to the concentration effect, but in the reverse direction. When the administration of nitrous oxide is discontinued, large volumes of the gas move to the alveoli, causing a temporary reduction in the amount of oxygen.

Summary of factors affecting various portions of the equilibrium curve

Having considered the various factors that influence the rate of equilibration between inspired anesthetic and ultimately the brain, it may be useful to summarize the influence of these various factors on portions of the equilibrium curve as shown in Fig. 27-1, right.

Factors of importance in relation to:
1. Initial slope
   (a) Cardiac output
   (b) Blood/air solubility coefficient
   (c) Alveolar ventilation
2. "Knee" of initial slope
   (a) Blood/air solubility coefficient
   (b) Concentration of inspired anesthetic
3. Secondary slope
   (a) Blood/tissue coefficients
   (b) Minor factors such as metabolism and diffusion through skin and into body cavities

Practical illustration of the blood/gas solubility coefficient for nitrous oxide[31]

If a closed flask contains 1 L. of blood and 1 L. of nitrous oxide at 37° C. with a nitrous oxide pressure of 1 atmosphere in both phases, then:

In the gas phase

Partial pressure of nitrous oxide	760 mm. Hg
Partial pressure of water vapor	47 mm. Hg
Total pressure	807 mm. Hg
Volume of nitrous oxide	1 L.

In the liquid phase

Partial pressure of nitrous oxide	760 mm. Hg
Partial pressure of water vapor	47 mm. Hg
Total pressure	807 mm. Hg
Volume of nitrous oxide	0.47 L.

The Ostwald solubility coefficient for nitrous oxide (blood/air) is then 0.47.

STAGES AND SIGNS OF ANESTHESIA

Very soon after the public introduction of ether by Morton in 1846 it was noted that a pattern of events occurred as the patient was anesthetized. This pattern is a fairly predictable progression of symptoms and signs due to increasing depth of anesthesia, which is reflected by changes in various systems of the body.

John Snow, regarded as the world's first full-time specialist in anesthesia, in 1848 published an account of this pattern,[52] which he divided into five degrees or stages.

From the time of John Snow until Arthur Guedel[23] published his account of the signs and stages of ether anesthesia in 1920, little advance was made in the description of this pattern of depression. Guedel's classic description is the one to which most people refer when they mention "the stages and signs of anesthesia." However, it should be remembered that the stages and signs of anesthesia as described by Guedel were a description of his observations of human beings who were receiving open-drop ether.

GUEDEL'S STAGES OF ETHER ANESTHESIA (WITH ARTUSIO'S MODIFICATION[1])

Stage I – Analgesia
Plane 1 – Normal memory and sensation
Plane 2 – Amnesia and partial analgesia
Plane 3 – Amnesia and analgesia
Stage II – Delirium
Begins with unconsciousness and ends with loss of eyelid reflex; purposeless movements may occur and hyperreaction to stimuli present; pupils widely dilated; reflex vomiting may occur
Stage III – Surgical anesthesia
Plane 1 – Sleep
Begins with loss of eyelid reflex and ends with eyes in resting position looking straight ahead; reflex swallowing present in light plane and maximum constriction of pupils present in deep plane; patient does not move and appears to be sleeping quietly
Plane 2 – Sensory loss
Begins when eyes come to rest and ends with onset of lower intercostal muscle paralysis; pupils begin to dilate and some skeletal muscle relaxation occurs; corneal reflex lost
Plane 3 – Muscle tone loss
Begins with onset of lower intercostal muscle paralysis and ends with complete intercostal muscle paralysis; marked skeletal muscle relaxation occurs, including beginning paralysis of diaphragm; pupils widely dilated, pupillary reflex to light lost, and lacrimation stops; laryngeal reflex becomes paralyzed
Plane 4 – Intercostal paralysis
Begins with onset of complete intercostal muscle paralysis and ends with complete diaphragmatic paralysis; corneal reflex lost and pupils maximally dilated; circulation depressed but still present
Stage IV – Medullary paralysis
Begins with complete respiratory paralysis which leads to complete circulatory failure

Although the general principles involved are similar, the description of the stages and signs of anesthesia with different agents cannot be the same because all general anesthetics do not have exactly the same effects on the human body. The stages of anesthesia are simply artificial divisions of the pattern of anesthetic depression according to signs produced by the action of the anesthetic on different tissues. The signs are ultimately produced by changes in the activity of end organs: skeletal muscle, smooth muscle, and glands.

In 1954 Artusio[1] subdivided Guedel's first stage for ether anesthesia into three discernible planes. However, these planes of anesthesia were not seen during the phase of induction but were found after deep anesthesia with ether had been lightened and the patient subsequently awakened.

The various levels of anesthesia can be extended into the toxic and fatal realm and the entire process divided into nine different levels: (1) clouded consciousness, (2) unconscious hyperactivity, (3) light surgical anesthesia, (4) moderate surgical anesthesia, (5) deep surgical anesthesia, (6) respiratory and circulatory collapse, (7) apparent death (reversible), (8) apparent death (partially reversible), and (9) death (irreversible).

METHODS OF ADMINISTRATION OF GENERAL ANESTHETICS

Since most of the general anesthetic drugs are gases or vapors, the most common route of administration of these drugs is through the respiratory tract.

From the practical point of view the requirements of a system for administering anesthetic drugs by inhalation are as follows: (1) source of oxygen, (2) source of general anesthetic drug, (3) mechanism for removal of carbon dioxide, and (4) mechanism for adequate ventilation.

The various systems for administering general anesthetics by the inhalation route have been given various names. The terms used for describing these various systems may be divided into two categories.

1. Mechanical
   (a) Open, semiopen, semiclosed, and closed
   (b) Circle and to-and-fro
2. Physiologic
   (a) Nonrebreathing
   (b) Partial rebreathing
   (c) Complete rebreathing

The open system for administering general anesthetics can be used with those drugs that can be dropped in liquid form through the air onto a vaporizing surface through which the patient breathes. This form is represented by the so-called ether cone or ether mask. The source of oxygen in this case is the ambient atmosphere. The source of drug might be any convenient container from which the liquid anesthetic could escape in drop form. Removal of carbon dioxide is accomplished by blowing it out through the mask in the same way that oxygen is breathed in from the ambient atmosphere through the mask. With this system there is obviously no means for mechanical assistance to respiration. One refinement in this method is to introduce a stream of oxygen underneath the mask in order to accomplish two purposes. The first is to increase the concentration of oxygen beneath the mask to normal or above. Since there is some trapping of gases exhaled, such as carbon dioxide, the concentration of oxygen beneath the mask tends to become lower than that of the ambient atmosphere. Second, the stream of oxygen tends to help in flushing out the carbon dioxide from beneath the mask, thus preventing hypercapnia. The semiopen method is one in which a towel or some other similar object is wrapped around the mask in order to make a more nearly perfect seal between the mask and the face of the patient. The reason for doing this is simply more nearly to ensure that the patient breathes gases that have come through the mask rather than those that leak in around its edges. This allows for more rapid induction because the concentration of the general anesthetic can be maintained at a higher level.

The closed system is one that the patient theoretically breathes from and back into without any contamination from the ambient atmosphere. Oxygen and anesthetic drugs must be supplied to the system, and carbon dioxide must be removed from the system. This system is called semiclosed when part of the contained gases are allowed to escape into the ambient atmosphere with each exhalation. The components of the closed system are as follows:

1. Gas tanks that contain oxygen and the anesthetic gases to be used
2. Flowmeters to measure the minute volume of these gases
3. Vaporizers to introduce the anesthetic vapors into the system
4. A carbon dioxide absorber
5. A rebreathing bag
6. Necessary connecting tubing
7. Unidirectional valves (required in the circle system only)

In the circle system these various components are arranged so that the gases and vapors flow in one direction only, and the patient breathes in and out of this circle at one point only. In the to-and-fro system these various components are arranged in a linear fashion, and the gases pass from one end to the other and back again, with the patient breathing in and out of the system at one end only. The diagrams shown in Fig. 27-3 should make these arrangements quite clear.

The physiologic description of these systems applies as follows. With the closed system there is complete rebreathing. With the semiclosed system there is partial rebreathing since part of the exhaled gases are lost to the atmosphere and consequently cannot be rebreathed.

To obtain a nonrebreathing system an arrangement completely different from the circle and to-and-fro systems must be used. As can be seen from the diagram in Fig. 27-3, C, the patient breathes out of the system but essentially not back into it. There are inherent in the valve, however, a few milliliters of dead space, which in the adult have no practical significance whatever but in the infant and smaller child may constitute a volume of significant rebreathing.

The last diagram in Fig. 27-3 represents a nonrebreathing system without a valve. This system is analogous to the ambient atmosphere but differs from it in two respects: (1) it contains an anesthetic atmosphere and (2) the exhaled gases are removed by means of the flushing action of high flow rates rather than by the dilution mechanism that normally exists.

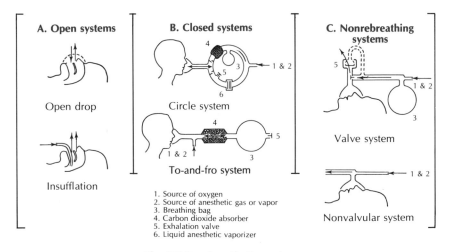

Fig. 27-3. Anesthetic systems.

POTENCY, EFFICACY, AND SAFETY OF GENERAL ANESTHETICS

Potency of a drug is usually expressed as activity per unit weight administered or activity per unit of concentration in blood or other fluid. Such methods of expressing potency would be impractical and meaningless for general anesthetics because no fixed dose is administered.

The minimal alveolar concentration (MAC) of anesthetic[13] has been used for quantitating the potency of general anesthetics. For example, the minimal alveolar concentrations of anesthetic required for preventing response to a painful stimulus in dogs (in volumes percent) were as follows:

Methoxyflurane	0.23	Fluroxene	6.0	Xenon	119.0
Halothane	0.87	Cyclopropane	17.5	Nitrous oxide	188.0
Diethyl ether	3.04				

Potency, of course, would be the reciprocal of the MAC, and as determined in this experiment, it correlated better with the oil/gas partition coefficient than any other physical constant.

Potency of a general anesthetic is often confused with its *efficacy*. Anesthetics differ not only in the MAC's required for producing their effect but also in the magnitude of their effect. For example, ether, cyclopropane, chloroform, and halothane, if administered in high enough concentration for a long enough period, can carry a patient through the four planes of Guedel's stage III and all the way to stage IV (medullary paralysis). Such anesthetics are occasionally referred to as 100% or complete anesthetics. On the other hand, nitrous oxide and ethylene can only take a patient down through plane 1 of stage III as long as their concentration in the inspired air does not exceed 80%, leading to hypoxia. Since plane 1 represents in a general way 25% of the planes in stage III, such weak anesthetics are sometimes referred to as 25% or incomplete anesthetics.

The safety of general anesthetics in terms of approximate therapeutic index is not very great. For example, the anesthetic blood concentration of ether is 120 mg./100 ml. and the lethal concentration is 180 mg./100 ml. What makes these agents safe enough in the hands of a competent anesthesiologist is *controllability*, or rapid elimination when the anesthetic is discontinued.

Individual features of the safety of the anesthetics will be discussed in relation to the various agents.

EFFECT ON PHYSIOLOGIC SYSTEMS

The study of anesthetic effects on physiologic systems is difficult because it is often not clear how much a certain effect attributed to an anesthetic may be caused by anoxia, hypercapnia, or an action secondary to central nervous system depression. This subject will be discussed briefly; the reader is advised to study review articles[65-67,71] for greater details.

NERVOUS SYSTEM

It is generally believed that anesthesia results from depression of the ascending reticular activating system in the brainstem.[65] The ascending activating system may be especially susceptible to anesthetics because of its abundant synapses or some special affinity. The loss of motor tone during anesthesia is largely a consequence of depression of the spinal cord. There is some difference of opinion on peripheral neuromuscular blockade caused by anesthetic concentrations of diethyl ether and by higher concentrations of some other anesthetics. d-Tubocurarine may be potentiated in its action not only by diethyl ether but also by cyclopropane, chloroform, and halothane.[65]

RESPIRATION

Respiratory depression is a common accompaniment of general anesthesia except in the case of diethyl ether, which is often referred to as a respiratory stimulant. This unusual effect of diethyl ether is not well understood. It appears to depress the respiratory center but may reflexly and through metabolic actions cause some stimulation.[65]

The respiratory depressant action of most anesthetics is probably related to depression of the reticular activating system and reduction of the sensitivity of the respiratory center to carbon dioxide.

Tachypnea may be observed not only with ether but also with trichloroethylene and halothane. It has been claimed that these agents sensitize the pulmonary stretch receptors.[65]

CIRCULATION

As a generality, all anesthetics depress the heart and the degree of depression is dependent on concentration.[65] Falling blood pressure is a common accompaniment of anesthesia, except that in the case of ether and cyclopropane there is a compensatory sympathoadrenal activation with demonstrable elevations of plasma norepinephrine.[65] The activation of the sympathetic system counteracts the direct depressant action of the anesthetics on the heart. In the absence of such activation, as in the case of halothane, there is a definite tendency for the blood pressure to fall.

Cardiac arrhythmias are quite common during anesthesia. The injection of epinephrine or norepinephrine is more likely to elicit arrhythmias in animals anesthetized with chloroform, cyclopropane, trichloroethylene, and halothane. Because experimental evidence indicates the danger of ventricular fibrillation, catecholamine injections are best avoided when these anesthetics are employed. The cyclopropane-epinephrine sequence is used in experimental pharmacology for testing antifibrillatory drugs.

Cyclopropane has the reputation of tending to produce arrhythmias with great frequency. It is quite likely that hypercapnia plays an important role in the causation of many of these arrhythmias.

MISCELLANEOUS EFFECTS

Metabolic acidosis may occur during anesthesia, and disturbances in carbohydrate metabolism have been reported, particularly following diethyl ether. In studies on acidosis, hypercapnia and sympathoadrenal activation with lactacidemia have received much attention. There is evidence that anesthetics may interfere with sugar transport into cells peripherally.[65]

Liver damage has been attributed to chloroform. With the introduction of several new halogenated anesthetics such as halothane, the possibility of hepatotoxicity has been carefully studied. Halothane seems to be exonerated as a hazardous hepatotoxic agent by consensus,[70] although some suspicion remains. Halothane may not be hepatotoxic in general, but in a very few individuals its apparent relationship to liver damage is difficult to dismiss.[28]

Nausea and vomiting in the postoperative period are seen more frequently with some anesthetics. Cyclopropane is one of the worst offenders; diethyl ether can also cause this troublesome complication. Halothane, in contrast to most other anesthetics, is not likely to cause nausea and vomiting.

BASIC MECHANISMS OF ANESTHETIC ACTION

The mechanism whereby anesthetics cause a reversible depression of neural activity has interested investigators for many years. While numerous theories have been proposed, most of them are purely descriptive. Some, however, are of considerable interest.

Meyer[33] and Overton[41] were impressed with the relationship between the solubility of anesthetics in oil compared with water, and they found some parallelism between lipid solubility and anesthetic action.

Quastel[49] showed inhibition of oxygen consumption in vitro by barbiturates and some other anesthetics. It is generally believed that biochemical theories based on overall oxygen consumption by anesthetics are not satisfactory. There is poor correlation between the ability of various compounds to depress oxygen consumption of the brain and their anesthetic potency.

Pauling[43] proposed that the gaseous anesthetics may form stable hydrate crystals or clathrates within the central nervous system. This theory is a radical departure from all previous ones in that it emphasizes an effect of anesthetics on water structure rather than on lipids or enzymes. Somewhat similar proposals have been made by others.[34]

The study of the MAC of various anesthetics required to produce a standard analgesic effect indicates again that the potency of various compounds correlates best with their oil/gas partition coefficient.[13] Anesthetics with high lipid solubility are effective at low alveolar concentrations. There is preliminary indication in these studies that anesthesia is produced when the various anesthetics reach a *certain relative saturation* of some lipid structure in the brain. Such a suggestion is in harmony with Ferguson's principle[17] (p. 10), which states that the potency of nonspecific drugs is dependent on the relative saturation of some cellular compartment or "biophase."

CLINICAL CHARACTERISTICS OF COMMONLY USED GENERAL ANESTHETICS

Clinical anesthesia is the result of the interaction of several factors: (1) the physical status of the patient, (2) the working requirements of the surgeon and the anesthesiologist, (3) the effects of available anesthetic drugs, (4) the efficiency of available equipment, and (5) the technical skill of the anesthetist or anesthesiologist. The anesthetic drugs do not overshadow the importance of the other factors, although in some situations one drug may be considered more suitable than others.

The use of general anesthetic agents may produce effects that are nonspecific and unrelated to the individual agent used. Fear and anticipation, interference with control mechanisms, stress reaction, and surgical trauma may all cause release of catecholamines and adrenal steroids, resulting in circulatory and metabolic changes. Decreased renal blood flow and urinary output as well as changes reflected in altered liver function

Table 27-2. Adverse effects of inhalation anesthetics

Adverse effect	Inhalation anesthetic
Myocardial depression and hypotension	Chloroform, halothane, methoxyflurane, ethyl chloride
Myocardial depression compensated by increased sympathetic activity	Ether, cyclopropane
Sensitization of the heart to catecholamines	Chloroform, halothane, cyclopropane, ethyl chloride, trichloroethylene
Liver damage	Chloroform, halothane, ethyl chloride, methoxyflurane, vinyl ether
Kidney damage	Chloroform, methoxyflurane, vinyl ether
Excessive salivation and respiratory secretions	Ether, vinyl ether
Potentiation of neuromuscular blocking drugs	Ether, halothane, methoxyflurane, cyclopropane
Convulsions in children	Vinyl ether, trichloroethylene

tests may result. It is as important to separate these nonspecific effects from the specific action of general anesthetics as it is to delineate the placebo effect from true pharmacologic action in other areas of clinical pharmacology.

INHALATION AGENTS—GASES
NITROUS OXIDE

$$N_2O$$

When administered with at least 20% oxygen, nitrous oxide is not a potent enough gas in most cases to produce full surgical anesthesia. It is therefore commonly used in combination with other drugs, for example, thiopental. The time required for induction and emergence is very short. Unless hypoxia supervenes during nitrous oxide anesthesia, there is no depression of circulation, respiration, or kidney or liver function. Nitrous oxide will not explode and would be a close approach to the ideal anesthetic if it produced good muscle relaxation and had sufficient potency. Muscle tone, however, is normal or increased, and full surgical anesthesia is not obtainable with 80% nitrous oxide except in very ill patients.

CYCLOPROPANE

$$CH_2$$
$$H_2C \triangle CH_2$$

Cyclopropane (trimethylene) is potent, but during induction it is often used in 50% concentration. During the maintenance phase, 10 to 20% is usually sufficient. Induction occurs in 1 to 2 minutes and emergence to clouded consciousness in 5 to 10 minutes, depending on the previous depth and duration of anesthesia.

During surgical anesthesia the pulse rate tends to slow and in light to moderate levels will respond to atropine. Total peripheral resistance is increased, and the myocardium is depressed. Release of catecholamines may be expected to produce serious arrhythmias. Postanesthetic "cyclopropane shock" has been shown to be related to accumulation of carbon dioxide and is prevented by maintaining adequate ventilation.

Marked respiratory depression is prone to occur with cyclopropane, especially when it is combined with other respiratory depressants such as thiopental and narcotics. Although this gas has a peculiar odor, few patients find it disagreeable during induction.

Skeletal muscle relaxation is adequate in surgical levels of anesthesia. In deeper levels the uterus is well relaxed also. Cyclopropane has no special effects on the kidney, liver, or metabolism other than those expected from the general anesthetic process.

The outstanding disadvantages of cyclopropane are that it is explosive and nausea and vomiting often occur during recovery.

ETHYLENE

$$CH_2=CH_2$$

Except for a slightly greater potency, ethylene has practically the same pharmacologic effects as nitrous oxide. In addition, it has two characteristics that make it a poor substitute for nitrous oxide: (1) it is explosive in concentrations used clinically and (2) it has a characteristically unpleasant odor. For these reasons many anesthesiologists do not use this drug at all.

INHALATION AGENTS — VOLATILE LIQUIDS
ETHYL ETHER

$$(C_2H_5)_2O$$

Ether is irritating to the respiratory mucosa, reflexly stimulating respiration. The direct effect on the respiratory center is probably depressant, an obvious effect during deep levels of anesthesia. Respiratory tract secretions are increased, especially when prophylactic atropine is not used.

The blood pressure, pulse, and cardiac rhythm are fairly normal during light to moderate levels of surgical anesthesia. The myocardium may be somewhat depressed, as is the case with cyclopropane, but this effect is normally counteracted by release of catecholamines. Total peripheral resistance is decreased. Although injected epinephrine causes arrhythmias, they do not tend to result in ventricular fibrillation.

Skeletal muscles and also the uterus are well relaxed in deeper levels of ether anesthesia. Liver and kidney effects are clinically similar to cyclopropane. Significant metabolic acidosis is not produced except in special circumstances.

Major disadvantages of ether are its explosiveness, frequency of nausea and vomiting during recovery, slow induction, and slow emergence. Because of its irritating effect, ether is difficult to inhale if used alone for induction.

VINYL ETHER

$$CH_2=CH—O—CH=CH_2$$

Vinyl ether (Vinethene) is very similar in its effects to ethyl ether. It differs from ether in two essential characteristics. First, durations of induction and emergence are very short. Second, liver damage is prone to occur after approximately 1/2 hour of anesthesia and is probably related to hypoxia. For these reasons vinyl ether is most commonly used for open-drop induction in children. It should seldom be used for periods longer than 10 or 15 minutes. Kidney damage and convulsions in children are hazards in the clinical use of vinyl ether.

TRICHLOROETHYLENE

$$CCl_2{=}CHCl$$

Trichloroethylene (Trilene) can be used to produce full surgical anesthesia. Induction and emergence times are relatively short. During surgical anesthesia with this drug, tachypnea and cardiac arrhythmias may occur. Therefore trichloroethylene is used in a manner somewhat similar to nitrous oxide, that is, in concentrations insufficient to produce unconsciousness but sufficient to produce analgesia. When it is used in concentrations below 1%, there is little effect upon the circulation or respiration. Trichloroethylene does not damage the liver or kidneys and in analgesic concentrations does not produce any skeletal muscle relaxation whatever. Arrhythmias are produced if epinephrine is injected during trichloroethylene anesthesia. The anesthetic may cause convulsions in children.

HALOTHANE

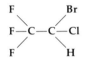

Halothane (Fluothane) is a potent vapor that is clinically very similar to chloroform except for less tendency to cause liver damage. The rate of induction is not much faster than with ether, but the rate of emergence is more rapid. In concentrations below 2% there is relatively little effect upon the circulation or respiration, but in greater concentrations the blood pressure tends to fall and respiratory minute volume decreases.

The main circulatory effects of halothane result from both its central actions[2] and its direct depression of the myocardium. Initially, hypotension and bradycardia can be reversed by atropine, but not in the deeper levels of anesthesia. Total peripheral resistance is decreased. *There is no reflex sympathoadrenal activation, as in the case of ether or cyclopropane, to counteract the depressant action on the heart.*

Halothane causes very little respiratory tract irritation to oppose its direct depressant effect on the respiratory center. Tachypnea may develop.

Skeletal muscle relaxation is adequate, and in deeper levels marked relaxation of the uterus occurs with halothane.

An important clinical feature of halothane is that it causes very little nausea and vomiting.

Although halothane anesthesia may be followed by hepatic failure,[6] this is rare and is probably not a direct effect of the anesthetic, such factors as hypoxia, hypercapnia, and ischemia probably being involved.[70] Suspicion remains that in a rare individual halothane may be causally connected with hepatic failure. Recurrent hepatitis attributable to halothane suggests sensitization or idiosyncrasy.[28]

The advantages of halothane are that it is easy to administer, it produces little nausea and vomiting, and it is nonexplosive. Its disadvantages are that it is expensive, it tends to depress respiration and circulation, and it may cause hepatic failure.

METHOXYFLURANE

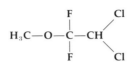

Methoxyflurane (Penthrane) is a potent nonexplosive anesthetic with such low vapor pressure that it is relatively difficult to vaporize, resulting in an unusual safety factor. Since induction and emergence are very slow, thiopental is usually employed for rapid induction, and the anesthetic is stopped 1/2 hour before the operation is to end. Its effects on circulation and respiration are similar to those of halothane.

The outstanding feature of this drug is the remarkable skeletal muscle relaxation that occurs in light anesthesia. This may be due to an action on the spinal cord.[38] Renal and hepatic damage may occur after the use of methoxyflurane, although this may be difficult to demonstrate in animal experiments.[8]

FLUROXENE

$$CF_3 - CH_2 - O - CH = CH_2$$

Fluroxene (Fluoromar) is a volatile liquid with an anesthetic potency similar to that of diethyl ether. Chemically it is 1,1,1-trifluoroethyl vinyl ether. For surgical anesthesia, fluroxene is used in 3 to 8% concentrations. It is flammable in air in concentrations of 4 to 12%. This anesthetic has not achieved widespread favor, although some anesthesiologists find it quite useful. It is potentially hepatotoxic.

CHLOROFORM

$$CHCl_3$$

Chloroform is a potent nonexplosive anesthetic with fairly rapid induction and emergence. Hypotension, arrhythmias, and respiratory depression are prone to occur, especially beyond light levels of anesthesia. It is not particularly irritating to breathe and seldom produces respiratory tract secretions. In the past many cases of severe liver damage and subsequent death have occurred following the use of chloroform. Undoubtedly many of these deaths could be explained on the basis of hypoventilation and its deleterious effects on the liver. However, chloroform, like most chlorinated hydrocarbons, seems to have a certain inherent capability to produce liver and kidney damage. For this reason it is seldom used today.

ETHYL CHLORIDE

$$CH_3 - CH_2Cl$$

Ethyl chloride is a potent drug that produces very rapid induction of anesthesia. It is a powerful circulatory and respiratory depressant, is difficult to control, and has resulted in many anesthetic fatalities. It is not a drug that can be safely used. It is hepatotoxic.

INTRAVENOUS AGENTS
FACTORS DETERMINING THE DURATION OF ACTION OF
INTRAVENOUS ANESTHETICS

It was previously held that the fat stores of the body were responsible for the relatively short action of the so-called ultrashort-acting barbiturates.[3, 5] However, it has been shown that aqueous tissues such as muscle, because of their high exposure, exert a far more profound influence on circulating levels during the initial portion of an anesthetic.[45] After approximately 1 hour, these tissues become saturated, and then fatty tissues, in spite of their low exposure rate, can exert an influence. By this time metabolic transformation also becomes important. The distribution and metabolism have been reviewed in considerable detail.[51]

Plasma levels of thiopental fall at a rate of approximately 10 to 15% per hour.[5] The metabolism is actually quite slow. Its metabolites may be excreted in the urine for days. Negligible amounts are found unchanged, and 10 to 25% may appear as thiopental carboxylic acid.[5]

THIOPENTAL

Thiopental (Pentothal) is a potent intravenous anesthetic. In a 2% solution it has a pH of approximately 10. Induction occurs in a matter of seconds, but postanesthetic emergence is often considerably delayed. The fact that thiopental has to be metabolized and redistributed in the tissues rather than excreted through the lungs accounts for the prolonged emergence phase. Large doses given clinically result in circulatory depression. Even small doses produce marked central respiratory depression. It results in no significant liver or kidney damage. In light levels of anesthesia, skeletal muscle tone is normal or increased, but in very deep levels of anesthesia, skeletal muscle relaxation occurs. This drug is commonly used to provide rapid, pleasant induction. It is followed by some other general anesthetic or may be used in combination with nitrous oxide for relatively short operations.

Thiopental is the thioanalog of pentobarbital (Nembutal). Thiamylal (Surital) is the thioanalog of secobarbital (Seconal). The clinical pharmacologic effects of thiopental and thiamylal are indistinguishable.

Several other barbiturates such as methitural (Neraval) and methohexital (Brevital) have been introduced, with claims for shorter awakening time and various other advantages over thiopental. To date no drug has shown sufficient advantage over thiopental to supplant it in clinical use.

HYDROXYDIONE

Hydroxydione (Viadril) is a steroid (21-hydroxy-pregnanedione sodium succinate) without hormonal effects. Sleep is very slowly induced and poor analgesia results. Hypotension and thrombophlebitis are prone to occur. The disadvantages associated with this drug outweigh its advantages, and therefore it has not received clinical acceptance.

KETAMINE HYDROCHLORIDE

A nonbarbiturate intravenous anesthetic, ketamine is related to phencyclidine (Sernylan) that was abandoned because of its psychotomimetic effects. Chemically ketamine is 2-chlorophenyl-2-methylamino-cyclohexanone.

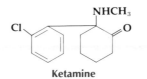

Ketamine

Ketamine is sometimes referred to as a "dissociative" anesthetic because the patient receiving it becomes unresponsive not only to pain but to the environment in general. Anesthesia is of short duration and is accompanied by blood pressure elevation, vivid dreams, hallucinations, and psychologic disturbances after recovery. The psychic reactions apparently are more likely to occur in children. Ketamine hydrochloride (Ketalar; Ketaject) is available in solutions containing 10 mg./ml. for intravenous and intramuscular injection.

RECTAL AGENTS

The rectal route is seldom used, even in children. Slow, irregular, and unpredictable absorption is characteristic of administration in this fashion. Tribromoethanol has been used as a rectally administered general anesthetic but is now obsolete.

PREANESTHETIC MEDICATION

In addition to the anesthetics themselves, a considerable number of drugs are used before and during surgical operations. The drugs given as preanesthetic medications have some definite indications, although some may have distinct disadvantages.

The justifications for using preanesthetic medications or anesthetic adjuncts are (1) to decrease anxiety, (2) to increase the effectiveness of an incomplete anesthetic such as nitrous oxide, (3) to reduce the amount of anesthetic needed, and (4) to antagonize or prevent undesirable actions of the anesthetics.

Among the most commonly used adjuncts are morphine and other narcotics, sedatives, hypnotics, and antianxiety agents, phenothiazines and nonphenothiazine antiemetics, skeletal muscle relaxants, anticholinergic drugs, antiarrhythmic drugs, and vasopressors. Most of these drugs have been discussed elsewhere. **Fentanyl citrate** (Sublimaze) is one of the strong narcotic analgesics having a short duration of action. It is used occasionally as a preanesthetic medication. It is a strong respiratory depressant, but its action is antagonized by the usual narcotic antagonists, nallorphine and levallorphan. Fentanyl is sometimes used in combination with **droperidol** (Inapsine), the combination (**Innovar**) being recommended to produce "*neuroleptanesthesia*," a concept that is difficult to define. Droperidol is a butyrophenone having the pharmacologic characteristics of a phenothiazine. Innovar, being a fixed-dose combination, is frowned on by many authorities. It may greatly increase the respiratory-depressant effects of barbiturates and related drugs, which must be used in reduced dosage when preceded by the administration of Innovar.

The most accepted preanesthetic medications are the following: a short-acting barbiturate such as pentobarbital or secobarbital the evening before the operation; morphine, 10 mg. subcutaneously 40 to 60 minutes before induction; and atropine, 0.65 mg. 45 to 60 minutes before induction.

All the drugs commonly used as preanesthetic medications have some disadvantages. Morphine and other narcotics tend to prolong the anesthetic state and may cause bronchial constriction in susceptible individuals. The barbiturates may contribute to postoperative excitement since they have no analgesic properties. Atropine, particularly when used *during* the operative procedure and with cyclopropane, can cause considerable arrhythmias and transient cardiac slowing. Despite these disadvantages, the use of a limited number of well-selected preanesthetic medications is justified.

References

1 Artusio, J. F.: Ether analgesia: A detailed description of the first stage of ether anesthesia in man, J. Pharmacol. Exp. Ther. 111:343, 1954.

2 Blackmore, W. P., Erwin, K. W., Wiegand, O. F., and Lipsey, R.: Renal and cardiovascular effects of halothane, Anesthesiology 21:489, 1960.

3 Brodie, B. B., Bernstein, E., and Mark, L. C.: The role of body fat in limiting the duration of action of pentothal, J. Pharmacol. Exp. Ther. 105:421, 1952.

4 Brodie, B. B., Burns, J. J., Mark, L. C., Lief, P. A., Bernstein, E., and Papper, E. M.: The fate of pentobarbital in man and dog and a method for its estimation in biological material, J. Pharmacol. Exp. Ther. 109:26, 1953.

5 Brodie, B. B., Mark, L. C., Papper, E. M., Lief, P. A., Bernstein, E., and Rovenstine, E. A.: The fate of thiopental in man and a method for its estimation in biological material, J. Pharmacol. Exp. Ther. 98:85, 1950.

6 Bunker, J. P., and Blumenfeld, C. M.: Liver necrosis after halothane anesthesia: cause or coincidence? New Eng. J. Med. 268:531, 1963.

7 Butler, T. G.: Theories of general anesthesia, Pharmacol. Rev. 2:121, 1950.

8 Cale, J. O., Parks, C. R., and Jenkins, M. T.: Hepatic and renal effects on methoxyflurane in dogs, Anesthesiology 23:248, 1962.

9 Davis, H. S., Collins, W. F., Randt, C. T., and Dillon, W. H.: Effect of anesthetic agents on evoked central nervous system responses: gaseous agents, Anesthesiology 18:634, 1957.

10 Davis, H. S., Dillon, W. H., Collins, W. F., and Randt, C. T.: Effect of anesthetic agents on evoked central nervous system responses: muscle relaxants and volatile agents, Anesthesiology 19:441, 1958.

11 Dundee, J. W., Knox, J. W., and Black, G. W.: Ketamine as an induction agent in anesthetics, Lancet 1:1370, 1970.

12 Eger, E. I., II.: Effect of inspired anesthetic concentration on the rate of rise of alveolar concentration, Anesthesiology 24:153, 1963.

13 Eger, E. I., II, Brandstater, B., Saidman, L. J., Regan, M. J., Severinghaus, J. W., and Munson, E. S.: Equipotent alveolar concentrations of methoxyflurane, halothane, diethyl ether, fluoxene, cyclopropane, xenon and nitrous oxide in the dog, Anesthesiology 26:771, 1965.

14 Ellis, S., and Wolfson, S. K.: Theories of anesthesia involving interference with oxygen metabolism: action of general anesthetics on the anaerobic turtle, J. Pharmacol. Exp. Ther. 106:284, 1952.

15 Epstein, R. M., Rackow, H., Salanitre, E., and Wolf, G.: Influence of the concentration effect on the uptake of anesthetic mixtures: the second gas effect, Anesthesiology 25:364, 1964.

16 Etsten, B., and Li, T.: Current concepts of myocardial function during anesthesia, Brit. J. Anaesth. 34:884, 1962.

17 Ferguson, J.: The use of chemical potentials as indices of toxicity, Proc. Roy. Soc. [Biol.] 127:387, 1939.

18 Forssmann, S., and Holmquist, C.: The relation between inhaled and exhaled trichlorethylene and trichloracetic acid excreted in the urine of rats exposed to trichlorethylene, Acta Pharmacol. 9:235, 1953.

19 French, J. D., and King, E. E.: Mechanisms involved in the anesthetic state, Surgery 38:228, 1955.

20 French, J. D., Verzeano, M., and Magoun, H. W.: A neural basis of the anesthetic state, Arch. Neurol. Psychiat. 69:519, 1953.

21 French, J. D., Verzeano, M., and Magoun, H. W.: An extra-lemniscial sensory system in the brain, Arch. Neurol. Psychiat. 69:505, 1953.

22 Gross, E. G., and Cullen, S. C.: The effects of anesthetic agents on muscular contraction, J. Pharmacol. Exp. Ther. 78:358, 1943.

23 Guedel, A.: Third stage ether analgesia: subclassification regarding significance of position and movements of eyeball, Amer. J. Surg. 34:53, 1920.

24 Haggard, H. W.: Absorption, distribution and elimination of ethyl ether. IV. Anesthetic tension of ether and physiological response to various concentration, J. Biol. Chem. 59:783, 1924.

25 Harris, T. A. B.: The mode of action of anesthetics, Edinburgh, 1951, E. & S. Livingstone, Ltd.

26 Katz, R. L.: Neuromuscular effects of diethyl ether and its interaction with succinylcholine and d-tubocurarine, Anesthesiology 27:52, 1966.

27 Kety, S. S.: Theory and applications of exchange of inert gas at lungs and tissues, Pharmacol. Rev. 3:1, 1951.

28 Klatskin, G., and Kimberg, D. V.: Recurrent hepatitis attributable to halothane sensitization in an anesthetist, New Eng. J. Med. 280:515, 1969.

29 Larrabee, M. G., and Holaday, D. A.: Depression of transmission through sympathetic ganglia during general anesthesia, J. Pharmacol. Exp. Ther. 105:400, 1952.

30 Larrabee, M. G., and Posternak, J. M.: Selective action of anesthetics on synapses and axons in mammalian sympathetic ganglia, J. Neurophysiol. 15:91, 1952.

31 Larson, C. P., Jr.: Solubility and partition coefficients. In Papper, E. M., and Kitz, R. J., editors: Uptake and distribution of anesthetic agents, New York, 1962, McGraw-Hill Book Co.

32 Manning, J. W., Cotten, M. D., Kelly, W. N., and Johnson, C. E.: Mechanism of cardiac arrhythmias induced by diencephalic stimulation, Amer. J. Physiol. 203:1120, 1962.

33 Meyer, H. H.: Zur Theorie der Alkoholmarkose. III. Mitt der Einfluss wechselnder Temperatur auf Wirkungstärke und Teilungskoefficient der Narkotika, Arch. Exp. Path. Pharmakol. 46:338, 1901.

34 Miller, S.: A theory of gaseous anesthetics, Proc. Nat. Acad. Sci. 47:1515, 1961.

35 Morris, L. E., and Feldman, S. A.: Influence of hypercarbia and hypotension upon liver damage following halothane anesthesia, Anaesthesia 18:32, 1963.

36 Moruzzi, G., and Magnoun, H. W.: Brainstem reticular formation and activation of the EEG, Electroenceph. Clin. Neurophysiol. 1:455, 1949.

37 Mullins, L. J.: Some physical mechanisms in narcosis, Chem. Rev. 54:289, 1954.

38 Ngai, S. H., and Hanks, E. C.: Effect of methoxyflurane on electromyogram, neuromuscular transmission, and spinal reflexes, Anesthesiology 23:158, 1962.

39 Ngai, S. H., and Papper, E. M.: Metabolic effects of anesthesia, Springfield, Ill., 1962, Charles C Thomas, Publisher.

40 Orcutt, F. S., and Waters, R. M.: Diffusion of nitrous oxide, ethylene, and carbon dioxide through human skin during anesthesia, including new method for estimating nitrous oxide in low concentrations, Anesth. Analg. 12:45, 1933.

41 Overton, E.: Studien uber die Narkose zugleich ein Beitrag zur algemeinen Pharmakologie, Jena, 1901, G. Fischer.

42 Panner, B. J., Freeman, R. B., Roth-Moyo, L. A., and Markowitch, W.: Toxicity following methoxyflurane anesthesia, J.A.M.A. 214:86, 1970.

43 Pauling, L.: A molecular theory of general anesthesia, Science 134:15, 1961.

44 Powell, J. F.: Trichlorethylene: absorption, elimination, and metabolism, Brit. J. Indust. Med. 2:142, 1945.

45 Price, H. L.: A dynamic concept of the distribution of thiopental in the human body, Anesthesiology 21:40, 1960.

46 Price, H. L.: General anesthesia and circulatory homeostasis, Physiol. Rev. 40:187, 1960.

47 Price, H. L., Linde, H. W., Jones, R. E., Black, G. W., and Price, M. L.: Sympathoadrenal response to general anesthesia in man and their relation to hemodynamics, Anesthesiology 20:563, 1959.

48 Price, H. L., and Widdicombe, J.: Actions of cyclopropane on carotid sinus baroreceptors and carotid body chemoreceptors, J. Pharmacol. Exp. Ther. 135:233, 1962.

49 Quastel, J. H.: Biochemical aspects of narcosis, Anesth. Analg. 31:151, 1952.

50 Raventos, J.: The action of fluothane—a new volatile anesthetic, Brit. J. Pharmacol. 11:394, 1956.

51 Richards, R. K., and Taylor, J. D.: Some factors influencing distribution, metabolism and action of barbiturates: a review, Anesthesiology 17:414, 1956.

52 Snow, J.: On chloroform and other anesthetics: their action and administration, London, 1848, John Churchill. Reprinted in Brit. J. Anaesth. 25:51, 1953.

53 Sollman, T.: A manual of pharmacology, ed 7, Philadelphia, 1948, W. B. Saunders Co.

54 Vandam, L. D., and Moore, F. D.: Adrenocortical mechanisms related to anesthesia, Anesthesiology 21:531, 1960.

55 Watland, D. C., Long, J. P., Pittinger, C. B., and Cullen, S. C.: Neuromuscular effects of ether, cyclopropane, chloroform, and fluothane, Anesthesiology 18:883, 1957.

56 Zauder, H. L., Massa, L. S., and Orkin, L. R.: Effects of general anesthetics on tissue oxygen "tensions," Anesthesiology 24:142, 1963.

Recent reviews

57 Alper, M. H., Flacke, W., and Krayer, O.: Pharmacology of reserpine and its implica-

tions for anesthesia, Anesthesiology **24**:524, 1963.

58 Bendixen, H. H., and Laver, M. B.: Hypoxia in anesthesia: a review, Clin. Pharmacol. Ther. **6**:510, 1965.

59 Bunker, J. P.: Final report of the national halothane study; editorial views, Anesthesiology **29**:231, 1968.

60 Dobkin, A. B., and Po-Giok Su, J.: Newer anesthetics and their uses, Clin. Pharmacol. Ther. **7**:648, 1966.

61 Dundee, J. W.: Clinical pharmacology of general anesthetics, Clin. Pharmacol. Ther. **8**:91, 1967.

62 Dykes, M. H. M., and Bunker, J. P.: Hepatotoxicity and anesthetics, Pharmacol. Physicians **4**(11):1, 1970.

63 Markee, S.: Pharmacologic considerations in the selection of a general anesthetic, Pharmacol. Physicians **2**(6):1, 1968.

64 Ngai, S. H., Mark, L. C., and Papper, E. M.: Pharmacologic and physiologic aspects of anesthesiology, New Eng. J. Med. **282**:479, 541, 1970.

65 Ngai, S. H., and Papper, E. M.: Anesthesiology, New Eng. J. Med. **269**:28, 1963.

66 Ngai, S. H., and Papper, E. M.: Anesthesiology, New Eng. J. Med. **269**:83, 1963.

67 Ngai, S. H., and Papper, E. M.: Anesthesiology, New Eng. J. Med. **269**:142, 1963.

68 Papper, E. M., and Kitz, R. J., editors: Uptake and distribution of anesthetic agents, New York, 1963, McGraw-Hill Book Co.

69 Stephen, C. R.: Anesthesia, 1972, Med. Coll. Va. Quart. **8**:100, 1972.

70 Summary of the national halothane study, J.A.M.A. **197**:775, 1966.

71 Vandam, L. D.: Anesthesia, Ann. Rev. Pharmacol. **6**:379, 1966.

28 Pharmacology of local anesthesia

GENERAL CONCEPT

Local anesthetics are drugs that are employed to produce a transient and reversible loss of sensation in a circumscribed area of the body. They achieve this effect by interfering with nerve conduction.

In 1884 Köller, who had studied *cocaine* with Sigmund Freud, introduced the drug into medicine as a topical anesthetic in ophthalmology. This was the beginning of the first era in the history of local anesthesia.

The second era began in 1904 with the introduction of *procaine* by Einhorn. This was the first safe local anesthesia suitable for injection. Procaine remained the most widely used local anesthetic until the introduction of *lidocaine* (Xylocaine), which is considered the agent of choice for infiltration at present. Other local anesthetics of importance are *tetracaine, mepivacaine, prilocaine,* and *bupivacaine*. All of these drugs are either esters or amides, and they differ from each other in their toxicity, metabolism, onset, and duration of action. Lidocaine, in addition to being an important local anesthetic, has important uses as an antiarrhythmic agent (p. 398).

Electrophysiologic studies indicate that the local anesthetics interfere with the rate of rise of the depolarization phase of the action potential. As a consequence the cell does not depolarize sufficiently after excitation to fire. Thus the propagated action potential is blocked by these drugs.

CLASSIFICATION OF LOCAL ANESTHETICS

Local anesthetics may be classified according to their chemistry or on the basis of their clinical usage.

ACCORDING TO CHEMISTRY

Local anesthetics are either esters or amides. They consist of an aromatic portion, an intermediate chain, and an amine portion. The aromatic portion confers lipophilic properties to the molecule, whereas the amine portion is hydrophilic. The ester or amide components of the molecule determine the characteristics of metabolic degradation. The esters are mostly hydrolyzed in plasma by pseudocholinesterase, whereas the amides are destroyed largely in the liver.

Esters of benzoic acid
    Cocaine
    Tetracaine (Pontocaine)
    Piperocaine (Metycaine)
    Hexylcaine (Cyclaine)
    Ethyl aminobenzoate (Benzocaine)
    Butacaine (Butyn)

Esters of *p*-aminobenzoic acid
    Procaine (Novocain)
    Butethamine (Monocaine)
    Chloroprocaine (Nesacaine)

Esters of meta-aminobenzoic acid
    Cyclomethycaine (Surfacaine)
    Metabutoxycaine (Primacaine)

Amides
  Lidocaine (Xylocaine)
  Dibucaine (Nupercaine)
  Mepivacaine (Carbocaine)
  Prilocaine (Citanest)

ACCORDING TO CLINICAL USAGE

Local anesthetics have several types of clinical applications, and their suitability for these varies with their pharmacologic properties. Some of these applications are (1) infiltration and block anesthesia, (2) surface anesthesia, (3) spinal anesthesia, (4) epidural and caudal anesthesia, and (5) intravenous anesthesia. In the following list the drugs of greatest interest are italicized.

Infiltration and block anesthesia: *procaine, chloroprocaine, hexylcaine, lidocaine,* mepivacaine, piperocaine, prilocaine, propoxycaine, and tetracaine; also, in dentistry: butethamine, metabutethamine, isobucaine, meprylcaine, and pyrrocaine

Surface anesthesia: *benzocaine, benoxinate, butacaine, butyl aminobenzoate, cocaine,* cyclomethycaine, dibucaine, dimethisoquin, diperodon, dyclonine, hexylcaine, lidocaine, phenacaine, piperocaine, pramoxine, proparacaine, and tetracaine; also, benzyl alcohol, phenol, and ethyl chloride

Spinal anesthesia (subarachnoid or intrathecal): *tetracaine,* procaine, dibucaine, lidocaine, mepivacaine, and piperocaine

Epidural and caudal anesthesia: *lidocaine, prilocaine, and mepivacaine;* also, procaine, chloroprocaine, piperocaine, and tetracaine

Intravenous anesthesia: *lidocaine and procaine* (seldom used for anesthesia but for other indications)

MODE OF ACTION OF LOCAL ANESTHETICS

Electrophysiologic studies indicate that the local anesthetics do not alter the resting membrane potential or threshold potential of nerves. They act on the rate of rise of the depolarization phase of the act on potential. Since depolarization does not reach the point at which firing occurs, propagated action potential fails to occur.

The effects of local anesthetics on ionic fluxes are of great interest, and recent studies emphasize the relationships between these drugs and the calcium ion with secondary effects on sodium fluxes. Although no detailed discussion will be attempted,[22] local anesthetic agents appear to compete with calcium for a site in the nerve membrane that controls the passage of sodium across the membrane. It is believed at present that calcium is bound to phospholipids in the cell membrane. A fair correlation could be found between local anesthetic potency and their ability to prevent the binding of calcium by phosphatidylserine in artificial membranes.

Experimental studies[1] indicate also that an increase in calcium concentration is able to overcome the nerve block produced by local anesthetics.

Active form of the local anesthetics

Problem 28-1. When the hydrochloride of a local anesthetic is injected, which is the active form, the uncharged base or the charged cation? When dealing with an intact isolated nerve, the local anesthetics such as lidocaine are more potent in an alkaline solution, suggesting the uncharged base as the active form.[26] On the other hand, when a desheathed nerve is used, the less alkaline preparations are more efficacious. It is believed at present that the uncharged base penetrates better across the nerve sheath, but it is the charged cation that exerts its pharmacologic effect.[26] The problem is complicated by the fact that the results are not applicable to all members of the series of local anesthetics.[22]

ACTION ON VARIOUS NERVE FIBERS

According to diameter, myelination, and conduction velocities, nerve fibers can be classified into three types—A, B, and C fibers.[7] The A fibers have a diameter of 1 to 20μ, are myelinated, and have conduction velocities up to 100 m./sec. Somatic motor and some sensory fibers fall into this classification. Blockade of these fibers results in skeletal muscle relaxation, loss of thermal and tactile sensation, proprioceptive loss, and loss of the sensation of sharp pain. B fibers vary in diameter from 1 to 3μ, are myelinated, and conduct at intermediate velocities. Preganglionic fibers fall into this group, and their blockade obviously results in autonomic paralysis. C fibers are usually under 1μ in diameter and are not myelinated, and conduction velocity is approximately 1 m./sec. Postganglionic fibers as well as more somatic sensory fibers fall into this classification. Blockade results in autonomic paralysis; loss of the sensation of itch, tickle, and dull pain; and loss of much of the thermal sensation.

Clinically the general order of loss of function is as follows: (1) pain, (2) temperature, (3) touch, (4) proprioception, and (5) skeletal muscle tone. If pressure is exerted on a mixed nerve, the fibers are depressed in somewhat the reverse order.

In summary, local anesthetic drugs depress the small, unmyelinated fibers first and the larger, myelinated fibers last. The time for the onset of action is shorter for the smaller fibers, and the concentration of drug required is less.

ABSORPTION, FATE, AND EXCRETION OF LOCAL ANESTHETICS

Absorption of the various local anesthetics is a function of the site of injection, the degree of vasodilation caused by the agent itself, the dose, and the presence of a vaso-constrictor in the solution. Epinephrine added to a procaine hydrochloride solution greatly increases its duration of action as an infiltration agent. The rate of absorption of lidocaine is greater than that of prilocaine, probably because of the vasodilator action of lidocaine.

The onset and duration of action of various local anesthetics as determined by a standardized ulnar block technique are shown in Table 28-1.

Local anesthetics of the ester type are hydrolyzed by plasma pseudocholinesterase. Those having the amide linkage are largely destroyed in the liver.

In man, procaine is broken down to p-aminobenzoic acid,[4] 80% of which is excreted

Table 28-1. Onset and duration of action of various local anesthetics determined by a standardized ulnar block technique*

Drug	Concentration	Relative potency	Onset in minutes	Duration of action in minutes
Procaine	1	1	7	19
Lidocaine	1	4	5	40
Mepivacaine	1	4	4	99
Prilocaine	1	4	3	98
Tetracaine†	0.25	16	7	135
Bupivacaine†	0.25	16	8	415

*Modified from Covino,[22] based on data from Albert.[3]
†Solutions contain epinephrine 1 : 200,000.

Table 28-2. Relative hydrolysis rates of local anesthetics by plasma esterase

Local anesthetic	Rate of hydrolysis
Piperocaine	6.5
Chloroprocaine	5.0
Procaine	1.0
Tetracaine	0.2
Dibucaine	0

in the urine, and diethylaminoethanol, 30% of which is excreted in the urine. Only 2% is excreted unchanged in the urine. Only 10 to 20% of lidocaine appears unchanged, the rest being metabolized, presumably mainly in the liver.[9]

Procaine is hydrolyzed in spinal fluid 150 times more slowly than in plasma, there being very little esterase present. The hydrolysis is due to the alkalinity of the spinal fluid and is approximately the same as with a buffer having the same pH.[6]

Lidocaine is metabolized in the liver by removal of one or both ethyl groups from the molecule. The resulting metabolites, monoethylglycinexylidide (MEGX) and glycinexilidine (GX), still have pharmacologic activity and may contribute to CNS toxicity.[18]

METHODS OF ADMINISTERING LOCAL ANESTHETICS

Local anesthetics may be administered by topical application, by infiltration of tissues to bathe fine nerve elements, by injection adjacent to nerves and their branches, and by injection into the epidural or subarachnoid spaces. Occasionally intravenous injections are utilized to control certain pain situations. The details of subarachnoid and epidural anesthesia are outside the intended scope of this discussion.

SYSTEMIC ACTIONS OF LOCAL ANESTHETICS

Local anesthetics exert their effect largely on a circumscribed area. Nevertheless, they are absorbed from the site of injection and may exert systemic effects, particularly on the cardiovascular system and the central nervous system and particularly when an excessive dose is utilized.

CARDIOVASCULAR EFFECTS

Since lidocaine is widely used as an antiarrhythmic drug, much has been learned about its effect on the heart, and this information is generally also applicable to the other local anesthetics. At nontoxic concentrations lidocaine alters or abolishes the rate of slow diastolic depolarization in Purkinje's fibers and may shorten the effective refractory period as well as the duration of the action potential. In toxic doses lidocaine decreases the maximal depolarization of Purkinje's fibers and reduces conduction velocity. Such doses may also have a direct negative inotropic effect.

The local anesthetics tend to relax the vascular smooth muscle, but cocaine can cause vasoconstriction by blocking the reuptake of norepinephrine.[22]

CENTRAL NERVOUS SYSTEM EFFECTS

Although the usual local anesthesia produces no central nervous system effects, increased doses may cause excitatory effects resulting in convulsions and eventually respiratory depression. It is believed on the basis of animal experiments that the local anesthetics may block inhibitory cortical synapses.[22] This leads to excitation. Larger doses depress both inhibitory and facilitory neurons leading to depression.

MISCELLANEOUS EFFECTS

Compared with their actions on the cardiovascular system and the central nervous system, the local anesthetics have few important additional effects. They may depress ganglionic transmission and neuromuscular transmission. These actions are unimportant unless some other potent agent is used concomitantly. For example, lidocaine may enhance the action of neuromuscular blocking agents.

VASOCONSTRICTORS AND LOCAL ANESTHETICS

Vasoconstrictors, particularly epinephrine, are commonly added to local anesthetic solutions that are to be used for infiltration or nerve block. The purpose is to prevent absorption of the drug and thereby prolong its action locally and reduce systemic reactions. Concentrations of epinephrine used for this purpose in local anesthesia vary from 2 to 10 μg/ml., or 1:500,000 to 1:100,000.

Although the addition of epinephrine to such drugs as procaine is sound, other drugs such as lidocaine, prilocaine, and mepivacaine may be used without the addition of vasoconstrictors.

Epinephrine may contribute to the systemic effects of local anesthetics and may be responsible for symptoms such as anxiety, tachycardia, and hypertension.

TOXICITY OF LOCAL ANESTHETICS

There are many popular misconceptions about toxicity of the local anesthetics. Procaine is considered extremely safe; yet tetracaine is considered extremely dangerous. Although tetracaine is ten times more toxic in animal studies than is procaine, when compared on a milligram basis, its potency is also ten times greater. When used clinically in concentrations one tenth that of procaine and in equal volumes, the clinical toxicity is the same. The ratio of toxicity to potency gives a clearer indication of relative toxicity: procaine 1:1 = tetracaine 10:10.

The majority of toxic reactions are due to overdosage. The figures given in Table 28-3 refer to maximum safe dosages, determined in milligrams per kilogram of body weight,

Table 28-3. Maximum safe dosages of local anesthetics administered to healthy adults without inadvertent intravascular or subarachnoid injection

Anesthetic	mg./kg. of body weight
4% cocaine	1 (topical)
1% procaine	10 (injection)
0.15% tetracaine	1 (injection)
1% lidocaine	5 (injection)

administered to healthy adults without inadvertent intravascular or subarachnoid injection.

In rare instances reactions occur in the form of apparently allergic manifestations such as skin wheals or bronchospasm. In actual practice the most common symptoms associated with administration of local anesthetics are not due to the local anesthetic drug at all. Emotional factors secondary to fear, anxiety, and pain produce symptoms in the majority of patients. Vasopressors such as epinephrine, added to the local anesthetic to slow absorption, are often used in sufficient quantities to produce systemic symptoms. Other toxic manifestations are tissue irritation and contact dermatitis.

In general the true pharmacologic signs of toxicity from local anesthetics are central nervous system stimulation followed by depression and peripheral cardiovascular depression. Salivation and tremor, convulsion, and coma, associated with hypertension and tachycardia and followed by hypotension, all occurring in a few minutes, represent the full-blown picture.

The treatment is symptomatic and essentially involves restoration of normal ventilation and circulation. Barbiturates in doses greater than hypnotic are effective in the *prevention* of central nervous system stimulation caused by local anesthetics.

CLINICAL CHARACTERISTICS OF COMMONLY USED LOCAL ANESTHETICS
COCAINE

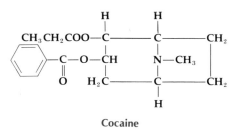

Cocaine

Cocaine is too toxic to be injected into the tissues and is therefore used only topically. It produces excellent topical anesthesia and vasoconstriction, which results in shrinkage of mucous membranes. Absorption from the urinary mucous membranes is rapid, and cocaine should not be used in this area. Some clinicians feel that vasoconstriction with 10% cocaine is better than with a 4% solution and that toxicity will be less with the stronger preparation because the cocaine will be more slowly absorbed. This may be dangerous, however. The vasoconstrictor effect of cocaine and potentiation by this local anesthetic of the actions of catecholamines are most likely consequences of inhibition of the uptake of catecholamines by adrenergic nerve terminals. Cocaine abuse is discussed on p. 312.

ETHYL AMINOBENZOATE

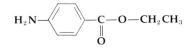

Ethyl aminobenzoate

Ethyl aminobenzoate (Benzocaine) is so poorly soluble that it is not absorbed from mucous membranes. Ointments containing 5 to 10% concentrations of ethyl aminobenzoate provide potent, safe topical anesthesia.

PROCAINE

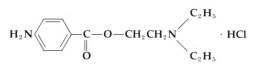

Procaine hydrochloride

Procaine (Novocain) is the standard against which all local anesthetics are compared. However, it has the disadvantage of producing poor topical anesthesia. Its duration of action is approximately 1 hour but can be significantly prolonged by the addition of epinephrine. Onset of anesthesia occurs rapidly. Afterward the patient often notes only the soreness produced by the needle used for injection. Procaine will block small to large nerve fibers in concentrations of 0.5 to 2%.

Chloroprocaine (Nesacaine) is a derivative of procaine that has a much shorter duration of action due to its more rapid hydrolysis. For this reason it has much less toxicity on intravenous injection.

LIDOCAINE

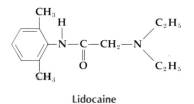

Lidocaine

Lidocaine (Xylocaine) may supplant procaine as the standard of comparison for local anesthetics. It is more potent and more versatile, being suitable not only for infiltration and nerve block but for surface anesthesia as well. This results in a rapid, potent anesthetic effect. It is used in concentrations of 0.5 to 2% and is more potent than equivalent solutions of procaine. Lidocaine has one other characteristic that distinguishes it from procaine and other local anesthetics — it very often produces sedation along with the local anesthesia. Lidocaine differs from most drugs in this group in being an amide rather than an ester. Lidocaine is metabolized in the liver by N-dealkylation Two of the metabolites still have pharmacologic activity and may contribute to toxic reactions in patients with altered metabolism.[18]

TETRACAINE

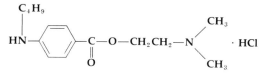

Tetracaine hydrochloride

369

The chief differences between tetracaine (Pontocaine) and procaine and lidocaine are tetracaine's longer time required for full onset of action (10 minutes or more), longer duration of action (approximately 50%), and greater potency. For injection anesthesia, tetracaine is available in 0.15% solution. For topical anesthesia it is used in 1 to 2% concentrations. Tetracaine should not be sprayed into the airway in concentrations greater than 2%. The total dose should be carefully calculated and probably should not, in this situation, exceed 0.5 mg./kg. of body weight. It is rapidly absorbed topically and has resulted in several fatalities from topical misuse. The chief disadvantage of tetracaine is slowness in onset of action.

MEPIVACAINE

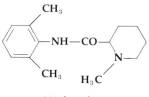

Mepivacaine

Mepivacaine (Carbocaine) has essentially the same clinical effects as lidocaine except for two particular points. It does not spread in the tissues quite as well, and its duration of action is longer.

DIBUCAINE

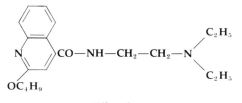

Dibucaine

Dibucaine (Nupercaine) is a very potent local anesthetic having a long duration of action. It is from ten to twenty times as active and toxic as procaine. As a consequence, it is employed in a more dilute solution for injection than procaine (0.05 to 0.1%). It is suitable for topical use and also for spinal anesthesia.

OTHER LOCAL ANESTHETICS

There are numerous other local anesthetics available that are very suitable for clinical use. However, the needs of most physicians can be met by the use of two or three different local anesthetics chosen for different purposes. Familiarity gained from frequent use of a few of these drugs will be reflected in fewer toxic reactions.

References

1 Aceves, J., and Machne, X.: The action of calcium and of local anesthetics on nerve cells, and their interaction during excitation, J. Pharmacol. Exp. Ther. 140:138, 1963.

2 Adriani, J.: Pharmacology of anesthetics, ed. 3, Springfield, Ill., 1952, Charles C Thomas, Publisher.

3 Albert, J., and Löfström, B.: Bilateral ulnar nerve blocks for the evaluation of local anesthe-

tic agents: tests with procaine, Xylocaine and Carbocaine, Acta Anesth. Scand. **5**:99, 1961.

4 Brodie, B. B., Lief, P. A., and Poet, R.: The fate of procaine in man following its intravenous administration and methods for the estimation of procaine and diethylaminoethanol, J. Pharmacol. Exp. Ther. **94**:359, 1948.

5 Crampton, R. S., and Oriscello, R. G.: Petit and grand mal convulsions during lidocaine hydrochloride treatment of ventricular tachycardia, J.A.M.A. **204**:201, 1968.

6 Foldes, F. F., and Aven, M. A.: The hydrolysis of procaine and 2-chloroprocaine in spinal fluid, J. Pharmacol. Exp. Ther. **105**:259, 1952.

7 Galley, A. H.: Caudal analgesia—clinical applications in vasospastic diseases of the legs and in diabetic neuropathy, Proc. Roy. Soc. Med. **45**:748, 1952.

8 Geddes, I. C.: A review of local anesthetics, Brit. J. Anaesth. **26**:208, 1954.

9 Gray, T. C., and Geddes, I. C.: A review of local anesthetics, J. Pharmacol. Physiol. **6**:89, 1954.

10 Hille, B.: Common mode of action of three agents that decrease the transient change in sodium permeability in nerves, Nature **210**: 1220, 1966.

11 Kalow, W.: Hydrolysis of local anesthetics by human serum cholinesterase, J. Pharmacol. Exp. Ther. **104**:122, 1952.

12 Nordqvist, P.: The action of histamine on procaine block in frog nerves, Acta Pharmacol. **8**.183, 1952.

13 Nordqvist, P.: The action of hyaluronidase on frog sciatic nerve with special reference to penetration of procaine, Acta Pharmacol. **8**:195, 1952.

14 Nordqvist, P.: Influence of acetylcholine, decamethonium, and histamine on frog nerves, Acta Pharmacol. **8**:233, 1952.

15 Pizzolato, P., and Renegari, O. J.: Histopathologic effects of long exposure to local anesthetics on peripheral nerves, Anesth. Analg. **38**:138, 1959.

16 Ritchie, J. M., and Greengard, P.: On the active structure of local anesthetics, J. Pharmacol. Exp. Ther. **133**:241, 1961.

17 Skou, J. C.: Local anesthetics; relation between blocking potency and penetration of a monomolecular layer of lipoids from nerves, Acta Pharmacol. **10**:325, 1954.

18 Strong, J. M., Parker, M., and Atkinson, A. J.: Identification of glycinexylidide in patients treated with intravenous lidocaine, Clin. Pharmacol. Ther. **146**:67, 1973.

19 Toman, J. E. P.: Neuropharmacology of peripheral nerve, Pharmacol. Rev. **4**:168, 1952.

Recent reviews

20 Adriani, J., and Zepernick, R.: Some recent studies on the clinical pharmacology of local anesthetics of practical significance, Ann. Surg. **158**:666, 1963.

21 Adriani, J., and Zepernick, R.: Clinical effectiveness of drugs used for topical anesthesia, J.A.M.A. **188**:711, 1964.

22 Covino, B. G.: Local anesthesia, New Eng. J. Med. **286**:975, 1035, 1972.

23 Foldes, F. F., Davidson, G. M., Duncalf, D., and Shigeo, K.: The intravenous toxicity of local anesthetic agents in man, Clin. Pharmacol. Ther. **6**:328, 1965.

24 de Jong, R. H., and Wagman, I. H.: Physiological mechanisms of peripheral nerve block by local anesthetics, Anesthesiology **24**:6484, 1963.

25 Luduena, F. P.: Duration of local anesthesia, Ann. Rev. Pharmacol. **9**:503, 1969.

26 Ritchie, J. M., and Greengard, P.: On the mode of action of local anesthetics, Ann. Rev. Pharmacol. **6**:405, 1966.

27 Shanes, A. M.: Drugs and nerve conduction, Ann. Rev. Pharmacol. **3**:185, 1963.

SECTION SIX

**DRUGS USED IN
CARDIOVASCULAR DISEASE**

Although many drugs exert an effect on the heart, five groups of agents will be discussed in this section either because they act selectively on the heart or because they are particularly useful in the treatment of cardiac disease: digitalis glycosides, antiarrhythmic drugs, coronary vasodilator drugs, anticoagulant drugs, and diuretic drugs. In addition, the hypocholesterolemic agents will be briefly discussed. Antihypertensive drugs were considered in Chapter 14.

29 Digitalis

It has a power over the motion of the heart to a degree yet unobserved in any other medicine, and this power may be converted to salutary ends.

WILLIAM WITHERING, 1785

GENERAL CONCEPT OF THE DIGITALIS EFFECT

Certain steroids and their glycosides have characteristic effects on the contractility and electrophysiology of the heart. Most of these glycosides are obtained from the leaves of the foxglove, *Digitalis purpurea* or *Digitalis lanata,* or from the seeds of *Strophanthus gratus.* These cardioactive steroids are widely used in the treatment of heart failure and in the management of certain arrhythmias. They are collectively referred to as digitalis.

Although catecholamines, methylxanthines, and glucagon also increase the contractility of the myocardium, digitalis must accomplish its effect by a unique mechanism and is by far the most important drug in the treatment of heart failure.

At the molecular level digitalis is a powerful inhibitor of sodium-potassium–adenosine triphosphatase (Na^+-K^+-ATPase). It is possible, although not proved, that the cardiac effects of the glycosides are a consequence of ATPase inhibition with changes in ion distribution.[74] This is most likely for the toxic effects of digitalis but not proved for the therapeutic effects.[70] ATPase inhibition would increase intracellular sodium at the expense of potassium and may secondarily affect calcium, which is believed to play a role in excitation-contraction coupling.[49, 65]

Digitalis exerts on the *electrophysiology* of the heart striking effects, which are not the same in all portions of the organ. Most significant are more rapid repolarization of the ventricles (shortened electrical systole) and, in higher concentrations, increased automaticity or increased rate of diastolic depolarization with appearance of ectopic activity. The A-V node is markedly affected by the glycosides. Digitalis slows conduction and prolongs the refractory period of this node.

Digitalis also exerts extracardiac effects, such as on the central nervous system. These extracardiac effects generally do not prevent the successful use of the drug for many years in patients subject to congestive failure.

Although digitalis is the most important drug in the treatment of heart failure, its use requires a good understanding of its pharmacology and the pathophysiology of heart disease. Digitalis poisoning is surprisingly common in current practice.[3, 74] The therapeutic index of the drug is small, and it is dangerous in certain circumstances. For example, either hypopotassemia or hypercalcemia greatly increase the possibility of fatal arrhythmias during digitalis administration.

DEVELOPMENT OF IDEAS ON DIGITALIS ACTION

The history of digitalis is a remarkable example of the discovery of an important drug in a folk remedy. William Withering,[53] having heard of a mixture of herbs that an old woman of Shropshire used successfully in the treatment of dropsy (congestive heart failure), suspected that its beneficial properties must have been caused by the fox-glove. In testing it in patients with congestive failure, Withering was greatly impressed with the diuretic effect of the foxglove and believed that the drug probably acted on the kidney. On the other hand, he also stated that the drug had a remarkable "power over the heart."

Subsequently, digitalis was tried in many different diseases, and several physicians both in France and in England were most impressed with the slowing of the heart rate caused by the foxglove. This was especially notable in patients with atrial fibrillation. James Mackenzie and Sir Thomas Lewis were of the opinion that the slowing effect on the ventricular rate, as seen in atrial fibrillation, was the main indication of the drug as well as its basic mode of action. There were other cardiologists, however, who believed that there was more to the digitalis effect.

Early pharmacologic studies performed on normal hearts failed to reveal possible beneficial effects of digitalis for reasons that will be discussed. Cattell and Gold, however, found an important effect on contractility of the cat papillary muscle.[14] This was an important contribution indicating that a reversal of failing contractility could be achieved with these glycosides under conditions that precluded actions on heart rate or heart size.

With the development of cardiac catheterization, the effects of digitalis on the heart and peripheral circulation became much better understood. The emphasis today

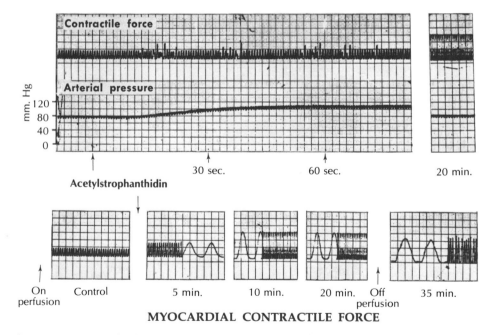

MYOCARDIAL CONTRACTILE FORCE

Fig. 29-1. Contractile force and arterial pressure recordings immediately and 20 minutes after injection of 1.4 mg. acetylstrophanthidin in a 28-year-old woman with an atrial septal defect. The lower tracings show contractile force recordings before injection and at intervals after acetylstrophanthidin. Note that the drug augments the contractile force of the nonfailing human heart and constricts the systemic vascular bed. (From Braunwald, E., Bloodwell, R. D., Goldberg, L. I., and Morrow, A. G.: J. Clin. Invest. **40**:52, 1961.)

is on the contractility-increasing actions of the drug, the finer mechanisms of which are the subject of intensive investigations. The possible role of the inhibition of $Na^+-K^+-ATPase$ and alteration in ion movements in the mediation of the effects of digitalis are of general interest. Thus a clinical observation on a folk remedy led to a highly useful therapeutic agent and to a research tool of great value to basic investigators.

EFFECTS OF DIGITALIS ON THE HEART

Digitalis increases the contractility of the heart muscle and influences its electrophysiologic properties such as conductivity, refractory period, and automaticity. It is increasingly recognized that the effectiveness of digitalis in the treatment of congestive failure is a consequence of its positive inotropic effect. On the other hand, some of its electrophysiologic influences make the drug highly useful in the treatment of a variety of arrhythmias.

Contractility is influenced by digitalis in both the normal and the failing heart. As shown in Fig. 29-1, it has been demonstrated in man by attaching a Walton-Brodie strain gauge arch to the right ventricular myocardium of patients undergoing cardiac surgery. It has also been shown in the isolated heart (Fig. 29-2).

Digitalis increases both the force and the velocity of myocardial contraction, and it shortens the duration of systole. It promotes more complete emptying of the ventricles and decreases the size of the heart in failure.

Problem 29-1. Although digitalis increases the contractility of the normal as well as the failing heart, its effect on cardiac output is much greater in congestive failure. In fact, its ability to increase cardiac output in normal individuals has been questioned for many years.

The explanation of this paradox is related to hemodynamic adjustments. In the normal individual, digitalis not only increases cardiac contractility but it also causes constriction of peripheral vessels. It may also decrease venous pressure and may slow the sinus rate. Under these circumstances no increase in cardiac output can be demonstrated despite the positive inotropic effect.

The situation is different in the failing heart. In patients with congestive failure, the peripheral resistance is already high because the falling cardiac output leads to increased sympathetic tone. Under these circumstances the positive inotropic effect of digitalis increases cardiac output because the tone of peripheral vessels is lowered due to decreased sympathetic tone.

Problem 29-2. Does digitalis increase the *efficiency* of the failing heart? It has been observed that digitalis will increase cardiac output in the failing heart without a corresponding increase in oxygen consumption. At first glance this could be interpreted as an increase in efficiency, since more work is performed by the heart per unit of oxygen consumed.[6]

The problem is much more complicated, however. The ventricular radius of the failing heart is reduced by digitalis. Oxygen consumption should be reduced as the ventricular radius becomes smaller. It is becoming clear that if heart size remained constant, digitalis would increase oxygen consumption as it increased contractility. On the other hand, the reduction of ventricular radius leads to a decrease in oxygen utilization, and the two effects cancel each other out.

ELECTROPHYSIOLOGIC EFFECTS

The electrophysiologic effects of digitalis provide the basis of its actions on *conductivity, refractory period,* and *automaticity*. These effects must be examined separately on the conducting tissue and the ventricular and atrial muscle cells. The problem is made complex by the existence of both *autonomic* and *direct* actions of the glycosides and by differences in the sensitivity of normal and diseased heart to the electrophysiologic effects of digitalis.

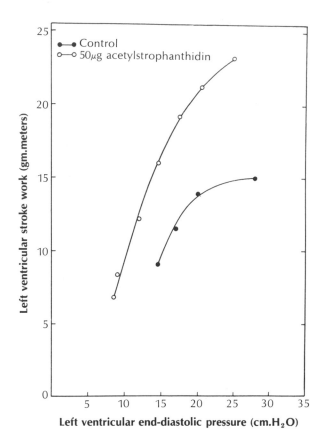

Fig. 29-2. Left ventricular function curves before and after injection of 50 µg acetylstro-phanthidin into the left coronary artery in the isolated supported heart preparation. Mean aortic pressure constant at 65 mm. Hg; heart rate constant at 162 beats/min. Stroke work was varied by varying stroke volume. In response to the injection of acetylstrophanthidin the ventricular function curve shifted upward and to the left; that is, myocardial contractility increased. (From Sarnoti, S. J., Gilmore, J. P., Wallace, A. G., Skinner, N. S., Mitchell, J. H., and Daggett, W. M.: Amer. J. Med. **37:**3, 1964.)

CONDUCTING TISSUE

The low-dose effects of digitalis in the atrioventricular conduction, which is slowed, are commonly referred to as *vagal effects,* since they are reversed by atropine. The direct effect of the drug not reversible by atropine becomes evident with higher doses.

A-V node conduction is prolonged by digitalis. Prolongation of the P-R interval and varying degrees of block are electrocardiographic evidences of this action when the supraventricular rate is slow.

A-V refractory period is also prolonged by digitalis. This action becomes important when the supraventricular rate is rapid, such as in atrial flutter and fibrillation when the purpose in using digitalis is to decrease the number of impulses reaching the ventricles.

Purkinje fibers and, to a lesser extent, ventricular muscle respond to digitalis with a

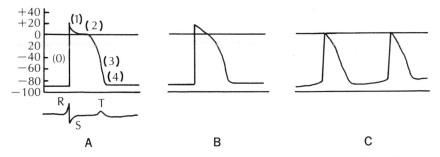

Fig. 29-3. Diagram of the effect of a digitalis glycoside on isolated Purkinje fibers. **A,** Control before digitalis. **B,** Decrease in duration of action potential as digitalis shortens the plateau. The refractory period in Purkinje fibers is shortened. **C,** Increased rate of diastolic depolarization with development of ectopic pacemaker activity. (Modified from Hoffman, B. F., and Singer, D. H.: Prog. Cardiovasc. Dis. 7:226, 1964, by permission of Grune & Stratton, Inc.)

shortening of the action potential, decreased refractory period, and the appearance of pacemaker activity as a result of increased rate of diastolic depolarization[74] (Fig. 29-3). Recent evidence suggests that increased automaticity is more likely if the fibers are stretched or potassium is low.[72] This fits the observation that in "healthy" hearts in young people, the predominant effect of digitalis is block, whereas in patients with cardiac disease, ventricular arrhythmias are common consequences of digitalis administration.

VENTRICULAR AND ATRIAL MUSCLE

In the ventricle, digitalis shortens the refractory period and the duration of the action potential. Thus the Q-T interval shortens. Isolated tissue studies show that low concentrations of digitalis increase contractility prior to a significant change in transmembrane action potential.[74]

In the atrium, the actions of digitalis are complicated by vagal effects. Digitalis may increase the release of acetylcholine and may also increase the sensitivity of the fibers to the released mediator.[31] In a normally innervated atrium without atropine, digitalis shortens the refractory period. On the other hand, in the denervated or atropine-treated atrium, digitalis may cause an increase in the refractory period.

EFFECT OF DIGITALIS ON THE HEART RATE

In normal individuals, digitalis has little effect on the heart rate. In congestive failure, digitalis slows the rapid sinus rhythm primarily by an indirect mechanism. The tachycardia in this case is a consequence of increased sympathetic activity brought about by decreased cardiac output. As digitalis increases cardiac output, the sympathetic drive to the sinoatrial node is reduced. Digitalis is not useful in the treatment of sinus tachycardia caused by fever and other conditions, since it has essentially no effect on the S-A node.

Other factors that may play a role in the cardiac slowing caused by digitalis are (1) prolongation of the refractory period of the A-V node when atrial rate is rapid, (2) slowing of A-V conduction (a partial block may be converted to complete block), and (3) reflex vagal stimulation elicited by digitalis. These mechanisms will be discussed further in connection with the antiarrhythmic drugs.

ELECTROCARDIOGRAPHIC EFFECTS

The effects of digitalis reflect the more rapid repolarization of the ventricle, changes in A-V nodal conduction and refractory period, and increased ectopic activity. They are characterized by S-T–segment depression, inversion of the T wave, shortened Q-T interval, prolongation of the P-R interval, A-V dissociation, and ventricular arrhythmias such as premature ventricular contractions, bigeminal rhythm, and ventricular fibrillation.

FUNDAMENTAL CELLULAR EFFECTS OF DIGITALIS

The exact mechanism of the positive inotropic effect of digitalis is unknown. It is generally believed that the drug has no important effects on intermediary metabolism, energy production, or the basic properties of the contractile proteins.

Digitalis has two striking effects that are probably related to its inotropic, electrophysiologic, and toxic actions. One is related to Na^+-K^+-ATPase inhibition, the other to calcium metabolism.

Even in low concentrations, the cardiac glycosides inhibit the Na^+-K^+-ATPase. It is believed by many investigators, although not proved, that the enzyme inhibition is related to the inotropic actions of digitalis. Others believe that the enzyme inhibition and alteration of the ionic movements may be more related to the toxic effects of digitalis. In any case, it is well established that hypopotassemia aggravates digitalis toxicity, whereas potassium administration is commonly used in the treatment of digitalis poisoning, particularly when a potassium deficit already exists.

There are many reasons to believe that some connection exists between the digitalis effect and calcium. The two drugs are synergistic[65] and calcium administration is dangerous in digitalized patients. Digitalis may increase the availability of intracellular calcium for the process of excitation-contraction coupling.

EXTRACARDIAC EFFECTS OF DIGITALIS

When used in therapeutic doses, the effects of digitalis are exerted largely on the heart. Some of the extracardiac effects may be important, however, as an aid to recognizing impending digitalis-induced cardiac toxicity.

The *gastrointestinal effects* manifest themselves commonly in the form of nausea and anorexia. These effects are central or reflex in origin when the purified glycosides are used. With powdered digitalis or digitalis tincture, a local effect contributes to nausea and anorexia. The intravenously administered glycosides exert their emetic effect by acting on the chemoreceptor trigger zone.[7]

The *neurologic effects* consist of blurred vision, paresthesias, and toxic psychosis. These symptoms are often misdiagnosed in elderly patients.

Endocrinologic changes such as gynecomastia occur rarely. Allergic reactions are extremely uncommon.

The *diuretic effect* is mostly a consequence of an improvement of renal circulation, although in large doses the various glycosides cause some inhibition of sodium reabsorption directly in the renal tubules.[35]

Some experiments suggest that an action of digitalis on the central nervous system contributes to arrhythmia and ventricular fibrillation.[13,45,48] For example, the intravenous administration of large doses of digitalis glycoside induces ventricular fibrillation in the dog. Ventricular fibrillation did not occur, however, after bilateral cardiac sympathectomy and ligation of the adrenal glands.[30] In some definitive experiments,[13] electrical activity was monitored in sympathetic, parasympathetic, and phrenic nerves before and after ouabain administration in cats. Ouabain increased traffic in these nerves. Spinal transection prevented these effects and increased the dose of ouabain needed for producing ventricular arrhythmias. It appears, then, that neural activation, probably at the level of the brainstem, plays a role in the development of ouabain-induced arrhythmias. Procedures that reversed or diminished neural influence, such as cord section or the administration of propranolol, prevented or reversed some of the cardiotoxicity of a digitalis glycoside.

SOURCES AND CHEMISTRY

The cardioactive steroids and their glycosides are widely distributed in nature. Since their effects on the heart are qualitatively the same, it is sufficient to utilize only a few of these in therapeutics. Some believe that most physicians would do well to utilize only one such as digoxin, an intermediate acting glycoside, which can be given orally or intravenously. Nevertheless, there are several digitalis glycosides in current use, and their sources and chemistry will be briefly summarized.

The glycosides most commonly used are obtained from the foxglove or *Digitalis purpurea, Digitalis lanata,* or the seeds of the African tree, *Strophanthus gratus.* The most important glycosides obtained from these plants are as follows:

Digitalis purpurea:	digitoxin
	digoxin
	digitalis leaf
Digitalis lanata:	digoxin
	lanatoside C
	deslanoside
Strophanthus gratus:	ouabain

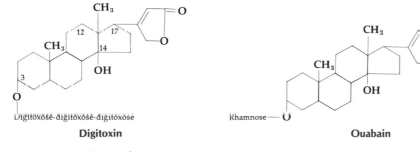

Digitoxin   **Ouabain**

(Digoxin differs only in
having an OH at C-12)

The structure of digitoxin is characterized by a steroid nucleus with an unsaturated lactone attached in the C-17 position. The three sugars attached to the C-3 position are unusual 20-deoxyhexoses. The molecule without the sugars is called an *aglycone* or *genin.* The steroidal structure and the unsaturated lactone are essential for the characteristic cardioactive effect. The removal of the sugars results in generally weaker and more evanescent activity.

Digoxin differs from digitoxin only in the presence of an OH at the C-12 position. Lanatoside C (Cedilanid) is the parent compound of digoxin and differs only from the latter by having an additional glucose molecule and an acetyl group on the oligosaccharide side chain. Removal of the acetyl group by alkaline hydrolysis yields the deslanoside, and the further removal of glucose by enzymatic hydrolysis gives digoxin.

Ouabain, obtained from the seeds of *Strophanthus gratus,* differs somewhat in its steroidal portion from the previously discussed compounds. Its aglycone is known as G-strophanthidin, and the sugar to which it is attached in the glycoside is rhamnose.

The various clinically useful glycosides and genins differ mainly in their pharmacokinetic characteristics, which are reflections of their water or lipid solubility, gastrointestinal absorption, metabolism, and excretion.[74] Digitoxin is highly lipid-soluble, digoxin is less so, and ouabain is water-soluble. As expected from their solubilities, digitoxin is completely absorbed from the gastrointestinal tract and persists in the body for a long time, having a half-life of 7 days. Digoxin is not as well absorbed and has a biologic half-life of 1.5 days. Ouabain, a highly polar compound, is not well absorbed from the gastrointestinal tract and has a short duration of action. (See Table 29-1.)

Digitoxin is highly bound to plasma proteins and is metabolized in the liver. It also undergoes enterohepatic circulation, being excreted in the bile and subsequently reabsorbed. Experimentally, hepatectomy increases the half-life of digitoxin, whereas renal failure increases the half-life of digoxin.

The essential feature of the pharmacokinetics of various digitalis compounds depends on the observation[63] that the total glycoside losses from the body are proportional to the total amount present; that is, the disappearance is a first-order reaction. The more glycoside there is in the body, the more is lost each day.

In the case of digoxin in a patient having normal renal function, the half-life of the drug is 1.6 days. This means that when such a patient is given a *loading dose* of digoxin, 65% of it will still be in the body one day later and 35% will be lost. Since the purpose

Table 29-1. Properties of digitalis preparations*

Preparation	Absorption G. I.	Onset of action†	Half-life‡	Peak effect	Excretion or metabolism	Digitalizing dose Oral	Digitalizing dose I. V.	Oral maintenance dose
Digoxin	75%	15-30 min.	36 hr.	1½-5 hr.	Renal: some G. I.	1.25-1.5 mg.	0.75-1.0 mg.	0.25-0.5 mg.
Digitoxin	95%	25-120 min.	5 days	4-6 days	Hepatic§	0.7-1.2 mg.	1.0 mg.	0.1 mg.
Ouabain	Unreliable	5-10 min.	21 hr.	½-2 hr.	Renal: some G. I.	—	0.3-0.5 mg.	—
Deslano-side	Unreliable	10-30 min.	33 hr.	1-2 hr.	Renal	—	0.8 mg.	—

*Modified from Smith, T. W.: New Eng. J. Med. **288**:721, 1973.
†I. V. administration.
‡For normal subjects.
§Enterohepatic circulation exists.

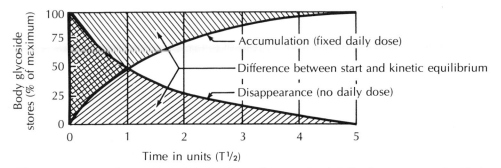

Fig. 29-4. Accumulation of a digitalis glycoside on a fixed daily dose compared with its disappearance after dosage is stopped. Time is expressed in units of half-times. (From Jeliffe, R. W.: Ann. Int. Med. **69**:703, 1968.)

of subsequent *maintenance doses* is to replace losses, the daily maintenance dose will be 35% of the loading dose. The loading dose is usually 0.75 to 1.5 mg. of digoxin given in three divided doses approximately 5 hours apart.[63] The loading dose sets the total glycoside in the body to a desired level. Since the glycoside disappears logarithmically, after 5 glycoside half-lives only one thirty-second of the loading dose remains in the body. The purpose of the maintenance doses, then, is to keep the total amount of glycoside at the desired level. In the case of digoxin, urinary losses represent 86% of the total loss, and changes in renal function will greatly influence its dosages.

If no loading dose is given and the patient is placed on a fixed daily maintenance dose, the body stores of the glycoside will accumulate until the amount that is lost daily equals the maintenance dose. The curve of accumulation is a mirror image of the disappearance curve, and kinetic equilibrium will be reached in approximately 5 half-lives. Ninety percent of maximum will be reached in 3.3 half-lives (Fig. 29-4).

PREPARATIONS OF DIGITALIS

Digoxin may be looked on as the prototype of digitalis glycosides. There are experts who believe that most physicians could limit themselves to this drug whenever a digitalis preparation is needed. Nevertheless, there are several glycosides in current use, which differ largely in speed of onset, duration of action, gastrointestinal absorption, and suitability for intravenous administration.

It is essential to remember that all digitalis glycosides exert the same qualitative effects on the myocardium and that the therapeutic to toxic ratios are the same. Some are clearly more dangerous than others by virtue of differences in their durations of action. The patient poisoned with acetylstrophanthidin is not in jeopardy for as long a period as is one with digitoxin.

The modern trend is to use pure glycosides rather than the older digitalis powdered leaf or other impure compounds, which must be standardized by bioassay. In the bioassay techniques, the unknown preparation is compared with a USP reference standard with regard to lethal potency on cats, frogs, or pigeons, or using the emetic effect on pigeons. The pure glycosides are measured spectrophotometrically.

Digoxin has an intermediate duration of action with a biologic half-life of about 36 hours. The compound may be administered orally or intravenously. When administered orally, about 75% of it is absorbed. Recent studies indicate[21] that there is considerable variation in bioavailability of digoxin tablets obtained from different manufacturers. Fortunately the products of the largest suppliers are reliable.

Gastrointestinal absorption of the drug is influenced not only by the source of the tablets. Patients with malabsorption syndromes may absorb digoxin poorly. Also, cholestyramine binds the drug, interferes with its absorption, and may cause a return of congestive heart failure.

Digoxin is excreted by glomerular filtration and is not significantly reabsorbed by the tubules. Only 20% of the drug is bound by plasma proteins. The loss of digoxin from the body takes place in an exponential fashion. In other words, the loss of the glycoside is proportional to the amount present in the body. The half-life of tritiated digoxin is 1.6 days, which increases to 4.4 days in anuric patients.[22,59]

Oral preparations of digoxin (Lanoxin) include tablets of 0.125, 0.25, and 0.5 mg., and an elixir of 0.05 mg./ml. It is also available in solution for injection, 0.1 and 0.25 mg./ml.

Just as digoxin, deslanoside (Cedilanid-D) is derived from D. lanata. It is similar in action to digoxin, and its usual digitalizing intravenous dose is 1.4 mg. Deslanoside is a derivative of lanatoside C (Cedilanid), which is poorly absorbed from the gastrointestinal tract and is rarely used. Deslanoside is essentially the injectable form of lanatoside C.

Digitoxin is the main active glycoside in digitalis leaf (D. purpurea). On a weight basis it is a thousand times as active as the powdered leaf, so that 1 mg. of digitoxin is equivalent to 1 Gm. of the leaf.

Digitoxin is the least polar of the useful cardiac glycosides, and it is highly bound to plasma proteins (97%). In contrast with digoxin, digitoxin is largely metabolized by the liver with renal excretion being a minor factor in its disposition. Digitoxin undergoes enterohepatic circulation and cholestyramine interferes with its reabsorption.

The physiologic half-life of digitoxin is approximately 5 to 7 days. Anuria prolongs the half-time to 8 days. This prolongation is obviously relatively less than in the case of digoxin, which depends much more on renal excretion for its elimination.

A patient on digitoxin therapy loses about 10% of the amount in the body in a day. The drug accumulates until the peak stores represent 10 times the daily maintenance dose. A loading dose is generally given at the beginning of treatment, since on a daily maintenance dose a long time would be required for full digitalization. Because of its slow metabolic degradation, its toxic effects continue for a long time after the drug is discontinued. This is one of the reasons for the increasing popularity of digoxin in preference to digitoxin, although there is no unanimity on this question. The metabolic degradation of digitoxin is accelerated by drugs that stimulate the activity of hepatic microsomal enzymes, such as phenobarbital.

Transition from digoxin to digitoxin in a patient may lead to difficulties because of their different pharmacokinetics.[63] Transition from digoxin maintenance to digitoxin maintenance would lead to underdigitalization, whereas changing from digitoxin to digoxin without careful adjustment of dosages may lead to digitalis poisoning.

Oral preparations of digitoxin (Crystodigin; Digitalin Nativelle; Purodigin) include oral tablets containing 0.05, 0.1, 0.15, and 0.2 mg.; elixir, 0.5 mg./ml.; injectable solution, 0.2 mg./ml.

Ouabain, a crystalline glycoside, is obtained from *Strophanthus gratus*. It is a highly polar glycoside, suitable for intravenous injection only, because it is poorly absorbed from the gastrointestinal tract. It is commonly used in experimental work. Its plasma half-life is 21 hours.

Gitalin is a mixture of glycosides obtained from *D. purpurea*. It has no advantages, although a more favorable therapeutic index has been claimed for it. This has also been denied.

Acetylstrophanthidin is an experimental drug of extremely short duration of action. It has been proposed for a therapeutic test to determine the completeness of digitalization. Its use should be reserved for the experts and for clinical investigations only.[27]

THERAPEUTIC INDICATIONS FOR DIGITALIS

Digitalis is the principal drug of choice in the treatment of congestive failure and in certain arrhythmias. Some of the latter indications are absolute and others are controversial.

Congestive failure

Congestive failure caused by a variety of underlying mechanisms responds well to digitalis treatment. By increasing contractility, the drug increases cardiac output and relieves the elevated ventricular pressures, pulmonary congestion, and venous pressure. Diuresis is brought about with relief of edema.

Controversy exists in relation to the use of digitalis in myocardial infarction with failure. The drug may aggravate the arrhythmias that commonly accompany the infarction. Some experts believe that this danger has been overemphasized.[26] Other areas of controversy relate to the prophylactic use of digitalis, which is avoided by most clinicians.

Arrhythmias

Arrhythmias of certain types represent important indications for the use of digitalis. Among these the most prominent are atrial fibrillation, atrial flutter, and paroxysmal atrial tachycardia.

Atrial fibrillation. The main purpose of using digitalis in atrial fibrillation in the absence of congestive failure is to slow the ventricular rate. This is achieved by the prolongation of the refractory period of the A-V node, which allows fewer of the supraventricular impulses to get through. Digitalis does not generally stop the atrial fibrillation itself.

Atrial flutter. In atrial flutter, the rapid atrial rate is accompanied by a 2:1 or 3:1 A-V block. Digitalis further increases the magnitude of the A-V block, thus slowing the ventricular rate. As to the atrial flutter itself, digitalis tends to convert flutter to fibrillation. This effect is probably a consequence of decreasing the refractory period of the atria. Occasionally, after flutter is converted to fibrillation by digitalis and the drug is stopped, normal sinus rhythm may result.

Paroxysmal atrial tachycardia. Paroxysmal atrial tachycardia often responds to increased vagal activity, which can be elicited by pressure on the carotid sinus. Digitalis may act by a similar mechanism, since it has a definite vagal effect. Shortening the refractory period of the atria is the probable electrophysiologic basis for stopping paroxysmal atrial tachycardia with digitalis.[74]

DIGITALIS POISONING

Intoxication with digitalis is common and hazardous. In a recent survey carried out in a general hospital, digitalis intoxication was found to be the most common adverse drug reaction.[34]

The symptoms of digitalis poisoning include both extracardiac and cardiac manifestations. In mild to moderate intoxication, the symptoms consist of anorexia, ventricular ectopic beats, and bradycardia. These may progress to nausea and vomiting, headache, malaise, and ventricular premature beats. In severe intoxication, the symptoms are characterized by blurring of vision, disorientation, diarrhea, ventricular tachycardia, and sinoatrial and atrioventricular block. This may progress to ventricular fibrillation.

There are several reasons for the frequency of digitalis intoxication. The therapeutic index of digitalis is low and highly variable in different patients. The common use of thiazide diuretics leads to hypopotassemia, which aggravates digitalis toxicity.

The development of methods for determining serum concentrations of digoxin and digitoxin by radioimmunoassay may be important in the prevention of some cases of digitalis intoxication (Fig. 29-5). It should be stressed, however, that such determinations should not replace good clinical judgment because numerous factors influ-

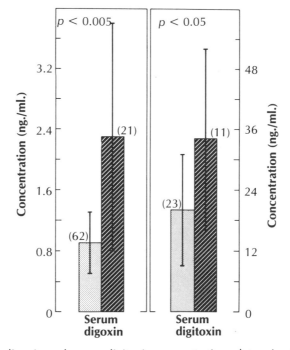

Fig. 29-5. Serum digoxin and serum digitoxin concentrations determined by radioimmunoassay. Stippled bars refer to patients without toxic effects, and crosshatched bars refer to patients with definite toxic effects. Numbers of patients are shown in parentheses. (From Beller, G. A., Smith, T. W., Abelmann, W. H., Haber, E., and Hood, W. B.: New Eng. J. Med. **284**:989, 1971.)

ence the significance of a given serum concentration. Some of these factors are the underlying heart disease, the serum concentration of potassium and magnesium, and endocrine factors.

The electrocardiographic changes observed in digitalis poisoning can be explained on the basis of the drug's electrophysiologic effects. Ventricular arrhythmias are related to increased automaticity (increased rate of diastolic depolarization). A-V dissociation is related to the actions of digitalis on conduction and refractory period at the A-V node. The lowering of the S-T segment and inversion of the T wave commonly observed after digitalis may reflect rapid repolarization of the ventricle and perhaps a change in the initiation of the repolarization process.

DRUG INTERACTIONS AND DIGITALIS INTOXICATION

In addition to the potassium-losing diuretics that predispose to digitalis toxicity, there are other drug interactions of clinical significance. Calcium (parenteral) and catecholamines or sympathomimetic drugs may promote ectopic pacemaker activity in digitalized patients. Barbiturates such as phenobarbital may accelerate the metabolism of digitoxin. Cholestyramine resin binds digitoxin in the intestine and thus interferes with its enterohepatic circulation. Digitalis can be used in reserpinized patients, since the glycosides still exert their characteristic cardiotonic effect. On the other hand, the administration of parenteral reserpine to a digitalized patient may cause arrhythmias, probably as a consequence of sudden catecholamine release.[9]

TREATMENT OF DIGITALIS POISONING

The most important measure in the treatment of digitalis poisoning is the discontinuation of the drug administration. Potassium chloride by mouth or by slow intravenous infusion may be helpful in stopping the ventricular arrhythmias. It should be remembered, however, that elevated potassium concentrations may aggravate A-V block, although potassium may improve it if serum potassium is low. It is believed by many investigators that the infusion of potassium in a digitalized patient may produce abnormally high serum concentrations because of the effect of the glycosides on the membrane ATPase in various tissues. Other drugs that are used occasionally in digitalis poisoning are the antiarrhythmic drugs such as diphenylhydantoin, lidocaine, and procainamide.

DIGITALIZATION AND MAINTENANCE

The principles behind the loading dose and the maintenance dose have already been discussed in relation to pharmacokinetics of digitalis (p. 382). For practical purposes, initial digitalization is accomplished by either a *rapid method* or a *cumulative (slow) method.*

In the rapid method, the estimated loading dose is administered in a single dose or in two or three divided doses given a few hours apart, depending on the response. In the cumulative method, smaller doses are employed at greater intervals until full digitalization takes place by cumulation. For example, digitoxin may be given for initial digitalization in a single dose of 1.2 or 0.4 mg. every 8 hours for 3 doses. This initial digitalization is followed in subsequent days by the maintenance dose, which in the case of digitoxin is 0.1 to 0.2 mg. daily.

For details on digitalizing and maintenance doses of the various glycosides see Table 29-1.

References

1 Allen, J. C., and Schwartz, A.: A possible biochemical explanation for the insensitivity of the rat to cardiac glycosides, J. Pharmacol. Exp. Ther. **168**:42, 1969.

2 Areskog, N. H.: Effects of two rapid acting cardiac glycosides on dog's heart-lung preparation, Acta Physiol. Scand. **55**:139, 1962.

3 Beller, G. A., Smith, T. W., Abelmann, W. H., Haber, E., and Hood, W. B.: Digitalis intoxication. A prospective clinical study with serum level correlations, New Eng. J. Med. **284**:989, 1971.

4 Bernstein, M. S., Neschis, M., and Collini, F.: Treatment of acute massive digtalis poisoning by administration of a chelating agent, New Eng. J. Med. **261**:961, 1959.

5 Bing, R. J., Choudhury, J. D., Michal, G., and Kako, K.: Myocardial metabolism, Ann. Intern. Med. **49**:1201, 1958.

6 Bing, R. J., and Danforth, W. H.: Physiology of the myocardium, J.A.M.A. **172**:438, 1960.

7 Borison, H. L.: Role of gastrointestinal innervation in digitalis emesis, J. Pharmacol. Exp. Ther. **104**:396, 1952.

8 Braunwald, E., Bloodwell, R. D., Goldberg, L. I., and Morrow, A. G.: Studies on digitalis. IV. Observations in man on the effects of digitalis preparations on the contractility of the nonfailing heart and on total vascular resistance, J. Clin. Invest. **40**:52, 1961.

9 Dick, H. L. H., McCawley, E. L., and Fisher, W. A.: Reserpine-digitalis toxicity, Arch. Intern. Med. **109**:503, 1962.

10 Doherty, J. E., Flanigan, W. J., Patterson, R. M., and Dalrymple, G. V.: The excretion of tritiated digoxin in normal human volunteers before and after unilateral nephrectomy, Circulation **50**:555, 1969.

11 Doherty, J. E., and Perkins, W. H.: Studies with tritiated digoxin in human subjects after intravenous administration, Amer. Heart J. **63**:528, 1962.

12 Friend, D. G.: Current concepts in therapy: cardiac glycosides, New Eng. J. Med. **266**:402, 1962.

13 Gillis, R. A., Raines, A., Sohn, Y. J., et al.: Neuroexcitatory effects of digitalis and their role in the development of cardiac arrhythmias, J. Pharmacol. Exp. Ther. **183**:154, 1972.

14 Gold, H.: Pharmacologic basis of cardiac therapy, J.A.M.A. **132**:547, 1946.

15 Gold, H., and Cattell, M.: Mechanism of digitalis action in abolishing heart failure, Arch. Intern. Med. **65**:263, 1940.

16 Gold, H., Kwit, N. T., Otto, H., and Fox, T.: On the vagal and extra-vagal factors in cardiac slowing by digitalis in patients with auricular fibrillation, J. Clin. Invest. **18**:429, 1939.

17 Gubner, R. S., and Kallman, H.: Treatment of digitalis toxicity by chelation of serum calcium, Amer. J. Med. Sci. **234**:136, 1957.

18 Hajdu, S.: Bioassay of cardiac active principles based on the staircase phenomenon of the frog heart, J. Pharmacol. Exp. Ther. **120**:90, 1957.

19 Heymans, C., Bouckaert, J. J., and Reginiers, P.: Sur le mecanisme reflèxe de la bradycardie provoquée par les digitaliques, C. R. Soc. Biol. **110**:572, 1932.

20 Hoffman, B. F., and Singer, D. H.: Effects of digitalis on electrical activity of cardiac fibers, Progr. Cardiovasc. Dis. **7**:226, 1964.

21 Huffman, D. H., and Azarnoff, D. L.: Absorption of orally given digoxin preparations, J.A.M.A. **222**:957, 1972.

22 Jeliffe, R. W.: An improved method of digoxin therapy, Ann. Intern. Med. **69**:703, 1968.

23 Kahn, J. B., Jr.: Effects of ribosides and related compounds on phosphate transport in incubated fresh and cold-stored human erythrocytes, J. Pharmacol. Exp. Ther. **120**:239, 1957.

24 Kahn, J. B., Jr., and Cohen, S. B.: Effects of ribosides and related compounds on cation transport in cold-stored human erythrocytes, J. Pharmacol. Exp. Ther. **120**:9, 1957.

25 Kreidberg, M. B., Chernoff, H. L., and Lopez, W. L.: Treatment of cardiac failure in infancy and childhood, New Eng. J. Med. **268**:23, 1963.

26 Lown, B., Klein, M. D., Barr, I., Hagemeijer, F., Kosowsky, B. D., and Garrison, H.: Sensitivity to digitalis drugs in acute myocardial infarction, Amer. J. Cardiol. **30**:388, 1972.

27 Lown, B., and Levine, S. A.: Current concepts in digitalis therapy, Boston, 1954, Little, Brown & Co.

28 McMichael, J., and Sharpey-Schafer, E. P.: The action of intravenous digoxin in man, Quart. J. Med. **13**:123, 1944.

29 Medical Letter on Drugs and Therapeutics **4**:75, 1962.

30 Mendez, C., Aceves, J., and Mendez, R.: The antiadrenergic action of digitalis on the refractory period of the A-V transmission system, J. Pharmacol. Exp. Ther. **131**:199, 1961.

31 Mendez, R., and Mendez, C.: The action of

cardiac glycosides on the refractory period of heart tissues, J. Pharmacol. Exp. Ther. **107**:24, 1953.

32 Moe, G. K., and Mendez, R.: The action of several cardiac glycosides on conduction velocity and ventricular excitability in the dog heart, Circulation **4**:729, 1951.

33 Morrow, D. H., Gaffney, T. E., and Braunwald, E.: Studies on digitalis. VIII. Effect of autonomic innervation and of myocardial catecholamine stores upon the cardiac action of ouabain, J. Pharmacol. Exp. Ther. **140**:236, 1963.

34 Nechay, B. R., and Nelson, J. A.: Renal ouabain-sensitive ATP-ase activity and Na$^+$ reabsorption, J. Pharmacol. Exp. Ther. **175**:717, 1970.

35 Ogilvie, R. I., and Ruedy, J.: An educational program in digitalis therapy, J.A.M.A. **222**:50, 1971.

36 Peters, H. P., and Visscher, M. B.: The energy metabolism of the heart in failure and the influence of drugs upon it, Amer. Heart J. **11**:273, 1936.

37 Rasmussen, K., Jervell, J., Storstein, L., and Gjerdrum, K.: Digitoxin kinetics in patients with impaired renal function, Clin. Pharmacol. Ther. **13**:6, 1972.

38 Robertson, D. M., Hollenhorst, R. W., and Callahan, J. A.: Ocular manifestations of digitalis toxicity, Arch. Ophthal. **76**:640, 1966.

39 Rose, O. A., Batterman, R. C., and DeGraff, A. C.: Clinical studies on digoxin, a purified digitalis glycoside, Amer. Heart J. **24**:435, 1942.

40 Rosenblum, H.: Maintenance of digitalis effects after rapid parenteral digitalization, J.A.M.A. **182**:192, 1962.

41 Sarnoff, S. J., Gilmore, J. P., Wallace, A. G., Skinner, N. S., Mitchell, J. H., and Daggett, W. M.: Effect of acetyl strophanthidin therapy on cardiac dynamics, oxygen consumption and efficiency in the isolated heart with and without hypoxia, Amer. J. Med. **37**:3, 1964.

42 Schmidt, D. H., and Butler, V. P.: Immunological protection against digoxin toxicity, J Clin. Invest. **50**:866, 1971.

43 Schwartz, A., Allen, J. C., and Harigaya, S.: Possible involvement of cardiac Na$^+$, K$^+$-adenosine triphosphatase in the mechanism of action of cardiac glycosides, J. Pharmacol. Exp. Ther. **168**:31, 1969.

44 Spann, J. F., Sonnenblick, E. H., Cooper, T., Chidsey, C. A., Willman, V. L., and Braunwald, E.: Studies on digitalis. XIV. Influence of cardiac norepinephrine stores on the response of isolated heart muscle to digitalis, Circulation Res. **19**:326, 1966.

45 Standaert, F. G., Levitt B., Roberts, J., and Raines, A.: Antagonism of ventricular arrhythmias induced by digitalis—a neural phenomenon, Europ. J. Pharmacol. **6**:209, 1969.

46 Stead, E. A., Jr.: The role of the cardiac output in the mechanisms of congestive failure, Amer. J. Med. **6**:232, 1949.

47 Stewart, H. J., and Cohn, A. E.: Studies on effect of action of digitalis on output of blood from heart; effect on output in normal human hearts; effect on output of hearts in heart failure with congestion in human beings, J. Clin. Invest. **11**:917, 1932.

48 Stickney, J. L., and Lucchesi, B. R.: The effect of sympatholytic agents on the cardiovascular responses produced by the injection of acetylstrophanthidin into the cerebral ventricles, Europ. J. Pharmacol. **6**:1, 1969.

49 Sulakhe, P. V., and Dhalla, N. S.: Excitation-contraction coupling in heart. VII. Calcium accumulation in subcellular particles in congestive heart failure, J. Clin. Invest. **50**:1019, 1971.

50 Szent-Györgyi, A.: Chemical physiology of contraction in body and heart muscle, New York, 1953, Academic Press, Inc.

51 Weissler, A. M., Snyder, J. R., Schoenfeld, C. D., and Cohen S.: Assay of digitalis glycosides in man, Amer. J. Cardiol. **17**:768, 1966.

52 Williams, J. F., Klocke, F. J., and Braunwald, E.: Studies on digitalis. XIII. A comparison of the effects of potassium on the inotropic and arrythmia-producing actions of ouabain, J. Clin. Invest. **45**:346, 1966.

53 Withering, W.: An account of the foxglove, and some of its medicinal uses; with practical remarks on dropsy, and other diseases, London, 1785, C. G. J. & J. Robinson. (Reprinted in Medical Classics **2**:305, 1937.)

54 Wollenberger, A.: The energy metabolism of the failing heart and the metabolic action of the cardiac glycosides, Pharmacol. Rev. **1**:311, 1949.

55 Wood, E. H., and Moe, G. K.: Correlation between serum potassium changes in the heart-lung preparation and the therapeutic and toxic effects of digitalis glycosides, Amer. J. Physiol. **129**:499, 1940.

56 Woodbury, L. A., and Hecht, H. H.: Effects of cardiac glycosides upon the electrical activity of single ventricular fibers of the frog heart, and their relation to the digitalis effect of the electrocardiogram, Circulation **6**:172, 1952.

Recent reviews

57 Briggs, A. H., and Holland, W. C.: The chemistry of heart failure and digitalis action, Connecticut Med. J. **26**:630, 1962.

58 Butler, V. P.: Digoxin: immunologic approaches to measurement and reversal of toxicity, New Eng. J. Med. **283**:1150, 1970.

59 Doherty, J. E.: The clinical pharmacology of digitalis glycosides; a review, Amer. J. Med. Sci. **255**:382, 1968.

60 Dunham, E. T., and Glynn, I. M.: Adenosine triphosphatase activity and the active movements of alkali metal ions, J. Physiol. **156**:274, 1961.

61 Edman, K. A. P.: Drugs and properties of heart muscle, Ann. Rev. Pharmacol. **5**:99, 1965.

62 Glynn, I. M.: The action of cardiac glycosides on ion movements, Physiol. Rev. **16**:381, 1964.

63 Jeliffe, R. W.: An improved method for replacing one digitalis glycoside with another, Med. Times **98**:105, 1970.

64 Katz, A. I., and Epstein, F. H.: Physiologic role of sodium-potassium-activated triphosphatase in the transport of cations across biologic membranes, New Eng. J. Med. **278**:253, 1968.

65 Koch-Weser, J.: Mechanism of digitalis action on the heart, New Eng. J. Med. **277**:417, 469, 1967.

66 Langer, G. A.: Ion fluxes in cardiac excitation and contraction and their relation to myocardial contractility, Physiol. Rev. **48**:708, 1968.

67 Langer, G. A.: The mechanism of action of digitalis, Hosp. Practice, p. 49, Aug., 1970.

68 Lee, K. S.: Relation of cations to the inotropic and metabolic actions of cardiac glycosides. In Wilbrandt, W., editor: New aspects of cardiac glycosides, First International Pharmacological Meeting, 1961, New York, 1963, Pergamon Press, Inc.

69 Marks, B. H.: Effects of drugs on the inotropic property of the heart, Ann. Rev. Pharmacol. **4**:155, 1964.

70 Marks, B. H., and Weissler, A. M.: Basic and Clinical Pharmacology of Digitalis: Proceedings of a Symposium, Springfield, Ill., 1972, Charles C Thomas, Publisher.

71 Mason, D. T.: The cardiovascular effects of digitalis in normal man, Clin. Pharmacol. Ther. **7**:1, 1966.

72 Rosen, M. R., Gelband, H., Merker, C., and Hoffman, B. F.: Mechanisms of digitalis toxicity: effects of ouabain on phase four of canine Purkinje fiber transmembrane potentials, Circulation **47**:681, 1973.

73 Skou, J. C.: Enzymatic basis for active transport of Na^+ and K^+ across cell membrane, Physiol. Rev. **45**:596, 1965.

74 Smith, T. W.: Digitalis glycosides, New Eng. J. Med. **288**:719, 942, 1973.

75 Sodeman, W. A.: Diagnosis and treatment of digitalis toxicity, New Eng. J. Med. **273**:35, 93, 1965.

76 Trautwein, W.: Generation and conduction of impulses in the heart as affected by drugs, Pharmacol. Rev. **15**:277, 1963.

77 West, T. C., and Toda, N.: Cardiovascular pharmacology, Ann. Rev. Pharmacol. **7**:145, 1967.

78 Wilbrandt, W., editor: New aspects of cardiac glycosides, First International Pharmacological Meeting, 1961, New York, 1963, Pergamon Press, Inc.

30 Antiarrhythmic drugs

GENERAL CONCEPT

The antiarrhythmic drugs are useful in the prevention and treatment of certain disorders of cardiac rhythm. The common arrhythmias are believed to arise as a consequence of electrophysiologic changes in the heart, and the antiarrhythmic drugs exert their effect by altering or normalizing the electrophysiologic disturbances.

Impulses in the heart are generated by one of two possible mechanisms[45]: (1) the spontaneous discharge of a pacemaker cell at a normal or abnormal site and (2) the re-entry mechanism. Experimental evidence indicates that the automaticity of Purkinje fibers is increased by epinephrine, isoproterenol, digitalis, or low potassium concentration.[50] On the other hand, *quinidine,* the prototype antiarrhythmic drug, or high potassium concentrations decrease automaticity in the same preparation.

In addition to quinidine, *procainamide* is often employed as an antiarrhythmic agent. *Lidocaine,* a local anesthetic, is widely used, particularly in coronary care units in the treatment of ventricular arrhythmias. *Diphenylhydantoin,* an anticonvulsant, may be useful in the treatment of arrhythmias induced by digitalis. *Propranolol,* a beta adrenergic blocking agent, and *potassium salts* also find application in the management of certain arrhythmias. *Bretylium,* an investigational adrenergic neuronal blocking drug, also has antiarrhythmic properties.

ELECTROPHYSIOLOGIC BASIS OF ANTIARRHYTHMIC ACTION

The properties of the heart muscle that are basically involved in arrhythmias are automaticity, conduction velocity, and the *refractory period.* Automaticity is related directly to the rate of diastolic depolarization. The velocity of conduction in atrial and ventricular muscle is about 0.3 m./sec. There is much slower conduction at the A-V node and the junctional fibers. On the other hand, Purkinje's fibers conduct impulses rapidly, at a velocity of 1.5 to 2.5 m./sec.[38] The *functional refractory period* is defined as the period during which an impulse from another part of the heart fails to excite an already excited portion of the heart muscle. The functional refractory period is of the order of 0.25 second. This is followed by a short period of a *relative refractoriness* lasting 0.05 second, during which the muscle becomes excitable to strong stimulation.

It is generally believed that most tachyarrhythmias are consequences of two basic mechanisms[43]: (1) disorders of impulse formation or increased automaticity and (2) disorders of impulse conduction. Disorders of impulse formation can be abolished by drugs that depress automaticity or the rate of diastolic depolarization (Fig. 30-1). Drugs that alter conduction velocity or the refractory period may arrest ectopic circus movements. Most tachyarrhythmias probably result from disorders of impulse formation or conduction or a combination of the two.[43]

Table 30-1. Effects of antiarrhythmic drugs*

Drug	Automaticity		Conduction velocity	Refractory period	Inotropic effect	Autonomic effects	Adverse effects
	Atrium	Ventricle					
Quinidine	↓	↓	↓	↑	↓	Vagolytic	Shock; hemolysis; thrombocytopenia; G. I.; cinchonism
Procainamide	↓	↓	↓	↑	↓	Vagolytic	Lupus; shock; G. I.; psychosis
Lidocaine	0	↓	0	↓	0	0	CNS depression; seizures; shock
Propranolol	↓	↓	↓	↓	↓↓	Beta blocking	Heart failure; bronchospasm; hypoglycemia; rash; G. I.
Diphenylhydantoin	↓	↓	↑	↓	0	0	Sedation; ataxia; gum changes; lymphoma; lupus; rash; folate deficiency; osteomalacia

*Modified from Wasserman, A. J., and Proctor, J. D.: Med. Coll. Va. Quart. **9**:53, 1973.

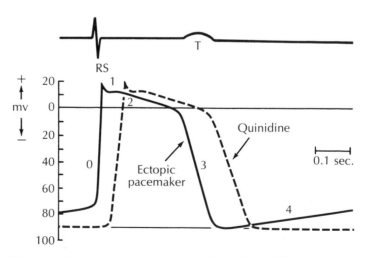

Fig. 30-1. Diagrammatic representation of the effect of quinidine on the transmembrane electrical potential of a spontaneously depolarizing conductive fiber in the ventricular myocardium. (Modified from Mason et al.: Clin. Pharmacol. Ther. **11**:460, 1970.)

The conditions necessary for reentry to occur are as follows[44]: (1) the conduction pathway must be blocked; (2) there must be slow conduction over an alternate route to a point beyond the block; and (3) there must be delayed excitation beyond the block. With a sufficient delay in excitation beyond the block, the tissue proximal to the site of block may be excited from the opposite direction and the circuit is then established.[44] It is easy to see that drugs which influence conduction velocity and refractory period can abolish a circus movement.

The effects of some antiarrhythmic drugs on the various properties of the heart muscle are summarized in Table 30-1.

An examination of Table 30-1 indicates that all the antiarrhythmic drugs depress automaticity in the ventricles and most do so in the atria. The decrease in the rate of diastolic depolarization by quinidine is shown in Fig. 30-1. The effects of antiarrhythmic drugs on conduction velocity and refractory periods are complex and will be discussed under the individual drugs.

It should be emphasized that the antiarrhythmic drugs are potentially dangerous, especially so if their pharmacology is not understood by the user. It is also clear that many arrhythmias do not require treatment and that antiarrhythmic drugs may do more harm than good.

ANTIARRHYTHMIC DRUGS
QUINIDINE

Quinidine is the dextrorotatory isomer of quinine and has the following structure:

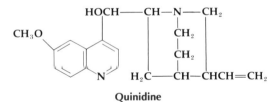

Quinidine

The introduction of quinidine into therapeutics is one of the classic stories of medical history. In 1914 the Viennese cardiologist Wenckebach[32] had a Dutch sea captain as a patient. The captain had a completely irregular pulse as a consequence of auricular fibrillation. Wenckebach described the situation in this way.

> He did not feel great discomfort during the attack, but, as he said, being a Dutch merchant, used to good order in his affairs, he would like to have good order in his heart business also, and asked why there were heart specialists if they could not abolish this very disagreeable phenomenon. On my telling him that I could promise him nothing, he told me that he knew himself how to get rid of his attacks, and as I did not believe him, he promised to come back the next morning with a regular pulse, and he did. It happens that quinine in many countries, especially in countries where there is a good deal of malaria, is a sort of drug for everything, just as one takes acetylsalicylic acid today if ones does not feel well or is afraid of having taken a cold. Occasionally, taking the drug during an attack of fibrillation, the patient found that the attack was stopped within from twenty to twenty-five minutes, and later he found that a gram of quinine regularly abolished his irregularity.*

Wenckebach began to use quinine in the treatment of auricular fibrillation. His

*From Beckman, H.: Treatment in general practice, Philadelphia, 1934, W. B. Saunders Co.

results were generally disappointing except in those patients in whom the arrhythmia was recent. He noted, however, that even when quinine failed to abolish fibrillation it had a "marked soothing action on the often terrific rate of the ventricle."

In 1918 Frey[8] tried drugs related to quinine in patients with auricular fibrillation and introduced quinidine, the dextro isomer of quinine, into cardiac therapy. During the succeeding years the antifibrillatory action of quinidine was confirmed, but its widespread use led to a number of sudden deaths.

Eventually it was recognized that there are definite contraindications to use of the drug. In the presence of conduction defects it may produce cardiac standstill and should be avoided. Once the mode of action of the drug was understood and contraindications to its use were recognized, quinidine obtained its present position in cardiac therapy.

Cardiac effects

Quinidine may be looked on as the prototype of the antiarrhythmic drugs. It decreases automaticity by reducing the rate of spontaneous diastolic depolarization (Fig. 30-1). It diminishes conduction velocity and prolongs the functional and effective refractory periods. Quinidine is sometimes referred to as a Group 1 antiarrhythmic drug, since it not only acts to decrease the rate of diastolic depolarization but also moves the threshold voltage toward zero. In this respect it resembles the actions of procainamide.

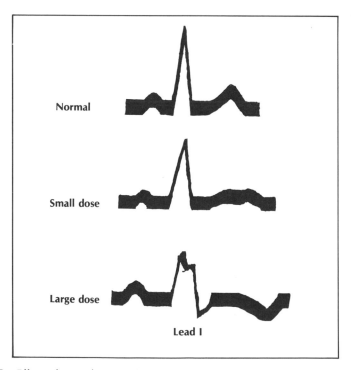

Fig. 30-2. Effect of quinidine on electrocardiogram. Note changes in P wave, QRS complex, and T wave at varying dosage levels. (From Burch, G. E., and Winsor, T.: A primer of electrocardiography, Philadelphia, 1960, Lea & Febiger.)

A complicating factor in the action of quinidine is its "vagolytic" or anticholinergic effect. This may counteract its direct effect and may explain the acceleration of heart rate that may be caused by the drug. The anticholinergic effect may also explain the paradoxical tachycardia that may be seen in some cases during the treatment of atrial flutter with block.

Quinidine probably exerts its fundamental action at the cell membrane, where it interferes with cation transfer. The drug apparently decreases membrane permeability to sodium. The antiarrhythmic actions of quinidine are further increased by potassium and are reduced in hypokalemia. The depressant effect of quinidine on contractility may be related to interference with calcium transport.

Electrocardiographic effects. Quinidine in higher doses prolongs the P-R, QRS, and Q-T intervals (Fig. 30-2). Widening of the QRS complex is related to slowing conduction in the His-Purkinje system and in the ventricular muscle. Changes in the Q-T interval and alteration in T waves are related to changes in repolarization. The direct effect of the drug on A-V conduction and refractoriness of the A-V system explains the prolongation of the P-R interval.

Extracardiac and adverse effects

Quinidine tends to depress all muscle tissue, including vascular smooth muscle and skeletal muscle. Particularly when injected intravenously, the drug can cause profound hypotension and shock. Its effect on skeletal muscle becomes particularly evident in patients with myasthenia gravis, in whom it causes profound weakness.

Cinchonism caused by quinidine is characterized by ringing of the ears and dizziness and is similar to what may be observed after the administration of quinine or salicylates.

Quinine poisoning

Quinidine thrombocytopenia appears to occur on an allergic basis. In a typical case, a patient taking quinidine for several weeks notices the development of petechial hemorrhages in the buccal mucous membranes. The symptoms disappear when the drug is discontinued and reappear after reinstitution of therapy. A positive Ackroyd test can usually be demonstrated in vitro.

Cardiotoxicity and its treatment

Quinidine may cause ventricular arrhythmias and even ventricular fibrillation. The so-called "quinidine syncope" is probably a consequence of ventricular fibrillation.[52]

It may seem paradoxical that an antiarrhythmic drug can cause ventricular arrhythmias. Since quinidine depresses automaticity, the clinically observed ventricular arrhythmias after excessive doses of quinidine are probably due to a reentry mechanism rather than to increased automaticity.[50]

Quinidine is particularly dangerous in patients having conduction defects. In such patients when conduction is further impaired and automaticity of the Purkinje system is depressed, the ventricles may not take over when A-V conduction fails, and cardiac standstill may ensue. The administration of the drug should be stopped when significant increases in P-R interval or QRS widenings supervene during treatment.

In addition to stopping the drug administration, quinidine intoxication is treated supportively with maintenance of blood pressure, oxygen, and bed rest. Sodium bicarbonate and sodium lactate have also been recommended.

Pharmacokinetics

When given orally, quinidine produces its peak effect in 2 to 4 hours. Its half-life is about 4 to 6 hours. Therapeutic plasma levels are 3 to 6 $\mu g/ml$.

About 10 to 50% of administered quinidine is excreted in unchanged form in the urine. The rest is transformed in the liver by hydroxylation. The amount excreted is influenced by the pH of the urine. Alkalinization with molar sodium lactate tends to decrease the excretion of quinidine, although it may improve some toxic effects of the drug.

Quinidine is bound to plasma proteins, a fact that may account for some lack of correlation between blood levels and therapeutic effect. Nevertheless, toxic manifestations correlate better with serum levels than with the dose of the drug.[43]

Drug interactions occur with quinidine and will be discussed in Chapter 58.

Preparations, methods of administration, and dose

Preparations of quinidine include the following: quinidine sulfate in tablets containing 200 and 300 mg. and timed-release tablets of 300 mg.; quinidine gluconate (Quinaglute) in tablets containing 300 mg.; and quinidine hydrochloride in solution for injection, 120 mg./ml., for intramuscular use.

The usual adult dosage of quinidine is 200 to 400 mg. three to five times daily for 1 to 3 days. Larger doses should be used only in the hospital.

Quinidine hydrochloride or gluconate are available for intramuscular injection. Intravenous administration is dangerous and should not be undertaken without monitoring the electrocardiogram.

Blood levels of quinidine have been studied by several investigators. A single dose of 200 to 400 mg. of quinidine sulfate given on an empty stomach will produce a plasma level of 2 to 4 mg./L. in about 2 hours. The level tends to decline fairly rapidly, and at the end of 24 hours little quinidine remains in the blood. If the same dose is given every 4 hours or at shorter intervals, definite accumulation occurs. It is the opinion of some investigators that there is a relationship between the height of the blood level of quinidine and success in converting auricular fibrillation.[27] The level necessary could not be predicted in a given patient, but most patients required 4 to 8 mg./L. This level is attained by deliberately producing a cumulation through the frequent administration of the drug.

PROCAINAMIDE

Development as cardiac drug

The commonly used local anesthetic procaine was shown by Mautz[18] in 1936 to elevate the threshold to electrical stimulation when applied to the myocardium of animals. In subsequent years thoracic surgeons and anesthesiologists frequently used topical procaine in surgery to reduce premature ventricular and atrial contractions during surgery. Procaine was even administered intravenously for this purpose.

The chemical structures of procaine and procainamide are shown below.

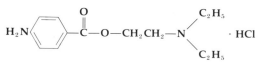

Procaine hydrochloride

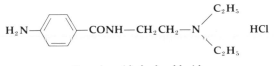

Procainamide hydrochloride

Encouraged by these studies, investigators studied the antifibrillatory activities of compounds related to procaine, including the effects of the two hydrolysis products of procaine, *p*-aminobenzoic acid and diethylaminoethanol. The most fruitful consequence of these studies was the finding that if the ester linkage in procaine was replaced by an amide linkage, the resulting compound had distinct advantages as an antiarrhythmic drug. The main advantages consist of greater stability in the body and fewer central nervous system effects. The greater stability results from the fact that the drug is an amide rather than an ester.

Cardiac effects

Procainamide is a typical Group 1 antiarrhythmic drug just like quinidine.[36] It decreases automaticity and shifts the threshold voltage of heart muscle toward zero. It lengthens the duration of the action potential and refractory period in atria and ventricles. It slows conduction in the atrium, A-V node, and ventricle. It decreases membrane responsiveness in atrial and ventricular muscle.

Generally, the effects of procainamide are similar to those of quinidine. Traditionally, procainamide has been preferred for ventricular arrhythmias, whereas quinidine was more commonly employed for atrial arrhythmias. However, there may not be a good basis for these preferences.[43] Nevertheless, procainamide is often preferred to quinidine when parenteral treatment is needed, since quinidine injections have caused catastrophic hypotension in some cases.

Procainamide is effective against a wide variety of atrial, A-V junctional, and ventricular arrhythmias. The drug is considered a poor choice against ventricular arrhythmias in patients with severe A-V conduction disturbances, since it may make conduction worse.[36] Although it is effective against digitalis-induced ventricular arrhythmias, its effects are considered too unpredictable.[36]

Pharmacokinetics

Procainamide may be given by intravenous injection, intravenous infusion, intramuscular injection, and the oral route. Large intravenous injections may cause severe hypotension. On the other hand, 100 mg. doses may be injected every 5 minutes for 4 to 8 doses without significant hypotension.[36]

The plasma concentration of procainamide falls rapidly after its intravenous injection because of its rapid redistribution into a large volume of distribution. The later rate of disappearance of the drug has a half-life of $3\frac{1}{2}$ hours.

About 60% of the drug is excreted in the urine and 25 to 30% is acetylated probably by the liver.

Intramuscular administration of procainamide has no great advantages over oral administration, unless the patient is unable to take the drug by mouth. When administered orally, effective plasma concentrations may be achieved in 15 minutes, with peak levels at 45 to 75 minutes. Absorption is essentially complete and its half-life in the body is $3\frac{1}{2}$ to 4 hours.[36]

Extracardiac effects and toxicity

Procainamide may cause a marked fall of blood pressure after the administration of large intravenous doses. This is probably a consequence of its action on vascular smooth muscle and on contractility of the myocardium although ganglionic blocking effects have also been described.[24] The drug has local anesthetic properties but is not useful for nerve block.

Nausea, anorexia, mental confusion, hallucinations, skin rashes, agranulocytosis, chills, and fever have been reported after the use of procainamide. A lupus erythematosus–like syndrome has also been observed in patients taking procainamide.[23]

LIDOCAINE

Lidocaine (Xylocaine) is currently widely used as an antiarrhythmic drug in coronary care units. It is effective against ventricular arrhythmias, but is ineffective against atrial fibrillation and flutter. The drug is also ineffective against atrial and A-V junctional tachycardias unless they are caused by digitalis. A major limitation of lidocaine results from the necessity of parenteral administration.

From an *electrophysiologic standpoint*, lidocaine is a Group 2 antiarrhythmic drug.[36] It suppresses automaticity in Purkinje fibers without altering the threshold potential. Lidocaine decreases the duration of the action potential in Purkinje's fibers and shortens the refractory period. It has essentially no effect on atrial muscle. Conduction velocity is either unaltered or may be actually increased. The drug does not prolong the QRS complex, since it does not alter conduction. Lidocaine does not affect the Q-T interval, since it does not prolong the duration of the action potential in the ventricles.

Pharmacokinetics

Lidocaine is used only by the parenteral route, by intravenous injection or constant rate infusion. By *intravenous injection* 0.5 to 1.5 mg./kg. of body weight may be given every 3 to 5 minutes for a total dosage of 200 to 300 mg. The minimal effective concentration of lidocaine in plasma is 1 to 2 μg/ml. After a single intravenous injection the concentration of lidocaine drops rapidly because of its redistribution in an apparent volume of about 120 L. After this initial distribution the rate of elimination of the drug is slow as a consequence of hepatic metabolism and renal excretion.[29] Less than 10% of a dose is excreted through the kidneys. For details on the hepatic metabolism and the formation of active metabolites, see Chapter 28.

The plasma half-life of lidocaine is about 2 hours. Since the half-life is short and the minimal effective concentration is low, lidocaine is occasionally administered by intravenous infusion, usually after some single intravenous injections.

Intramuscular injection of lidocaine is still experimental, although some investigators advocate it for the prophylaxis of ectopic rhythms in impending myocardial infarction. However, intramuscular injection is controversial. A special 10% solution and a dose of 4 mg./kg. injected into the deltoid muscle will produce a plasma level of 1 μg/ml. in 5 minutes. This level will persist for 90 to 120 minutes with a peak of 3.3 μg/ml. in 15 minutes after the injection.[36]

Preparations

Lidocaine hydrochloride (Xylocaine hydrochloride) is available in solutions for injection of 5, 10, 15, and 20 mg./ml.

DIPHENYLHYDANTOIN

The antiepileptic drug diphenylhydantoin (Dilantin) was found to decrease ventricular arrhythmias in dogs after coronary ligation in 1950.[14] More recently it has become widely used as an antiarrhythmic drug especially in digitalis-induced tachyarrhythmias, which may be its only real indication.[52]

The effects of diphenylhydantoin on the heart are summarized in Table 30-1. The drug decreases automaticity, but its actions on conduction velocity and refractory period are the opposite of those of quinidine. Diphenylhydantoin has no negative inotropic effects.

The effective level of diphenylhydantoin for antiarrhythmic activity is about 6 to 18 μg/ml., which is about the same as for its anticonvulsant effectiveness.

Pharmacokinetics

Diphenylhydantoin is absorbed slowly when given by mouth and peak levels are not obtained for several hours. The drug should not be given intramuscularly, since its absorption is erratic.[52] The drug is metabolized by liver microsomal enzymes, being parahydroxylated. The disappearance of diphenylhydantoin does not follow first-order kinetics because of saturation of the microsomal enzymes at therapeutic serum levels. With this reservation, it is useful to know that within the usual therapeutically effective concentration, serum levels fall to one half in 18 to 24 hours.

Dosage

For oral administration to obtain a prompt effect, diphenylhydantoin may be administered in a dose of 1000 mg. the first day, 500 to 600 mg. the second and third day, and 400 to 500 mg. thereafter.[52]

Diphenylhydantoin may be injected intravenously when urgent indications exist. Fifty to 100 mg. may be given at 5-minute intervals until a therapeutic effect, a toxic effect, or a total of 1000 mg. is given.

Preparations

Diphenylhydantoin sodium (Dilantin sodium) is available in capsules containing 100 mg. It is also available as a powder to make a solution for injection, 50 mg./ml.

PROPRANOLOL

The beta adrenergic blocking agent propranolol (Inderal) acts on the heart by two mechanisms: (1) it opposes the action of catecholamines released by sympathetic fibers and (2) it has a direct effect characterized by the reduction of the rate of diastolic depolarization, decreased conduction velocity, decreased refractory period, and decreased inotropic state.[52]

The major disadvantage of the beta blockers is cardiac depression. It is the belief of competent investigators that propranolol should only be used as an antiarrhythmic drug when the arrhythmia is caused by adrenergic mechanisms. The drug should be avoided in patients with myocardial disease except in special situations in which other therapies have failed.

Dosage

Propranolol may be given orally or intravenously. The oral dose is 10 to 30 mg. three to four times a day. Intravenously 1 to 2 mg. may be given every 5 minutes without exceeding 10 mg.

BRETYLIUM TOSYLATE

Bretylium tosylate is an investigational antiarrhythmic drug that has been used before as an adrenergic neuronal blocking antihypertensive agent. The clinical usefulness of bretylium tosylate is unclear, although it may find some place in the management of severe ventricular tachyarrhythmias.

POTASSIUM

Elevated potassium concentrations in the plasma tend to reduce conduction velocity and shorten the refractory period. They also decrease automaticity. The cardiac actions of potassium are more marked on Purkinje fibers and on atrial muscle cells than on the A-V node. For this reason, potassium is more likely to cause intraventricular block than atrioventricular block.

Altered potassium concentrations have a great influence on digitalis toxicity. Also, elevated potassium concentrations reduce the response of the heart to electrical stimulation and interfere with the effectiveness of pacemakers.

SELECTION OF DRUGS IN TREATMENT OF CARDIAC ARRHYTHMIAS

There are several principles that should be remembered before selecting a drug for the treatment of a cardiac arrhythmia. (1) Many arrhythmias do not require drug treatment. (2) Most antiarrhythmic drugs can be dangerous. (3) Cardioversion (DC countershock) has changed many of the indications for the use of antiarrhythmic medications.

With these limitations, the use of antiarrhythmic drugs in various arrhythmias will be briefly summarized.

SUPRAVENTRICULAR ARRHYTHMIAS
Paroxysmal atrial tachycardia

Paroxysmal atrial tachycardia may occur in otherwise normal individuals. It may terminate spontaneously but may recur. It may also occur as a manifestation of digitalis toxicity.

Increased vagal influences may terminate the tachycardia without the use of drugs, and pressure on the carotid sinus is often employed for this purpose. Methacholine has been used for terminating an acute attack but it may cause alarming reactions, such as profound hypotension. Digitalis and quinidine may be used either for terminating an acute attack or for the prevention of recurrences.

Atrial flutter

Digitalis is the most important drug in the treatment of atrial flutter. It acts primarily by increasing the degree of atrioventricular block, thereby decreasing the ventricular rate. As to the flutter itself, digitalis tends to convert it to fibrillation. The explanation resides in the ability of digitalis to shorten the refractory period in the atrial muscle.[45] Occasionally quinidine is used for the conversion of flutter to normal sinus rhythm. In this case digitalis should be employed first to prevent excessive tachycardia, a consequence of the vagolytic action of quinidine. Cardioversion finds increasing usefulness in the treatment of atrial flutter.

Atrial fibrillation

Digitalis is the most important drug in the treatment of atrial fibrillation. It does not convert atrial fibrillation to normal sinus rhythm, but it slows the ventricular rate by increasing atrioventricular block and it corrects cardiac failure if it is present. Quinidine can convert atrial fibrillation to normal sinus rhythm, but the newer tendency is to use cardioversion for this purpose. Even when DC countershock is employed, quinidine may be helpful in preventing the recurrence of atrial fibrillation.

VENTRICULAR ARRHYTHMIAS

Occasional premature ventricular contractions generally do not require drug treatment. On the other hand, ventricular tachycardia may be a serious condition that requires intensive treatment. Although DC countershock is now commonly used for stopping ventricular tachycardia, it should not be employed if the arrhythmia is caused by digitalis.

The selection of antiarrhythmic drugs for the treatment of ventricular tachycardia is undergoing changes as newer drugs are being studied. Traditionally, quinidine and procainamide have been used. Currently, lidocaine is extremely popular, particularly in coronary care units. Propranolol or diphenylhydantoin may be useful in digitalis-induced ventricular tachycardia. Finally, bretylium tosylate is being used as an investigational drug in some cases of ventricular tachycardia, but its exact place in therapeutics is impossible to state at this time.[3]

References

1 Armitage, A. K.: The influence of potassium concentration on the action of quinidine and of some antimalarial substances on cardiac muscle, Brit. J. Pharmacol. 12:74, 1957.

2 Beckman, H.: Treatment in general practice, Philadelphia, 1934, W. B. Saunders Co.

3 Bernstein, J. G., and Koch-Weser, J.: Effectiveness of bretylium tosylate against refractory ventricular arrhythmias, Circulation 45:1024, 1972.

4 Bolton, F. G.: Thrombocytopenic purpura due to quinidine: serologic mechanisms, Blood 11:547, 1956.

5 Cheng, T. O.: Atrial flutter during quinidine therapy of atrial fibrillation, Amer. Heart J. 52:273, 1956.

6 Conn, R. D.: Diphenylhydantoin sodium in cardiac arrhythmias, New Eng. J. Med. 272:277, 1965.

7 Dawes, G. S.: Experimental cardiac arrhythmias and quinidine-like drugs, Pharmacol. Rev. 4:43, 1952.

8 Frey, W.: Weitere Erfahrungen mit Chinidin bei absoluter Herzunregelmässigkeit, Klin. Wchnschr. 55:849, 1918.

9 Frieden, J.: Antiarrhythmic drugs. VII. Lidocaine as an antiarrhythmic agent, Amer. Heart J. 79:713, 1965.

10 Gertler, M. M., Kream, J., Hylin, J. W., Robinson, H., and Neidle, E. G.: Effect of quinidine on intracellular electrolytes of the rabbit heart, Proc. Soc. Exp. Biol. Med. 92:629, 1956.

11 Gold, H., Modell, W., and Price, L.: Combined actions of quinidine and digitalis on the heart: an experimental study, Arch. Intern. Med. 50:766, 1932.

12 Grossman, J. I., Lubow, L. A., Frieden, J., et al.: Lidocaine in cardiac arrhythmias, Arch. Intern. Med. 121:396, 1968.

13 Harris, A. S., Estandia, A., Ford, T. J., Jr., and Tillotson, R. F.: Quinidine lactate and gluconate in the suppression of ectopic ventricular tachycardia associated with myocardial infarction, Circulation 4:522, 1951.

14 Harris, A. S., and Kokernot, R. H.: Effects of diphenylhydantoin sodium (Dilantin sodium) and phenobarbital sodium upon ectopic ventricular tachycardia in acute myocardial infarction, Amer. J. Physiol. 163:505, 1950.

15 Harrison, D. C., Griffin, J. R., and Fiene, T. J.: Effects of beta adrenergic blockade with propranolol in patients with atrial arrhythmias, New Eng. J. Med. 27:410, 1965.

16 Holland, W. C., and Klein, R. L.: Effect of temperature, Na and K concentration, and quinidine on transmembrane flux of K^{42} and

incidence of atrial fibrillation, Circulation Res. **6**:516, 1958.

17 Johnson, E. A., and McKinnon, M. G.: The differential effect of quinidine and pyrilamine on the myocardial action potential at various rates of stimulation, J. Pharmacol. Exp. Ther. **120**:460, 1957.

18 Koch-Weser, J.: Antiarrhythmic prophylaxis in ambulatory patients with coronary heart disease, Arch. Intern. Med. **129**:763, 1972.

19 Koch-Weser, J., and Klein, S. W.: Procainamide dosage schedules, plasma concentrations and clinical effects, J.A.M.A. **215**:1454, 1971.

20 Koch-Weser, J., Klein, S. W., Foo-Canto, L. L., Kastor, J. A., and DeSanctis, R. W.: Antiarrhythmic prophylaxis with procainamide in acute myocardial infarction, New Eng. J. Med. **281**: 1253, 1969.

21 Manning, J. W., Cotten, M. D., Kelly, W. N., and Johnson, C. E.: Mechanism of cardiac arrhythmias induced by diencephalic stimulation, Amer. J. Physiol. **203**:1120, 1962.

22 Mautz, F. R.: The reduction of cardiac irritability by the epicardial and systemic administration of drugs as a protection in cardiac surgery, J. Thorac. Surg. **5**:612, 1936.

23 Paine, R.: Procainamide hydrocholoride and lupus erythematosus, J.A.M.A. **194**:23, 1965.

24 Paton, W. D. M., and Thompson, J. W.: Procaine amide, Brit. Med. J. **1**:991, 1953.

25 Prinzmetal, M., Rakita, L., Borduas, J. L., Flamm, E., and Goldman, A.: The nature of spontaneous auricular fibrillation in man with comments on the action of anti-arrhythmic drugs, J.A.M.A. **157**:1175, 1955.

26 Rosenblueth, A., and Garcia Ramos, J.: Estudino sobre el flutter y la fibrillación, Arch. Inst. Cardiol. Mex. **17**:441, 1947.

27 Scherf, D.: Studies on auricular tachycardia caused by aconitine administration, Proc. Soc. Exp. Biol. Med. **64**:233, 1947.

28 Sokolow, M., and Edgar, A. L.: Blood quinidine concentrations as guide in treatment of cardiac arrhythmias, Circulation **1**:576, 1950.

29 Strong, J. M., Parker, M., and Atkinson, A. J.: Identification of glycinexylidide in patients treated with intravenous lidocaine, Clin. Pharmacol. Ther. **14**:67, 1973.

30 Unger, A. H., and Sklaroff, H. J.: Fatalities following intravenous use of sodium diphenylhydantoin for cardiac arrhythmias, J.A.M.A. **200**:335, 1967.

31 Wedd, A. M., Blair, H. A., and Warner, R. S.: The action of procaine amide on the heart, Amer. Heart J. **42**:399, 1951.

32 Wenckebach, K. F.: Die unregelmässige Herz-

tätigkeit und ihre klinische Bedeutung, Leipzig, 1914, W. Engelmann.

Recent reviews

33 Bassett, A. L. and Hoffman, B. F.: Antiarrhythmic drugs: electrophysiological actions, Ann. Rev. Pharmacol. **11**:143, 1971.

34 Bellet, S.: Atrial fibrillation, J.A.M.A. **189**:419, 1964.

35 Bigger, J. T.: Antiarrhythmic drugs in ischemic heart disease, Hosp. Practice, p. 69, Nov. 1972.

36 Bigger, J. T., and Giardina, E.-G. V.: The pharmacology and clinical use of lidocaine and procainamide, Med. Coll. Va. Quart. **9**:65, 1973.

37 Escher, D. J. W., and Furman, S.: Emergency treatment of cardiac arrhythmias, J.A.M.A. **214**: 2028, 1970.

38 Guyton, A. C.: Textbook of medical physiology, ed. 4, Philadelphia, 1971, W. B. Saunders Co.

39 Hayes, A. H.: The actions and clinical use of the newer antiarrhythmic drugs, Rational Drug Ther. **6**:1, July 1972.

40 Hoffman, B. F., and Cranefield, P. F.: The physiological basis of cardiac arrhythmias, Amer. J. Med. **37**:670, 1964.

41 Hoffman, B. F., Cranefield, P. F., and Wallace, A. G.: Physiological basis of cardiac arrhythmias. I and II, Mod. Conc. Cardiovasc. Dis. **35**:103, 1966.

42 Kayden, H. J.: Pharmacology of procaine amide, Amer. Heart J. **70**:423, 1965.

43 Mason, D. T., Spann, J. F., Zelis, R., and Amsterdam, E. A.: The clinical pharmacology and therapeutic applications of the antiarrhythmic drugs, Clin. Pharmacol. Ther. **11**:460, 1970.

44 Moe, G.: Reentry, Med. Coll. Va. Quart. **9**:33, 1973.

45 Moe, G. K., and Mendez, C.: Physiologic basis of premature beats and sustained tachycardias, New Eng. J. Med. **288**:250, 1973.

46 Moe, R. A., and Abrams, W. B.: The "ideal" antiarrhythmic drug. In Brest, A. N., and Moyer, J. H., editors: Cardiovascular drug therapy, New York, 1965, Grune & Stratton, Inc.

47 Morrelli, H. F., and Melmon, K. L.: Pharmacologic basis for the clinical use of antiarrhythmic drugs, Pharmacol. Physicians **1**(7):1, 1967.

48 Sodeman, W. A.: Diagnosis and treatment of digitalis toxicity, New Eng. J. Med. **273**:93, 1965.

49 Sokolow, M., and Perloff, D.: Clinical pharmacology and use of quinidine, Progr. Cardiov. Dis. **3**:316, 1961.

50 Surawicz, B.: Ventricular tachyarrhythmias, Med. Coll. Va. Quart. **9**:48, 1973.

51 Trautwein, W.: Generation and conduction of impulses in the heart as affected by drugs, Pharmacol. Rev. **15**:277, 1963.

52 Wasserman, A. J., and Proctor, J. D.: Pharma cology of antiarrhythmias: quinidine, beta-blockers, diphenylhydantoin, bretylium, Med. Coll. Va. Quart. **9**:53, 1973.

31 Antianginal drugs

GENERAL CONCEPT

It is an old empirical observation that amyl nitrite (1867) and nitroglycerin (1879) relieve the pain of angina pectoris. Since nitrates and nitrites dilate blood vessels, including the coronary arteries, the role of coronary vasodilatation in the relief of angina has been generally assumed.

The problem is much more complex, however. Angina results from an imbalance between oxygen demand and supply in ischemic areas of the myocardium. Drugs may improve angina theoretically by reducing the demand or by increasing the supply of oxygen. There is increasing evidence for a reduction of demand by an action on the peripheral circulation as a primary mechanism for the antianginal effect of the nitrates and nitrites. On the other hand, drugs that increase myocardial oxygen demand, such as the catecholamines, have adverse effects in patients with coronary disease.

The simple view that coronary vasodilatation is sufficient to explain the antianginal effect of the rapidly acting nitrites has been made untenable by the discovery of drugs (e.g., dipyridamole) that are potent coronary vasodilators but are not effective as antianginal drugs.

In addition to the short-acting nitrites and nitrates, there are several longer-acting drugs. These prevent anginal attacks also when administered sublingually. However, their prophylactic value when administered orally is controversial.

The use of propranolol, a beta adrenergic blocking agent, is a new approach to angina that emphasizes the importance of reduction of cardiac work in relief of angina.

METHODS OF STUDY

The effect of drugs on the coronary circulation has been studied by many different methods. Because of the intimate connection between cardiac work and coronary blood flow, the most meaningful methods are the ones that allow an estimate of both.

Coronary blood flow can be measured in anesthetized animals by means of a rotameter attached to the coronary sinus. In man the nitrous oxide method has been used for the same purpose. If cardiac output and oxygen consumption are measured simultaneously, a good estimate of the effects of a drug on the flow/work ratio may be obtained.

A clinical method has been used by Russek and co-workers[24] for estimating the effectiveness of a coronary vasodilator in patients subject to angina pectoris. In this method the patient is made to perform an exercise tolerance test, the Master two-step test, in which he ascends and descends a stair for forty steps in a given time. The appearance of precordial pain and T-wave inversion in the electrocardiogram are considered indicative of myocardial ischemia. When the test is repeated following the administration of a presumed coronary vasodilator, both manifestations of myocardial ischemia should be prevented or delayed in appearance. If a drug prevents the pain but not the T-wave changes, it is assumed that it has an analgesic effect without influencing myocardial ischemia.

Coronary blood flow has also been studied in patients, by means of the nitrous oxide method, under conditions in which the actions of the drugs on cardiac output, systemic blood pressure, and myocardial oxygen consumption could also be determined.[34]

CORONARY VASODILATORS
NITRATES AND NITRITES

A variety of nitrites and nitrates are useful in medicine because of their relaxing effect on various smooth muscles. The coronary blood vessels are so susceptible to this action that minute doses can cause an increase in coronary blood flow.

Chemistry and preparations

The clinically useful nitrites and nitrates exert qualitatively similar effects. The most interesting compounds in the group and their formulas are as follows:

Nitrates

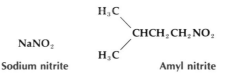

The highly effective representative of this group is glyceryl trinitrate, or nitroglycerin. Its effects will be described as those of a prototype, and all other nitrites and nitrates will be discussed by comparison.

Effects of nitroglycerin

If a patient suffering from an attack of angina pectoris places a small 0.3 mg. tablet of nitroglycerin under his tongue, the attack frequently subsides in a matter of minutes. Furthermore, the drug is often effective if taken prophylactically before the performance of some task that ordinarily produces angina.

This is not a placebo effect. Although a large proportion of patients suffering from angina pectoris claim benefit from placebo tablets, a significantly greater number derive benefit from nitroglycerin. Furthermore, if a patient between anginal attacks is asked to perform a standard exercise tolerance test such as the Master two-step test, he may develop precordial pain and T-wave inversion on the electrocardiogram, generally interpreted as consequences of myocardial ischemia. If the same patient has received prophylactic nitroglycerin, he is often protected against both the pain and the electro-cardiographic alterations during exercise.

The simplest interpretation of this remarkable effect of nitroglycerin would be that the drug improves blood flow to ischemic areas in the myocardium by dilating coronary vessels. This interpretation, however, appears to be untenable.

Problem 31-1. Would nitroglycerin administered directly into a coronary artery relieve angina? This has been tested by two clinical investigators.[8] In 25 patients undergoing cardiac catheterization as possible candidates for revascularization surgery, 0.075 mg. of nitroglycerin was injected into the left coronary artery through the angiographic catheter at a time when angina was induced by pacing. The intracoronary injection was ineffective despite a significant increase in coronary sinus blood flow in many of the patients. Intravenous injection of 0.2 mg. of nitroglycerin relieved the angina that was unaffected by the preceding intracoronary injection. This study indicates that it is the action of nitroglycerin on the systemic circulation that is responsible for its antianginal effect.

The antianginal effect of nitroglycerin is believed to result from reduction of venous tone, diminished venous return, some peripheral arterial dilatation, and to a questionable extent from dilatation of those coronary arteries that are capable of responding to the drug.[32]

In addition to the coronary vessels, certain other vascular areas are quite susceptible to the action of nitrites. The skin vessels of the face and neck, the so-called blush areas, may be markedly dilated. Meningeal vessels are dilated also, and this is the probable cause of the headache that may be produced by the nitrites.

Table 31-1. Effect of nitrites and beta blocking drugs on myocardial oxygen requirements and supply*

	Nitrites	Beta blockade
Determinants of myocardial oxygen requirements		
Heart rate	↑	↓ †
Left ventricular pressure	↓	↓ †
Left ventricular volume and radius	↓	↑
Velocity of contraction	↑	↓ †
Systolic ejection period	↓	↑
Determinants of myocardial oxygen supply		
Coronary vascular bed	↑ †	↓

* Courtesy Dr. Lawrence Cohen.
† Most significant effects.

Effects of nitroglycerin and nitrites on other smooth muscles

Probably all smooth muscles can be made to relax by the nitrites, and some minor therapeutic applications of this effect have been made. The biliary tract can be relaxed with sublingual nitroglycerin, as evidenced by a measured decrease in biliary pressure. The nitrites also can relax the ureter. Though they have been shown to relax the bronchial smooth muscle, much more effective medications are available for this purpose.

Comparison of nitroglycerin with other nitrites and nitrates

Amyl nitrite is a volatile liquid that is available in small glass pearls containing 0.2 ml. These are crushed in a handkerchief by the patient and inhaled. Amyl nitrite has a short onset of action, less than 1 minute, but its duration of action is also short, not exceeding 10 minutes. It is particularly prone to cause cutaneous vasodilatation, marked lowering of systemic pressure, and even syncope and tachycardia. In addition, its odor is objectionable, particularly when used by ambulatory patients. For these reasons nitroglycerin is preferred.

Sodium nitrite has more toxicologic than therapeutic importance. Although its smooth muscle effects are similar to those of other nitrites, its irritant effects on the gastric mucosa and its tendency to produce methemoglobin make it unsuitable as a coronary vasodilator.

A number of organic nitrates and nitrites have been prepared for the purpose of obtaining a nitroglycerin-like effect with a longer duration of action. The best known preparations and their doses are erythrityl tetranitrate tablets of 15 to 30 mg., mannitol hexanitrate tablets of 16 or 32 mg., pentaerythritol tetranitrate in 10 mg. tablets, and triethanolamine trinitrate diphosphate tablets of 2 mg. Isosorbide dinitrate (Isordil) is available in the form of sublingual (5 mg.), oral (10 mg.), and sustained-release (40 mg.) tablets. Isosorbide dinitrate (Isordil) administered sublingually (2.5 to 5 mg.) is about as effective as nitroglycerin given by the same route. Its duration of action is about 2 hours, being similar to nitroglycerin in this respect also.

A puzzling situation exists with regard to the longer-acting nitrates. They should theoretically have great advantages in the management of angina, and some clinical reports, particularly with pentaerythritol tetranitrate (Peritrate), indicate beneficial effects on the basis of the exercise tolerance test.[24,25] Nevertheless, few clinicians can achieve results comparable to those obtained with the use of the short-acting compounds nitroglycerin or amyl nitrite. Also, tolerance may develop to their effects.

Tolerance to vascular actions of nitrites

It is common experience that when nitrites are administered to a patient for several days the dosage must be increased in order to maintain the desired vascular effects. Tolerance also develops in production of headache by nitrites. The exact mechanism of tolerance is not known, and it fortunately disappears if the drug is discontinued for a few days, the patient again becoming susceptible not only to the vascular effects but also to the headache.

Toxic effects of nitrites and nitrates

The toxic effects of nitrites and nitrates are generally predictable from known pharmacologic actions of these compounds. Severe fall of blood pressure with syncope, headaches, glaucoma, and elevated intracranial pressure can result from excessive dosage or unusual susceptibility of the patient. In addition, the nitrites can produce methemoglobinemia by oxidizing the iron of the hemoglobin molecule from the ferrous to the ferric state. This ability is used to advantage in the treatment of cyanide poisoning.[4]

Nitrite poisoning may be acute or chronic. It may result from the therapeutic or accidental intake of nitrites or from the ingestion of some nitrate that may be converted to nitrites by intestinal bacteria, as has occurred following the ingestion of bismuth subnitrate. Increasing attention is paid to the fact that well water in some rural areas may contain enough nitrate to cause chronic intoxication with methemoglobinemia. Chronic poisoning due to nitrates and nitrites is an industrial hazard, particularly in the explosives industry.

Metabolism of organic nitrates

Organic nitrates are changed in the body to nitrites.[17] Blood levels of nitrites, however, do not correlate well with antianginal activity.[3,14] It has been suggested that coronary dilator activity depends upon the intact molecule of the organic nitrate and not upon reduction to nitrite. Thus isosorbide dinitrate, although it did not undergo hydrolysis and reduction, evoked increased coronary blood flow in the perfused rabbit heart.[11]

The degradation of nitroglycerin occurs primarily in the liver[16] by means of a glutathione-dependent organic nitrate reductase. The activity of the liver is largely responsible for the ineffectiveness of orally administered nitrates compared with the sublingually given tablets.

Therapeutic aims in use of nitrites and nitrates

The most important use of these compounds is in the management of angina pectoris. These drugs have been used in the treatment of hypertensive cardiovascular disease but have been replaced by more effective and less hazardous forms of medication. They may be used occasionally in biliary colic and ureteral spasm.

PAPAVERINE AND RELATED DRUGS

Papaverine is an alkaloid of opium. Its formula indicates that it is a benzylisoquinoline compound, differing from the morphine group of opium alkaloids both chemically and pharmacologically. Papaverine is not a narcotic and is not addictive.

Papaverine hydrochloride is available for oral administration and for injection. The average dose is 100 mg.

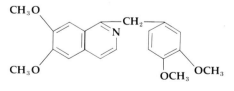

Papaverine

The main pharmacologic effect of papaverine is smooth muscle relaxation. In addition, it has a moderate quinidine-like effect on the heart.

The coronary vasodilator properties of papaverine are well documented. Eckenhoff and Hafkenschiel[6] in 1947 found it to be more effective than the nitrites in causing increased coronary blood flow in dogs. By electrocardiographic monitoring in patients, Russek and co-workers[24] found that papaverine improved exercise tolerance.

Despite this impressive background, papaverine is not nearly so effective as nitroglycerin in the management of angina pectoris. The reasons for this discrepancy between experimental work and clinical experience are quite puzzling.

In addition to its action on coronary vessels, papaverine is capable of relaxing other arteries. It has been widely used in vasospasm accompanying peripheral arterial embolism, pulmonary embolism, and cerebrovascular thrombosis.

When the drug is injected intravenously, its quinidine-like effects may be dangerous. Sudden death has resulted from such a procedure.

The chemist has not been able to improve significantly upon papaverine by slight alterations in its structure. One such drug whose effects are very similar to those of papaverine is dioxyline (Paveril).

AMINOPHYLLINE AND OTHER THEOPHYLLINE COMPOUNDS

The effects of aminophylline and other theophylline salts on the coronary circulation are quite controversial. The xanthines, particularly theophylline, tend to dilate smooth muscles and cause increased coronary blood flow in various experimental preparations. At the same time, theophylline increases the work of the heart, and much of the increase in coronary blood flow may be secondary to this effect.

In angina patients the evidence for the usefulness of theophylline compounds is quite conflicting. Several investigators have been unable to demonstrate any benefit from theophylline in reducing the incidence of anginal attacks.[8,13] It is advisable not to rely on this drug when choosing a coronary vasodilator for the management of angina pectoris. The myocardial stimulant effect of theophylline is likely to be a disadvantage in the presence of defective coronary blood supply.

The greatest usefulness of aminophylline is in the treatment of bronchial asthma. It is used occasionally also as an adjunct to certain diuretics such as the mercurials.

OTHER DRUGS

Ethyl alcohol has the undeserved reputation of being a coronary vasodilator. Studies of Russek and associates[23] show that although the drug can prevent pain in angina patients following the standard exercise test, it does not prevent electrocardiographic changes in the T waves and RS-T segments. The conclusion seems to be that alcohol acts on the brain rather than on the coronary arteries.

MAO inhibitors have been advocated by some investigators for the management of angina. If they are useful at all, their action probably does not depend on an increase in coronary blood flow but perhaps on lowering of pressure. The excitatory effects they may produce are dangerous in a patient whose coronary blood flow is deficient.

Dipyridamole (Persantine), or 2,6-bis(diethanolamino)-4,8-dipiperidinopyrimido-[5,4-d]pyrimidine, has been introduced for coronary insufficiency. It is claimed that the drug has dual action, dilating coronary arteries and also influencing myocardial metabolism. Interestingly, although the drug is claimed to increase the oxygen supply to the heart, it is of little or no value in the treatment of angina pectoris.[5] Dipyridamole inhibits platelet aggregation, an action discussed on p. 420.

ANTIANGINAL DRUGS
CLINICAL PHARMACOLOGY

The overall impression of clinical pharmacologists may be summarized by saying that nitroglycerin is an excellent antianginal drug, particularly for prophylactic therapy.[14] Other coronary vasodilators are recommended by some investigators, but their usefulness is questioned by others. Some of the long-acting nitrates may be effective when given sublingually but are impotent when given orally. This, of course, is true for nitroglycerin as well.

The experimental use of beta adrenergic blocking agents as antianginal drugs represents a radically new approach to the problem.[10] Propranolol must be used cautiously because it may induce congestive failure and hypotension. It may also increase airway resistance in asthmatic patients. The beta blockers reduce the oxygen requirement of the heart and may be effective for 6 hours. Newer beta blockers such as practolol, sotalol, and alprenolol may be more selective than propranolol and have been used in the United Kingdom.

References

1 Albaum, H. G., Tepperman, J., and Bodansky, O.: A spectrophotometric study of the competition of methemoglobin and cytochrome oxidase for cyanide in vitro, J. Biol. Chem. **163**:641, 1946.

2 Amsterdam, E. A., Gorlin, R., and Wolfson, S.: Evaluation of long-term use of propranolol in angina pectoris, J.A.M.A. **210**:103, 1969.

3 Cass, L. J., and Cohen, J. D.: The correlation of pain relief with blood nitrate levels in angina pectoris when treated with pentaerythritol tetranitrate, Curr. Ther. Res. **3**:23, 1961.

4 Chen, K. K., Rose, C. L., and Clowes, G. H. A.: Comparative values of several antidotes in cyanide poisoning, Amer. J. Med. Sci. **188**:767, 1934.

5 DeGraff, A. C., and Lyon, A. F.: Evaluation of dipyridamole (Persantin), Amer. Heart J. **65**:423, 1963.

6 Eckenhoff, J. E., and Hafkenschiel, J. H.: The effect of nikethamide on coronary blood flow and cardiac oxygen metabolism, J. Pharmacol. Exp. Ther. **91**:362, 1947.

7 Epstein, S. E.: Treatment of angina pectoris by electrical stimulation of the carotid sinus nerves; results in 17 patients with severe angina, New Eng. J. Med. **280**:971, 1969.

8 Ganz, W., and Marcus, H. S.: Failure of intracoronary nitroglycerin to alleviate pacing-induced angina, Circulation **46**:880, 1972.

9 Gold, H., Kwit, N. T., and Otto, H.: Xanthines (theobromine and aminophyline) in treatment of cardiac pain, J.A.M.A. **108**:2173, 1937.

10 Hamer, J.: The effect of propranolol (Inderal) in angina pectoris, Brit. Med. J. **2**:720, 1964.

11 Krantz, J. C., Lu, G. G., Bell, F. K., and Cascorbi, H. F.: Nitrites. XIX. Studies of the mechanism of action of glyceryl trinitrate, Biochem. Pharmacol. **2**:1095, 1962.

12 Levine, S. A.: Some notes concerning angina pectoris, J.A.M.A. **171**:1838, 1960.

13 Master, A. M., Jaffe, H. L., and Dack, S.: The drug treatment of anginal pectoris due to coronary artery disease, Amer. J. Med. Sci. **197**:774, 1939.

14 Modell, W.: Clinical pharmacology of antianginal drugs, Clin. Pharmacol. Ther. **3**:97, 1962.

15 Needleman, P.: Tolerance to the vascular effects of glyceryl trinitrate, J. Pharmacol. Exp. Ther. **171**:98, 1970.

16 Needleman, P., Blehm, D. J., Harkey, A. B., Johnson, E. M., and Lang, S.: The metabolic pathway in the degradation of glyceryl trinitrate, J. Pharmacol. Exp. Ther. **179**:347, 1971.

17 Needleman, P., and Krantz, J. C., Jr.: The biotransformation of nitroglycerin, Biochem. Pharmacol. **14**:1225, 1965.

18 Raab, W.: The sympathogenic biochemical trigger mechanism of angina pectoris. Its therapeutic suppression and long-range prevention, Amer. J. Cardiol. **9**:576, 1962.

19 Rinzler, S. H.: Assessment of antianginal agents, Clin. Pharmacol Ther. **3**:505, 1962.

20 Rowe, G. G., Chelius, C. J., Afonso, S., Gurtner, H. P., and Crumpton, C. W.: Systemic and coronary hemodynamic effects of erythrityl tetranitrate, J. Clin. Invest. **40**:1217, 1961.

21 Russek, H. I.: Propranolol and isosorbide dinitrate synergism in angina pectoris, Amer. J. Cardiol. **21**:44, 1968.

22 Russek, H. I., and Howard, J. C.: Glyceryl trinitrate in angina pectoris, J.A.M.A. **189**:108, 1964.

23 Russek, H. I., Naegele, C. F., and Regan, F. D.: Alcohol in the treatment of angina pectoris, J.A.M.A. **143**:355, 1950.

24 Russek, H. I., Urbach, K. F., Doerner, A. A., and Zohman, B. L.: Choice of a coronary vasodilator drug in clinical practice, evaluation of effects by electrocardiographic tests, J.A.M.A. **153**:207, 1953.

25 Russek, H. I., Zohman, B. L., and Dorset, V. J.: Objective evaluation of coronary vasodilator drugs, Amer. J. Med. Sci. **229**:46, 1955.

26 Sjoerdsma, A., Axelrod, J., Shofer, R., King, W. M., and Davidson, J. D.: Fate of papaverine, Fed. Proc. **154**:58, 1956.

27 Winbury, M. M., Howe, B. B., and Hefner, M. A.: Effect of nitrates and other coronary dilators on large and small coronary vessels; an hypothesis for the mechanism of action of nitrates, J. Pharmacol. Exp. Ther. **168**:70, 1969.

Recent reviews

28 Friend, D. G.: Angina pectoris therapy, Clin. Pharmacol. Ther. **5**:385, 1964.

29 Haddy, F. J.: Physiology and pharmacology of the coronary circulation and myocardium, particularly in relation to coronary artery disease, Amer. J. Med. **47**:274, 1969.

30 Mason, D. T., Spann, J. F., Zelis, R., and Amsterdam, E. A.: Physiologic approach to the treatment of angina pectoris, New Eng. J. Med. **281**:1225, 1969.

31 Melville, K. I.: The pharmacological basis of antianginal drugs, Pharmacol. Physicians **4**:1, March, 1970.

32 Oglesby, P.: Angina pectoris, Rational Drug Ther. **6**:1, Dec., 1972.

33 Rowe, G. G.: Effects of drugs on the coronary circulation of man, Clin. Pharmacol. Ther. **7**:547, 1966.

34 Winbury, M. M.: Experimental approaches to the development of antianginal drugs, **3**:2, 1964.

32 Anticoagulant drugs

GENERAL CONCEPT

Anticoagulants are widely used in the prevention and treatment of deep venous thrombosis and pulmonary embolism and in some other thromboembolic diseases. Since thrombosis is probably initiated by platelet adhesion and aggregation and is completed by the coagulation mechanism with fibrin formation, anticoagulant drugs may interrupt this chain of events at several points.

Heparin interferes with the formation of fibrin by inhibiting thrombin and some earlier steps in the coagulation mechanism. The coumarin and indandione oral anticoagulants antagonize the functions of vitamin K and cause a delayed decrease in prothrombin and factors VII, IX, and X.

Theoretically, inhibitors of platelet aggregation and adhesion should have a favorable effect in the prevention of thrombosis. Dipyridamole and a number of other drugs are effective in vitro, but further experience is needed for demonstrating their in vivo usefulness.

There are additional approaches to the treatment of thrombosis. Streptokinase and urokinase activate plasminogen and may dissolve some intravascular thrombi. The venom of the Malayan pit viper causes fibrinogen depletion by direct conversion of fibrinogen to fibrin. Its use is experimental.

Heparin is antagonized by protamine sulfate and coumarin anticoagulants by vitamin K. Heparin therapy may be monitored by whole blood–clotting time, whereas the coumarin and indandione anticoagulants require prothrombin time determinations, most commonly by the Quick one-stage procedure.

CLOTTING PROCESS AND ITS SUSCEPTIBILITY TO DRUG ACTION

A schematic picture of current views of coagulation is as follows:

Phase I—Formation of activated thromboplastin
Interaction of Hageman factor, glasslike surface, antihemophilic factor, Christmas factor, plasma thromboplastin antecedent, platelets, and calcium lead to plasma thromboplastin; plasma thromboplastin may be acted upon by tissue thromboplastin, Stuart factor (factor X), and serum prothrombin conversion accelerator (SPCA or factor VII) in the presence of calcium to form activated thromboplastin.

Phase II—Activated thromboplastin

$$\text{Prothrombin} \xrightarrow{\text{Calcium and proaccelerin (factor V)}} \text{Thrombin}$$

Phase III—Thrombin

$$\text{Fibrinogen} \xrightarrow{\hspace{4cm}} \text{Fibrin}$$

Calcium
Plasma accelerator

Phase IV — Fibrinolysin (plasmin)
Fibrin ——————————————————————→ Lysed fibrin

The clotting process according to this scheme may be divided into four stages. Thromboplastin is generated in the first stage, thrombin in the second, and fibrin in the third. The fourth stage is that of fibrin and fibrinolysin. A more up-to-date scheme of coagulation is shown in Fig. 32-1, and the blood coagulation factors are listed on p. 000.

Coagulation is vulnerable to drug action at several points. In vitro, inactivation of calcium by oxalate, citrate, or ethylenediaminetetraacetic acid (EDTA) will prevent clotting. This approach is not effective in vivo because ionized calcium levels sufficiently low to accomplish an anticoagulant effect are incompatible with life. Heparin and similar highly charged molecules can block clotting both in vitro and in vivo.

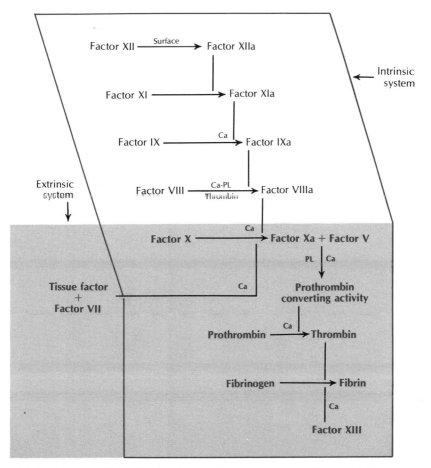

Fig. 32-1. Scheme of blood coagulation. Reactions enclosed by solid lines are of the "intrinsic system," whereas those within the color box are of the "extrinsic system." **PL,** Phospholipid; **Ca,** calcium. (From Williams, W. J.: Resident Staff Physician **15:**39, 1969.)

Blood coagulation factors*

Factor	I	Fibrinogen
Factor	II	Prothrombin
Factor	III	Tissue factor, tissue thromboplastin, thrombokinase
Factor	IV	Calcium
Factor	V	Proaccelerin, labile factor, plasma Ac-globulin
Factor	VI	
Factor	VII	Proconvertin, stable factor, serum prothrombin conversion accelerator (SPCA)
Factor	VIII	Antihemophilic globulin (AHG), antihemophilic factor (AHF)
Factor	IX	Plasma thromboplastin component (PTC), Christmas factor
Factor	X	Stuart-Prower factor
Factor	XI	Plasma thromboplastin antecedent (PTA), antihemophilic factor C
Factor	XII	Hageman factor
Factor	XIII	Fibrin-stabilizing factor, fibrinase

* Modified from Williams, W. J.: Resident Staff Physician **15:**39, 1969.

Finally, compounds that block the production of some of the proteins that are essential in the scheme will prevent clotting in vivo but not in the test tube. This is the mode of action of the coumarins.

ANTICOAGULANTS
HEPARIN

This naturally occurring anticoagulant was discovered in Howell's[17] laboratory in 1916 and was named heparin because it was thought to be predominantly localized in the liver. Actually it is known today that heparin is confined largely in mast cells, which appear to be highly concentrated in the liver of certain species but not in the human being.

From a chemical standpoint, heparin is a sulfated mucopolysaccharide composed of repeating units of sulfated glucosamine and glucuronic acid. Its molecular weight is about 20,000. It is a strong acid and is available in the form of its sodium salt. The chemical formula of heparin follows:

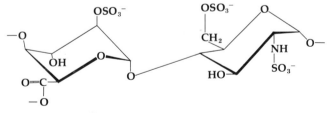

Configuration of disaccharides in heparin

Anticoagulant effect

Heparin inhibits clotting both in vitro and in vivo. Its most important action is as an antithrombin factor, and some of its other actions are probably a consequence of this as well. The antithrombin effect requires the presence of a plasma cofactor, which appears to be either an albumin or a lipoprotein. Heparin alone, without the plasma cofactor, will not block the interaction of purified thrombin and fibrinogen in the test tube.

In addition to this effect on thrombin, heparin inhibits the conversion of prothrombin to thrombin and has an antithromboplastic effect. It is possible that both of these actions are a consequence of a primary antithrombin action.

The fundamental action of heparin is not understood but is doubtless related in some way to the strong electronegative charge of the molecule. Organic bases such as toluidine blue and protamine sulfate inhibit the effect of heparin, probably because they combine with it to form additional compounds in which the electronegative charge is neutralized.

Lipemia-clearing effect

Injected heparin has the remarkable ability of decreasing the turbidity of plasma following alimentary hyperlipemia.[13] Interest in this phenomenon has been growing steadily. The current status of the problem has been reviewed by Robinson and French.[29]

When heparin is added in vitro to lipemic plasma, it causes no clearing. On the other hand, when lipemic plasma is added to clear plasma from an animal that has received heparin, clearing takes place.

The actual clearing factor appears to be a lipase that catalyzes the hydrolysis of triglycerides. The triglycerides of plasma are associated with proteins in the chylomicrons. Neutral fats that are split off by the enzyme from the chylomicrons are gradually dissolved in the plasma. Probably through the same mechanism, the β-lipoproteins, which are of high molecular weight and low density, are transformed into α-lipoproteins of lower molecular weight and high density.[12]

The clearing factor is present in various tissues and appears to be released from its binding sites by heparin. Heparin is most probably an integral part of the lipase and may provide a link between enzyme and substrate.

The lipemia-clearing effect of heparin requires much smaller doses than those necessary for significant anticoagulant action. Lipemia is cleared by doses of less than 1 μg/kg. in the rat and as little as 2 mg. in man. Larger doses of heparin, however, will release greater enzyme activity.

Administration and dosage

Heparin is not absorbed from the gastrointestinal tract. In order to obtain an anticoagulant effect the sodium salt of heparin is injected intravenously or subcutaneously.

The usual intravenous dose of heparin is an initial 5000 units, followed by doses of 5000 to 10,000 units every 4 hours for a total of 25,000 units daily. Recent studies indicate that small subcutaneous doses of 5000 units may be useful in the prevention of deep vein thrombosis.[10]

Commercial preparations of heparin are bioassayed on the basis of anticoagulant action in comparison with a standard preparation. One hundred USP units corresponds to about 1 mg. of heparin.

Preparations

Heparin sodium USP is available as a suspension for injection, 1000, 5000, 10,000, 20,000, and 40,000 units/ml., and as a gel for repository injection, 20,000 units/ml.

Toxicity

Except for its anticoagulant effect, heparin is quite inert pharmacologically. An intravenous injection of 5 mg./kg. is used routinely in experimental animals, and this large quantity has no significant effects on blood pressure, heart rate, or respiration.

In its clinical use heparin may promote bleeding from open wounds and mucous membranes, especially when dosage is excessive. Some believe that cerebral hemorrhage may be precipitated in susceptible patients. Elderly women are especially susceptible to heparin.[20]

In man, long-term heparin treatment may result in osteoporosis.[19] Also, symptoms suggesting hypersensitivity and inhibition of aldosterone secretion have been reported.

Heparin antagonists

The effects of heparin overdosage will last only a relatively short time because the drug is metabolized in a few hours. If hemorrhage threatens during even a short waiting period, true chemical antidotes are available.

— **Protamine sulfate** will combine with heparin milligram for milligram to block its anticoagulant effect both in the test tube and in the patient.

Toluidine blue and **hexadimethrine** (Polybrene) have also been used clinically as heparin antagonists but are now considered obsolete.

Metabolism and excretion

After intravenous injection, blood levels of heparin decline exponentially with a half-life of about 1 hour. Although most of the heparin is metabolized in the body, as much as 50% of a large intravenous dose may be excreted in the urine.[47]

Synthetic heparin substitutes

A variety of sulfated polysaccharides exert an anticoagulant effect and have lipemia-clearing activities, but most of these have serious toxic effects. Alginic acid sulfate (Paritol) is prone to produce anaphylactoid reactions. Pectin sulfate (Treburon) has caused alopecia. Dextran sulfates are being investigated as possible heparin substitutes, but there is good evidence that they can cause histamine release.

COUMARIN AND INDANDIONE ANTICOAGULANTS
Development

The story of the introduction of the coumarin compounds into therapeutics is unusually interesting. It has been known for many years that cattle can develop a hemorrhagic disease when they eat spoiled sweet clover. It has also been known that the hemorrhages are caused by lowered prothrombin levels in the animals. In 1941 Link[25] and associates at the University of Wisconsin showed that a coumarin compound was responsible for this hemorrhagic disease of cattle. They synthesized bishydroxycoumarin (Dicumarol), which has been used quite extensively in clinical practice and was the forerunner of a number of coumarin and indandione derivatives.

The various coumarin anticoagulants act by the same basic mechanism. They inhibit the formation of prothrombin, factor VII (proconvertin), factor IX (Christmas), and factor X (Stuart-Power factor).

The coumarin anticoagulants include, in addition to bishydroxycoumarin (Dicumarol), warfarin sodium (Coumadin sodium), warfarin potassium (Athrombin-K), acenocoumarol (Sintrom), phenprocoumon (Liquamar). The indandione derivatives are phenindione (Danilone, Eridione, Hedulin), diphenadione (Dipaxin) and anisindione (Miradon).

The chemical formulas of certain coumarin and indandione drugs are shown below.

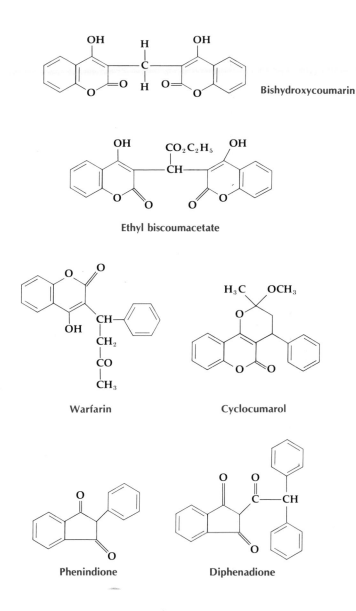

Bishydroxycoumarin

Ethyl biscoumacetate

Warfarin

Cyclocumarol

Phenindione

Diphenadione

Mode of action

There is a characteristic delay in the action of these compounds. This is understandable because the normal prothrombin content of the plasma must decline before the evidence of deficient synthesis can manifest itself. The coumarin compounds vary in speed of onset and duration of action, probably because of their varying speeds of absorption and metabolic degradation.

The administration of vitamin K can reverse the coumarin-induced hypoprothrombinemia. This fact and the structural similarities between these compounds suggest that the coumarins act as antimetabolites of vitamin K.

The exact mode of action of the coumarin anticoagulants is not known. Recent studies suggest that these drugs inhibit the transport of vitamin K to its site of action in liver cells.[26]

Individual variations in susceptibility and importance of laboratory tests

There is great individual variation in susceptibility to the coumarin anticoagulants. The variation is a consequence of many factors. Absorption from the intestine, metabolic transformation, diet, and genetically conditioned resistance[25] may all contribute.

Prothrombin concentration during coumarin therapy is measured by comparing the prothrombin time of the patient's plasma with that of normal plasma. In the usual one-stage prothrombin test, thromboplastin is added to citrated plasma at 37° C. Calcium chloride is then added in excess and the time for clotting is recorded. It is known now that the test measures not only prothrombin but also such other components as factor VII.

During therapy with the coumarin drugs it is desirable to maintain prothrombin concentration at 20% of normal, and dosage is adjusted in order to achieve this aim. Without such laboratory control, use of the coumarins would be dangerous. Severe depression of prothrombin concentration may be associated with bleeding, which can manifest itself as microscopic hematuria or even such severe bleeding as cerebral hemorrhage. Some investigators feel that the bleeding cannot be explained simply on the basis of depression of prothrombin levels, and they also postulate increased fragility of capillaries and venules.

Comparison of various coumarins and indandiones

The drugs in this group differ in potency, absorption, and metabolic transformation. Their varying potency is reflected in the dosage recommended for obtaining comparable depressions in prothrombin concentration (Table 32-1).

Vitamin K as antidote to prothrombin-depressant drugs

Two methods are available for counteracting the action of the coumarin drugs and their congeners: fresh whole blood transfusion and use of vitamin K preparations.

Among the most effective antidotes for coumarin poisoning is phytonadione (vitamin K_1; Mephyton), which is water soluble and may be administered intravenously in doses of 100 to 200 mg. Vitamin K_1 oxide and phytonadione are administered as emulsions. When used in large doses as antidotes, the vitamin K preparations have prolonged action and prevent reinstitution of coumarin or indandione therapy for as long as 2 weeks. Some advocate the use of much smaller doses for this reason. Vitamin K preparations have no effect on the anticoagulant action of heparin.

Table 32-1. Average doses of various coumarin and indandione anticoagulants

Preparation	Average initial dose (mg.)	Average maintenance dose (mg.)
Bishydroxycoumarin (Dicumarol)	300	100–200
Warfarin sodium (Coumadin sodium)	60	10
Cyclocumarol (Cumopyran)	1,000	25–50
Acenocoumarin (Sintrom)	15–25	2–10
Phenprocoumon (Liquamar)	20–30	1–5
Phenindione (Hedulin; Danilone)	100–200	25–50
Diphenadione (Dipaxin)	20–30	15

CLINICAL PHARMACOLOGY AND DRUG INTERACTIONS

Anticoagulants are of probable therapeutic benefit in a variety of clinical conditions, and they may possibly be effective in others. Rheumatic heart disease with embolism, deep vein thrombosis, transient cerebral ischemic attacks, and insertion of prosthetic cardiac valves represent probable indications. More controversial uses include myocardial infarction, acute coronary insufficiency, and disseminated intravascular thrombosis.[47]

Heparin is the most effective and safest anticoagulant. On the other hand, the necessity for frequent injections and its high cost are disadvantages. Disadvantages of the coumarins and the indandiones are delay in action and need for careful laboratory control for adjustment of dosage.

Phenindione has caused serious toxic effects such as agranulocytosis and liver damage. Many clinical investigators in this country prefer the coumarins and find that warfarin is one of the best from the standpoint of ease of regulation. According to one survey, there is no justification for the preference of heparin over warfarin for anticoagulation following myocardial infarction.[51] It is a good rule for the physician to use the anticoagulant with which he is thoroughly familiar and only if he has facilities for one-stage prothrombin time determinations.

Drug interactions in the clinical use of coumarin anticoagulants are of great importance. (See also Chapter 58.) Some drugs stimulate the metabolic degradation of the coumarins and thus decrease their effectiveness. Other drugs increase the effectiveness of the anticoagulants by blocking their metabolism or by interfering with their binding to plasma proteins.

Drug effects on the response to coumarin anticoagulants are as follows:

Drugs that increase the effect of coumarin anticoagulants

Antibiotics affecting the intestinal flora	Disulfiram
Phenylbutazone and some other acidic drugs	Androgenic anabolic steroids
	Methylphenidate
Salicylates (large doses)	Propylthiouracil
Chloral hydrate	d-Thyroxine
Clofibrate	

Drugs that decrease the effect of coumarin anticoagulants

Barbiturates	Glutethimide
Ethchlorvynol	Griseofulvin

Coumarin potentiation of other drugs

Tolbutamide	Diphenylhydantoin

FIBRINOLYSIN

Blood has the inherent capacity of dissolving clots by means of the fibrinolytic system. There are reasons to believe that this system functions under normal circumstances to remove minor fibrin depositions that occur in small vessels. Clotted blood may be injected repeatedly into rabbits without being demonstrable at autopsy. It is presumably dissolved through fibrinolysis.

The present state of the problem of fibrinolysin has been reviewed extensively by Sherry and associates.[33] Fibrinolysin, also called plasmin by some investigators, is a proteolytic enzyme that attacks a variety of proteins but has a great affinity for fibrinogen or fibrin. A schematic representation of the human fibrinolytic system is shown below.

Plasminogen or profibrinolysin	$\xrightarrow{\text{Activators Kinases}}$	Plasmin or fibrinolysin	$\xrightarrow{\text{Inhibitors}}$	Inactive enzyme

Fibrin or $\longrightarrow$ Split products
other proteins

(with a downward arrow from "Plasmin or fibrinolysin" toward Split products)

Plasminogen, or profibrinolysin, occurs in plasma as the inactive precursor of fibrinolysin. Among those substances that may activate it directly or indirectly in the human being is streptokinase.

Streptokinase-streptodornase (Varidase) is a mixture of enzymes used topically for dissolving blood clots (streptokinase) and the viscous nucleoproteins of pus (streptodornase). It is useful in evacuating the contents of hemothorax and empyema and as an aid in surgical debridement.

Adverse effects to the enzyme mixture include fever and local irritation. Active hemorrhage is a contraindication to its use. The usefulness of streptokinase-streptodornase in the form of buccal tablets or the intramuscular route for a systemic anti-inflammatory effect is not certain.

Streptokinase-streptodornase is available as a powder for topical use containing 100,000 units of streptokinase and 25,000 units of streptodornase per vial. Streptokinase-streptodornase should not be injected intravenously because of hazardous impurities present in the preparation.

Epsilon-aminocaproic acid (Amicar) inhibits plasminogen activators and to a lesser extent plasmin. The drug has been used to decrease hemorrhage associated with certain surgical procedures. In one study it lowered fibrinolytic activity and suppressed urokinase excretion in cirrhotic patients at a dosage of 10 Gm. daily for 7 days.[24]

Urokinase, the naturally occurring activator of the fibrinolytic enzyme system in human urine, is being investigated. It has many advantages over bacterial products such as streptokinase, although its preparation is quite difficult. Preliminary results in pulmonary embolism are promising.[36]

Fibrinolysin (human) (Thrombolysin) is a product of the actions of streptokinase on human fibrinolysin. It has been used in thromboembolic diseases except those involving the cerebral and coronary vessels. Its effectiveness is difficult to evaluate.

Of great pharmacologic interest is the experimental finding that various vasoactive drugs, particularly vasodilators, can cause enhancement of fibrinolysis.[15] It appears likely that blood vessels possess a fibrinolytic activator[3]; perhaps vasoactive drugs cause release of an activator from the vessel walls.

INHIBITORS OF PLATELET FUNCTION: DIPYRIDAMOLE

There is increasing interest in drugs that inhibit platelet aggregation and adhesiveness and thus might prevent thrombus formation. The vasodilator drug dipyridamole (Persantine) was found (1965) to inhibit platelet aggregation in vitro. Dipyridamole inhibits in vitro the platelet aggregation effect of adenosine diphosphate and this first stage of norepinephrine-induced aggregation.[7] There are several other compounds, including aspirin, prostaglandin E_1, and pyrazole drugs,[28] that influence platelet function in vitro and may prevent platelet aggregation induced by collagen.

The in vivo effectiveness of these drugs in the prevention of thrombosis is under intense investigation. Dipyridamole may reduce the incidence of thromboembolic phenomena in patients with artificial heart valves.[17] Although this area of investigation is of great interest, much further work is needed before the in vivo effectiveness of antiplatelet drugs is clearly established.

References

1 Advisory Committee on Coagulation Products: Investigations of fibrinolysis and labeling changes in fibrinolysin products, J.A.M.A. 180:536, 1962.

2 Allen, J. G., Sanderson, M., Milham, M., Kirschon, A., and Jacobson, L. O.: Heparinemia (?). An anticoagulant in the blood of dogs with hemorrhagic tendency after total body exposure to roentgen rays, J. Exp. Med. 87:71, 1948.

3 Astrup, T., and Buluk, K.: Thromboplastic and fibrinolytic activities in vessels of animals, Circ. Res. 13:253, 1963.

4 Brodie, B. B., Weiner, M., Burns, J. J., Simson, G., and Yale, E. K.: The physiological disposition of ethyl biscoumacetate (Tromexan) in man and a method for its estimation in biological material, J. Pharmacol. Exp. Ther. 106:453, 1952.

5 Burns, J. J., Weiner, M., Simson, G., and Brodie, B. B.: The biotransformation of ethyl biscoumacetate (Tromexan) in man, rabbit and dog, J. Pharmacol. Exp. Ther. 108:33, 1953.

6 Cronkite, E. P.: The hemorrhagic syndrome of acute ionizing radiation illness produced in goats and swine by exposure to the atomic bomb at Bikini, 1946, Blood 5:32, 1950.

7 Cucuianu, M. P., Nishizawa, E. E., and Mustard, J. F.: Effect of pyrimido-pyrimidine compounds on platelet function, J. Lab. Clin. Med. 77:958, 1971.

8 Fletcher, A. P., Alkjaersig, N., and Sherry, S.: The maintenance of a sustained thrombolytic state in man: induction and effects, J. Clin. Invest. 38:1096, 1959.

9 Friedberg, C. K.: Should we abandon anticoagulant therapy in acute myocardial infarction? J.A.M.A. 180:307, 1962.

10 Gallus, A. S., Hirsch, J., Tuttle, R. J., Trebilbock, R., O'Bryan, S. E., Carroll, J. J., Minden, J. H., and Hudecki, S. M.: Small subcutaneous doses of heparin in prevention of venous thrombosis, New Eng. J. Med. 288:545, 1973.

11 Glynn, M. F., Murphy, E. A., and Mustard, J. F.: Platelets and thrombosis, Ann. Intern. Med. 64:715, 1966.

12 Graham, D. M., Lyon, T. P., Gofman, J. W., Jones, H. B., Yankley, A., Simonton, J., and White, S.: Blood lipids and human atherosclerosis: influence of heparin upon lipoprotein metabolism, Circulation 4:666, 1951.

13 Hahn, P. F.: Abolishment of alimentary lipemia following injection of heparin, Science 98:19, 1943.

14 Harlan, W. R., Jr., Winesett, P. S., and Wasserman, A. J.: Tissue lipoprotein lipase in normal individuals and in individuals with exogenous hyperglyceridemia and the relationship of this enzyme to assimilation of fat, J. Clin. Invest. 46:239, 1967.

15 Holemans, R.: Enhancement of fibrinolysis in the dog by injection of vasoactive drugs, Amer. J. Physiol. 208:511, 1965.

16 Hollander, W., and Chobanian, A.: The effects of an inhibitor of cholesterol biosynthesis, triparanol (MER-29), in subjects with and without coronary artery disease, Boston Med. Quart. 10:1, 1959.

17 Howell, W. H.: The purification of heparin and its chemical and physiological reactions, Bull. Hopkins Hosp. 42:199, 1928.

18 Hunter, R. B., and Tudhope, G. R.: Mode of action of Tromexan, Lancet 1:821, 1953.

19 Jaffee, M. D., and Willis, P. W., III: Multiple fractures associated with long-term sodium heparin therapy, J.A.M.A. 193:158, 1965.

20 Jick, H., Slone, D., Borda, I. T., and Shapiro, S.: Efficacy and toxicity of heparin in relation to age and sex, New Eng. J. Med. 279:284, 1968.

21 Jorpes, J. E.: Heparin in the treatment of thrombosis: an account of its chemistry, physiology, and application in medicine, ed. 2, London, 1946, Oxford University Press.

22 Kazmier, F. J., Spittell, J. A., Thompson, J. J., and Owen, C. A.: Effect of oral anticoagulants on factors VII, IX, X, and II, Arch. Intern. Med. 115:667, 1965.

23 Lee, C. C., Trevoy, L. W., Spinks, J. W. T., and Jaques, L. B.: Dicumarol labeled with C14, Proc. Soc. Exp. Biol. Med. 74:151, 1950.

24 Lewis, J. H., and Doyle, A. P.: Effects of epsilon aminocaproic acid on coagulation and fibrinolytic mechanisms, J.A.M.A. 188:56, 1964.

25 Link, K. P.: The anticoagulant from spoiled sweet clover hay, Harvey Lect. 39:162, 1944.

26 Lowenthal, J., and Birnbaum, H.: Vitamin K and coumarin anticoagulants: dependence of anticoagulant effect on inhibition of vitamin K transport, Science 164:181, 1969.

27 O'Reilly, R. A., Aggeler, P. M., Hoag, M. S., Leong, L. S., and Kropatkin, M. L.: Hereditary transmission of exceptional resistance to cou-

marin anticoagulant drugs, New Eng. J. Med. **271**:809, 1964.

28 Packham, M. A., Warrior, E. S., Glynn, M. F., Senyi, A., and Mustard, J. F.: Alteration of the response of platelets to surface stimuli by pyrazole compounds, J. Exp. Med. **126**:171, 1967.

29 Robinson, D. S., and French, J. E.: Heparin, the clearing factor, lipase, and fat transport, Pharmacol. Rev. **12**:241, 1960.

30 Salzman, E. W., Harris, W. H., and DeSanctis, R. W.: Anticoagulation for prevention of thromboembolism following fractures of the hip, New Eng. J. Med. **275**:122, 1966.

31 Seaman, A. J., Griswold, H. E., Reaume, R. B., and Ritzmann, L.: Long-term anticoagulant prophylaxis after myocardial infarction, New Eng. J. Med. **281**:115, 1969.

32 Sellers, E. M., and Koch-Weser, J.: Potentiation of warfarin-induced hypoprothrombinemia by chloral hydrate, New Eng. J. Med. **283**:827, 1971.

33 Sherry, S., Fletcher, A. P., and Alkjaersig, N.: Fibrinolysis and fibrinolytic activity in man, Physiol. Rev. **39**:343, 1959.

34 Spinks, J. W. T., and Jaques, L. B.: Tracer experiments in mammals with Dicumarol labeled with carbon[14], Nature **166**:184, 1950.

35 Stirling, M., and Hunter, R. B.: Pharmacology of bis 3-3'-(4-oxycoumarinyl) ethyl acetate (Tromexan), Lancet **2**:611, 1951.

36 Tow, D. E., Wagner. H. N., and Holmes, R. A.: Urokinase in pulmonary embolism, New Eng. J. Med. **277**:1161, 1967.

37 Vietti, T. .J., Stephens, J. C., and Bennett, K. R.: Vitamin K_1 prophylaxis in the newborn, J.A.M.A. **176**:791, 1961.

38 Weiner, M., Shapiro, S., Axelrod, J., Cooper, J. R., and Brodie, B. B.: The physiological disposition of Dicumarol in man, J. Pharmacol. Exp. Ther. **99**:409, 1950.

39 Wright, I. S., Marple, C. D., and Beck, D. F.: Myocardial infarction: its clinical manifestations and treatment with anticoagulants. A study of 1031 cases, New York, 1954, Grune & Stratton, Inc.

Recent reviews

40 Coon, W. W., and Willis, P. W.: Some side effects of heparin, heparinoids, and their antagonists, Clin. Pharmacol. Ther. **7**:379, 1966.

41 Deykin, D.: The use of heparin; current concepts, New Eng. J. Med. **280**:937, 1969.

42 Deykin, D.: Warfarin therapy, New Eng. J. Med. **283**:691, 801, 1970.

43 Ebert, R. V.: Long-term anticoagulant therapy after myocardial infarction, J.A.M.A. **207**:2263, 1969.

44 Fletcher, A. P., and Sherry, S.: Thrombolytic agents, Ann. Rev. Pharmacol. **6**:89, 1966.

45 Gaston, L. W.: The blood clotting factors, New Eng. J. Med. **270**:236, 290, 1964.

46 Jorpes, J. E.: Heparin: its chemistry, pharmacology, and clinical use, Amer. J. Med. **33**:692, 1962.

47 Ogston, D., and Douglas, A. S.: Anticoagulant and thrombolytic drugs, Drugs **1**:228, 1971.

48 O'Reilly, R. A., and Aggeler, P. M.: Determinants of the response to oral anticoagulant drugs in man, Pharmacol. Rev. **22**:35, 1970.

49 Quick, A. J.: Control of anticoagulant therapy, Arch. Intern. Med. **111**:232, 1963.

50 Ratnoff, O. D.: Epsilon aminocaproic acid — a dangerous weapon, New Eng. J. Med. **280**:1124, 1969.

51 Sodium heparin versus sodium warfarin in acute myocardial infarction (cooperative study), J.A.M.A. **189**:555, 1964.

52 Weiner, M.: The rational use of anticoagulants, Pharmacol. Physicians **1**(11):1, 1967.

33 Diuretic drugs

GENERAL CONCEPT

Diuretics are drugs that increase the net renal excretion of solute and water. The renal tubule utilizes numerous transport processes for the reabsorption of most of the glomerular filtrate. Diuretics inhibit some of these transport processes, and their site of action within the nephron determines the quantitative and qualitative influence they exert on water and solute excretion.

Although the *mercurial diuretics* are looked on by many as having mainly historical interest, they still have important clinical uses. They produce predictable diuresis without excessive potassium loss and are given by intramuscular injection.

The *carbonic anhydrase inhibitors* are somewhat ineffective in edematous states but are used in other conditions, such as glaucoma and as adjuncts in conditions in which alkaline urine may be of benefit.

The *thiazide diuretics* are administered orally and are especially useful in hypertensive patients with congestive failure. They have disadvantages such as the induction of hypokalemic alkalosis, occasional hyperglycemia, and hyperuricemia.

Furosemide and *ethacrynic acid* are powerful diuretics, and their potent action requires close supervision of the patient.

The *osmotic diuretics* such as mannitol are effective in restoring glomerular filtration after transient hypotension. They must be injected intravenously.

Spironolactone and *triamterene* conserve potassium. They are not potent when used alone but may increase the degree of diuresis obtained by other drugs.

DIURETICS
Development of major diuretics

The diuretic action of inorganic mercury salts such as calomel has been known for centuries, but the discovery that organic mercurials are highly potent in reducing edema came accidentally from their former use in the treatment of syphilis. One compound, merbaphen (Novasurol), was noted to have a powerful diuretic action. The story of the mercurial diuretics is summarized by Vogl.[47] Numerous compounds were subsequently introduced, and until recently they largely dominated the field in treating edema of cardiac origin.

The development of the carbonic anhydrase inhibitors was an outgrowth of investigations on sulfanilamide. It was observed that sulfanilamide tended to produce metabolic acidosis. Pitts and co-workers[38] traced this effect to inhibition of the acidification of urine. This observation, coupled with knowledge that the compound was an inhibitor of carbonic anhydrase, led to the hypothesis that other inhibitors of this enzyme might prove to be useful diuretics. Synthetic work in this direction led to the introduction of acetazolamide.

Further work on carbonic anhydrase inhibitors produced other compounds such as chlorothiazide, which has additional effects in decreasing tubular reabsorption of electrolytes. These compounds were found to be highly effective in management of both congestive failure and hypertensive cardiovascular disease. Because of their effectiveness and ease of administration by the oral route, they have essentially replaced all other diuretics for major clinical uses.

More recently, two very powerful diuretics were introduced. One, furosemide, is a sulfonamide and is related to the thiazides. The other, ethacrynic acid, is chemically unrelated to the other diuretic drugs.

Since the most important action of the diuretics is to block the tubular reabsorption of sodium in the kidney, it is necessary to describe current concepts of the renal handling of sodium before the site of action of diuretics is discussed.

Renal handling of sodium

Under normal circumstances the kidney regulates sodium balance by adjusting the excretion of salt to the varying dietary intake. Intake of sodium chloride may vary from 0 to more than 200 mEq./day, and the normal kidney will accommodate its daily output correspondingly, thus maintaining a fairly constant *volume* of extracellular fluid.

Since most of the sodium filtered through the glomeruli is reabsorbed in the tubules and most diuretics act by blocking reabsorption, it is essential to examine this process in some detail.

The filtered load of sodium is the product of its concentration in the filtrate times the glomerular filtration rate (GFR), thus:

$$\textbf{Filtered load} = \textbf{Plasma concentration} \times \textbf{GFR}$$

and

$$\textbf{Tubular reabsorption} = \textbf{Filtered load} - \textbf{Amount excreted}$$

There is much evidence to indicate that tubular reabsorption adjusts itself to the filtered load, which is to say that it adjusts itself to the glomerular filtration rate (GFR). The intrinsic property of the nephron that leads to increased tubular reabsorption as the GFR increases, and lowered reabsorption with a falling GFR, is termed glomerulotubular balance.[60] Experimental verification of this concept has been achieved by micropuncture studies of the proximal tubule. Since inulin is filtered by the glomerulus and is not reabsorbed in the tubules, measurement of its concentration in proximal tubular fluid (TF) in comparison with its concentration in plasma (P) indicates the magnitude of the fractional reabsorption of water and solutes. Actual measurements indicate that the ratio TF/P remains constant despite widely varying GFR's,[60] which proves that the fractional reabsorption in the proximal tubule accommodates to varying GFR's.

In addition to the glomerulotubular balance, other factors contribute to the regulation of sodium reabsorption. Aldosterone stimulates sodium reabsorption in the distal tubule. The secretion of aldosterone is responsive to alterations in extracellular volume, the receptors for sensing changes in volume being located in the juxtaglomerular apparatus of the kidney.[60] Renin released from this site determines the level of angiotensin II, which stimulates the output of aldosterone.[59, 60]

Glomerulotubular balance and aldosterone do not account completely for regu-

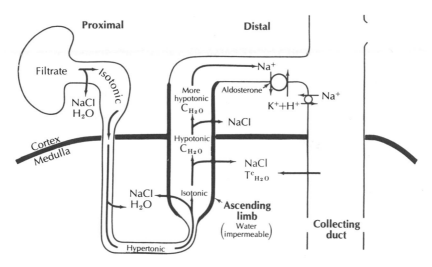

Fig. 33-1. Anatomic and functional subdivisions of the nephron. (From Seldin, D. W., Eknoyan, G., Suki, W., and Rector, F. C., Jr.: In Proceedings of the Third International Congress on Nephrology, vol. 1, Basel, 1967, S. Karger.)

lation of sodium reabsorption. A *third factor* is revealed by experiments in which saline loading in dogs could cause an increase in the excretion of sodium not explicable simply by alterations in GFR or aldosterone secretion. The nature of this third factor is not understood.

In edematous states a reduced GFR results in greater fractional reabsorption of sodium by the tubules. This may be the most important factor in glomerulonephritis, where edema is associated with elevated plasma volume. In cardiac failure or hypoalbuminemia, on the other hand, if plasma volume is reduced, hypersecretion of aldosterone contributes to sodium retention.

Diuretics and renal handling of sodium

The effectiveness of diuretics depends on the potency of their inhibitory effect on sodium reabsorption and their site of action within the nephron. Their effectiveness also depends on endogenous factors that contribute to sodium reabsorption.[75]

The anatomic and functional subdivisions of the nephron are shown schematically in Fig. 33-1. Sodium reabsorption in the proximal tubule may be measured by micropuncture in rats and dogs and is about 70% of the filtered load. Indirect methods must be used for the estimation of sodium reabsorption at other segments of the nephron.

The site of action of a diuretic is inferred from the following relationships[75]:

1. *Proximal tubular site*—greater fractional delivery than normal from this site, as revealed by micropuncture studies
2. *Ascending limb of Henle's loop*—inhibition of free-water clearance with or without evidence for inhibition of free-water reabsorption
3. *Distal tubule and collecting duct*—reduction of potassium and hydrogen excretion at a given rate of sodium excretion

Drugs used in cardiovascular disease

Free-water clearance (C_{H_2O}) is defined by the following equation:

$$C_{H_2O} = \underline{V} - \frac{U_{mOsm}}{P_{mOsm}} \times \underline{V}$$

where $\underline{V}$ represents the urine flow in milliliters per minute, and U_{mOsm} and P_{mOsm} represent the solute concentration of the urine and plasma in milliosmoles per kilogram of water. The free-water clearance is negative during antidiuresis. This negative value is designated $T^c_{H_2O}$, or free-water clearance reabsorption.[23]

Free water is found only in urine that is hypoosmotic relative to plasma. Free water may be defined as "that fraction of the water of hypoosmotic urine which must be subtracted in order to make the urine isoosmotic."[56] It is formed in the ascending limb of the loop of Henle where sodium and an anion are reabsorbed without carrying water with them. C_{H_2O} must be studied in hydrated animals to ensure the absence of circulating antidiuretic hormone. On the other hand, free-water reabsorption, to be maximal, requires the presence of large amounts of circulating antidiuretic hormone (that is, hydropenia and antidiuresis).

Drugs that block reabsorption of sodium in the proximal tubule are expected to increase C_{H_2O} because they promote the passage of large volumes of isosmotic urine through the ascending limb. Drugs that act by blocking reabsorption of sodium in the ascending limb should reduce C_{H_2O}.

On the basis of these assumptions it may be inferred that some of the more important diuretics act at the following sites:

1. *Chlorothiazide and related drugs* inhibit C_{H_2O}, suggesting an action on the ascending limb, perhaps the cortical diluting segment.[75]
2. *Furosemide and ethacrynic acid* inhibit both C_{H_2O} and $T^c_{H_2O}$, suggesting an action on the medullary diluting segment of the ascending limb.
3. *Mercurial diuretics* in very high doses act like furosemide and ethacrynic acid. Morphologic studies suggest a proximal tubular effect. They probably act at many sites.[56]
4. *Carbonic anhydrase inhibitors* act at the exchange sites of the distal tubule. The same is true for spironolactone and triamterene, drugs that antagonize aldosterone.

Table 33-1. Functional subdivisions of various renal segments*

Segment	% Na reabsorbed	C_{H_2O}	$T^c_{H_2O}$	K secretion
Proximal	70	—	—	—
Ascending limb of inner medullary segment	≧ 10	—	—	—
Medullary diluting segment	5	+	+	—
Cortical diluting segment	10	+	—	—
Distal	5	±	—	+
Collecting duct	1–2	±	—	+

* From Seldin, D. W., Eknoyan, G., Suki, W., and Rector, F. C., Jr.: In Proceedings of the Third International Congress on Nephrology, vol. 1, Basel, 1967, S. Karger.

Brief summary of renal physiology

In the *proximal convoluted tubule*, 70 to 80% of the glomerular filtrate is reabsorbed. Sodium is reabsorbed by an active process,[20] and water follows passively, with the result that the tubular fluid remains isosmotic with plasma. The location of the sodium pumping mechanism may be at the interstitial border of the cells. Active reabsorption of chloride in the thick medullary limb of Henle has recently been postulated.[41]

In the *ascending limb of the loop of Henle*, sodium and chloride are absorbed without water.[75] The ascending limb then consists of *diluting segments*, both medullary and cortical.

In the *distal tubules and collecting ducts*, about 7% of the filtered sodium is reabsorbed, potassium is secreted, and the urine is acidified. This is the site of action of the antidiuretic hormone and of aldosterone.

MERCURIAL DIURETICS

After their intramuscular injection, the mercurials produce copious diuresis in edematous states as a consequence of combining with SH groups in the ascending limb of Henle. Diuresis begins in 30 to 60 minutes and becomes maximal in 2 to 3 hours. The delay is probably caused by plasma protein binding.

Effect on renal handling of water and electrolytes

Mercurials increase the excretion of sodium and chloride. Output of the latter is in excess of the former, the difference being partly made up by H^+ and K^+. As a consequence, the urine contains relatively more chloride than sodium, whereas the plasma tends to become alkalotic. The main effect of the mercurials is probably on the thick ascending limb of Henle.

Factors influencing effectiveness

The organic mercurials are believed to release mercury ions in the renal tubular cells. The ionization of mercury is influenced by the hydrogen ion concentration, being greater at an acid pH.[26] In accordance with this view, acidosis promotes the effectiveness of the mercurials, whereas alkalosis inhibits it.

Hypochloremic alkalosis, which may be induced by prolonged mercurial therapy, opposes the action of the mercurials. Acidifying salts and potassium chloride then promote their effectiveness. Other factors that inhibit mercurial diuresis are reduced glomerular filtration, salt-retaining adrenal steroids, hyposmolarity of plasma, and dimercaprol (BAL).

Methods of administration and metabolism

Mercurial diuretics are usually administered by the intramuscular route and are effective and safe when given in this manner. There is little excuse for intravenous injection, since there is the possibility of cardiac toxicity.

Mercurial diuretics are available also for subcutaneous and oral administration, but their subcutaneous injection can cause local reaction, and the oral route may produce severe gastric irritation. Also, results are not predictable following oral administration. Intramuscular injection is by far the best method of administration.

The mercurials are excreted fairly rapidly by renal tubular secretion and also in the feces.[49] Most of the mercury of a single injection is expelled in less than 24 hours, but a small percentage remains in the body, presumably in the kidney, for 1 to 3 days. Consequently, doses should not be given frequently because they may have a cumulative toxic effect. This is not likely to occur if injections are not given oftener than twice a week and if renal function is fairly good.

Toxicity

When properly used, mercurial diuretics are quite safe. Their safety is a consequence of their selective localization in the kidney, where their concentration may be 100 times greater than in plasma. Cardiac toxicity develops only following intravenous injection, which may be considered an improper use.

True mercury poisoning may develop if the diuretics are given in excessive doses or too frequently. The most frequent cause of mercury poisoning with diuretics is their administration to patients whose renal blood flow is severely impaired.

Comparison of various mercurial diuretics

The structural formulas of the commonly used mercurials mersalyl (Salyrgan), mercaptomerin (Thiomerin), mercurophylline (Mercuzanthin), mercumatilin (Cumertilin), chlormerodrin (Neohydrin), and meralluride (Mercuhydrin) follow:

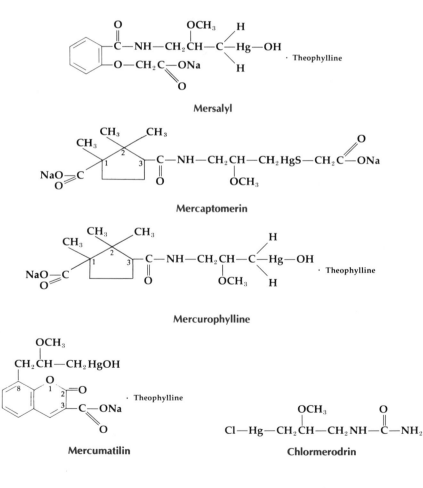

Mersalyl

Mercaptomerin

Mercurophylline

Mercumatilin

Chlormerodrin

428

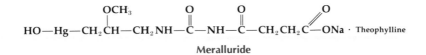

Meralluride

With the exception of chlormerodrin, which is intended for oral use, all these preparations are injectable and, with the exception of mercaptomerin also, are combined with theophylline to promote their absorption from the intramuscular depot site.

These injectable preparations are usually given intramuscularly in doses of 1 to 2 ml., each milliliter containing approximately 40 mg. Hg.

CARBONIC ANHYDRASE INHIBITORS

Although obsolete as diuretics, the carbonic anhydrase inhibitors are employed in the treatment of other conditions such as glaucoma. They represent interesting examples of the therapeutic application of enzyme inhibitors.

The discovery of carbonic anhydrase was a consequence of studies on CO_2 transport in the blood. Its discovery provided an explanation of the fact that blood traversing the pulmonary capillaries loses its CO_2 in less than 1 second, whereas in the test tube the hydration and dehydration of CO_2 take at least 100 times longer. The enzymatic catalysis of the reaction of carbon dioxide and water to form carbonic acid $(CO_2 + H_2O \rightarrow H \cdot HCO_3)$ was clearly shown by 1932. Details of this work were given by Roughton[42] in 1935.

The carbonic anhydrase enzyme was found to be present in high concentration in the red cell, the gastric mucosa, the pancreas, and the renal cortex. Its presence in the gastric mucosa led to the suggestion that it may play a role in the elaboration of hydrogen ions for gastric juice.

When sulfanilamide was introduced into therapeutics, its use was observed to lead to the development of acidosis, a drop in plasma CO_2, a rise in urinary pH, and a loss of Na^+, K^+, and H_2O into the urine. The compound was also demonstrated to be a specific inhibitor of carbonic anhydrase.[31] The role of H^+ transport in renal acidification was established by Pitts and co-workers.[38]

Further studies on the sulfonamides have shown that their carbonic anhydrase inhibition is associated with a free $-SO_2NH_2$ group. The various sulfonamides that were later introduced as chemotherapeutic agents contained substitutions in the sulfonamide nitrogen to inhibit their action on carbonic anhydrase.

A large number of sulfonamides were synthesized for the purpose of finding potent inhibitors of carbonic anhydrase. This work led to the development of acetazolamide (Diamox) and eventually to the discovery of the chlorothiazide diuretics, which have additional diuretic actions not explained by their inhibitory effect on carbonic anhydrase. The structure of acetazolamide is shown along with that of sulfanilamide for comparison.

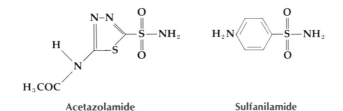

Acetazolamide   Sulfanilamide

429

Mode of action

The carbonic anhydrase inhibitors block the catalysis of the reaction $CO_2 + H_2O \rightleftarrows H \cdot HCO_3$. Even though the enzyme is widely distributed in the body, therapeutic doses of acetazolamide exert their principal effect on the kidney. Effects on other systems are also demonstrable, particularly when large doses of the drug are given.

Renal effects of acetazolamide

When acetazolamide is administered to a patient or a dog at a dose level of 5 mg./kg., the following changes may be seen in the electrolyte pattern of the urine: Na^+ is markedly increased; K^+ is markedly increased; Cl^- is not significantly affected; HCO_3^- is markedly increased; and NH_4^+ and titratable acidity are decreased.

These effects are explicable on the basis of what is known about the role of H^+ transport in renal acidification, the drug slowing the rate of H^+ generation through its inhibitory action on the hydration of CO_2.

Hydrogen ion transport plays three important roles in the renal handling of electrolytes.

1. H^+ can exchange for Na^+ in the tubular fluid. This process results in sodium reabsorption and increased titratable acidity.
2. H^+ transport is involved in the reabsorption of bicarbonate (Fig. 33-2). It exchanges for tubular Na^+ and combines with HCO_3 to form H_2CO_3, which then spontaneously decomposes to CO_2 and H_2O. The net effect of these reactions is that sodium bicarbonate is reabsorbed and hydrogen ion is eliminated.
3. H^+ transport is involved in ammonium excretion.

With these mechanisms in mind, the effects of acetazolamide on urinary pH and electrolyte output become understandable. Na^+ output is increased because its exchange for H^+ is limited by the decreased availability of H^+. For the same reason bicarbonate output is increased and titratable acidity is decreased.

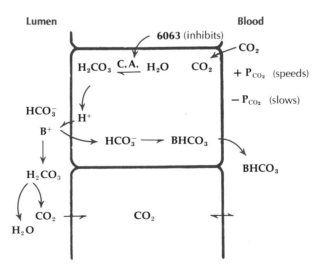

Fig. 33-2. Schema of processes involved in the reabsorption of bicarbonate-bound base by renal tubules. 6063 = a carbonic anhydrase inhibitor. (From Dorman, P. J., et al.: J. Clin. Invest. **33**:88, 1954.)

Since an acid urine favors the diffusion of NH_3 from the tubular cell, the lowering of ammonium excretion is probably caused by the more alkaline urine produced by the carbonic anhydrase inhibitors through their inhibition of H^+ secretion.

The increased excretion of potassium has an ingenious explanation.[3,4] There is a great deal of evidence to suggest that the renal tubules can exchange either H^+ or K^+ for luminal Na^+. Furthermore, a reciprocal relationship seems to exist between H^+ and K^+, depending on their availability. When the generation of H^+ is blocked by the carbonic anhydrase inhibitor, the exchange of Na^+ for K^+ predominates. This would explain the increased output of potassium following acetazolamide.

Extrarenal effects of acetazolamide

Carbonic anhydrase is present in organs other than the kidney, and its inhibition may influence other systems in the body. Prolonged use of the compound can result in systemic acidosis. This is, however, largely a consequence of its renal action.

When very large doses of acetazolamide are given to experimental animals, the secretion of hydrochloric acid may be diminished. The doses for obtaining this effect are so large that it can have no therapeutic importance.

Carbonic anhydrase is present in red cells, but therapeutic doses of acetazolamide do not interfere with the transport of carbon dioxide in the blood. The carbonic anhydrase inhibitors may have a central nervous system effect, causing drowsiness and disorientation in some patients. A favorable action has been claimed in the treatment of epilepsy, although the mode of action of the drug in this case is not clear. It may be a consequence of the acidosis, which has been reported to have a beneficial effect in epilepsy.

Glaucoma is the main indication for the use of carbonic anhydrase inhibitors. The aqueous humor has a high concentration of bicarbonate, and the beneficial effect of the carbonic anhydrase inhibitors may be related to an action on the secretion of bicarbonate.

Newer carbonic anhydrase inhibitors

Ethoxzolamide (Cardrase) is similar in action to acetazolamide. It is administered in doses of 62.5 to 250 mg. one or more times daily. Its administration should be intermittent rather than continuous.

Dichlorphenamide (Daranide) is one of the most potent carbonic anhydrase inhibitors. The dose must be individualized and may range from 25 to 100 mg.

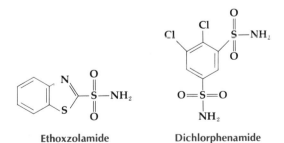

Ethoxzolamide   Dichlorphenamide

THIAZIDE DIURETICS

One of the most important developments in the diuretic field has been the introduction of chlorothiazide (Diuril) and its derivatives.[6] The discovery of the thiazide diuretics is an outgrowth of studies on the carbonic anhydrase inhibitors. The thiazides have some inhibitory actions on carbonic anhydrase. They differ from the parent compounds in having additional effects on sodium reabsorption. Although they tend to cause loss of potassium, uric acid retention, and some impairment of carbohydrate tolerance, they have become very popular in the treatment of edematous states and also as antihypertensive medications.

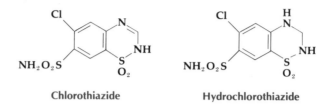

Chlorothiazide   Hydrochlorothiazide

Renal effects

The characteristic effects of the thiazide diuretics are as follows:
1. Increased excretion of sodium and potassium as well as chloride and water but no significant primary effect on acid-base balance; diuretic effectiveness also independent of acid-base alterations
2. A maximal capability of inhibiting the reabsorption of 5 to 10% of the amount of sodium and chloride filtered by the glomeruli
3. An antihypertensive effect, based probably (but not certainly) on a primary diuretic action
4. Decreased urinary volume in patients with diabetes insipidus

The thiazides are secreted by the renal tubules.[7] The transport mechanism involved is the same as for the penicillins or p-aminohippurate. Thiazides competitively depress the secretion of penicillin, whereas probenecid depresses the clearance of the thiazides, also competitively. The cumulation of the thiazides in the kidney may explain their selective effect on the organ.

Chlorothiazide can cause a significant reduction in urine volume when administered to patients having diabetes insipidus. The mechanism of this apparently paradoxical effect is not completely understood, but there is no reason to believe that there is any similarity between the actions of thiazides and the antidiuretic hormone.

Antihypertensive action

During the early clinical trials of chlorothiazide, it was observed that addition of this new medication to other antihypertensive therapy resulted in a significant additional fall of blood pressure.[50]

Further observations indicated that chlorothiazide alone had a significant antihypertensive action in addition to potentiating the effect of many other drugs.[58]

The nondiuretic congener of the thiazides, *diazoxide*, lowers blood pressure without having a renal effect. This is often used as an argument for some undefined action of the thiazides, perhaps on vascular smooth muscles. It is more likely, however, that the diuretic effect does play an important role in the lowering of the blood pressure by the thiazides.

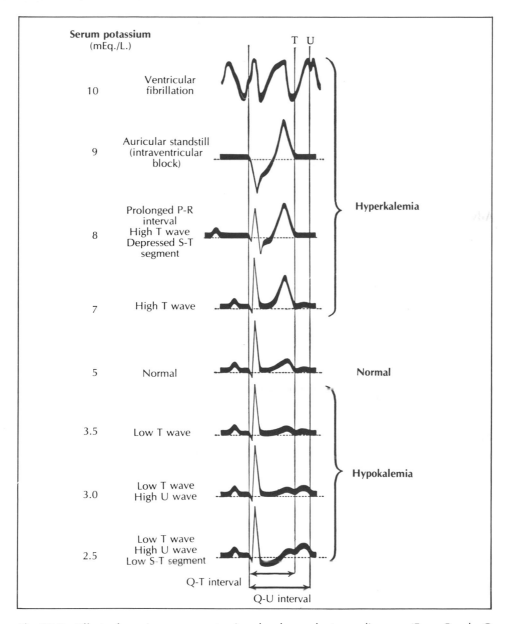

Fig. 33-3. Effect of varying serum potassium levels on electrocardiogram. (From Burch, G. E., and Winsor, T.: A primer of electrocardiography, Philadelphia, 1960, Lea & Febiger.)

Toxic effects

The major side effects of the thiazides are as follows:
1. Hypokalemia
2. Hyperuricemia
3. Aggravation of diabetes mellitus[52]

Hypokalemia may require the administration of potassium chloride or the combined use of a thiazide and a drug that blocks the sodium-potassium exchange mechanism. Triamterene is used occasionally for this purpose. The correlations between serum potassium and the electrocardiogram are shown in Fig. 33-3.

The mechanism of hyperuricemia is not known with certainty. The thiazide diuretics and uric acid may compete for the same tubular secretory mechanism, but this may not be the explanation of uric acid retention.[9] Hyperuricemia may produce acute attacks of gout. Probenecid counteracts this effect of the thiazides and does not interfere with their antihypertensive effect.[19]

In rare instances the thiazide diuretics can cause skin reactions, thrombocytopenic purpura, and agranulocytosis.

Adverse effects of potassium supplements

A number of patients taking hydrochlorothiazide in the form of enteric-coated capsules that also contained potassium chloride developed ulcerations of the small bowel.[28] Thorough study of this problem led to the tentative conclusion that this adverse effect was caused by this particular form of potassium chloride. Perhaps the small intestine is highly susceptible to the effect of a concentrated solution of potassium chloride, which would result from the dissolution of an enteric-coated capsule reaching that site.

Other potassium salts such as gluconate are also widely used by patients who are on thiazide therapy. Recent evidence indicates that if hypopotassemia is associated with hypochloremic alkalosis, only potassium *chloride* is effective in restoring normal acid-base balance.[25]

Comparison of the various thiazide diuretics

Examination of the formulas of the various thiazide diuretics shows that they are very closely related to each other and to chlorthalidone, which is not truly a benzothiadiazine.

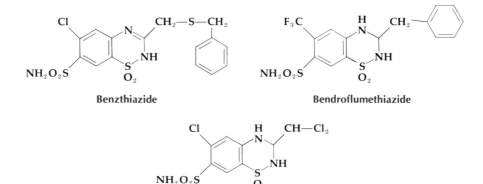

Benzthiazide

Bendroflumethiazide

Trichlormethiazide

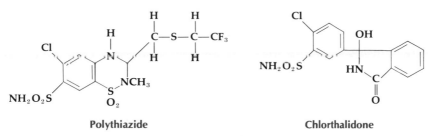

Polythiazide   Chlorthalidone

Flumethiazide (Ademol) has the same structural formula as chlorothiazide, except that F_3C replaces Cl.

Hydroflumethiazide (Saluron) has the same structural formula as hydrochlorothiazide, except that F_3C replaces Cl.

There is some confusion about the relative advantages of one thiazide over another, promoted perhaps by commercial competition. It is often said, for example, that one thiazide is more potent than another. This is certainly true if *potency* is defined as activity per unit weight, as reflected in the various dosages given in Table 33-2. A different picture appears if the diuretic *efficacy* of these drugs is compared on the basis of what percentage of the filtered sodium is excreted under their maximal influence. If looked upon in this manner, the percentage for most thiazides is about 10. For the newer sulfonamide furosemide it may be as high as 30. For ethacrynic acid the figure is about 20.

FUROSEMIDE AND ETHACRYNIC ACID

These highly potent diuretics have many similar properties and indications, although they are quite different chemically. Furosemide is a sulfonamide related to the thiazides. Ethacrynic acid was developed on the basis of rational drug design. Since the mercurials owe their diuretic action to an affinity for sulfhydryl groups, the chemist combined an unsaturated ketone, which tends to combine with sulfhydryl groups, and an aryloxyacetic acid, which is known to concentrate in the kidney. The result was ethacrynic acid.

Both drugs are not only more potent than the thiazides but also have a greater

Table 33-2. Comparable daily doses and duration of action of thiazide diuretics

Preparation	Dose (mg.)	Duration of action (hours)
Chlorothiazide (Diuril)	1,000	9
Hydrochlorothiazide (HydroDiuril)	100	15
Hydroflumethiazide (Saluron)	100	21
Benzthiazide (ExNa)	100	15
Methyclothiazide (Enduron)	5–10	more than 24
Bendroflumethiazide (Naturetin)	5–10	more than 18
Trichlormethiazide (Naqua)	4–8	more than 24
Polythiazide (Renese)	4–8	more than 24
Chlorthalidone (Hygroton) (not a thiazide but resembles one)	200	more than 24
Quinethazone (Hydromox) (not a thiazide but resembles one)	50–100	21

efficacy. They promote the excretion of a higher percentage of filtered salt than is the case for other diuretics. This percentage is of the order of 20 to 30, compared with 10 for the thiazides.

It is believed that furosemide and ethacrynic acid exert their major action on the ascending limb of the loop of Henle (p. 426).

Similarities and differences with the thiazides

Except for their much greater efficacy, furosemide and ethacrynic acid resemble the thiazides in their pharmacology. Both drugs are excreted unchanged into the urine. Their mechanism of excretion is the organic acid secretory system of the proximal tubules. Since uric acid is secreted by the same mechanism, both drugs tend to cause retention of urate. Probenecid is useful in preventing hyperuricemia caused by these drugs. Interestingly, the uricosuric agent prevents the secretion of the diuretics by the proximal tubule and prolongs their action, but it does not prevent their diuretic effectiveness.

Both furosemide and ethacrynic acid cause potassium loss and impaired glucose tolerance. Potassium loss is greatly augmented in the presence of increased aldosterone secretion. Under these circumstances the potassium-retaining diuretics triamterene or spironolactone are useful adjuncts to furosemide or ethacrynic acid therapy.

The greatest dangers associated with the use of furosemide or ethacrynic acid are excessive diuresis with circulatory collapse and severe hypokalemia. Ototoxicity has also been described after the use of these diuretics.

Preparations and dosage

Furosemide (Lasix) is available for oral administration in tablets containing 40 mg. and in solution for injection, 10 mg./ml.

The usual oral dosage for adults initially is 40 to 80 mg., which may be increased gradually. Excessive doses may cause hypotension and vascular collapse. Dosage for intravenous administration in adults is 20 to 40 mg., given slowly. The same dosage may be used for intramuscular administration. The immediate diuretic effect may be an advantage in the treatment of acute pulmonary edema and hypertensive crisis.

Preparations of **Ethacrynic acid** (Edecrin) include tablets containing 25 and 50 mg. for oral administration and, for injection, Edecrin sodium powder, 50 mg.

The usual dosage by mouth for adults is 50 mg. initially, with careful adjustment subsequently. The intravenous dose is 50 mg. for adults, or 0.5 mg./kg. The rapid and potent diuretic action may be useful, just as that of furosemide, in the treatment of acute pulmonary edema and hypertensive crisis. The drug may cause hypotension, vascular collapse, potassium depletion, hyperuricemia, and transient deafness.

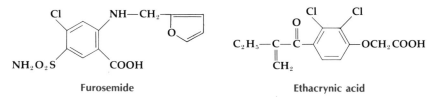

Furosemide   Ethacrynic acid

TRIAMTERENE AND SPIRONOLACTONE

The diuretics triamterene and spironolactone are seldom used alone. They are important in combination with other diuretics to reverse hypokalemia or antagonize the action of aldosterone.

Triamterene is not a true aldosterone antagonist; nevertheless, it causes some sodium excretion associated with potassium retention. Spironolactone is a competitive inhibitor of aldosterone. Thus it blocks the reabsorption of sodium in exchange for potassium and hydrogen. The different mechanisms of action of triamterene and spironolactone are evident by the demonstration that a combination of the two drugs has a greater effect than the sum of the maximal actions of the drugs when given alone.[66]

Triamterene (Dyrenium) is supplied in capsules containing 100 mg. Dosage must be carefully regulated, but the usual dose is 100 mg. twice daily. The drug is contraindicated in severe kidney disease and in the presence of hyperkalemia. Triamterene and a thiazide diuretic are sometimes used in the same patient. The rationale for using such a combination is that the natriuresis resulting from thiazide therapy promotes a compensatory aldosterone secretion. Aldosterone tends to antagonize the sodium-excreting action of the thiazide, while aggravating potassium loss. Addition of triamterene provides the opposite effect.

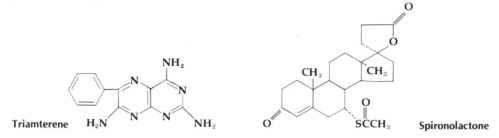

Triamterene   Spironolactone

Spironolactone (Aldactone) is supplied in 25 mg. tablets. The daily dosage is 50 to 100 mg. The main contraindication to the use of the drug is hyperkalemia.

Mannitol

Mannitol is not reabsorbed by the tubules and may be considered to be the prototype of the osmotic diuretics. Its site of action is the proximal tubule leading to a greater delivery of sodium and chloride to the loop of Henle. The drug must be injected intravenously.

Mannitol is available as a 25% solution for intravenous injection in 50 ml. containers. It is also available as a 5, 10, 15, and 20% solution in 1,000 ml. containers. In addition to its use as a diuretic adjunct, mannitol finds some usefulness in neurosurgery for reduction of cerebrospinal fluid pressure and for the reduction of intraocular pressure. It is contraindicated in patients with severe renal disease.

MINOR DIURETICS
Xanthines

The previously discussed major diuretics primarily affect the tubular reabsorptive processes of the kidney. The xanthines—theophylline, theobromine, and caffeine— have a combined effect on renal hemodynamics and tubular reabsorptive capacity. This dual action may have real advantages in some clinical situations, but the overall potency of these compounds is very much less than that of the mercurials or chlorothiazide. As a consequence, the xanthines are occasionally useful as adjuncts to mercurial diuretics.

Of the three xanthines, theophylline is the most potent diuretic. Its structure is as follows:

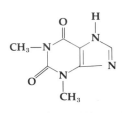

Theophylline

The ability of theophylline to inhibit tubular reabsorption of electrolytes has been shown experimentally.[48] It is most effective when injected intravenously as one of its soluble salts, *aminophylline*. In addition, the compound increases cardiac output and can produce increased glomerular filtration. When aminophylline and a mercurial are administered simultaneously, the combined diuretic effect is greater than what could be expected from one of these drugs alone.[49] This may be advantageous when the effectiveness of mercurials is decreased as a result of impaired glomerular filtration.

Ammonium chloride

Ammonium salts produce metabolic acidosis because ammonium is converted to urea by the liver, thus leaving an excess of chloride.

The renal tubules respond to metabolic acidosis by increasing their production of ammonia from glutamine and other amino acids. There is a delay of several hours to days, however, before the kidney can fully develop this capacity to form ammonia. During this period of delay, sodium in the urine is excreted in combination with chloride, and true diuresis ensues. Once the kidney is able to produce nearly as much ammonia as the amount ingested, the diuretic action of ammonium chloride ceases because chloride in tubular urine can then be balanced with ions of ammonium rather than sodium. Thus refractoriness to ammonium chloride diuresis develops within a few days.

Ammonium chloride is seldom used by itself as a diuretic, but it is helpful in potentiating the action of the mercurials.

Ammonium chloride is administered in large doses, 6 to 10 Gm./day. It can cause considerable gastric irritation, and for this reason enteric-coated tablets are occasionally used. The compound is given intermittently in order to avoid development of refractoriness. It may induce hepatic coma in liver disease, in which case L-lysine monohydrochloride may be substituted.

References

1 Anderson, W. A. D., and Bethea, W. R.: Renal lesion following administration of hypertonic solutions of sucrose, J.A.M.A. **114**:1983, 1940.

2 Bank, N., Koch, K. M., Aynedjian, H. S., and Aras, M.: Effect of changes in renal perfusion pressure on the suppression of proximal tubular sodium reabsorption due to saline loading, J. Clin. Invest. **48**:271, 1969.

3 Berliner, R. W.: Renal secretion of potassium and hydrogen ions, Fed. Proc. **11**:695, 1952.

4 Berliner, R. W., Kennedy, T. J., Jr., and Orloff, J.: Relationship between acidification of the urine and potassium metabolism, Amer. J. Med. **11**:274, 1951.

5 Berliner, R. W., Levinsky, N. G., Davidson, D. G., and Eden, M.: Dilution and concentration of the urine and the action of antidiuretic hormone, Amer. J. Med. **24**:730, 1958.

6 Beyer, K. H.: The mechanism of action of chlorothiazide, Ann. N. Y. Acad. Sci., **71**:363, 1958.

7 Beyer, K. H., and Baer, J. E.: Physiological basis for the action of newer diuretic agents, Pharmacol. Rev. **13**:517, 1961.

8 Brickman, A. S., Massry, S. G., and Coburn, J. W.: Changes in serum and urinary calcium during treatment with hydrochlorothiazide; studies on mechanisms, J. Clin. Invest. **51**:945, 1972.

9 Bryant, J. M., Yü, T. F., Berger, L., Schwartz, N., Torosdag, S., Fletcher, L., Fertig, H., Schwartz, M. S., and Quan, R. B. F.: Hyperuricemia induced by the administration of chlorthalidone and other sulfonamide diuretics, Amer. J. Med. 33:408, 1962.

10 Calesnick, B., Christensen, J. A., and Richter, M.: Absorption and excretion of furosemide-S^{35} in human subjects, Proc. Soc. Exper. Biol Med. 123:17, 1966.

11 Cannon, P. J., Ames, R. P., and Laragh, J. H.: Methylenebutyryl phenoxyacetic acid. Novel and potent natriuretic and diuretic agent, J.A.M.A. 185:854, 1963.

12 Cornish, A. L., McClellan, J. T., and Johnston, D. H.: Effects of chlorothiazide on the pancreas, New Eng. J. Med. 265:673, 1961.

13 Davidow, M., Kakaviatos, N., and Finnerty, F. A.: Intravenous administration of furosemide in heart failure, J.A.M.A. 200:824, 1967.

14 Davies, B. M. A., and Yudkin, J.: Role of glutaminase in the production of urinary ammonia, Nature 167:117, 1951.

15 Dirks, J. H., Cirksena, W. J., and Berliner, R. W.: Effects of saline infusion on sodium reabsorption by proximal tubule of dog, J. Clin. Invest. 44:1160, 1965.

16 Edmonds, C. J.: An aldosterone antagonist and diuretics in the treatment of chronic oedema and ascites, Lancet 1:509, 1960.

17 Farah, A., and Kruse, R.: The relation of mercurial diuresis to cellular protein-bound sulfhydryl changes in renal cells, J. Pharmacol. Exp. Ther. 130:13, 1960.

18 Farah, A., and Maresh, G.: The influence of sulfhydryl compounds on diuresis and renal and cardiac circulatory changes caused by mersalyl, J. Pharmacol. Exp. Ther. 92:73, 1948.

19 Freis, E. D., and Sappington, R. F.: Long-term effect of probenecid on diuretic-induced hyperuricemia, J.A.M.A. 198:127, 1966.

20 Giebisch, G.: Measurements of electrical potentials and ion fluxes in single renal tubules, Circulation 21:879, 1960.

21 Ginsberg, D. J., Saad, A., and Gabuzda, G. J.: Metabolic studies with the diuretic triamterene in patients with cirrhosis and ascites, New Eng. J. Med. 271:1229, 1964.

22 Hagedorn, C. W., Kaplan, A. A., and Hulet, W. H.: Prolonged administration of ethacrynic acid in patients with renal disease, New Eng. J. Med. 272:1152, 1965.

23 Heinemann, H. O., Demartini, F. E., and Laragh, J. H.: The effect of chlorothiazide on renal excretion of electrolytes and free water, Amer. J. Med. 26:853, 1959.

24 Kagawa, C. M., Cella, J. H., and Von Arman, C. G.: Action of new steroids in blocking effect of aldosterone and desoxycorticosterone on salt, Science 126:1015, 1957.

25 Kassirer, J. P., Berkman, P. M., Lawrenz, D. R., and Schwartz, W. B.: The critical role of chloride in the correction of hypokalemic alkalosis in man, Amer. J. Med. 38:172, 1965.

26 Kessler, R. H., Lozano, R., and Pitts, R. F.: Studies on structure-diuretic activity relationships of organic compounds of mercury, J. Clin. Invest. 36:656, 1957.

27 Komorn, R. M., and Cafruny, E. J.: Ethacrynic acid: diuretic property coupled to reaction with sulfhydryl groups in renal cells, Science 143:133, 1964.

28 Lawrason, F. D., Alpert, E., Mohr, F. L., and McMahon, F. G.: Ulcerative-obstructive lesions of the small intestine, J.A.M.A. 191:641, 1965.

29 Levinsky, N. G., and Lalone, R. C.: Mechanism of sodium diuresis after saline infusion in the dog, J. Clin. Invest. 42:1261, 1963.

30 Liddle, G. W.: Sodium diuresis induced by steroidal antagonists of aldosterone, Science 126:1016, 1957.

31 Mann, T., and Keilin, D.: Sulfanilamide as a specific inhibitor of carbonic anhydrase, Nature 146:164, 1940.

32 Martz, B. L.: A diuretic assay utilizing normal subjects, Clin. Pharmacol. Ther. 3:340, 1962.

33 Mathog, R. H., and Klein, W. J.: Ototoxicity of ethacrynic acid and aminoglycoside antibiotics in uremia, New Eng. J. Med. 280:1223, 1969.

34 Mudge, G. H., Ames, A., III, Foulks, J., and Gilman, A.: Effect of drugs on renal secretion of potassium in dog, Amer. J. Physiol. 161:151, 1950.

35 Parfitt, A. M.: Chlorothiazide-induced hypercalcemia in juvenile osteoporosis and hyperparathyroidism, New Eng. J. Med. 281:55, 1969.

36 Pitts, R. F.: Some reflections on mechanisms of action of diuretics, Amer. J. Med. 24:745, 1958.

37 Pitts, R. F.: The physiological basis of diuretic therapy, Springfield, Ill., 1959, Charles C Thomas, Publisher.

38 Pitts, R. F., Alexander, R. S., and Fagan, K.: The nature of the renal tubular mechanism for acidifying the urine, Amer. J. Physiol. 144:239, 1945.

39 Pitts, R. F., Krück, F., Lozano, R., Taylor, D. W., Heidenreich, O. P. A., and Kessler, R. H.: Studies on the mechanism of diuretic action of chlorothiazide, J. Pharmacol. Exp. Ther. 123:89, 1958.

40 Ramos, G., Rivera, A., and Pena, J. C.: Mechanism of the antidiuretic effect of saluretic drugs, Clin. Pharmacol. Ther. 8:557, 1967.

41 Rocha, A. S., and Kokko, J. P.: Sodium chloride and water transport in the medullary thick ascending limb of Henle: evidence for active chloride transport, J. Clin. Invest. 52:612, 1973.

42 Roughton, F. J. W.: Recent work on carbon dioxide transport by the blood, Physiol. Rev. 15:241, 1935.

43 Shenkin, H. A., Goluboff, B., and Haft, H.: The use of mannitol for the reduction of intracranial pressure in intracranial surgery, J. Neurosurg. 19:897, 1962.

44 Stahl, W. M.: Effect of mannitol on the kidney: changes in intrarenal hemodynamics, New Eng. J. Med. 272:381, 1965.

45 Suki, W., Rector, F. C., Jr., and Seldin, D. W.: The site of action of furosemide and other sulfonamide diuretics in the dog, J. Clin. Invest. 44:1458, 1965.

46 Timmerman, R. J., Springman, F. R., and Thomas, R. K.: Evaluation of furosemide, a new diuretic agent, Curr. Ther. Res. 6:88, 1964.

47 Vogl, A.: The discovery of the organic mercurial diuretics, Amer. Heart J. 39:881, 1950.

48 Walker, A. M., Schmidt, C. F., Elsom, K. A., and Johnston, C. G.: Renal blood flow of unanesthetized rabbits and dogs in diuresis and antidiuresis, Amer. J. Physiol. 118:95, 1937.

49 Weston, R. E., Escher, D. J. W., Grossman, J., and Leiter, L.: Mechanisms contributing to unresponsiveness to mercurial diuretics in congestive failure, J. Clin. Invest. 31:901, 1952.

50 Wilkins, R. W.: New drugs for hypertension with special reference to chlorothiazide, New Eng. J. Med. 257:1026, 1957.

51 Wirz, H.: Kidney, water and electrolytes, Ann. Rev. Physiol. 23:577, 1961.

52 Wolff, F. W., Parmley, W. W., White, K., and Okun, R.: Drug-induced diabetes: diabetogenic activity of long-term administration of benzothiadiazines, J.A.M.A. 185:568, 1963.

Recent reviews

53 Baer, J. E., and Beyer, K. H.: Renal pharmacology, Ann. Rev. Pharmacol. 6:261, 1966.

54 Beyer, K. H.: Electrolyte adjustments in modern diuretic therapy, Pharmacol. Physicians 1(8):1, 1967.

55 Bricker, N. S.: The control of sodium excretion with normal and reduced nephron populations, Amer. J. Med. 43:313, 1967.

56 Cafruny, E. J.: The site and mechanism of action of mercurial diuretics, Pharmacol. Rev. 20:89, 1968.

57 Earley, L. E.: Diuretics, New Eng. J. Med. 276:966, 1967.

58 Earley, L. E., and Orloff, J.: Thiazide diuretics, Ann. Rev. Med. 15:149, 1964.

59 Ehrlich, E. N.: Aldosterone, the adrenal cortex and hypertension, Ann. Rev. Med. 19:373, 1968.

60 Frazier, H. S.: Renal regulation of sodium balance, New Eng. J. Med. 279:868, 1968.

61 Gantt, C. L.: Diuretic therapy, Rational Drug Ther. 6:1, Aug. 1972.

62 Giebisch, G.: Coupled ion and fluid transport in the kidney, New Eng. J. Med. 287:913, 1972.

63 Giebisch, G.: Renal tubular transfer of sodium, chloride, and potassium, Amer. J. Med. 36:643, 1964.

64 Gottschalk, C. W.: Osmotic concentration and dilution of the urine, Amer. J. Med. 36:670, 1964.

65 Haber, E.: Recent developments in pathophysiologic studies of the renin-angiotensin system, New Eng. J. Med. 280:148, 1969.

66 Kessler, R. H.: The use of furosemide and ethacrynic acid in the treatment of edema, Pharmacol. Physicians 1(9):1, 1967.

67 Kessler, R. H.: The treatment of noncardiac edema, Pharmacol. Physicians. 2(7):1, 1968.

68 Landon, E. J., and Forte, L. R.: Cellular mechanisms in renal pharmacology, Ann. Rev. Pharmacol. 11:171, 1971.

69 Milne, M. D.: Renal pharmacology, Ann. Rev. Pharmacol. 5:119, 1965.

70 Mudge, G. H.: Renal pharmacology, Ann. Rev. Pharmacol. 7:163, 1967.

71 Orloff, J., and Burg, M.: Kidney, Ann. Rev. Physiol. 33:83, 1971.

72 Orloff, J., and Handler, J. S.: The cellular mode of action of antidiuretic hormone, Amer. J. Med. 36:686, 1964.

73 Pitts, R. F.: Renal production and excretion of ammonia, Amer. J. Med. 36:720, 1964.

74 Schwartz, W. B., and Relman, A. S.: Effects of electrolyte disorders on renal structure and function, New Eng. J. Med. 276:383, 452, 1967.

75 Seldin, D. W., Eknoyan, G., Suki, W., and Rector, F. C., Jr.: The physiology of modern diuretics. In Proceedings of the Third International Congress on Nephrology, vol. 1, Basel 1967, S. Karger.

76 Steinmetz, P. R.: Excretion of acid by the kidney—functional organization and cellular aspects of acidification, New Eng. J. Med. 278:1102, 1968.

77 Thurau, K.: Renal hemodynamics, Amer. J. Med. 36:698, 1964.

78 Weiner, I. M., and Mudge, G. H.: Renal tubular mechanisms for excretion of organic acids and bases, Amer. J. Med. 36:743, 1964.

79 Welt, L. G., Sachs, J. R., and Gitelman, H. J.: Electrolyte and mineral metabolism, Ann. Rev. Pharmacol. 6:77, 1966.

34 Pharmacologic approaches to atherosclerosis

Arteriosclerotic cardiovascular disease appears to be a multifactorial disease in which hyperlipidemia is one of the causative factors. Pharmacologic approaches to the disease are generally aimed at altering hyperlipidemia. Several epidemiologic studies[30] indicate that dietary changes that lower serum lipids also decrease the development of arteriosclerotic cardiovascular disease. There is every reason to believe that pharmacologic agents may be able to accomplish the same effect.

Among the hyperlipidemic drugs, *clofibrate* decreases cholesterol synthesis and probably inhibits lipoprotein release from the liver. *Cholestyramine* binds bile acids and leads to lowered serum cholesterol. *Dextrothyroxine* increases the catabolism of cholesterol by the liver. *Nicotinic acid* may inhibit free fatty acid release from adipose tissue and lowers cholesterol synthesis. *Sitosterols* interfere with cholesterol absorption. *Female sex hormones* have complex effects on serum lipids and are not generally effective in hyperlipoproteinemias. *Polyunsaturated fatty acids,* recommended by many authorities in the dietary management of atherosclerosis, remain controversial from the standpoint of both their mode of action and their effectiveness.

CLOFIBRATE

Clofibrate (*p*-chlorophenoxyisobutyrate; Atromid S) is becoming the most important lipid-lowering drug, and favorable results have been reported in the long-term treatment of hyperlipidemia.[3] It was first used in combination with, or as a vehicle for, androsterone, which is known to decrease cholesterol synthesis in the liver. Further studies revealed that clofibrate alone, when administered orally in doses of 500 mg. four times daily, will lower the concentration of triglycerides, lipoproteins, and cholesterol in plasma within a few weeks.

The mode of action of clofibrate is probably related to an inhibition of hepatic cholesterol synthesis and to a decrease in the rate of lipoprotein release from the liver.[2, 30] The drug is useful in types III, IV, and V hyperlipidemias and is less effective in type II.

Side effects of clofibrate administration include gastrointestinal upset and increased sensitivity to coumarin anticoagulants.

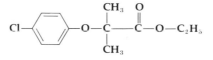

Clofibrate

Clofibrate is available in 500 mg. capsules. The usual dose is one capsule four times a day.

CHOLESTYRAMINE

Cholestyramine (Questran; Cuemid) is a quaternary ammonium anion exchange resin that binds bile acids in the intestinal lumen, exchanging them for chloride. Since the resin is not absorbed, it promotes the excretion of bile acids. Increased fecal excretion of bile acids may lower serum cholesterol because there is a continual conversion of the sterol to bile acids, which are in large part reabsorbed under normal circumstances. Cholestyramine is used primarily for the relief of pruritus associated with biliary tract obstruction. The drug may interfere with the absorption of numerous drugs and fat-soluble vitamins.[7]

Cholestyramine may be useful in type II hyperlipoproteinemia. Side effects of the drug include constipation and nausea. A similar drug, **Colestipol**,[8] is being investigated.

Cholestyramine is available in granular form. It is administered in doses of 4 Gm. three times a day.

DEXTROTHYROXINE

It is generally known that a reciprocal relationship exists between thyroid function and serum cholesterol. Among the thyroxine analogs that have been synthesized, dextrothyroxine (Choloxin) has received the most attention in the treatment of hyperlipoproteinemias. It is estimated the levothyroxine is ten to twenty times as calorigenic as dextrothyroxine, but the latter has about 20% of the hypocholesterolemic action of levothyroxine.

Dextrothyroxine may reduce serum cholesterol levels by promoting the hepatic conversion of cholesterol to bile acids. The drug may be useful in types II and III hyperlipoproteinemias.

Side effects of dextrothyroxine are a consequence of its metabolic stimulating action. They include angina and arrhythmias. In the large Coronary Drug Research Project,[20] dextrothyroxine at 6 mg./day produced sufficient adverse effects and suspicion of excess mortality that the drug was eliminated from the study.

NICOTINIC ACID

When given in large doses of 1.5 to 8 Gm./day, nicotinic acid has been found useful in hyperlipoproteinemias of types II, III, IV, and V. The drug acts by several mechanisms. It inhibits free fatty acid release from adipose tissue, and it may inhibit cholesterol synthesis in the liver at an early stage. The usefulness of nicotinic acid is greatly limited by its side effects. Flushing, pruritus, gastrointestinal complaints, and disturbances in liver function are frequent during the administration of nicotinic acid.

SITOSTEROLS

Absorption of cholesterol from the gastrointestinal tract is interfered with by certain plant sterols, known as sitosterols (Cytellin). These sterols are not significantly absorbed but have many disadvantages. They must be administered frequently and they are unpalatable. As a consequence they have not become widely used.

FEMALE SEX HORMONES

Although estrogens may lower serum cholesterol, they elevate serum triglycerides. Studies of women taking oral contraceptives often reveal an elevation of serum triglycerides.

Some reports claimed that conjugated estrogenic substances (Premarin) increased the chances of survival of men having coronary disease.[16] Other studies in which ethinyl estradiol was used, failed to show any benefit in patients who had had a previous myocardial infarction.[27]

POLYUNSATURATED FATTY ACIDS

Vegetable oils such as corn oil or safflower oil that contain a very high concentration of polyunsaturated fatty acids will reduce serum cholesterol in a majority of persons when used in place of saturated fats.[14] The mechanism whereby polyunsaturated fats accomplish this is not certain. The possibilities that have been considered are (1) by influencing absorption and transport of cholesterol or (2) by influencing synthesis and catabolism of the sterol.[9]

The unsaturated fats do not promote fecal excretion of cholesterol despite early claims to the contrary.[15] It is likely that the lowering of plasma cholesterol is a consequence of redistribution.

CLASSIFICATION AND MANAGEMENT OF HYPERLIPOPROTEINEMIAS

Atherosclerosis is common and severe in some types of hyperlipoproteinemia, and the aim of management is to lower the concentration of lipids. The use of lipid-lowering agents depends on the type of hyperlipoproteinemia. The Frederickson classification[22] recognizes five different lipoprotein patterns, which are designated *types I* through *V.*

Type I This type is characterized by elevated chylomicrons with normal beta lipoproteins. None of the drugs is useful in its treatment, although reduction of dietary fat may be helpful.

Type II Patients in this group have elevated serum cholesterols and normal triglycerides. In addition to a low cholesterol diet and substitution of polyunsaturated fats for saturated ones, the following drugs are helpful: clofibrate, dextrothyroxine (Choloxin), nicotinic acid, and cholestyramine.

Type III Patients in this group show abnormalities in the composition of their lipoproteins. Response to diet and drugs is much better than in type II patients. Clofibrate is effective, and dextrothyroxine and nicotinic acid are also useful.

Type IV Patients in this group are usually obese and show a prebeta band on electrophoresis. Diet therapy with carbohydrate restriction, the use of polyunsaturated fats, and clofibrate are effective therapeutic measures.

Type V This group has the characteristics of a combination of types I and IV. Weight reduction, clofibrate, and nicotinic acid are recommended.

References

1 Ahrens, E. H., Jr., Hirsch, J., Insull, W., Jr., Tsaltas, T. T., Blomstrand, R., and Peterson, M. L.: Dietary control of serum lipids in relation to atherosclerosis, J.A.M.A. **164**:1905, 1957.

2 Avoy, D. R., Swyryd, E. A., and Gould, R. G.: Effects of *p*-chlorophenoxyisobutyryl ethyl ester (CPIB) with and without androsterone on cholesterol biosynthesis in rat liver, J. Lipid Res. **6**:369, 1965.

3 Berkowitz, D.: Treatment of hyperlipidemia with clofibrate, J.A.M.A. **218**:1002, 1971.

4 Best, M. M., and Duncan, C. H.: Effects of clofibrate and dextrothyroxine singly and in combination on serum lipids, Arch. Intern. Med. **118**:97, 1966.

5 Boyd, G. S.: Effect of linoleate and estrogen on cholesterol metabolism, Fed. Proc. 21:86, 1962.

6 Christensen, N. A., Achor, R. W. P., Berge, K. G., and Mason, H. L.: Nicotinic acid treatment of hypercholesteremia, J.A.M.A. 177:546, 1961.

7 Gallo, D. G., Bailey, K. R., and Sheffner, A. L.: The interaction between cholestyramine and drugs, Proc. Soc. Exp. Biol. Med. 120:60, 1965.

8 Glueck, C. J., Ford, S., Scheel, D., and Steiner, P.: Colestipol and cholestyramine resin, J.A.M.A. 222:676, 1972.

9 Goldsmith, G. A.: Mechanisms by which certain pharmacologic agents lower serum cholesterol, Fed. Proc. 21:81, 1962.

10 Hollander, W., and Chobanian, A.: The effects of an inhibitor of cholesterol biosynthesis, triparanol (MER-29), in subjects with and without coronary artery disease, Boston Med. Quart. 10:1, 1959.

11 Oliver, M. F., and Boyd, G. S.: Influence of reduction of serum lipids on prognosis of coronary heart disease, Lancet 2:499, 1961.

12 Oliver, M. F., Roberts, S. D., Hayes, D., Pantridge, J. F., Suzman, M. M., and Bersohn, I.: Effect of atromid and ethylchlorophenoxyisobutyrate on anticoagulant requirements, Lancet 1:143, 1963.

13 Parsons, W. B., Jr.: Studies on nicotonic acid use in hypercholesterolemia, Arch. Intern. Med. 107:653, 1961.

14 Portman, O. W., and Stare, F. J.: Dietary regulation of serum cholesterol levels, Physiol. Rev. 39:407, 1959.

15 Spritz, N., Ahrens, E. H., Jr., and Grundy, S.: Sterol balance in man as plasma cholesterol concentrations are altered by exchanges of dietary fats, J. Clin. Invest. 44:1482, 1965.

16 Stamler, J.: Effectiveness of estrogens for the long-term therapy of middle-aged men with a history of myocardial infarction. In Seventh Hahnemann Symposium on Coronary Heart Disease, New York, 1963, Grune & Stratton, Inc.

17 Steiner, A., Howard, E. J., and Algun, S.: Importance of dietary cholesterol in man, J.A.M.A. 181;186, 1962.

18 Wilens, S. L., and Plair, C. M.: Blood cholesterol, nutrition, and atherosclerosis, Arch. Intern. Med. 116:373, 1965.

Recent reviews

19 The Coronary Drug Project Research Group: The coronary drug project, J.A.M.A. 214:1303, 1970.

20 The Coronary Drug Project Research Group: The coronary drug project, J.A.M.A. 220:996, 1972.

21 Fredrickson, D. S., and Lees, R. S.: Familial hyperlipoproteinemia. In Stanbury, J. B., Wyngarden, J. B., and Fredrickson, D. S., editors: The metabolic basis of inherited disease, New York, 1965, McGraw-Hill Book Co.

22 Fredrickson, D. S., Levy, R. I., and Lees, R. S.: Transport in lipoproteins: an integrated approach to mechanisms and disorders, New Eng. J. Med. 276:34, 94, 148, 215, 273, 1967.

23 Garattini, S., and Paoletti, R.: Drugs in lipid metabolism, Ann. Rev. Pharmacol. 3:91, 1963.

24 Goldsmith, G. A.: Highlights on the cholesterol-fats, diets, and atherosclerosis problem, J.A.M.A. 176:783, 1961.

25 Lees, R. S., and Wilson, D. E.: The treatment of hyperlipidemia, New Eng. J. Med. 284:186, 1971.

26 Lown, B., Portman, O. W., and Stare, F. J.: Some comments on the use of agents which lower serum cholesterol, Clin. Pharmacol. Ther. 3:421, 1962.

27 Malinow, M. R.: Hormones and atherosclerosis, Advances Pharmacol. 2:211, 1963.

28 Pinter, K. G., and Van Itallie, T. B.: Drugs and atherosclerosis, Ann. Rev. Pharmacol. 6:251, 1966.

29 Steinberg, D.: Chemotherapeutic approaches to the problem of hyperlipidemia, Advances Pharmacol. 1:59, 1962.

30 Weiss, P.: The treatment of hyperlipidemia, Rational Drug Ther. 6:1, Sept., 1972.

31 Wessler, S., and Avioli, L. A.: Classification and management of familial hyperlipoproteinemia, J.A.M.A. 207:929, 1969.

SECTION SEVEN

DRUG EFFECTS ON THE RESPIRATORY AND GASTROINTESTINAL TRACTS

35 Drug effects on the respiratory tract

Numerous drugs, along with other measures, contribute to the effective management of pulmonary disorders, particularly in chronic obstructive lung disease. The *bronchodilators* are helpful in opening blocked airways; the *mucolytic drugs* aid in altering the characteristics of respiratory tract fluid; the *antibiotics* are useful in dealing with infections; the *corticosteroids* reduce the inflammatory process. In addition to these useful drug effects, the hazardous nature of sedative drugs and oxygen at high concentration is increasingly recognized. It is also becoming clear that the lung is a metabolic organ which contributes to the elaboration and destruction of a variety of endogenous compounds of great pharmacologic activity. Drug-induced pulmonary diseases are receiving increased attention also.

The groups of drugs that will be discussed at this point are the bronchodilators, expectorants, and mucolytic agents. In addition, the current concepts on the metabolic functions of the lung of pharmacologic interest and drug-induced pulmonary diseases will also be considered.

PHARMACOLOGY OF BRONCHIAL SMOOTH MUSCLE

Numerous drugs are capable of causing contraction or relaxation of the bronchial smooth muscle. The more important ones are enumerated in Tables 35-1 and 35-2.

The bronchial constrictors listed in Table 35-1 are of experimental interest only and have no therapeutic importance. Histamine and methacholine are said to have a greater constrictor effect in asthmatics than in normal individuals, and these compounds are sometimes used by clinical investigators for testing the potency of bronchodilator drugs.

The bronchodilator drugs listed in Table 35-1 vary greatly in their importance in current therapeutics. Atropine and other anticholinergics are avoided in the treatment of obstructive lung disease for several reasons. Not only are these drugs ineffective

Table 35-1. Drugs acting on bronchial smooth muscle

Causing contraction	Causing relaxation or opposing contraction
Acetylcholine and related drugs	Atropine and other anticholinergic drugs
Histamine	Antihistaminics
Beta adrenergic blockers	Beta adrenergic agonists
Alpha adrenergic agonists	Dimethylxanthine (theophylline)
Slow-reacting substance of anaphylaxis	Inhibitors of the immunologic release of mediators of anaphylaxis
Bradykinin	Prostaglandins E
Prostaglandin $F_{2\alpha}$	Antagonists of slow-reacting substance of anaphylaxis and prostaglandins F

447

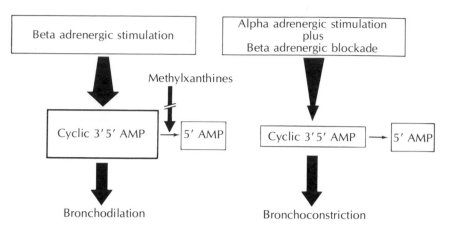

Fig. 35-1. Bronchodilation and bronchoconstriction as influenced by cyclic 3'5' AMP tissue concentrations. (Schematic representation of a working hypothesis. For details see Problem 35-2, p. 449).

except against administered cholinergic agents, but they also tend to cut down on bronchial secretions. Inspissated mucus produced by the anticholinergic drugs aggravates attacks of bronchial asthma. Several drugs mentioned in Table 35-1 are of experimental interest only, so that for all practical purposes the therapeutically useful bronchodilators are limited to the beta adrenergic agonists and the methylxanthines.

BETA ADRENERGIC AGONISTS AND METHYLXANTHINES AS BRONCHODILATORS

The effectiveness of epinephrine, sympathomimetic drugs, and theophylline derivatives such as aminophylline in bronchial asthma has been known for many years. Increased knowledge of the mode of action of these compounds is of more recent origin, and schemes of their influence on the bronchi are shown in Fig. 35-1.

With the postulation of alpha and beta receptors[6] it became clear that the beta receptor agonists and the methylxanthines or phosphodiesterase inhibitors are especially potent in dilating the bronchial smooth muscle. It is most likely that the effectiveness of both groups of drugs is based on their common property of increasing the levels of cyclic AMP in the smooth muscle of the bronchioles (Fig. 35-1).

The pure, direct-acting beta adrenergic agonist isoproterenol has become one of the most widely used bronchodilators. Its administration by a specially constructed inhaler has contributed to its popularity. It has some disadvantages, however. As expected from its pharmacology, isoproterenol causes considerable cardiac stimulation and its action is short. Furthermore, it has been suggested[11] that the use of isoproterenol may have contributed to the annual increase in mortality of asthmatics in England and Wales. The deaths have been attributed to various causes, such as alterations in the viscosity of bronchial secretions, decreased arterial oxygen tensions, and increased ventricular irritability with arrhythmias.[11]

With the postulation by Lands[6] of two types of beta adrenergic receptors, efforts have been directed at synthesizing drugs that would have a more specific effect on the bronchial smooth muscle and would also have a more prolonged action, thus avoiding the disadvantages of isoproterenol.

Lands termed β_1 those receptors responsible for cardiac stimulation and lipolysis, whereas those responsible for bronchodilatation and vasodepression were referred to as β_2. If two types of beta receptors indeed exist, it should be possible to synthesize beta agonists that have marked bronchodilator activity without much cardiac stimulation. A drug related to isoproterenol, salbutamol, appears to have such characteristics.

Problem 35-1. Is it possible to increase bronchodilator activity without a corresponding increase in cardiac stimulant effect in beta adrenergic agonists? Salbutamol and isoproterenol were compared on asthmatic subjects and in normal individuals in a double-blind trial to compare bronchodilator and cardiovascular activity.[12]

Aerosols containing salbutamol (100 γg per inhalation) or isoproterenol (500 γg per inhalation) were provided for a double-blind trial in identical containers. Forced expiratory spirograms were analyzed for forced expiratory volume in 1 second (F.E.V.$_1$) and forced vital capacity (F.V.C.) as well as by other criteria. Heart rate was measured from a continuous electrocardiogram.

In asthmatic subjects the F.E.V.$_1$ showed a similar increase with both drugs initially, but 3 and 4 hours later the values were significantly higher for salbutamol. Heart rate did not increase with salbutamol but showed a rise with isoproterenol. In normal subjects, salbutamol produced a small increase in heart rate, whereas isoproterenol increased heart rate on the average by 33 beats a minute and caused palpitation.

It may be concluded from this clinical study that for comparable bronchodilator activity salbutamol produces much less cardiac stimulation. It appears, then, that the beta receptors in the bronchial smooth muscle and the heart are somewhat different. Animal experiments[4] point to the same conclusion.

Since beta adrenergic receptors mediate bronchodilation, the question remains: are there alpha adrenergic receptors in the bronchial smooth muscle and do they have any function in drug effects?

Problem 35-2. Do alpha adrenergic receptors play a role in drug-induced bronchoconstriction? In a recent experimental study,[7] isolated strips of human bronchi were tested for their response to a variety of drugs. The bronchodilating effect of epinephrine was abolished by propranolol. After beta receptor blockade, epinephrine produced bronchoconstriction. However, the dose of epinephrine required for the constrictor effect was 10 times greater than the dose that caused bronchial dilatation prior to beta receptor blockade. The constriction caused by epinephrine could be abolished by phentolamine, an alpha adrenergic blocking drug. It may be concluded from this study and from other evidence that alpha adrenergic agonists may cause bronchoconstriction in high doses. Such bronchoconstriction becomes evident after the beta receptors are blocked. Whether the alpha receptor–mediated bronchoconstriction has any clinical significance remains to be demonstrated. It is not known, for example, if it is related to tachyphylaxis to epinephrine, the so-called *epinephrine fastness* in asthmatics.

Although the adrenergic drugs are most effective, the methylxanthines such as theophylline and its double salt aminophylline are useful. This is especially true in patients in whom some contraindication exists to the adrenergic drugs or in those who are tolerant to them. Intravenously administered aminophylline may be effective in terminating an asthmatic attack.

In addition to the adrenergic drugs and the methylxanthines, the adrenal corticosteroids are used in severe asthma. The mode of action of the corticosteroids remains unknown, although it is probably related to their antiinflammatory effect. Several other drugs are used experimentally as bronchodilators, such as the prostaglandins of the E series. Other drugs are useful in combination with bronchodilators, such as disodium cromoglycate (p. 660) and the mucolytic agents that will be discussed later (p. 451).

ADVERSE EFFECTS OF BRONCHODILATORS

Epinephrine and isoproterenol have all the cardiovascular side effects predictable from their pharmacology, and patients may manifest tachycardia, palpitations, and arrhythmias. Ephedrine, which acts by releasing endogenous catecholamines, crosses the blood-brain barrier and causes nervousness and wakefulness in addition to the peripheral sympathomimetic effects.

Orally administered theophylline or aminophylline causes gastric irritation, and these drugs are irregularly absorbed from the gastrointestinal tract. It is claimed that theophylline in 20% alcohol is less likely to cause gastric irritation and is better absorbed. Aminophylline suppositories are irregularly absorbed and may lead to rectal irritation. Intravenously administered aminophylline may lead to central nervous system stimulation and convulsions.

INDIVIDUAL BRONCHODILATORS

Epinephrine is highly effective in the treatment of acute asthma. It may be injected subcutaneously for a short duration of action, intramuscularly, or as a suspension in oil. It may be administered as an inhalant. When issued frequently, it may produce tachyphylaxis, the mechanism of which is not understood. Perhaps it is a rebound phenomenon.

Ephedrine is highly useful in the prevention and treatment of asthma. It is effective when given orally, and it has a duration of action that lasts several hours. It acts by releasing endogenous catecholamines, and tachyphylaxis may develop to its continued use. Central nervous system stimulation is a common side effect caused by ephedrine. For this reason there are combinations of ephedrine and phenobarbital available. The latter is usually present in doses too small to counteract the wakefulness caused by ephedrine. The usual dosage of ephedrine for adults is 15 to 50 mg., which may be given as often as every hour if needed. **Pseudoephedrine hydrochloride** (Sudafed) is an active stereoisomer of ephedrine used in a manner similar to the latter.

Isoproterenol as the hydrochloride or sulfate is administered preferably by inhalation. The drug may also be given intravenously. Sublingual tablets of the drug are available, but absorption of these is irregular. Cardiovascular side effects are common after the administration of isoproterenol. Sudden death has occurred under these circumstances.

Protokylol hydrochloride (Caytine) is similar to isoproterenol in its action and may be given orally. It also has a more prolonged effect.

Salbutamol is one of a series of selective stimulants of the $beta_2$ receptors. Its cardiovascular effects are less than its bronchodilator actions, and the duration of action of the drug is considerably greater than that of isoproterenol. Other selective beta stimulants are **metaproterenol sulfate,** known previously as orciprenaline terbutaline sulfate, and **soterenol hydrochloride.** These selective beta stimulants are still experimental in the United States.

Aminophylline (theophylline ethylenediamine) may be administered by slow intravenous injection, orally, or rectally. Its absorption from the gastrointestinal tract is variable. Irritation of the rectum may result from suppositories. Excessive blood levels such as may occur from intravenous injections may lead to convulsions, shock, and death. About 85% of aminophylline is theophylline. For blood levels of theophylline after its intravenous injection, see Mitenko and Ogilvie.[7a]

Oxtriphylline (Choledyl) is the choline salt of theophylline, containing 64% theophylline. It is more soluble than theophylline and may be better absorbed after oral administration.

Dyphylline (Dilor, Lufyllin, Neothylline) is 7(2,3-dihydroxypropyl) theophylline, a neutral derivative. It corresponds to 70% anhydrous theophylline. It is more soluble than the parent compound and is less irritating. It may even be injected by the intramuscular route.

Theophylline sodium glycinate is similar in its indications and uses to aminophylline. It contains 51% theophylline.

Theophylline is available also as an elixir (Elixophyllin), which contains 80 mg./15 ml. in 20% alcohol.

EXPECTORANTS AND MUCOLYTIC DRUGS

Although widely used, the expectorants and mucolytic drugs hardly constitute one of the brilliant chapters of pharmacology. These drugs presumably alter the viscosity of the sputum, change the volume of respiratory tract fluid, and facilitate expectoration. The mode of action of some of these drugs is understood. In many cases, however, there is much doubt about their mechanism of action and their effectiveness.

Acetylcysteine (Mucomyst) reduces the viscosity of sputum, presumably by depolymerizing mucopolysaccharides. It is used by nebulization or by instillation into the trachea. Acetylcysteine may cause bronchospasm and irritation of the upper respiratory tract and the mouth. The drug reacts with rubber and metals.

Terpin hydrate is a volatile oil that is believed to act on the bronchial secretory cells. It is commonly employed as a vehicle for cough mixtures in the form of the elixir.

A number of expectorants are believed to stimulate respiratory tract secretion by a reflex through irritation of the stomach. These include **potassium iodide, syrup of Ipecac, glyceryl guaiacolate, and ammonium chloride.** Proof for the effectiveness of these drugs is hard to find.

Pancreatic dornase is pancreatic deoxyribonuclease that hydrolyzes the deoxyribonucleoprotein of purulent sputum and thereby reduces its viscosity.

It is the belief of competent authorities that the inhalation of nebulized water, sodium chloride solutions, and hygroscopic agents may be more valuable than the use of other inhalants in the treatment of diseases of the respiratory tract complicated by difficulties in expectoration.

ELABORATION AND DESTRUCTION OF PHARMACOLOGIC AGENTS BY THE LUNGS

It is increasingly recognized that lungs are involved in the elaboration and destruction of a variety of pharmacologic agents. Histamine has long been known to be present in high concentration in the mast cells of the lungs, and its release by anaphylaxis has been studied by many workers.

In addition to histamine, other pharmacologic agents are released during anaphylaxis. According to a study on the perfused guinea pig lung,[13] in addition to histamine, the lipid slow-reacting substance, prostaglandins, serotonin, and certain polypeptides such as bradykinin may also be released or elaborated.

The prostaglandins are receiving much attention for a number of reasons. The

451

lungs are a major site of prostaglandin synthesis. In addition, mechanical stimulation of the lungs or simply hyperinflation[8] may lead to increased synthesis or release of prostaglandins. The significance of this is still not clear. In addition to the prostaglandins, a number of peptides such as bradykinin and others[13] may be elaborated by the lungs.

The potential of the lung for synthesizing hormonal agents is best seen in cases of bronchogenic carcinoma, which may lead to endocrine syndromes with elaboration of many different polypeptide hormones.

The lungs are highly efficient in inactivating a number of pharmacologically active compounds. PGE and PGF are rapidly removed and inactivated during one circulation through the lungs. Bradykinin is almost completely removed in one circulation through the lungs. This is achieved by kininases, which act on the nonapeptide by splitting off the C-terminal amino acid residue or a C-terminal dipeptide.

The conversion of angiotensin I to angiotensin II takes place mainly in the lungs. The converting enzyme is present in high concentrations in these organs. It is believed that the rapid conversion of angiotensin I by the lungs takes place in the plasma membrane of the capillary endothelial cells. It is of great interest that bradykinin is inactivated, but angiotensin is activated by the lung. It has been suggested[5] that one enzyme, a dipeptide hydrolase, is responsible for both of these activities.

DRUG-INDUCED PULMONARY DISEASES

No discussion of drug effects on the respiratory tract would be complete without mentioning the drug-induced pulmonary diseases. For a detailed discussion of this, Rosenow[9] should be consulted.

Drugs may influence pulmonary function directly or indirectly. An example of a direct adverse effect is oxygen toxicity. Drugs alter pulmonary function indirectly by various mechanisms. Sedative drugs are an important cause of acute ventilatory failure. Pulmonary edema may be caused by salt and water overload or by depression of cardiac output. Intravenous medications causing thrombophlebitis contribute to pulmonary embolism. Finally, drug allergies may cause bronchospasm.

The directly acting drugs that may induce pulmonary disease encompass a variety of classes, such as inhalants, cancer chemotherapeutic agents, analgesics, antimicrobial drugs, and a miscellaneous category.

INHALANTS

Several inhalants may lead to altered pulmonary function. They include oxygen, acetylcysteine, and isoproterenol. In addition, aspiration of mineral oil and iodinated oils used for bronchography can lead to adverse effects.

It may seem surprising that **oxygen** is toxic in high concentrations, but the tendency of premature infants to develop retrolental fibroplasia and blindness after the prolonged administration of the gas at greater than 40% concentration is well documented. In addition, adults who inhale oxygen at greater than 60% concentrations may develop pulmonary irritation, congestion, atelectasis, and decreased vital capacity. Central nervous system changes manifested by paresthesias also occur. The pulmonary toxic effect of oxygen in man under hyperbaric conditions has been studied in great detail.[3] Breathing oxygen at 2 atmospheres, symptoms began within 3 to 8 hours and consisted of mild tracheal irritation and decreased vital capacity. After 8 to 10 hours, symptoms were characterized by uncontrollable coughing, dyspnea at rest, and a tracheobronchial burning sensation. Recovery of vital capacity occurred generally in 1 to 3 days.

Mineral oil, when aspirated, causes acute or chronic pneumonitis. **Iodinated oils** employed in bronchography may have adverse effects on a pulmonary reserve that is already impaired.

The bronchoconstrictor effect of acetylcysteine has already been mentioned (p. 451). **Isoproterenol** has been implicated by association in cases of sudden death in asthmatics. It has been suggested that in some individuals the drug is converted to 3-methoxyisoproterenol, which is a weak antagonist of the beta adrenergic receptor. **Disodium cromoglycate** may also cause some bronchospasm when given by nebulization.

CANCER CHEMOTHERAPEUTIC AGENTS

Cancer chemotherapeutic agents may in some cases cause pulmonary diseases. Diffuse pulmonary disease has been associated with the use of **busulfan** and **cyclophosphamide.**[9] **Methotrexate** has also been implicated in some cases of pulmonary disease.

ANALGESICS

The narcotic analgesics **heroin** and **methadone** may produce pulmonary edema by mechanisms that are obscure (p. 301). **Propoxyphene** poisoning has also been associated with pulmonary edema.

Aspirin may cause bronchoconstriction in some individuals. Although this is often referred to as aspirin allergy, its immunologic basis is unlikely. Often the aspirin-sensitive person fails to show similar reactions to sodium salicylate, whereas he may react to chemically unrelated anti-inflammatory drugs such as indomethacin. The mechanism of this "aspirin hypersensitivity" remains a mystery.

ANTIMICROBIAL DRUGS

A variety of antimicrobial drugs may cause pulmonary diseases. **Nitrofurantoin** administration may lead to a pleuropneumonic reaction. **Sulfonamides** may cause vasculitis, which may include the pulmonary vessels. Sulfonamides, para-amino salicylate, and penicillin may produce pulmonary infiltration with eosinophilia, usually referred to as "Löffler's syndrome." The **aminoglycosides** may cause muscle weakness, which with involvement of respiratory muscles may lead to respiratory paralysis. **Polymyxin B** given by aerosol can cause bronchospasm. This antibiotic is a well-known histamine releaser.

MISCELLANEOUS DRUGS CAUSING PULMONARY DISEASE

Methysergide can produce chronic pleural effusion. **Corticosteroids** may lead to the development of opportunistic pulmonary infections, particularly *pneumocystis carinii* pneumonia. The **ganglionic blocking agents** have been involved in some pulmonary diseases, which are now largely of historical interest, since the drugs are rarely used at present.

A critical review of drug-induced pulmonary diseases is difficult because much of the available information is based on clinical observations and not on actual experiments. The purpose of this brief summary is simply to call attention to the existence of drug-induced pulmonary diseases. Familiarity with the existence of such diseases may not only promote their accurate recognition but may also help in designing experiments that may elucidate the mechanisms involved.

References

1 Bianco, S., Griffin, J. P., Kamburoff, P. L., and Prime, F. J.: The effect of thymoxamine on histamine induced bronchospasm in man, Brit. J. Dis. Chest 66:27, 1972.

2 Choo-Kang, Y. F. J., Simpson, W. T., and Grant, I. W. B.: Controlled comparison of the bronchodilator effects of three β-adrenergic stimulant drugs administered by inhalation to patients with asthma, Brit. Med. J. 2:287, 1969.

3 Clark, J. M., and Lambertsen, C. J.: Rate of development of pulmonary O_2 toxicity in man during O_2 breathing at 2.0 Ata, J. Appl. Physiol. 30:739, 1971.

4 Hinds, L., and Katz, R. L.: Dissociation of tracheobronchial and cardiac effects of some beta-adrenergic stimulants, Anesthesiology 34:445, 1971.

5 Igic, R., Erdos, E. G., Yeh, H. S. J., Sorrells, K., and Nakajima, T.: The angiotensin I converting enzyme of the lung, Circ. Res. 31(supp. 2):51, 1972.

6 Lands, A. M., Arnold, A., McAnliff, J. P., et al.: Differentiation of receptor systems activated by sympathomimetic amines, Nature 214:597, 1967.

7 Mathé, A. A., Aström, A., and Persson, N. A.: Some bronchoconstricting and bronchodilating responses of human isolated bronchi: evidence for the existence of α-adrenoceptors, J. Pharm. Pharmacol. 23:905, 1971.

7a Mitenko, P. A., and Ogilvie, R. I.: Rational intravenous doses of theophylline, New Eng. J. Med. 289:600, 1973.

8 Piper, P., and Vane, J. R.: The release of prostaglandins from lung and other tissues, Ann. N. Y. Acad. Sci. 180:363, 1971.

9 Rosenow, E. C.: The spectrum of drug-induced pulmonary disease, Ann. Intern. Med. 77:977, 1972.

10 Sjoerdsma, A.: Relationships between alterations in amine metabolism and blood pressure, Cir. Res. 9:734, 1961.

11 Speizer, F. E., Doll, R., and Heaf, P.: Observations on recent increase in mortality prone asthma, Brit. Med. J. 1:339, 1968.

12 Tattersfield, A. E., and McNicol, M. W.: Salbutamol and isoproterenol; a double-blind trial to compare bronchodilator and cardiovascular activity, New Eng. J. Med. 281:1323, 1969.

13 Vane, J. R.: Mediators of the anaphylactic reaction, in identification of asthma, Ciba Foundation Study Group No. 38, Edinburgh, 1971, Churchill Livingstone.

14 Vane, J. R.: Prostaglandins and the aspirin-like drugs, Hosp. Practice 7:61, 1972.

Recent reviews

15 Barton, A. D., and Lourenco, R. V.: Bronchial secretions and mucociliary clearance, Arch. Intern. Med. 131:140, 1973.

16 Miller, W. F.: Aerosol therapy in acute and chronic respiratory disease, Arch. Intern. Med. 131:148, 1973.

36 Drug effects on the gastrointestinal tract

Drugs that exert a useful effect on the gastrointestinal tract may be best grouped according to their therapeutic indications. Since the most common medical problems in relation to the gastrointestinal tract are the management of peptic ulcer, constipation, diarrhea, and deficiencies of digestive factors, the various drugs used in gastroenterology will be discussed under the following headings: anticholinergics, antacids, and cathartics, laxatives, and antidiarrheal agents. The histamine H_2 receptor antagonists, still experimental, were discussed on p. 202.

ANTICHOLINERGICS

In peptic ulcer, smooth muscle spasm and the action of hydrochloric acid are in some way related to pain and perhaps to perpetuation of the ulcer. The anticholinergics are used to reduce smooth muscle spasm, and many contribute to reduction of hydrochloric acid secretion. These drugs are tertiary or quaternary amines basically related to atropine. Their pharmacology has been discussed previously (Chapter 9).

The advantages claimed for quaternary anticholinergics are lessened central nervous system side effects and the likelihood of their having some ganglionic blocking action in addition to their ability to block the vagus through a peripheral anticholinergic effect.

While large doses of the anticholinergic drugs can block gastrointestinal motility and hydrochloric acid secretion, clinical use of these drugs is hampered by the many anticholinergic side effects such as blurring of vision, dryness of the mouth, and difficulties in micturition.

Belladonna preparations and atropine have long been used in the treatment of peptic ulcer. They decrease gastric peristalsis but influence only basal gastric hydrochloric acid secretion. The decreased gastric motility, however, may allow the neutralizing action of administered antacids to be maintained for a longer time. These preparations also relieve spasm and pain.

Some of the most commonly used antispasmodics are propantheline (Pro-Banthine), diphemanil (Prantal), oxyphenonium (Antrenyl), penthienate (Monodral), tricyclamol (Co-Elorine), methscopolamine bromide (Pamine), dicyclomine (Bentyl), and glycopyrrolate (Robinul). Although none of these drugs is perfect,[19] their administration to the point of tolerance along with antacids provides dramatic relief of pain in ulcer patients.

GASTRIC ANTACIDS

Neutralization of gastric hydrochloric acid as a primary aim in the treatment of peptic ulcer was first advocated by Sippy (1923), although antacids such as calcium carbonate and sodium bicarbonate had been used for many years for indigestion.

The presence of acid gastric juice is considered a hindrance to healing of an ulcer and may actually contribute to symptoms such as pain. The pH of the gastric juice is normally between 1 and 2, and the purpose of antacid medication is to raise the pH to about 4 without producing systemic alkalosis. Complete neutralization is considered undesirable because it inhibits pepsin and may actually increase secretion of gastric hydrochloric acid. Calcium carbonate is especially potent in causing the so-called "acid rebound."

Gastric antacids are generally classified as *systemic* and *nonsystemic*, depending on the amount of systemic absorption of the cation responsible for the neutralization of gastric hydrochloric acid. Sodium bicarbonate (baking soda) is the only systemic antacid that has been used medically. It is now entirely abandoned except for its use by the lay public. Sodium bicarbonate is a very effective and rapid-acting neutralizer of gastric acid. Its disadvantage is that systemic absorption of the sodium ion causes alkalosis, which is characterized by elevated CO_2 content and pH of the plasma, loss of appetite, weakness, mental confusion, and, rarely, tetany. Renal insufficiency and calcinosis have been described in patients who have been taking systemic antacids for·long periods of time.

The gastric antacids preferred at present are the drugs whose cationic portion is not absorbed from the intestine and that raise the pH of the gastric contents only to about 4. These drugs are often referred to as *nonsystemic buffer antacids*. Various aluminum and magnesium salts have this property.

The value of antacids is reduced by their short duration of action, which in turn is caused by gastric emptying. On the other hand, the duration of action of an antacid may be as long as 3 hours if it is given 1 hour after eating.[4]

Inhibition of gastric secretion by H_2 receptor antagonists is of great experimental interest. Burimamide and metiamide were discussed on p. 202.

NONSYSTEMIC GASTRIC ANTACIDS
Aluminum hydroxide gel and dihydroxyaluminum aminoacetate

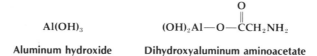

$$Al(OH)_3 \qquad\qquad (OH)_2Al-O-\overset{\overset{\textstyle O}{\textstyle \|}}{C}CH_2NH_2$$

Aluminum hydroxide   **Dihydroxyaluminum aminoacetate**

Aluminum hydroxide gel (Amphojel) is a colloidal suspension that is available in a liquid preparation or in tablets. In the acid stomach, aluminum chloride is formed, but in the alkaline intestine, aluminum hydroxide is again formed and the chloride reabsorbed. As a consequence, no alteration in systemic acid-base balance occurs. This drug has been widely used in liquid and tablet form and also by continuous drip through a gastric tube in treating peptic ulcer.

Aluminum hydroxide gel will raise the pH of the stomach contents to only about 4. Its only disadvantages are a constipating effect and the possibility of causing some loss of phosphate in the feces. The former difficulty may be prevented by the addition of certain magnesium salts. The phosphate loss is not likely to be serious with moderate doses in patients receiving an adequate diet. However, aluminum phosphate gel may be used, which will obviate this difficulty, although it has a lesser capacity to neutralize acid. The binding of phosphate by aluminum salts may be beneficial in the management of patients with renal phosphatic calculi.[13]

Dihydroxyaluminum aminoacetate is comparable to aluminum hydroxide gel on the basis of available clinical experience. In the test tube the buffering action of this antacid in a solid form is comparable to that of liquid preparations of aluminum hydroxide gel. There is not enough clinical evidence to allow a clear-cut decision on the possible superiority of one of these drugs over the others.

Magnesium trisilicate

Magnesium trisilicate is another nonsystemic buffer antacid. In the stomach the drug is changed to magnesium chloride and silicon dioxide. In the alkaline intestine, magnesium remains as the carbonate, whereas chloride is reabsorbed. Silicon dioxide may coat the ulcer and may also function as an adsorbent in the intestinal tract.

In contrast to the aluminum salts, magnesium trisilicate not only does not cause constipation but in large doses may even produce some diarrhea. In many very popular preparations, aluminum hydroxide gel and magnesium trisilicate are combined in a single tablet. One of the most popular contains 0.5 Gm. of magnesium trisilicate and 0.25 Gm. of aluminum hydroxide. Apparently some silica may be absorbed, since in rare cases kidney stones containing silicon compounds have been reported.[7]

Other nonabsorbed antacids

Magnesium oxide, magnesium hydroxide, and calcium carbonate are gastric antacids that differ from the previous group in that they can elevate the pH of the gastric contents to 7 or above. An 8% aqueous suspension of magnesium hydroxide is widely known as milk of magnesia. These preparations are not absorbed from the intestine and will not cause systemic alkalosis. The magnesium salts are quite laxative, whereas the calcium carbonate is constipating.

Magaldrate (Riopan) is a hydrated magnesium aluminate, a buffer-antacid that is not absorbed. Among advantages claimed for it is its low sodium content. Some of the commonly used antacids have a surprising amount of sodium, a disadvantage in some patients.

CATHARTICS, LAXATIVES, AND ANTIDIARRHEAL AGENTS

Drugs that promote or inhibit intestinal evacuation were at one time among the most important therapeutic agents. Concepts concerning the significance and management of constipation and diarrhea have changed considerably during the past few decades and have led to diminished importance for this group of drugs.

Constipation, when not due to organic causes, is generally attributed today to poor dietary habits, lack of bulk-producing foods, and inattention to the stimulus for defecation. Correction of these poor habits will often take care of the problem of chronic constipation without the necessity of prescribing laxatives.

Nevertheless, cathartics and laxatives have some valid uses in medicine. Soft stools and lack of straining during defecation are desirable after hemorrhoidectomy and in persons with myocardial infarction. Cathartics are also prescribed for the purpose of speeding the elimination of various toxic materials such as some of the anthelmintics. By itself, however, chronic constipation should not be an indication for continual use of cathartics.

In diarrheal states the correction of fluid and electolyte changes are today considered to be the primary therapeutic goal. Small doses of opiates in the form of paregoric (camphorated tincture of opium) or codeine may be employed to slow intestinal motility. Astringents and adsorbents are also used but are not very effective. Determination of the cause of the diarrheal state—whether bacterial, parasitic, or toxic—is most important, and the specific cause should be corrected whenever possible.

Cathartics may be classified on the basis of their mode of action as follows:

1. Bulk cathartics—magnesium sulfate, magnesium hydroxide, sodium sulfate, sodium phosphate, methylcellulose, psyllium seeds, agar, and other nonabsorbed salts and hydrophilic colloids
2. Irritant cathartics—anthraquinone compounds such as cascara sagrada, aloe, senna, rhubarb, castor oil, and phenolphthalein
3. Surface-active agents—dioctyl sodium sulfosuccinate

Bulk cathartics

Bulk cathartics promote intestinal evacuation because they are not significantly absorbed from the intestine. As a consequence, they retain a considerable amount of water, distend the colon, and promote the expulsion of liquid stools.

Magnesium sulfate is widely used in medicine. It is generally administered in doses of 15 Gm. Little of it is absorbed under normal circumstances, and the effects of the small amount absorbed are minimized by rapid renal excretion. If there is prolonged intestinal retention of the drug and renal function is simultaneously impaired, some systemic effects such as central nervous system depression may occur. It may be estimated that 15 Gm. of magnesium sulfate requires 400 ml. of water in order to make an isotonic solution. If the drug is given in a more concentrated form, it will abstract water from the tissues.

Magnesium hydroxide, usually administered as magnesia magma (milk of magnesia), is considerably more pleasant than the bitter sulfate. It is also considerably less effective.

The hydrophilic colloids are not absorbed from the gastrointestinal tract and retain considerable quantities of water. They are widely used, but simple dietary measures such as inclusion of prunes and bran-containing cereals can generally serve the purpose equally well.

Irritant cathartics

Anthraquinone cathartics, also known as emodin compounds, are commonly used in proprietary mixtures and less frequently by the medical profession. The active principles in such drugs as cascara, aloe, senna, and rhubarb are glycosides of anthracene compounds. Their effect is exerted on the large intestine, and there is usually a delay of about 6 to 8 hours in obtaining defecation following the use of these compounds. Injected emodin drugs produce an effect in less than an hour. Therefore the delay in their action may be due to the time required for their reaching the large bowel, although other explanations have also been advanced.

The formula of emodin is as follows:

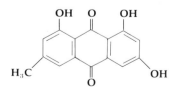

Emodin

Anthraquinone cathartics are partially absorbed from the intestine and may cause discoloration of the urine. One of the breakdown products, chrysophanic acid, behaves as an indicator, being yellow in acid urine and changing to red upon alkalinization.

The highly irritant, drastic cathartic resins such as jalap and podophyllum have no valid use in the treatment of constipation. The same may be said of croton oil.

Phenolphthalein is also more commonly used in proprietary preparations than on a physician's prescription. The history of the discovery of the cathartic action of phenolphthalein is interesting. It was used for making adulterated wine in Hungary, and its cathartic properties were soon appreciated.

There is a delay of some 6 to 8 hours in the cathartic action of phenolphthalein, although the time may be less in children. The drug is believed to act on the large intestine, its exact mode of action being unknown. It is partially absorbed, and although its toxicity is low, it can cause very undesirable skin eruptions and persistent discoloration. The phenomenon of fixed eruption caused by phenolphthalein probably has a true allergic basis because the involved areas of skin flare up again when doses of phenolphthalein are taken that would exert no effect in a normal person.

Oxyphenisatin and its acetate salt are related to phenolphthalein. They can cause hepatic damage and should not be used.

Castor oil is obtained from the seeds of *Ricinus communis*, or castor bean. The oil itself is nonirritating, but when it is hydrolyzed in the intestine to ricinoleic acid, a cathartic effect is produced. This action is exerted especially on the small intestine. The usual dose of castor oil is 15 ml.

Bisacodyl (Dulcolax) in the form of oral tablets and suppositories appears to be useful for bowel evacuation. It stimulates the contraction of the large intestine and is apparently not absorbed from the intestine.

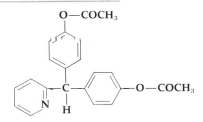

Bisacodyl

Bisacodyl is believed to initiate motility in the colon by a stimulant effect on parasympathetic nerve endings. The drug finds increasing applications in preparing patients for x-ray studies. Its use has made enemas unnecessary in some patients prior to operations.

Preparations of bisacodyl (Dulcolax) include enteric-coated tablets containing 5 mg. that should be swallowed whole and suppositories containing 10 mg. The suppositories should not be used in patients in whom absorption may be facilitated by the presence of fissures or ulcerations.

SURFACE-ACTIVE AGENTS

Dioctyl sodium sulfosuccinate (Doxinate; Colace) was introduced as a fecal softener. The drug acts as a dispersing or wetting agent and appears to be inert from a pharmacologic standpoint. It is used in daily doses of 10 to 20 mg. in children and in larger doses in adults.[16]

ANTIDIARRHEAL AGENTS

The management of diarrhea is based on elimination of the cause when possible and administration of proper fluids and electrolytes. In addition, a variety of absorbent compounds are employed, largely on an empirical basis. Some of these are bismuth subcarbonate, kaolin, activated charcoal, and pectin. Considerably more effective in stopping diarrhea and making the patient comfortable are the opiates. It should be kept in mind, however, that the narcotics may obscure the diagnosis. This is a serious disadvantage if the diarrhea is due to a major organic disease that may be curable, such as amebic dysentery. The camphorated tincture of opium (paregoric) has been used traditionally in the treatment of diarrhea. The usual dose is 4 ml. Codeine sulfate may be used also in doses of 16 to 32 mg. It is important to keep in mind that the opiates represent only symptomatic treatment, and efforts for detecting and correcting the underlying disturbances should not be neglected.

The opiate-like drug **diphenoxylate** (with atropine sulfate as Lomotil) has considerable efficacy as an antidiarrheal agent. A relatively low daily dosage (2.5 to 7.5 mg.) usually gives good results. Diphenoxylate has been particularly recommended for chronic diarrhea when the more addictive opiates are undesirable.[2] Each Lomotil tablet and each 5 ml. of liquid contains 2.5 mg. diphenoxylate and 0.025 mg. of atropine sulfate.

Cholestyramine may be an effective antidiarrheal agent whenever there is malabsorption of bile acids that contribute to the diarrhea. Such conditions include ileal resection[8] or the irritable bowel syndrome.[12] Cholestyramine therapy proved ineffective in tropical diarrhea in Vietnam.[10]

References

1 Alvarez, W. C.: An introduction to gastroenterology, New York, 1940, Paul B. Hoeber, Inc.

2 Barowsky, H., and Schwartz, S. A.: Method for evaluating diphenoxylate hydrochloride: comparison of its antidiarrheal effect with that of camphorated tincture of opium, J.A.M.A. **180**:1058, 1962.

3 Chapman, W. P., Wyman, S. M., Mora, L. O., Gillis, M. A., and Jones, C. M.: Barium studies on the comparative action of banthine, tincture of belladonna, and placebos on the motility of the gastrointestinal tract in man, Gastroenterology **23**:234, 1953.

4 Fordtran, J. S., and Collyns, J. A. H.: Antacid pharmacology in duodenal ulcer—effect of antacids on postcibal gastric acidity and peptic activity, New Eng. J. Med. **274**:921, 1966.

5 Gill, B. F.: Observations on the effect of orally administered atropine on the gastric response to insulin in patients with duodenal ulcer, Gastroenterology **19**:331, 1951.

6 Hammerlund, E. R., and Rising, L. W.: A further study of the comparative buffering capacities of various commercially available gastric antacids, J. Med. Pharm. Ass. **41**:295, 1952.

7 Herman, J. R., and Goldberg, A. S.: New type of urinary calculus caused by antacid therapy, J.A.M.A. **174**:1206, 1960.

8 Hofmann, A. F., and Poley, J. R.: Cholestyramine treatment of diarrhea associated with ileal resection, New Eng. J. Med. **281**:397, 1969.

9 Kirsner, J. B.: Current status of therapy in peptic ulcer, J.A.M.A. **166**:1727, 1958.

10 McCloy, R. M., and Hofmann, A. F.: Tropical diarrhea in Vietnam—a controlled study of cholestyramine therapy, New Eng. J. Med. **284**:139, 1971.

11 McHardy, G., and Balart, L. A.: Jaundice and oxyphenisatin, J.A.M.A. **211**:83, 1970.

12 Rowe, G. G.: Control of diarrhea by cholestyramine administration, Amer. J. Med. Sci. **255**:84, 1968.

13 Shorr, E., and Carter, A. C.: Aluminum gels in management of renal phosphatic calculi, J.A.M.A. **144**:1549, 1950.

14 Texter, E. C., Smith, H. W., and Barborka, C. L.: Evaluation of newer anticholinergic agents, Gastroenterology **30**:772, 1956.

15 Thomas, J. E.: The autonomic nervous system in gastrointestinal disease, J.A.M.A. **157**:209, 1955.

16 Wilson, J. L., and Dickinson, D. G.: Use of dioctyl sodium sulfosuccinate (aerosol O. T.) for severe constipation, J.A.M.A. **158**:261, 1955.

Recent reviews

17 Christensen, J.: The controls of gastrointestinal movements: some old and new views, New Eng. J. Med. **285**:85, 1971.

18 Grady, G. F., and Keusch, G. T.: Pathogenesis of bacterial diarrheas, New Eng. J. Med. **285**:831, 891, 1971.

19 Ingelfinger, F. J.: Anticholinergic therapy of gastrointestinal disorders, New Eng. J. Med. **268**:1454, 1963.

20 Kirsner, J. B.: Facts and fallacies of current medi-

cal therapy for uncomplicated duodenal ulcer, J.A.M.A. **187**:123, 1964.

21 Kirsner, J. B., Rubio, C. E., Mlynaryk, P., and Reed, P. I.: Problems in the evaluation of gastrointestinal drugs, Clin. Pharmacol. Ther. 3:510, 1962.

22 Roth, J. L. A.: Role of drugs in production of gastroduodenal ulcer, J.A.M.A. **187**:418, 1964.

23 State, D.: Gastrointestinal hormones in the production of peptic ulcer, J.A.M.A. **187**:410, 1964.

SECTION EIGHT

DRUGS THAT INFLUENCE METABOLIC AND ENDOCRINE FUNCTIONS

37 Insulin, glucagon, and oral hypoglycemic agents

GENERAL CONCEPT

Insulin, the hormone elaborated by the beta cells of the pancreas, is a key regulator of metabolic processes. Although its action on carbohydrate metabolism has received the most attention, its absolute or relative deficiency results in many other serious metabolic consequences. *Glucagon,* the hormone produced by the alpha cells of the pancreatic islets, has some actions such as glycogenolysis and hyperglycemia that are opposed to those of insulin. The ratio of the two hormones may determine their overall effect on the liver. Glucagon has positive inotropic effects on the heart, probably as a consequence of stimulating cyclic AMP production. The *hypoglycemic sulfonylureas* promote the release of insulin from the beta cells. *Phenformin* is also used occasionally for lowering the blood sugar in diabetics, but the drug acts by some mechanism other than the promotion of insulin release.

Insulin is elaborated in the beta cells as part of a larger peptide known as *proinsulin.* The release of insulin is stimulated not only by glucose but also by certain amino acids, gastrointestinal hormones, ketone bodies, and alpha receptor blockers such as phentolamine. Inhibitors of insulin release include alpha adrenergic agonists such as norepinephrine and epinephrine, unusual sugars (mannoheptulose), and diazoxide. The action of insulin is exerted on specific receptors in cell membranes.

INSULIN
Development of current concepts

In 1889 the surgical removal of the pancreas in the dog was shown to result in experimental diabetes[46] and in 1922 insulin was isolated from a dog's pancreas.[1] The introduction of insulin revolutionized the treatment of diabetes and greatly prolonged the lives of juvenile diabetic patients. Subsequent work was directed at developing injectable forms of insulin that would delay the absorption of the hormone and would thereby prolong its action in the body. Protamine zinc insulin[16] and other insulin protein complexes were introduced. Finally, NPH insulin and the lente insulins received wide clinical application because their administration only once each day proved very convenient.

Studies on insulin and diabetes were facilitated by the demonstration that alloxan could selectively destroy the beta cells of the pancreas.[10] This discovery provided a simple method for making experimental animals diabetic, compared with the previous and more laborious procedure of almost complete pancreatectomy.

Hand in hand with these investigations, work has proceeded on the chemistry and mode of action of insulin. The chemical structure of this protein hormone was established by Sanger and co-workers in 1954.[37] More recently, insulin has been synthesized.[57]

Although the overall effects of insulin in terms of lowering of blood sugar, glycogen

465

synthesis, and glucose utilization have been established for many years, its basic mode of action was considerably more difficult to postulate. An effect on hexokinase has been suggested by certain experiments.[8] Subsequent work could not be reconciled with the direct influence of insulin on hexokinase, although the enzyme may be influenced indirectly. Much greater attention has been paid to the fact that insulin may affect sugar transport in certain tissues.[19,20,24] According to this concept, the primary action of insulin is promoting the entry of sugars into certain cells. The enzymatic machinery would be secondarily affected, of course, by the change in the availability of substrates.

Studies on insulin were greatly aided by methods for determining the concentration of the hormone. This can be done by measuring its influence on glucose uptake by the isolated diaphragm of the rat[14] or by immunoassay.

In addition to its effect on glucose entry into muscle and fat, insulin exerts important influences on the liver.[28,29] In this organ, insulin inhibits the hepatic release of glucose and regulates directly or indirectly the level of certain enzymes such as those involved in gluconeogenesis and glycolysis. However, in the liver the effect of insulin is not simply on the entry of glucose into cells.

Glucagon, the hormone produced by the alpha cells of the pancreatic islets, is looked on by many as a physiologic antagonist to insulin.[67] In large doses, glucagon causes glycogenolysis and hyperglycemia. It also promotes gluconeogenesis in the liver from amino acids. Hypoglycemia results in high glucagon and low insulin levels, a hormonal ratio that favors glycogenolysis and gluconeogenesis. The ingestion of carbohydrates produces high insulin and low glucagon levels. Such a ratio would favor glycogen deposition, glycolysis, and fat synthesis.[53] A protein meal leads to the elevation of both insulin and glucagon concentrations. Under these conditions blood sugar remains normal, since the increased peripheral utilization of glucose (insulin) is balanced by hepatic glycogenolysis and gluconeogenesis.

Glucagon is available as the hydrochloride for the treatment of insulin reactions. It is administered subcutaneously or intramuscularly in doses of 0.5 to 2 mg.[64] Glucagon has some uses also as a cardiac drug. It has a positive inotropic effect probably mediated by increased cyclic AMP production. Its positive inotropic action differs from those of the catecholamines in that it is not accompanied by ventricular irritability or increased peripheral resistance.[33] Glucagon may be useful in the treatment of acute heart failure.[33]

The release of insulin from the beta cells by glucose and certain amino acids as well as by drugs and the influence of catecholamines in insulin release are problems of great current interest and will be discussed separately.

Insulin deficiency and diabetes

Although there is little doubt that experimental insulin deficiency produces the general picture of diabetes, the problem of clinical diabetes is not so easily explained except in young people—so-called juvenile type of diabetics. Many adult diabetics appear to have normal plasma levels of insulin according to precise immunoassay techniques. Furthermore, diabetics adequately treated with insulin still develop the vascular complications of the disease. Electron microscopy reveals thickening of the basement membranes of various blood vessels in diabetics and prediabetics, an alteration that could not be due to simple insulin deficiency. Some authorities believe that diabetes is a genetic disorder that affects the blood vessels and causes disruption of pancreatic beta cell regulation, leading to relative or actual deficiency of insulin.

B Chain

$$
\begin{array}{c}
\quad\quad \overset{NH_2}{|} \overset{NH_2}{|} \\
Phe \cdot Val \cdot Asp \cdot Glu \cdot His \cdot Leu \cdot Cy \cdot Gly \cdot Ser \cdot His \cdot Leu \cdot Val \cdot Glu \cdot Ala \cdot Leu \cdot Tyr \cdot Leu \cdot Val \cdot Cy \cdot Gly \cdot Glu \cdot Arg \cdot Gly \cdot Phe \cdot Phe \cdot Tyr \cdot Thr \cdot Pro \cdot Lys \cdot Ala \\
\;1\;\;\;\;2\;\;\;\;3\;\;\;\;4\;\;\;\;5\;\;\;\;6\;\;\;\;7\;\;\;\;8\;\;\;\;9\;\;\;10\;\;11\;\;12\;\;13\;\;14\;\;15\;\;16\;\;17\;\;18\;\;19\;\;20\;\;21\;\;22\;\;23\;\;24\;\;25\;\;26\;\;27\;\;28\;\;29\;\;30
\end{array}
$$

A Chain

$$
\begin{array}{c}
\quad\quad\quad\quad NH_2 \;\; S \quad\quad\quad\quad\quad\quad NH_2 \quad\quad NH_2 \;\; S \;\; NH_2 \\
Gly \cdot Ileu \cdot Val \cdot Glu \cdot Glu \cdot Cy \cdot Cy \cdot Ala \cdot Ser \cdot Val \cdot Cy \cdot Ser \cdot Leu \cdot Tyr \cdot Glu \cdot Leu \cdot Glu \cdot Asp \cdot Tyr \cdot Cy \cdot Asp \\
\;1\;\;\;\;2\;\;\;\;3\;\;\;\;4\;\;\;\;5\;\;\;\;6\;\;\;7\;\;\;\;8\;\;\;9\;\;\;10\;\;11\;\;12\;\;13\;\;14\;\;15\;\;16\;\;17\;\;18\;\;19\;\;20\;\;21
\end{array}
$$

Chemistry and standardization

The complete amino acid sequence of insulin has now been worked out.[37,38] The molecule consists of two chains of polypeptides, the A and B chains, joined by two disulfide bridges. In addition, the A chain contains another disulfide bridge. Insulins of various animal species have similar biologic activity and differ only in the sequence of three amino acids in the A chain. When the disulfide bonds are broken by reduction, the biologic activity of insulin disappears. The molecule contains a total of 48 amino acids, as shown above.

Proinsulin, the biosynthetic precursor of insulin, is a single-chain polypeptide. Its molecular weight is about 1.5 times that of insulin. Cleavage of proinsulin occurs within the beta cells, resulting in insulin and the connecting fragment known C-peptide.[44,65]

Insulin is *standardized* on the basis of its ability to lower the blood sugar in experimental animals, usually in the rabbit. An international unit of insulin should lower the blood sugar to 45 mg./100 ml. when injected into a fasting 2 kg. rabbit. The international standard insulin contains 22 IU/mg.

Insulin release and metabolism

Electron microscopic studies indicate that insulin is present in *beta* cells of the pancreas in a particulate form.[59] The most important stimulus for insulin release is *glucose,* but there are many other factors that can increase or decrease the release of insulin.

Factors that *promote* the release of insulin are *glucose, leucine, arginine* or a mixture of amino acids, *glucagon, ketone bodies, sulfonylureas, gastrin, secretin, pancreozymin, isoproterenol,* and *alpha-receptor blockers,* such as phentolamine.

Factors that *inhibit* the release of insulin are *norepinephrine* and *epinephrine*[35] (alpha adrenergic effects), unusual sugars such as *mannoheptulose,* and *diazoxide*[30,39] (p. 170).

Once released, insulin reaches the liver first, where much of it is retained.[29] Mechanisms involved in the ultimate destruction are not well known, but apparently both enzymatic and nonenzymatic processes are at play. There probably is not a specific insulin-binding protein in plasma.[51]

The subcutaneous injection of regular insulin produces almost immediate lowering of blood sugar. The lowest value is reached in about 3 hours, and a return to normal or above may be expected in about 6 hours. At the other end of the spectrum, protamine zinc insulin has a slow onset of action, and it may not exert much effect for the first 6 hours. It also has a long duration of action, probably from 24 to 36 hours. As a consequence, some cumulative effect may occur from daily injections of protamine zinc insulin.

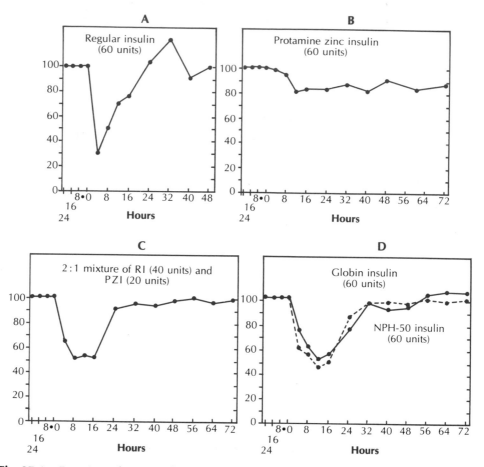

Fig. 37-1. Duration of action of various insulin preparations. (Modified from Rohr, J. H., and Colwell, A. R.: Proc. Amer. Diabetes Ass. **8**:37, 1948.)

The action of NPH insulin is similar to a 2:1 mixture of regular insulin and protamine zinc insulin. The abbreviation stands for *neutral protamine Hagedorn*. The preparation is almost neutral, contains a small quantity of protamine, and was developed by Hagedorn and co-workers.

The effects of these various insulins on the blood sugar are shown in Fig. 37-1. The purpose of the various additions to insulin is to delay absorption from the subcutaneous site of injection. Clearly the suspension should never be injected intravenously.

Mode of action

When insulin is injected into a normal or diabetic individual, the following changes may be observed in the blood chemistry: (1) blood sugar decreases, (2) blood pyruvate and lactate increase, (3) inorganic phosphate decreases, and (4) potassium decreases.

Lowering of the blood sugar may be explained on the basis of an increased uptake of sugar by tissues such as muscle and fat. There is evidence indicating a decreased hepatic output of glucose through the action of insulin.[28] It has been shown by hepatic vein catheterization in man that the injection of insulin causes decreased hepatic output of glucose.[2, 28]

Increases in blood pyruvate and lactate are generally attributed to the increased rate of glucose utilization. As more glucose-6-phosphate is produced, more will pass through the various triose states to pyruvate and lactate.

Fall of inorganic phosphate levels may be assumed to reflect the increased rate of phosphorylation of glucose, which results in greater consumption of phosphate. Finally, for reasons that are not well understood, whenever glycogen is deposited in the liver, potassium is also deposited. This would explain the *lowering of plasma potassium.*

In addition to these effects, insulin causes a fall in free amino acids in the plasma. It has also been shown that the incorporation of ^{35}S-labeled methionine into muscle was reduced in diabetic dogs but could be restored to normal with insulin. Thus insulin has an effect on protein metabolism also.

In the absence of insulin there is a failure in the synthesis of fatty acids. This has been demonstrated in both the diabetic animal and in vitro studies using liver slices.[4,6] It is believed that this effect of insulin on lipid metabolism is not a direct one but a consequence of a decreased rate of glycolysis, since the feeding of fructose to a diabetic patient restores lipogenesis to normal. Whereas fatty acid synthesis is deficient in the absence of insulin, cholesterol synthesis is increased.[42] The accumulation of ketone bodies is a well-known consequence of the diabetic state. Although not completely understood, it is attributed by some investigators to the accumulation of acetoacetyl coenzyme A resulting from the increased breakdown of fats and lack of its utilization for lipogenesis.[42]

Fundamental action

It has been suspected for many years that the primary action of insulin must be exerted at an initial stage of glucose metabolism. One of the reasons for this belief is the

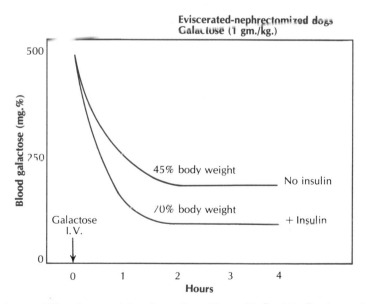

Fig. 37-2. Permeability theory of insulin action. (From Stadie, W. C.: Amer. J. Med. Sci. **229**:233, 1955; based on data from Goldstein, M. S., Henry, W. L., Huddlestun, B., and Levine, R.: Amer. J. Physiol. **173**:207, 1953.)

observation that the diabetic person can utilize efficiently whatever glycogen he has in his tissues.

The first enzymatic step in the utilization of glucose is as follows:

$$\text{Glucose} + \text{ATP} \xrightarrow[\text{Hexokinase}]{} \text{Glucose-6-phosphate} + \text{ADP}$$

The widely held permeability theory of insulin action is based on experiments in which the distribution of nonutilizable sugars such as galactose was studied in the hepatectomized dog. Under these conditions the injection of insulin resulted in lowering of the blood level of galactose, as shown in Fig. 37-2. The sugar became distributed in 70% of the body weight. The implication of this finding was that insulin caused the intracellular penetration of a sugar that is not phosphorylated or otherwise utilized in the hepatectomized animal.[23, 24] Many subsequent studies, even in vitro, have confirmed the idea that insulin promotes penetration of glucose and other sugars into muscle and fat.

It appears likely from studies on the red cell that a nonlipid-soluble compound such as glucose is transported across the cell membrane through some carrier mechanism.[32] Certain tissues such as muscle differ from erythrocytes in having a superimposed mechanism that opposes the penetration of glucose. This appears to be the site at which insulin acts. As a consequence, insulin promotes the entry of glucose into skeletal and heart muscle, fat, and leukocytes, whereas it is not required for sugar transport into the red cells, brain, or liver.

Factors that influence action

There are many factors that influence the action of insulin and alter the requirements of the diabetic individual. Hormones of the anterior pituitary gland, adrenal cortex, adrenal medulla, and thyroid gland have important influences. Also, the patient's diet, muscular exercise, hepatic disease, infection, and other stressful situations modify the response to insulin through hormonal and sometimes through unknown mechanisms. Finally, hypoglycemia following insulin overdosage has an adverse influence on subsequent insulin requirements.

All these factors increase the insulin requirements, except muscular exercise, which increases the utilization of sugar even in the absence of insulin.

In some instances, antibodies to insulin and other plasma factors may explain high degrees of resistance to the action of the hormone.

Special attention has been paid to the interactions of the pituitary and adrenal hormones with insulin. The ameliorating effect of hypophysectomy[17] and adrenalectomy[25] on experimental diabetes has been shown in classic experiments. Growth hormone, cortisone, and epinephrine can cause impairment of glucose utilization. It is believed that these hormones do not directly compete with insulin in glucose permeability. They may diminish phosphorylating capacity, or in the case of epinephrine they may cause the accumulation of glucose-6-phosphate, which secondarily may oppose glucose uptake.[19]

Preparations and clinical uses

Several preparations of insulin isolated from beef and pork pancreas are commonly used. The available preparations of insulin are of various types: crystalline zinc insulin (regular; CZI) protamine zinc insulin (PZI), neutral protamine Hagedorn insulin (NPH), Lente insulins, and extemporaneous mixtures.

Crystalline zinc insulin (regular; CZI) is an acidic protein having an isoelectric point of 5.3. The presence of zinc is a consequence of using the metal in the purification process. The absorption of regular insulin from the subcutaneous tissues is rapid, leading to peak activity in 2 to 4 hours. Regular crystalline insulin is available in solutions containing 40, 80, and 100 units/ml. A preparation that is clear in appearance is suitable for subcutaneous or intravenous administration.

Protamine zinc insulin (PZI) is very insoluble at pH 7.4 because of an excess of the basic protein, protamine, present in the concentration of 1.25 mg./100 units. When injected subcutaneously, PZI forms a depot from which it is absorbed very slowly. It should never be injected intravenously. PZI is available in solutions containing 40 and 80 units/ml.

Neutral protamine Hagedorn insulin (NPH) is an intermediate-acting insulin that contains only 0.5 mg. of protamine/100 units, nearly a stoichiometric amount. NPH is also known as isophane insulin suspension. Its peak effect occurs in 6 to 12 hours, and its duration of action is about 24 hours. It is available in solution containing 40 and 80 units/ml.

Lente insulins are slow acting without containing protamine. Their insolubility results from the addition of excess zinc in acetate rather than phosphate buffer. Under these conditions insoluble complexes of zinc-insulin form. Adjustments of pH yield crystalline or amorphous preparations. The amorphous form is absorbed more quickly and is referred to as Semilente; the crystalline form is called Ultralente. A mixture containing 70% Ultralente and 30% Semilente forms Lente insulin, which has absorption characteristics very similar to those of NPH insulin. Prompt insulin zinc suspension (Semilente insulin), insulin zinc suspension (Lente insulin) and extended insulin zinc suspension (Ultralente insulin), all containing 40 and 80 units/ml., are available.

Extemporaneous mixtures of the various insulins may create problems, particularly when regular insulin and PZI are mixed, because of the excess protamine in the latter. On the other hand, the various Lente insulins may be combined in various proportions to provide greater flexibility.

In the chronic management of diabetes some of the delayed absorption preparations such as NPH insulin are preferred at the present time. The details of determining the insulin requirement and diet therapy of individual patients are not within the scope of this discussion.

The greatest usefulness of regular insulin is in those situations in which the hormone must be administered intravenously. In diabetic acidosis and coma, very large doses of regular insulin, even up to hundreds of units, may have to be administered by the intravenous route.

Adverse effects

Complications of insulin therapy include hypoglycemia, local reactions, lipodystrophy, fluid retention, and visual disturbances. Also, systemic allergic reactions and insulin resistance due to the development of antibodies may occur.

Hypoglycemia is the greatest danger because of its catastrophic effects on the brain. Lipodystrophy results from the absorption of subcutaneous fat at the site of injection.

ORAL ANTIDIABETIC DRUGS
HYPOGLYCEMIC SULFONYLUREA COMPOUNDS

The introduction of the hypoglycemic sulfonylurea compounds represents a notable development in the management of diabetes. Laubatières[26, 27] observed in 1942 in France that certain sulfonamides, when administered experimentally to patients suffering from typhoid fever, produced symptoms and signs of hypoglycemia. Extensive investigations done subsequently in many laboratories established the fact that certain sulfonylureas can indeed produce hypoglycemia in normal animals but not in those made diabetic through the administration of alloxan. The most commonly used preparations in the United States are tolbutamide, chlorpropamide, acetohexamide, and tolazamide.

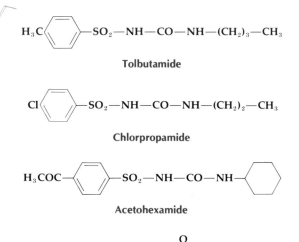

Tolbutamide

Chlorpropamide

Acetohexamide

Tolazamide

Mode of action

Despite earlier arguments to the contrary, the pancreas is essential for the hypoglycemic action of the sulfonylureas.[12, 18] The degree of granulation of the islet cells is related to the insulin content of the pancreas, and the sulfonylureas cause a decrease in the granulation of the beta cells.[7]

If the sulfonylureas act by promoting the release of insulin from the beta cells, they would be expected to be ineffective in the juvenile diabetic patient whose pancreas is grossly deficient in insulin. This is indeed the case. The greatest usefulness of these drugs is in the management of the maturity-onset type of diabetes in which the pancreas still contains substantial quantities of insulin.

Advantages of the hypoglycemic sulfonylureas over insulin in the management of diabetes are as follows:

1. *Ease of administration.* The sulfonylureas are taken in tablet form, whereas insulin must be injected.
2. *Endogenous release.* Release of insulin by the sulfonylureas resembles the physiologic process in that the hormone first reaches the liver, where much of it is

retained and exerts an effect on hepatic output of glucose. In contrast, injected insulin floods the peripheral tissues before it reaches the liver.

3. *Less allergic reaction.* Patients who are allergic to exogenous insulin obtained from animal sources or who have antibodies against such insulins may be managed more satisfactorily by promoting endogenous insulin release by means of the sulfonylureas.

The disadvantages of sulfonylurea therapy have to do with the relatively rare toxic and sensitizing properties of these drugs.

The tolbutamide controversy

In a recent cooperative study at twelve university medical centers a group of more than 800 diabetics were followed on one of four treatment schedules for 3 to 8 years. During that time 89 patients died, 61 of them from heart attacks or other cardiovascular causes. Thirty of the deaths occurred in the tolbutamide-treated group. The findings were interpreted as an indication that diet and tolbutamide therapy are no more effective than diet alone in prolonging life or even that diet and tolbutamide may be less effective than diet and insulin or diet alone insofar as cardiovascular mortality is concerned. Because of these findings, it has been recommended to physicians that sulfonylurea agents be used only in patients with adult-onset, nonketotic diabetes that cannot be controlled by diet or weight loss and in whom the use of insulin is impractical.

Many competent diabetologists have criticized the study and the conclusions on the basis of deficiencies in design, and it is quite possible that a more extensive study would not support the same conclusions. Until such information is available, some caution in the use of the sulfonylureas is advisable.

Preparations and clinical uses

The major characteristics of the oral hypoglycemic drugs are shown in Table 37-1.

Adverse effects

Hypoglycemia with sulfonylureas is generally not as great a danger as that after the use of insulin, but it may be serious and of long duration. An intolerance to alcohol similar to the disulfiram (Antabuse) reaction may occur, and gastrointestinal and allergic skin reactions have been reported.

Table 37-1. Characteristics of oral hypoglycemic drugs

Chemical type	Name	Half-life (hours)	Duration of action (hours)	Tablet size (mg.)
Sulfonylurea	Tolbutamide (Orinase)	4–6	6–12	500
	Acetohexamide (Dymelor)	6–8	12–24	250, 500
	Chlorpropamide (Diabenese)	30–36	60	100, 250
	Tolazamide (Tolinase)	7	10–14	100, 250
Biguanide	Phenformin hydrochloride (DBI)	3	4 6	25
	Phenformin hydrochloride, timed-release (DBI-TD)	3	8–14	50 (capsules)

PHENFORMIN

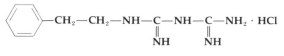

Phenformin hydrochloride

Certain biguanides, particularly phenformin (phenethylbiguanide; DBI), have received attention in the management of diabetes. The drug lowers blood sugar by potentiating the action of endogenous and exogenous insulin, particularly on adipose tissue.[55] As might be expected, phenformin is ineffective in the juvenile diabetic who lacks insulin. The drug exerts its effect within 4 hours and is eliminated in less than 24 hours.

Phenformin is not recommended for diabetic complications such as diabetic coma, where insulin is indispensable. The drug has numerous contraindications—severe hepatic and renal disease, for example. It should be avoided in pregnant women. Phenformin may cause ketosis and both reversible and irreversible lactic acidosis. Side effects of the drug, which are largely gastrointestinal, include nausea, vomiting, metallic taste in the mouth, and diarrhea. In view of the many contraindications and disagreeable side effects, phenformin is a somewhat difficult drug to use. Furthermore, there is no evidence for the drug's ability to prevent the vascular complications of diabetes.[58]

CLINICAL PHARMACOLOGY OF ORAL HYPOGLYCEMIC DRUGS

Extensive clinical experience indicates that the sulfonylureas just discussed are of about equal effectiveness in the treatment of adult-onset ketosis-resistant diabetics. These drugs differ from each other mainly in duration of action and in recommended dosage.

These drugs should not be relied upon for patients who develop the disease before they are 30 years of age. The same holds true for any diabetic who develops one of the complications of the disease such as coma, infection, or gangrene. The sulfonylureas should probably not be used for pregnant women or patients with uremia.

Drug interactions complicate the clinical use of the sulfonylureas. Tolbutamide is strongly bound to plasma proteins, where it can displace bishydroxycoumarin, thus leading to an increased anticoagulant effect.[48] The interactions of tolbutamide and anticoagulants in patients may be quite complex. Although some reports indicate that administration of tolbutamide to patients on bishydroxycoumarin therapy resulted in an increased anticoagulant effect,[5] others find that diabetic patients on long-term tolbutamide treatment reacted normally to bishydroxycoumarin and warfarin.[63] Perhaps the order of administration is important.[48] Thiazide diuretics oppose the action of the sulfonylureas.[15]

References

1 Banting, F. G., and Best, C. H.: The internal secretion of the pancreas, J. Lab. Clin. Med. 7:251, 1922.

2 Bearn, A. G., Billing, B. H., and Sherlock, S.: The response of the liver to insulin in normal subjects and in diabetes mellitus: hepatic vein catheterization studies, Clin. Sci. 11:151, 1952.

3 Brotherton, P. M., Grieveson, P., and McMartin, C.: A study of the metabolic fate of chlorpropamide in man, Clin. Pharmacol. Ther. 10:505, 1969.

4 Chaikoff, I. L.: Metabolic blocks in carbohydrate metabolism in diabetes, Harvey Lect. 47:99, 1951.

5 Chaplin, H., and Cassell, M.: Studies on the possible relationship of tolbutamide to Dicumarol in anticoagulant therapy, Amer. J. Med. Sci. **235**:706, 1958.

6 Chernick, S. S., and Chaikoff, I. L.: Two blocks in carbohydrate utilization in liver of diabetic rat, J. Biol. Chem. **188**:389, 1951.

7 Colwell, A. R., Jr., Colwell, J. A., and Colwell, A. R., Sr.: Intrapancreatic perfusion of the antidiabetic sulfonylureas, Metabolism **5**:727, 1956.

8 Cori, C. F.: Enzymatic reactions in carbohydrate metabolism, Harvey Lect. **41**:253, 1947.

9 Dear, H. D., Buncher, C. R., and Sawayama, T.: Changes in electrocardiogram and serum potassium values following glucose ingestion, Arch. Intern. Med. **124**:25, 1969.

10 Dunn, J. S., and McLetchie, N. G. B.: Experimental alloxan diabetes in rat, Lancet **2**:383, 1943.

11 Fajans, S. S., Floyd, J. C., Jr., Knopf, R. F., Rull, J., Guntsche, E. M., and Conn, J. W.: Benzothiadiazine suppression of insulin release from normal and abnormal islet tissue in man, J. Clin. Invest. **45**:481, 1966.

12 Fritz, I. B., Morton, J. V., Weinstein, M., and Levine, R.: Studies on the mechanism of action of sulfonylureas, Metabolism **5**:744, 1956.

13 Gellhorn, A., and Benjamin, W.: Insulin action in alloxan diabetes modified by actinomycin D, Science **146**:1166, 1964.

14 Gemill, C. L.: The effect of insulin on the glycogen content of isolated muscles, Bull. Hopkins Hosp. **66**:232, 1940.

15 Goldner, M. G., Zarowitz, H., and Akgun, S.: Hyperglycemia and glycosuria due to thiazide derivative administered in diabetes mellitus, New Eng. J. Med. **262**:403, 1960.

16 Hagedorn, H. D., Jensen, B. N., Krarup, N. B., and Wodstrup, I.: Protamine insulinate, J.A.M.A. **106**:177, 1936.

17 Houssay, B. A.: Hypophysis and metabolism, New Eng. J. Med. **214**:961, 1936.

18 Houssay, B. A., Penhos, J. C., Teodosio, N., Bowkett, J., and Apelbaum, J.: Action of the hypoglycemic sulfonyl compounds in hypophysectomized, adrenalectomized, and depancreatized animals, Ann. N. Y. Acad. Sci. **71**:12, 1957.

19 Kipnis, D. M.: Regulation of glucose uptake by muscle: functional significance of permeability and phosphorylating activity, Ann. N. Y. Acad. Sci. **82**:354, 1959.

20 Kipnis, D. M., Helmreich, E., and Cori, C. F.: Studies of tissue permeability: distribution of glucose between plasma and muscle, J. Biol. Chem. **234**:165, 1959.

21 Krall, L. P.: The biguanides: their role in this

era of the precise tool, Ann. N. Y. Acad. Sci. **82**:603, 1959.

22 Lacy, P. E., and Hartroft, W. S.: Electron microscopy of the islets of Langerhans, Ann. N. Y. Acad. Sci. **82**:287, 1959.

23 Levine, R., and Goldstein, M.: On the mechanism of action of insulin, Recent Progr. Hormone Res. **11**:343, 1955.

24 Levine, R., Goldstein, M., Huddlestun, B., and Klein, S. P.: Action of insulin on the permeability of cells to free hexoses, as studied by its effect on the distribution of galactose, Amer. J. Physiol. **163**:70, 1950.

25 Long, C. N. H., and Lukens, F. D. W.: The effects of adrenalectomy and hypophysectomy upon experimental diabetes in the cat, J. Exp. Med. **63**:465, 1936.

26 Loubatières, A.: L'utilisation des certaines substances sulfamidées dans le traitement du diabéte sucré experimental: Recherches personnelles (1942–1946), Presse Med. **63**:1701, 1955.

27 Loubatières, A.: The hypoglycemic sulfonamides: history and development of the problem from 1942 to 1955, Ann. N. Y. Acad. Sci. **71**:4, 1957.

28 Madison, L. L., Combes, B., Adams, R., and Strickland, W.: The physiological significance of the secretion of endogenous insulin into the portal circulation. III. Evidence for a direct, immediate effect of insulin on the balance of glucose across the liver, J. Clin. Invest. **39**:507, 1960.

29 Madison, L. L., and Unger, R. H.: The physiologic significance of the secretion of endogenous insulin into the portal circulation: comparison of the effects of glucagon-free insulin administered via the portal vein and via peripheral vein on the magnitude of hypoglycemia and peripheral glucose utilization, J. Clin. Invest. **37**:631, 1958.

30 Mereu, T. R., Kassoff, A., and Goodman, A. D.: Diazoxide in the treatment of infantile hypoglycemia, New Eng. J. Med. **275**:1455, 1966.

31 Mirsky, I. A., and Broh-Kahn, R. H.: Inactivation of insulin by tissue extracts: distribution and properties of insulin inactivating extracts (insulinase), Arch. Biochem. **20**:1, 1949.

32 Park, C. R., Reinwein, D., Henderson, M. J., Cadenas, E., and Morgan, H. E.: The action of insulin on the transport of glucose through the cell membrane, Amer. J. Med. **26**:674, 1959.

33 Parmely, W. W., Glick, G., and Sonnenblick, E. H.: Cardiovascular effects of glucagon in man, New Eng. J. Med. **279**:12, 1968.

34 Perley, M., and Kipnis, D. M.: Effect of gluco-

corticoids on plasma insulin, New Eng. J. Med. **274**:1237, 1966.

35 Porte, D., Jr.: A receptor mechanism for the inhibition of insulin release by epinephrine in man, J. Clin. Invest. **46**:86, 1967.

36 Renold, A. E., Marble, A., and Fawcett, D. W.: Action of insulin on deposition of glycogen and storage of fat in adipose tissue, Endocrinology **46**:55, 1950.

37 Ryle, A. P., Sanger, F., Smith, L. F., and Kitai, R.: The disulphide bonds of insulin, Biochem. J. **60**:541, 1955.

38 Sanger, F., and Thompson, E. O. P.: Aminoacid sequence in the glicyl chain of insulin, Biochem. J. **53**:353, 1953.

39 Seltzer, H. S., and Allen, E. W.: Inhibition of insulin secretion in "diazoxide-diabetes," Diabetes **14**:439, 1965.

40 Seltzer, H. S., and Allen, E. W.: Hyperglycemia and inhibition of insulin secretion during administration of diazoxide and trichlormethiazide in man, Diabetes **18**:19, 1969.

41 Shultz, K. T., Neelon, F. A., Nilsen, L. B., and Lebovitz, H. E.: Mechanism of postgastrectomy hypoglycemia, Arch. Intern. Med. **128**:240, 1971.

42 Siperstein, M. D.: Interrelationships of glucose and lipid metabolism, Amer. J. Med. **26**:685, 1959.

43 Stadie, W. C.: Current concepts of the action of insulin, Physiol. Rev. **34**:52, 1954.

44 Steiner, D. F., Hallund, O., Rubenstein, A., Cho, S., and Bayliss, C.: Isolation and properties of proinsulin, intermediate forms, and other minor components from crystalline bovine insulin, Diabetes **17**:725, 1968.

45 Villar-Palasi, C., and Larner, J.: Insulin-mediated effect on the activity of UDPG-glycogen transglucosylase of muscle, Biochim. Biophys. Acta **39**:171, 1960.

46 Von Mering, J., and Minkowski, O.: Diabetes mellitus nach Pankreas Extirpation, Centralbl. Klin. Med. **10**:393, 1889.

47 Weber, G., and Cantero, A.: Effect of Orinase on hepatic enzymes involved in glucose-6-phosphate utilization, Metabolism **7**:333, 1958.

48 Welch, R. M., Harrison, Y. E., Conney, A. H., and Burns, J. J.: An experimental model in dogs for studying interactions of drugs with bishydroxycoumarin, Clin. Pharmacol. Ther. **10**:817, 1969.

Recent reviews

49 Arky, R. A., and Knopp, R. H.: Evaluation of islet-cell function in man, New Eng. J. Med. **285**:1130, 1971.

50 Berson, S. A., and Yalow, R. S.: Plasma insulin in health and disease, Amer. J. Med. **31**:874, 1961.

51 Berson, S. A., and Yalow, R. S.: Insulin in blood and insulin antibodies, Amer. J. Med. **40**:676, 1966.

52 Bressler, R., and Galloway, J. A.: The insulins, Rational Drug Therapy **5**:1, May, 1971.

53 Cahill, J. F.: Glucagon, New Eng. J. Med. **288**:157, 1973.

54 Davidoff, F. F.: Oral hypoglycemic agents and the mechanism of diabetes mellitus, New Eng. J. Med. **278**:148, 1968.

55 Duncan, L. J. P., and Clarke, B. F.: Pharmacology and mode of action of the hypoglycemic sulphonylureas and diguanides, Ann. Rev. Pharmacol. **5**:151, 1965.

56 Johnson, R. D.: The management of coma in the diabetic patient — hypoglycemia, ketoacidosis, and the hyperosmolar state, Pharmacol. Physicians **2**(5): 1968.

57 Katsoyannis, P. G.: The chemical synthesis of human and sheep insulin, Amer. J. Med. **40**:652, 1966.

58 Knatterud, G. L., Meinert, C. L., Klimt, C. R. Osborne, R. K., and Martin, D. B.: Effects of hypoglycemic agents on vascular complications in patients with adult-onset diabetes. IV. A preliminary report on phenformin results, J. A. M. A. **217**:777, 1971.

59 Lacy, P. E.: The pancreatic beta cell, New Eng. J. Med. **276**:187, 1967.

60 Levine, R.: The action of insulin at the cell membrane, Amer. J. Med. **40**:691, 1966.

61 Levine, R., and Mahler, R.: Production, secretion, and availability of insulin, Ann. Rev. Med. **15**:413, 1964.

62 Madsen, J.: Extrapancreatic and intrapancreatic action of antidiabetic sulphonylureas; a review, Acta Med. Scand. (supp.) **476**:110, 1067.

63 Poucher, R. L., and Vecchio, T. J.: Absence of tolbutamide effect on anticoagulant therapy, J.A.M.A. **197**:1069, 1966.

64 Sokal, J. E.: Glucagon — an essential hormone, Amer. J. Med. **41**:331, 1966.

65 Steiner, D. F.: Proinsulin, Triangle **11**:51, 1972.

66 Unger, R. H.: Glucagon physiology and pathophysiology, New Eng. J. Med. **285**:443, 1971.

67 Unger, R. H., and Lefebre, P. J.: Glucagon: molecular physiology, clinical and therapeutic implications, New York, 1972, Pergamon Press, Inc.

38 Adrenal steroids

GENERAL CONCEPT

Since the observation by Hench in 1949 of a dramatic response to cortisone in a patient with rheumatoid arthritis, adrenal steroids and synthetic corticosteroids have become widely used and sometimes overused in medicine. *Cortisone* and related corticosteroids owe their popularity to their anti-inflammatory effect. More rarely, these drugs are useful for substitution therapy in adrenal insufficiency, which is often iatrogenic.

Aldosterone, the main mineralocorticoid of the adrenal gland, is largely of research interest. On the other hand, the *aldosterone antagonists* have important therapeutic applications.

DEVELOPMENT OF IDEAS CONCERNING ADRENAL STEROIDS

The adverse effects of destruction of the adrenal glands have been recognized ever since the original observations of Sir Thomas Addison. It has also been known for many years that the experimental removal of the adrenal cortices is incompatible with life. In most species, death following such an operation occurs within a week unless treatment is begun with extracts of adrenal cortex, pure steroids, or salt.

During the decade following 1930 there was an intensive search for the active principles that could account for the essential role of the adrenal glands. In 1937 Reichstein and von Euw[26] prepared deoxycorticosterone synthetically and later demonstrated it in the adrenal glands. Although this steroid had powerful effects on salt and water metabolism and became useful in the management of Addison's disease, it was obvious that extracts of adrenal cortex also contained some other compounds that could influence not only salt metabolism but also the handling of carbohydrates and proteins as well. Among the many steroids that were being isolated were some that indeed had marked glucocorticoid activity, as opposed to the mineralocorticoid deoxycorticosterone.

World War II stimulated interest in the glucocorticoids, previously isolated by Kendall at the Mayo Clinic. It was suspected that such compounds might be valuable in the treatment of shock and exhaustion,[28] although the scarcity of these compounds did not permit their evaluation in the human being. Intense efforts were made to synthesize amounts of the glucocorticoids adequate for clinical trial.

A milestone in the history of the adrenal steroids was the report of Hench and collaborators[16] on the effectiveness of cortisone and corticotropin in rheumatoid arthritis. Hench had been impressed for years with the potential reversibility of rheumatoid arthritis on the basis of the observation that patients tended to improve when jaundiced and also during pregnancy. It seemed possible that these improvements were associated with the production or retention of some "antirheumatic substance." Although Hench planned to try cortisone (compound E of Kendall) as early as 1941, it was not until 1948 that partial synthesis provided sufficient material for a clinical trial.

Results of the clinical trials in rheumatoid arthritis were dramatic, and soon cortisone and also corticotropin were found to cause symptomatic improvement in an amazing number of disease conditions. It was recognized at the same time that cortisone was not a cure for these many diseases. It seemed to "provide the susceptible tissues with a shieldlike buffer against the irritant."[15]

Although cortisol was largely responsible for the glucocorticoid activity of adrenal extracts, it was suspected that the amorphous fraction of such extracts still contained some material whose mineralocorticoid activity was much greater than that of deoxycorticosterone. The compound responsible for this was isolated in 1953 and was named *aldosterone.*

Subsequent research on the glucocorticoids led to the development of a variety of new steroids that have significantly greater anti-inflammatory potency than cortisone, although their influence on carbohydrate metabolism generally parallels their anti-inflammatory activity. A significant advantage of the newer steroids such as prednisone, methylprednisolone, triamcinolone, and dexamethasone is that these anti-inflammatory steroids exert little effect on renal sodium reabsorption while still possessing potent anti-inflammatory activity.

PITUITARY-ADRENAL RELATIONSHIPS
CORTICOTROPIN

Corticotropin (adrenocorticotropic hormone; ACTH) from the anterior pituitary stimulates adrenal steroid synthesis from cholesterol and is necessary for normal cortical structure and function. Although ACTH stimulates primarily the formation of glucocorticoids, it has a basic influence on the formation of all adrenal steroids.

ACTH release from the anterior pituitary is promoted by polypeptides isolated from the hypothalamus, sometimes referred to as corticotropin-releasing factor (CRF).

Regulation of ACTH release is determined largely by the influence of cortisol levels on CRF production through a negative feedback. Stressful stimuli, including drugs such as epinephrine, can override the feedback inhibition and elevate cortisol blood levels. In addition to these important regulatory influences, there is a diurnal variation in ACTH release that will be discussed subsequently.

The basic effect of ACTH on the adrenal cortex is mediated by cyclic AMP. Adenosine-3',5'-cyclophosphate acts similarly to ACTH both in vitro and on the perfused dog adrenal gland, whereas phosphorylase activity of beef adrenal slices is increased by ACTH.[43] ACTH may stimulate steroid synthesis by the system involving adenyl cyclase.

The polypeptide ACTH was isolated from the anterior pituitary and eventually synthesized. Human ACTH consists of thirty-nine amino acids, but not all amino acids are essential for biologic activity since the first nineteen (counting from the N-terminal end) are sufficient for stimulating cortisol production. The first thirteen amino acids in ACTH are the same as those in α-MSH (melanocyte-stimulating hormone), so it is not surprising that ACTH exerts an effect on melanocytes.

Preparations of ACTH are available for intravenous and intramuscular administration. Oral administration is ineffective. When injected intravenously, ACTH is rapidly destroyed in a matter of minutes. For this reason the hormone is administered either by intravenous infusion or by the intramuscular route as a repository ACTH injection

USP or sterile ACTH zinc hydroxide suspension USP. In the latter preparation, slow absorption is achieved by the addition of zinc hydroxide, while in the former preparation, gelatin retards absorption. Neither is suitable for intravenous use. Some preparations of ACTH injection USP are available for intravenous injection.

ACTH has few, if any, therapeutic uses. The glucocorticoids are much more convenient for the treatment of rheumatic or allergic diseases. Although it has been suggested that ACTH injections may not cause as much adrenal atrophy, this is doubtful.

ACTH has some valid uses in the diagnosis of disturbed adrenocortical function. An intravenous infusion of the hormone will result in an increase in the excretion of cortisol metabolites if the adrenal glands are normal or hyperplastic.

Lowering of the 11-oxygenated (11-oxy) adrenal steroids in the body promotes ACTH release by removal of the negative feedback. An interesting application of this knowledge is a test for anterior pituitary function by means of metyrapone (Fig. 38-1).

Metyrapone (Metopirone) inhibits the 11-beta hydroxylation in the biosynthesis of cortisol, corticosterone, and aldosterone. The decrease in these 11-oxy steroids leads to intense ACTH release from the anterior pituitary in normal individuals. Under these circumstances ACTH stimulates the production of precursors of the 11-oxy steroids, 11-deoxyhydrocortisone (compound S) and 11-deoxycorticosterone (DOC). The metabolites of these steroids, 17-hydroxycorticosteroids and 17-ketogenic steroids, may be measured in the urine. In deficient anterior pituitary function, metyrapone administration will not increase these urinary metabolites.

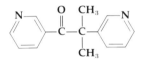

Metyrapone

In adults, metyrapone is administered orally in doses of 750 mg. every 4 hours for six doses. Urinary steroids are determined in the following 24 hours.

The metyprapone test is useless if adrenocortical function is defective. This is ascertained previously by determining the influence of ACTH infusion on steroid

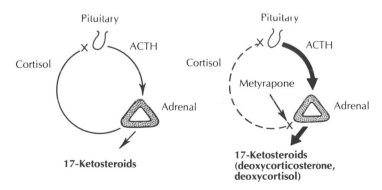

Fig. 38-1. Pituitary-adrenal feedback system and its inhibition by metyrapone. (Modified from Coppage, W. S., Jr., Island, D., Smith, M., and Liddle, G. W.: J. Clin. Invest. **38:**2101, 1959.)

output in the urine. Although the metyrapone test is still experimental, it is a remarkable example of the utilization of a new drug for probing body chemistry.

ANDROGENS

In addition to the glucocorticoids and aldosterone, the adrenal cortex produces androgenic steroids such as dehydroepiandrosterone. The production of androgenic steroids is greatly increased in the adrenogenital syndrome, in which an enzymatic defect channels much of the steroid production toward androgens. Exogenous glucocorticoid administration tends to depress the androgen output through pituitary inhibition.

ADRENAL SUPPRESSANTS

Certain toxic compounds such as amphenone B and the insecticide tetrachlorodiphenylethane (DDD) may damage the adrenal cortex. Amphenone B blocks several hydroxylations in addition to the one inhibited by metyrapone.

GLUCOCORTICOIDS
CORTISOL AND CORTICOSTERONE

Cortisol (hydrocortisone) and corticosterone are the principal glucocorticoids of the adrenal cortex. The structural formulas of these steroids are as follows:

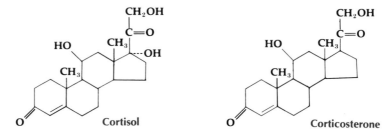

In the human adrenal cortex, cortisol predominates, whereas in some species such as the rat, corticosterone has greater quantitative importance. Human adrenal glands contain 2.3 to 5.5 μg of cortisol per gram of wet tissue.[18] In the plasma of normal subjects its concentration is about 8 μg/100 ml.[5] The rate of secretion shows a characteristic rhythm or diurnal variation. Secretion begins in the early hours of the morning, before the individual awakens, and gradually declines toward late evening. The reasons for this anticipatory secretion before daily activities begin are not known. Normal daily output of cortisol in man is about 25 mg.

Secretion of cortisol is greatly stimulated by ACTH. This is a direct effect, since even perfused adrenal glands produce more glucocorticoid when ACTH is added to the perfusate. Stressful situations promote adrenal glucocorticoid output by causing ACTH release. Many drugs exert similar effects, epinephrine being a prime example.[22,23] Interestingly, emotional stress and anxiety may be more important than physical stress.[17]

PHARMACOLOGIC EFFECTS

The effects of cortisol are exerted on the metabolism of carbohydrates, proteins, and fat; on electrolyte and water metabolism, inflammatory processes, inhibition of fibroblast proliferation, and increase in collagen breakdown; on stimulation of erythropoiesis and the production of platelets, reduction of the number of lymphocytes and eosinophils, and muscle strength and muscle wasting (depending on the dose); on the mental state and cerebral excitability, gastric acid production, bone formation, blood pressure, and immunologic processes.

Effect on carbohydrate, protein, and fat metabolism. It is quite likely that all these actions are a consequence of one basic metabolic action of the hormone, but at the present state of knowledge it is more convenient to describe these effects separately.

Cortisol increases gluconeogenesis and also tends to inhibit peripheral glucose utilization. As a consequence, it causes marked accumulation of glycogen in the liver and can produce hyperglycemia and glycosuria. Because of these effects, it tends to aggravate diabetes and may bring out an insulin-resistant disturbance of carbohydrate metabolism in latent diabetes.

The hormone corrects the disturbances of carbohydrate metabolism seen in adrenalectomized animals or in patients having Addison's disease, as shown in Table 38-1. Adrenalectomy improves experimental diabetes.[16]

Actinomycin and puromycin inhibit the actions of cortisol on glycogen deposition in the liver and synthesis of hepatic gluconeogenic enzymes. These results suggest that cortisol exerts its effect by stimulating the formation of certain enzyme proteins, which in turn depend on a certain RNA species.[13, 47]

Cortisol not only promotes the breakdown of proteins but also tends to inhibit their anabolism or synthesis. When large doses of the hormone are administered to children and young animals, they fail to grow and wounds heal much more slowly. Inhibition of antibody production in some species may also be a consequence of an antianabolic action.[12]

Little is known about the basic action of cortisol on fat metabolism. Unusual accumulations of fat (buffalo hump) occur in the patient treated with glucocorticoids. The adrenal glucocorticoids promote fat mobilization[4] and exert complex effects on ketone metabolism.[10] Cortisol has a *permissive* effect on free fatty acid release from adipose tissue by catecholamines.

Effect on electrolyte and water metabolism. Although the glucocorticoids exert much less effect on renal handling of electrolytes than do deoxycorticosterone and aldosterone, administration of cortisol or cortisone still results in increased sodium

Table 38-1. Effects of bilateral adrenalectomy

Circulatory	Decreased blood pressure
	Decreased blood volume
	Hyponatremia, hypochloremia, hypoglycemia, and hyperkalemia
	Increased nonprotein nitrogen
Renal	Increased excretion of sodium and chloride
	Decreased excretion of potassium
Digestive	Loss of appetite, nausea, and vomiting
Muscular	Weakness
	Decreased sodium and increased potassium and water in muscle
Miscellaneous	Decreased resistance to all forms of stress
	Hypertrophy of lymphoid tissue and thymus
	Death unless treatment is instituted

retention, increased potassium excretion, and hypokalemic alkalosis in patients on prolonged treatment. On the other hand, patients with Addison's disease cannot be kept in electrolyte balance with glucocorticoids alone.

The adrenalectomized animal cannot excrete a large water load. Cortisone will restore this particular function.

In addition to an influence on renal handling of electrolytes, adrenal steroids may influence the distribution of electrolytes between cells and extracellular fluid.[6]

Calcium metabolism is also affected by cortisol. It promotes the renal excretion of calcium, and it may reduce calcium absorption from the intestine.

Anti-inflammatory action. Most of the clinical uses of the glucocorticoids and of ACTH may be attributed to the remarkable ability of the steroids to inhibit the inflammatory process.

The anti-inflammatory action of these hormones can be demonstrated in experimental animals. Such laboratory techniques as the granuloma pouch and the reaction to an implanted cotton pellet have been valuable in the development and testing of the newer anti-inflammatory steroids.

In the granuloma pouch technique an air pocket is produced in the subcutaneous tissue and an irritant oil such as croton oil is injected. Inflammatory exudate accumulates in the pouch during the succeeding days. The injection of the anti-inflammatory steroids into the pouch or their systemic use can markedly inhibit the inflammatory process and reduce the volume of the exudate. In another procedure a cotton pellet is inserted into the subcutaneous tissue. The inflammatory process that develops will result in an increase in the weight of the pellet. The anti-inflammatory steroids will prevent this increase in weight by inhibiting the inflammatory process.

The *mechanism of the anti-inflammatory action* of the corticosteroids remains mysterious, although there is no lack of theories on this subject. The anti-inflammatory action has been attributed to suppression of migration of polymorphonuclear leukocytes, suppression of reparative processes and functions of fibroblasts, reversal of enhanced capillary permeability, and lysosomal stabilization.

Problem 38-1. Since there are both steroidal and nonsteroidal anti-inflammatory drugs, do they act by the same mechanism? This is not likely for several reasons. Clinical experience indicates that the corticosteroids are much more effective in asthma, whereas the nonsteroidal drugs are efficacious in rheumatoid arthritis. Experimentally, the nonsteroidal anti-inflammatory drugs such as aspirin or indomethacin inhibit prostaglandin synthesis, whereas cortisone has no such effect.

Relationships between anti-inflammatory and antiallergic actions. The remarkable effectiveness of the anti-inflammatory steroids in the treatment of a variety of allergic diseases such as bronchial asthma, urticaria, angioneurotic edema, and many others that may have an allergic component raises the important question of their mode of action in these conditions.

Theoretically this antiallergic effect may be due to an influence on immune mechanisms or may be an expression of the nonspecific anti-inflammatory action of these compounds. Although much attention has been paid to the fact that intensive steroid pretreatment can inhibit the Arthus phenomenon and antibody synthesis in the rabbit,[12] there is little evidence to indicate that a similar inhibition of antibody formation can explain the fairly rapid therapeutic effect of the glucocorticoids in human allergies. It appears more likely that the antiallergic effects are simply another manifestation of the nonspecific anti-inflammatory action of the adrenal glucocorticoids.

Miscellaneous effects. The cortisone-like steroids exert a striking effect on the number of circulating eosinophils. These elements may completely disappear from the blood following the administration of the glucocorticoids or upon the injection of ACTH.[31]

In addition to the eosinopenic effect, cortisone produces a marked decrease in circulating lymphocytes and an involution of lymphoid tissue.

There is little doubt that cortisone exerts effects on the central nervous system. Euphoria and other behavioral abnormalities may occur that cannot be explained by the clinical improvement of the primary disease. There is also evidence that glucocorticoid treatment may lower convulsive thresholds.[33]

The glucocorticoids improve muscle strength in adrenalectomized animals. On the other hand, they can cause muscle weakness in prolonged treatment, which is perhaps due to potassium loss and other metabolic actions on the muscle.

Prolonged administration of cortisone and related drugs inhibits the secretion of ACTH and leads eventually to an atrophy of the adrenal cortex. This problem has received much attention recently on the basis of clinical observations which indicate that stress, particularly associated with surgery, may be catastrophic in patients whose adrenal cortex is unresponsive as a result of previous hormonal treatment.[1]

It is of great interest that suitable modifications of dosage schedules may prevent adrenal atrophy during prolonged administration of glucocorticoids.[14,29] Thus, when the total 48-hour dosage was administered in a single dose every other day, prednisone proved efficacious, and side effects and adrenal suppression were reduced. Intermittent dosage regimens may be very important in children who ordinarily fail to grow on long-term corticosteroid therapy.

The effect of corticosteroid treatment on infections is quite complex.[30] Animal experiments suggest that cortisone exerts an adverse effect on the course of a variety of experimental infections, particularly fungal diseases. It must be remembered, however, that very large doses of the steroids are used in such experiments. With reasonable doses, antibody production is not decreased, opsonins remain normal, and leukocytes ingest and destroy microorganisms, even in experimental infections. In human beings, varicella and herpes of the eye may be more severe and fungal diseases may develop after prolonged steroid therapy. On the other hand, there is every reason to believe that the danger of using corticosteroids in infections has been exaggerated. Infection must be looked upon as an added factor, rather than as an absolute contraindication, when the risks of using corticosteroids are appraised.[47]

Excessive doses of glucocorticoids after prolonged administration produce the various manifestations of Cushing's disease, including moon face, hirsutism, acne, amenorrhea, osteoporosis, muscle wasting, variable hypernatremia and hypokalemia, hypertension, aggravation of diabetes mellitus, necrotizing arteritis in rheumatoid patients, aggravation of peptic ulcer, psychotic manifestations, and adrenal atrophy. The *most serious* systemic complications that may result from the clinical use of high doses of steroids are the diabetogenic and ulcerogenic effect; dissolution of supporting tissues such as bone, muscle, and skin; the hypertensive effect; and impairment of defense mechanisms against serious infections.[35]

METABOLISM

Cortisone and other synthetic corticosteroids are absorbed rapidly and completely from the gastrointestinal tract. After oral administration, maximal plasma concentrations are reached in 1 or 2 hours. Hepatic degradation of the corticosteroids leads to a fairly rapid fall in plasma levels so that after 8 hours only 25% of the peak value can be demonstrated and the active drugs disappear completely in about 12 hours.[36]

Drugs that promote the activity of microsomal enzymes in the liver tend to accelerate the metabolism of the corticosteroids. These drugs, which include phenobarbital, diphenylhydantoin, and others, may make it necessary to increase the dosage of the corticosteroids.

PREPARATIONS AND CLINICAL USES

Cortisol is available in oral tablets containing 10 or 20 mg. It is also available for intravenous injection and in various lotions and ointments for topical application.

Cortisone is used almost entirely in the tablet form or in suspension for intramuscular injection.

The large number of diseases in which cortisone and cortisol have been tried may be classified as follows on the basis of the degree of beneficial effect that may be expected from existing experience.

Favorable responses		Transient beneficial effects
Addison's disease	Acute bursitis	Acute leukemia
Hypopituitarism	Acute rheumatic fever	Multiple myeloma
Adrenogenital syndrome	Acute gouty arthritis	Lymphosarcoma
Severe bronchial asthma	Acquired hemolytic anemia	Chronic lymphatic
Acute ocular inflammations	Severe atopic dermatitis	leukemia
Rheumatoid arthritis	Acute lupus erythematosus	
	Severe penicillin reactions	

Certain principles may be derived from the accumulated experience in the therapeutic use of the adrenal steroids.

1. These drugs do not cure any disease. They do not represent replacement therapy, as does insulin in diabetes, except in the rare cases of Addison's disease or induced hypoadrenocorticism.
2. The anti-inflammatory adrenal steroids are particularly useful in disease processes that occur in episodes and so require no extended therapy. They are also very useful in conditions in which topical application may suffice.
3. Every effort should be made to use other drugs or procedures before prolonged steroid treatment is undertaken. With continued use, hyperadrenocorticism resembling Cushing's syndrome may be inevitable. Cessation of treatment with these steroids may precipitate acute exacerbations of various diseases. Their suppression of the function of the adrenal glands may represent a serious danger if the patient meets with stressful situations.
4. Despite their many disadvantages, the adrenal glucocorticoids are of great therapeutic importance in self-limiting diseases and in chronic disabling processes that fail to respond to any other treatment. The systemic use of these drugs is always a calculated risk that is often worth taking in the presence of incapacitating and otherwise incurable disease.

COMPARISON OF VARIOUS GLUCOCORTICOIDS

Several glucocorticoids have been introduced into therapeutics on the basis of having anti-inflammatory potency greater than cortisol without also having a corresponding increase in their tendency to retain sodium.

The chemical relationships among these newer glucocorticoids may be summarized in comparison with the structural formula of cortisone.

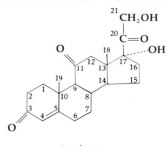

Cortisone

Cortisol has the same structural formula as cortisone except that OH is in position 11.

Prednisone (Meticorten) is the same as cortisone except that there is a double bond between positions 1 and 2.

Prednisolone (Meticortelone) is the same as prednisone except that OH is in position 11.

Methylprednisolone (Medrol) is the same as prednisolone except that CH_3 is in position 6.

Triamcinolone (Aristocort) is the same as prednisolone except that F (alpha) is in position 9 and there is an additional alpha OH in position 16.

Dexamethasone (Decadron) is the same as triamcinolone except that alpha CH_3 instead of OH is in position 16.

Betamethasone (Celestone) is the same as dexamethasone except that CH_3 is in position 16 beta instead of in alpha.

Fludrocortisone (9-alpha-fluorohydrocortisone) is the same as cortisol except that alpha F is in position 9.

Paramethasone (Haldrone) is the same as dexamethasone except that alpha F moves to position 6.

The introduction of prednisone and prednisolone into therapeutics was of great practical importance since their high anti-inflammatory action was not coupled with a correspondingly high sodium-retaining potency. This separation of effects allowed the physician to use these compounds without special salt-free diets and potassium supplementation.

Methylprednisolone and triamcinolone are even more potent than prednisolone with regard to anti-inflammatory effects. Dexamethasone is extremely active as an anti-inflammatory steroid, but, despite some early claims, there is no evidence that its effects on carbohydrate metabolism are not in proportion to its other actions.

Whereas the lack of sodium retention caused by these newer steroids is a significant advantage, increasing anti-inflammatory potencies have little importance as long as some of the adverse effects increase in parallel fashion.

The daily doses reflect the various potencies of these steroids (Table 38-2).

The possible advantages of increased potency are somewhat counterbalanced also by the lack of extensive experience concerning unusual adverse effects of these newer compounds.

The synthetic analogs of cortisol are usually administered in the form of oral tablets. Suspensions of some of the drugs are available for intramuscular and intra-articular

Table 38-2. Comparison of potencies of various steroids

Steroid	Anti-inflammatory potency	Daily dose (mg.)	Sodium retention
Cortisone acetate (Cortone)	0.8	50-100	0.8
Cortisol (Cortef)	1	50-100	1
Prednisone (Meticorten)	2.5	10-20	0.8
Prednisolone (Meticortelone)	3	10-20	0.8
Methylprednisolone (Medrol)	4	10-20	0
Triamcinolone (Aristocort)	5	5-20	0
Dexamethasone (Decadron)	20	0.75-3	0
Paramethasone (Haldrone)	6	4-6	0
Betamethasone (Celestone)	20	0.6-3	0
Deoxycorticosterone (DOC)	0	1-3	10-25
Fludrocortisone (Florinef)	12	0.1	100
Aldosterone	0.2		250

administration. Although they are of low solubility, water-soluble preparations of some of the steroids are available for intravenous use, such as the succinates or 21-phosphates.

MINERALOCORTICOIDS
ALDOSTERONE

Aldosterone is the main mineralocorticoid of the adrenal cortex. Extensive studies have been carried out on the role of this hormone in health and disease. A new disease entity, *primary aldosteronism*, has been described as a consequence of such studies.[7] Despite the great interest of such investigations, aldosterone has no therapeutic importance since deoxycorticosterone is available for the correction of electrolyte abnormalities in adrenal insufficiency.

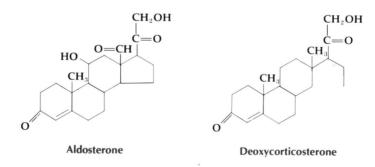

Aldosterone   Deoxycorticosterone

Aldosterone has an oxygen atom in position 11 and produces some effect on carbohydrate metabolism. However, its salt-retaining potency is so great and its concentration in the blood so small in relation to cortisol that its physiologic function must have little to do with organic metabolism.

Release of aldosterone is promoted by a decrease in circulating blood volume. Stimulation of aldosterone release by angiotensin is of great interest and suggests a connection between aldosterone secretion and the kidney with its juxtaglomerular apparatus.[3] This problem is discussed in Chapter 14. ACTH is necessary for aldosterone synthesis, but the final modulation of its production must be under the influence of other humoral factors, perhaps angiotensin.

Conditions in which aldosterone production is increased are as follows:

1. Primary aldosteronism, characterized by arterial hypertension, muscular weakness, tetany, hypokalemic alkalosis, negative potassium balance, hypomagnesemia, high serum sodium levels, and alkaline urine. This may be caused by adenoma or hyperplasia of the adrenal glands.
2. Secondary hyperaldosteronism, occurring in renal artery constriction with hypertension, malignant hypertension, pregnancy and toxemia of pregnancy, cirrhosis of the liver, nephrotic edema, and less certainly in essential hypertension. In many patients with congestive heart failure, aldosterone output is within normal limits.

Aldosterone antagonists

Spironolactone (Aldactone) and triamterene antagonize aldosterone at the level of the renal tubules.

Spironolactone is a synthetic steroid that competes with aldosterone for the distal tubular receptor involved in sodium-potassium exchange. Triamterene, on the other hand, does not compete with aldosterone but has a direct effect on the renal tubules. Both drugs favor sodium excretion and potassium retention (p. 436).

DEOXYCORTICOSTERONE

Deoxycorticosterone acetate is available in solution in sesame oil for intramuscular injection. There are also microcrystalline suspensions of deoxycorticosterone trimethyl acetate for the same purpose. Pellets are also available for subcutaneous implantation, which allows release of the steroid over a period of several months.

The main effect of deoxycorticosterone is exerted on the renal tubules. It promotes increased reabsorption of sodium and loss of potassium. Prolonged, intensive treatment with deoxycorticosterone in experimental animals can produce hypertension and necrotic changes in the heart and skeletal muscle. It is believed that these actions are due to potassium loss and sodium retention.[8]

References

1 Abbott, W. E., Krieger, H., and Level, S.: The role of ACTH, cortisone and hydrocortisone in surgery, Ann. Intern. Med. 43:702, 1955.
2 Baker, B. L., and Adams, G. D.: The physiology of connective tissue, Ann. Rev. Physiol. 17:61, 1955.
3 Bartter, F. C., Casper, A. G. T., Delea, C. S., and Slater, J. D. H.: On the role of the kidney in control of adrenal steroid production, Metabolism 10:1006, 1961.
4 Bogdonoff, M. D., Estes, E. H., Jr., Friedberg, S. J., and Klein, R. F.: Fat mobilization in man, Arch. Intern. Med. 55:328, 1961.
5 Bondy, P. K., and Altrock, J. R.: Estimation of the rate of release of adrenal 17-hydroxy-corticosteroids in the human being by the venous catheter technique with a method for determining plasma 17-hydroxycorticosteroids, J. Clin. Invest. 32:703, 1953.
6 Bush, I. E.: Chemical and biological factors in the activity of adrenal steroids, Pharmacol. Rev. 14:317, 1962.
7 Conn, J. W.: Presidential address. Painting background: primary aldosteronism, a new clinical syndrome, J. Lab. Clin. Med. 45:3, 1955.
8 Darrow, D. C., and Miller, H. C.: Production of cardiac lesions by repeated injections of desoxycorticosterone acetate, J. Clin. Invest. 21:601, 1942.

9 Dorfman, R. I.: Adrenocortical steroids in humans: metabolism and generalizations. In Wolstenholme, G. E. W., and Millar, E. C. P., editors: The human adrenal cortex, Ciba Foundation, Colloquia On Endocrinology, vol. 8, Boston, 1955, Little, Brown & Co.

10 Engel, F. L.: The influence of the endocrine glands on fatty acid and ketone body metabolism, Amer. J. Clin. Nutr. 5:417, 1957.

11 Gann, D. S., Mills, I. H., and Bartter, F. C.: On the hemodynamic parameter mediating increase in aldosterone secretion in the dog, Fed. Proc. 19:605, 1960.

12 Germuth, F. G., Jr., Oyama, J., and Ottinger, B.: Mechanism of action of 17-hydroxy-11-dehydrocorticosterone (compound E) and of adrenocorticotropic hormone in experimental hypersensitivity in rabbits, J. Exp. Med. 94:139, 1951.

13 Greengard, O., Weber, G., and Singhal, R. L.: Glycogen deposition in the liver induced by cortisone: dependence on enzyme synthesis, Science 141:160, 1963.

14 Harter, J. G., Reddy, W. J., and Thorn, G. W.: Studies on an intermittent corticosteroid dosage regimen, New Eng. J. Med. 269:591, 1963.

15 Hench, P. S.: Introduction: cortisone and ACTH in clinical medicine, Mayo Clin. Proc. 25:474, 1950.

16 Hench, P. S., Slocumb, C. H., Barnes, A. R., Smith, H. L., Polley, H. L., and Kendall, E. C.: The effects of adrenal cortical hormone 17-hydroxy-11-dehydro-corticosterone (compound E) on the acute phase of rheumatic fever, Mayo Clin. Proc. 24:277, 1949.

17 Hill, S. R., Goetz, F. C., Fox, H. M., Murawski, B. J., Krakauer, L. J., Reifenstein, R. W., Gray, S. J., Reddy, W. J., Hedberg, S. E., St. Mark, J. R., and Thorn, G. W.: Studies on adrenocortical and psychological response to stress in man, Arch. Intern. Med. 97:269, 1956.

18 Hudson, P. B., and Lombardo, M. E.: Analysis of human adrenal vein blood and adrenal glands for steroidal substances, J. Clin. Endocr. 15:324, 1955.

19 Ingle, D. J., Nezamis, J. E., and Morley, E. H.: Comparative values of adrenal steroids and extract by continuous intravenous injections in sustaining the ability of adrenalectomized rats to work, Endocrinology 50:1, 1952.

20 Kadowitz, P. J., and Yard, A. C.: Influence of hydrocortisone on cardiovascular responses to epinephrine, Europ. J. Pharmacol. 13:281, 1971.

21 Liddle, G. W., Duncan, L. E., Jr., and Bartter, F. C.: Dual mechanism regulating adreno-cortical function in man, Amer. J. Med. 21:380, 1956.

22 Long, C. N. H.: Regulation of ACTH secretion, Recent Progr. Hormone Res. 7:75, 1952.

23 Long, C. N. H., Katzin, B., and Fry, E.: The adrenal cortex and carbohydrate metabolism, Endocrinology 26:309, 1952.

24 Long, C. N. H., and Lukens, F. D. W.: The effects of adrenalectomy and hypophysectomy upon experimental diabetes in the cat, J. Exp. Med. 63:465, 1936.

25 Mills, L. C.: Corticosteroids in endotoxic shock, Proc. Soc. Exp. Biol. Med. 138:507, 1971.

26 Reichstein, T., and von Euw, J.: Constituents of the adrenal cortex: isolation of substance Q (desoxycorticosterone) and R with other materials, Helv. Chim. Acta 21:1181, 1938.

27 Schayer, R. W., Smiley, R. L., and Davis, K. J.: Inhibition by cortisone of the binding of new histamine in rat tissues, Proc. Soc. Exp. Biol. Med. 87:590, 1954.

28 Selye, H.: General adaptation syndrome and diseases of adaptation, J. Clin. Endocr. 6:117, 1946.

29 Soyka, L. F., and Saxena, K. M.: Alternate-day steroid therapy for nephrotic children, J.A.M.A. 192:225, 1965.

30 Sparberg, M., and Kirsner, J. B.: Steroid therapy and infections, J.A.M.A. 188:680, 1964.

31 Thorn, G. W.: The eosinophil, ACTH, epinephrine and stress, Amer. J. Med. 14:139, 1953.

32 Walton, J., Watson, B. S., and Ney, R. L.: Alternate-day vs shorter interval steroid administration, Arch. Intern. Med. 126:601, 1970.

33 Woodbury, D. M., and Sayers, G.: Effect of adrenocorticotrophic hormone, cortisone and desoxycorticosterone on brain excitability, Proc. Soc. Exp. Biol. Med. 75:398, 1950.

Recent reviews

34 David, D. S., Grieco, M. H., and Cushman, P.: Adrenal glucocorticoids after twenty years, J. Chronic Dis. 22:637, 1970.

35 Editorial: Pharmacologic effects of adrenal corticosteroids, New Eng. J. Med. 273:875, 1965.

36 Fries, J. F., and McDevitt, H. O.: Systemic corticosteroid therapy in rheumatic diseases, Rational Drug Ther. 6:1, Nov. 1972.

37 Gaunt, R., Chart J. J., and Renzi, A. A.: Interactions of drugs with endocrines, Ann. Rev. Pharmacol. 3:109, 1963.

38 Greaves, M. W.: The pharmacological basis for the rational use of topically applied corticosteroids, Pharmacol. Physicians 3(10):1, 1969.

39 Harrison, T. S., Chawla, R. C., and Wojtalik, R. S.: Steroidal influences on catecholamines, New Eng. J. Med. **279**:136, 1968.

40 Liddle, G. W.: Clinical pharmacology of the anti-inflammatory steroids, Clin. Pharmacol. Ther. **2**:615, 1961.

41 Melby, J. C.: Assessment of adrenocortical function, New Eng. J. Med. **285**:735, 1971.

42 O'Malley, B. W.: Mechanisms of action of steroid hormones, New Eng. J. Med. **284**:370, 1971.

43 Schwyzer, R.: Chemistry and metabolic action of nonsteroid hormones, Ann. Rev. Biochem. **33**:259, 1964.

44 Smelik, P. G., and Sawyer, C. H.: Pharmacological control of adrenocortical and gonadal secretions, Ann. Rev. Pharmacol. **2**:313, 1962.

45 Sparberg, M., and Kirsner, J. B.: Steroid therapy and infections, J.A.M.A. **188**:680, 1964.

46 Thorn, G. W.: Clinical considerations in the use of corticosteroids, New Eng. J. Med. **274**:775, 1966.

47 Weber, G., Singhal, R. L., and Stamm, N. B.: Actinomycin: inhibition of cortisone-induced synthesis of hepatic gluconeogenic enzymes, Science **142**:390, 1963.

39 Thyroid hormones and antithyroid drugs

GENERAL CONCEPT

A normal person produces about 80 μg of thyroxine and 50 μg of triiodothyronine in 24 hours. Alterations in the output of these thyroid hormones result in important changes in oxygen consumption, cardiovascular function, cholesterol metabolism, neuromuscular activity, and cerebral function. Growth and development are also seriously affected when the production of thyroid hormones is deficient.

THYROID HORMONES
NATURE AND SYNTHESIS

The thyroid gland removes inorganic iodine from the plasma and forms a number of iodinated amino acids that are held in colloid form in a large molecular protein known as thyroglobulin. If thyroglobulin is hydrolyzed, a variety of iodinated amino acids can be isolated from the hydrolysate. Thyroxine was first isolated in 1915 by Kendall,[15] and its structure was established in 1926 by Harington and Barger.[13] Triiodothyronine has also been isolated and structurally identified.[11,12] In addition to these highly active compounds, their probable precursors, monoiodotyrosine and diiodotyrosine, have also been identified in hydrolysates of thyroglobulin.

The nature of the circulating thyroid hormone has been established with a fair degree of certainty. The circulating organic iodine compounds are bound to a globulin of plasma but may be extracted by butanol and other organic solvents. The level of this protein-bound iodine (PBI) correlates well with other evidence of thyroid function. It is quite certain that this PBI of plasma is not thyroglobulin. As a matter of fact, the release of thyroglobulin from the thyroid gland is distinctly abnormal and may provoke an antibody response.[30]

There is good evidence to indicate that most of PBI is thyroxine, with minor quantities of triiodothyronine.[11,23] Thyroxine, then, is believed to be the principal hormonal product of the thyroid gland.

STEPS IN SYNTHESIS OF THYROXINE

The structural formulas of the various organic iodine compounds of the thyroid gland are shown at the top of p. 491.

The following steps may be distinguished in the elaboration of thyroxine: (1) concentration of inorganic iodide (iodide trapping), (2) oxidation of iodide to free iodine or hypoiodite, (3) formation of monoiodotyrosine and diiodotyrosine, and (4) coupling of two diiodotyrosines to form thyroxine, or tetraiodothyronine.

The ability of the thyroid gland to concentrate iodide can be demonstrated if the rapid formation of organic iodine compounds is simultaneously blocked by such antithyroid drugs as propylthiouracil or methimazole. Under these conditions the concen-

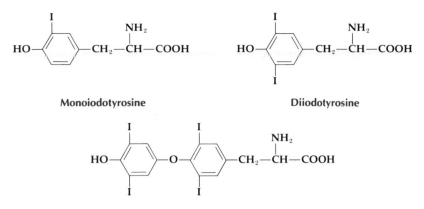

Monoiodotyrosine   **Diiodotyrosine**

Tetraiodothyronine

tration of iodide in the gland may be 30 to 200 times greater than that in plasma. This iodide-trapping mechanism can be blocked by thiocyanate or perchlorate.

The oxidation of iodide to free iodine is believed to be an enzymatic step that may be blocked by antithyroid drugs of the thiourea or thioamide type.

It is believed that tyrosine is iodinated while it is attached in peptide linkage to thyroglobulin. The release of thyroxine from the storage protein probably involves the activity of a proteolytic enzyme.

Iodine cycle

Some of the features of the metabolism of iodine are shown schematically in Fig. 39-1.

The daily intake of iodine is about 150 μg. This quantity plus about 70 μg from the daily thyroxine secretion and degradation enter the inorganic pool of iodine. The thyroid gland takes up about 70 μg of iodine a day. The rest is removed by renal ex-

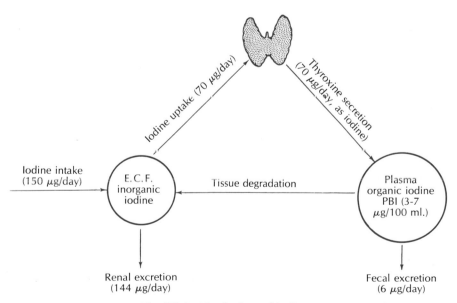

Fig. 39-1. Metabolism of iodine.

cretion, except for small quantities excreted in the feces. Thus the thyroid gland and the kidney compete with each other with respect to the clearance of inorganic iodide.

EFFECTS

A deficiency of thyroid hormones results in decreased metabolic rate, alterations in growth and development, disturbances in water and electrolyte metabolism, altered functions of the central nervous system, skeletal muscles, and circulation, and changes in cholesterol metabolism. Clinical conditions that may be attributed to thyroid deficiency are cretinism and myxedema of the adult and juvenile types.

The actions of the thyroid hormones may be exerted on the following functions[3]:
1. Calorigenesis and thermoregulation
2. Metabolism of lipids, proteins, and carbohydrates
3. Reproduction
4. Growth and development
5. Cardiovascular system
6. Water and electrolyte handling
7. Nervous system

An excess of thyroid hormones produces many of the symptoms and signs of thyrotoxicosis such as nervousness and mental instability, tachycardia, elevated pulse pressure, sweating, and hypersusceptibility to epinephrine. The basal metabolic rate is elevated, the plasma PBI is above normal limits, and radioactive iodine uptake by the thyroid is increased.

The basic mechanism of action of the thyroid hormones is not understood. One of the puzzling observations is that the hormone has no effect on oxygen consumption in vitro, although an elevated metabolic rate can be induced in vivo by thyroxine administration.

Certain in vitro studies indicate that thyroxine can uncouple oxidative phosphorylation in intact mitochondrial systems. These observations are of interest because dinitrophenol, another potent calorigenic drug, is a known uncoupling agent.

Puromycin, a drug that blocks protein synthesis, was found to reverse the hypermetabolism induced in rats by the previous administration of thyroxine, suggesting that the calorigenic effect of thyroxine is a consequence of its effect on protein synthesis.[26] This may be another example of the increasing number of hormonal effects being attributed to RNA and protein synthesis.

THYROXINE AND CATECHOLAMINES

It is a common belief in medicine that hyperthyroidism makes patients more sensitive to epinephrine. With the availability of numerous catecholamine depleters and adrenergic blocking agents, the traditional view of a thyroxine-catecholamine synergism could be reexamined.

Reserpine and guanethidine have beneficial effects on the symptoms of thyrotoxicosis.[7,41] In exogenous hyperthyroidism, guanethidine caused a return of heart rate to control values and a disappearance of palpitation and tremor.[9] The drug had no effect on serum cholesterol, body weight, or PBI levels. The amelioration of the symptoms of hyperthyroidism by catecholamine-depleting agents would fit the hypothesis that some end organs are more susceptible to the amines or that the metabolism is altered.

Although many of the manifestations of hyperthyroidism resemble those of sympathetic hyperactivity, the exact relationship between thyroxine and catecholamines is not understood. The catecholamine depleting drugs are useful in the treatment of some manifestations of hyperthyroidism, but other forms of treatment described subsequently are much more important.[33]

THYROTROPIC HORMONE

The activities of the thyroid gland are greatly influenced by the thyrotropic hormone of the anterior lobe of the pituitary body, which promotes the synthesis and release of thyroxine by the thyroid gland. It has been demonstrated that hypophysectomy depresses the following phases of ^{131}I metabolism in rat thyroids: the total uptake of ^{131}I, the iodide-concentrating capacity, the rate of formation of monoiodotyrosine, diiodotyrosine, and thyroxine, and the rate of appearance of thyroxine in plasma.[20] It has been suggested on the basis of these findings that the thyrotropic hormone exerts a very general effect on the thyroid gland, which may involve enzyme synthesis.

The rate of secretion of the thyrotropic hormone is normally inhibited by increased levels of thyroxine or triiodothyronine. When the synthesis of thyroxine is inhibited by the goitrogenic drugs, the thyroid gland becomes enlarged and its vascularity is increased, changes attributed to increased levels of circulating thyroid-stimulating hormone as a consequence of lower thyroxine levels.

The role of the thyrotropic hormone in the causation of exophthalmos is not clear. Some investigators believe that this may be an extrathyroidal effect of the hormone. Severe exophthalmos may be precipitated by thyroidectomy. This is usually explained as a result of removal of a negative feedback or as a consequence of the ability of the thyroid to destroy the thyroid-stimulating hormone. Later clinical experience seems contrary to this view, and it is now suggested that control of hyperthyroidism should not be delayed for fear of progression of the eye changes.[31]

There is evidence for a role of a long-acting thyroid stimulator (LATS) in Graves' disease.[39] This substance is unrelated to thyrotropin in regard to chemistry or source. It is a 7S gamma globulin and its mode of action is not understood. If it is an antibody, it may act against some constituent of the thyroid that normally exerts an inhibitory action on the gland. Even more recent evidence indicates the immune factors participate in the pathogenesis of toxic diffuse goiter, and LATS may only be one of the manifestations of such a process.[44]

CLINICAL USES AND PREPARATIONS

Indications for the use of thyroid preparations include hypothyroidism and conditions in which suppression of thyrotropin secretion is desirable. These include nontoxic goiter and chronic thyroiditis (Hashimoto's disease). Thyroid preparations also have various diagnostic uses. Their employment in the treatment of obesity and dysmenorrhea is not based on good evidence.

Several preparations are available when treatment with thyroid hormones is indicated.

Thyroid USP is the cleaned, dried, and powdered thyroid gland of animals used for food by man. It is standardized only by chemical and not biologic assay. It should contain 0.17 to 0.23% of iodine in organic combination. Variability in response may result from reliance on chemical assay alone.

Preparations include tablets containing 15, 30, 60, 120, 200, 250, and 300 mg. and enteric-coated tablets of 30, 60, 120, and 200 mg.

Thyroid extract (Proloid) is a purified extract of the thyroid gland, assayed chemically and biologically. It is available in tablets containing 15, 30, 60, 100, 200, and 300 mg.

Levo-thyroxine sodium (Synthroid sodium) is the synthetic sodium salt of levo-thyroxine, with actions and uses similar to those of thyroid extract except that it may be injected intravenously in emergencies such as myxedema coma.[43] The potency of 0.1 mg. of levo-thyroxine is equal to that of 60 mg. of thyroid USP from the standpoint of a clinical response.

Preparations include tablets containing 0.025, 0.05, 0.1, 0.15, 0.2, and 0.3 mg. and powder to make injectable solution, 0.05 mg./ml.

Liothyronine sodium (Cytomel) is the synthetic sodium salt of levo-triiodothyronine. It may be injected intravenously in myxedema coma, for which it is the drug of choice. Other uses are similar to those of thyroid extracts. The potency of 0.025 mg. of liothyronine sodium is equivalent to that of 60 mg. of thyroid USP.

Preparations include tablets containing 5, 25, and 50 μg and powder to make injectable solution, 114 μg/ml.

Liotrix (Euthyroid; Thyrolar) is a mixture of levo-thyroxine sodium and liothyronine sodium in the ratio of 4:1.

THYROXINE ANALOGS

Certain thyroxine analogs are being studied on an experimental basis. It is claimed that some selectivity can be achieved with regard to cholesterol lowering as compared with calorigenic action. Further work is necessary before the usefulness of the various thyroxine analogs is clearly established. Two of these analogs are triiodothyroacetic acid (TRIAC) and 3,3'-diiodothyronine.

ANTITHYROID DRUGS

The development of the antithyroid drugs is the result of a series of interesting experimental observations. Perhaps the first indication of antithyroid action was the finding that rabbits on a cabbage diet developed goiter.[25] Numerous studies followed on the antithyroid principles in plants of the *Brassica* genus. Interest in this field was further stimulated when it was found that rats on sulfaguanidine administration also developed hyperplastic thyroid glands.[18] A systematic study of this problem[1] led eventually to the clinical trial of thiourea and thiouracil in thyrotoxicosis.

CLASSIFICATION

Drugs that depress thyroid function can be placed in one of several categories on the basis of their mode of action.

Inhibitors of thyroxine synthesis
Thiourea
Thiouracil
Propylthiouracil
Methylthiouracil
Methimazole
Miscellaneous amines and sulfur compounds

Inhibitors of iodide trapping
Thiocyanates
Perchlorate
Drugs whose mode of action is uncertain
Iodides
Drugs that destroy thyroid tissue
Radioactive iodine (^{131}I)

INHIBITORS OF THYROXINE SYNTHESIS

Drugs in this category do not prevent the iodine-concentrating ability of the thyroid gland but block formation of the iodinated amino acids. These drugs inhibit thyroid peroxidase, the iodide-oxidizing enzymes. They block the reactions that require free iodine.

When these inhibitors of thyroxine formation are administered to man or experimental animals, the preformed thyroxine continues to be secreted. However, thyroxine secretion diminishes as the stored organic iodine becomes exhausted because of a lack of resynthesis. This brings forth increased secretion of the thyroid-stimulating hormone, which produces a hyperplastic, highly vascularized thyroid gland that has a greatly increased capacity for iodide trapping. The individual becomes myxedematous.

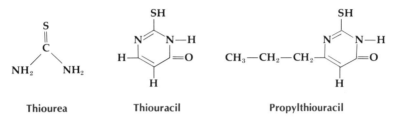

| Thiourea | Thiouracil | Propylthiouracil |

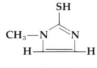

Methimazole

Thiouracil was the first antithyroid drug used extensively. Its use led to numerous cases of drug allergy and agranulocytosis, and it was soon replaced by propylthiouracil. This drug is used in doses of 50 to 100 mg. three or four times a day in tablet form. It causes allergic reactions and blood dyscrasias much less frequently than does thiouracil and is one of the most popular antithyroid drugs. Methylthiouracil has about the same potency as propylthiouracil but is less desirable in view of the more frequent allergic side effects observed following its use. Methimazole (Tapazole) is a highly potent antithyroid drug with a long duration of action. It is used in the form of 5 to 10 mg. tablets, which are administered three times a day.

Activity

Considering thiouracil as 100, the activity of these drugs in man is compared as follows:

Thiouracil	100
6-N-Propylthiouracil	75
6-Methylthiouracil	100
Methimazole	1,000

Metabolism

All these thioamide drugs are absorbed rapidly from the gastrointestinal tract. They are also excreted and metabolized fairly rapidly, necessitating frequent administration. The distribution of thiouracil in the body is unequal,[27] several organs, including the thyroid gland, containing more of the drug than the average of other tissues.

Clinical applications

Propylthiouracil and some other thioamide drugs are becoming very important in the initial treatment of thyrotoxicosis. Several days may elapse before their action becomes manifest, but eventually they induce a euthyroid state in most patients. They also maintain such a state long enough for many spontaneous remissions to occur. Characteristically these drugs increase the size and vascularity of the thyroid gland.

The usual daily oral dosages for adults of the inhibitors of thyroxine synthesis are 200 to 300 mg. of propylthiouracil, 15 to 30 mg. of methimazole (Tapazole), and 200 mg. of methylthiouracil.

INHIBITORS OF IODIDE TRAPPING

Drugs such as thiocyanate, perchlorate, and nitrate can block the iodide-concentrating ability of the thyroid. Perchlorate has undergone clinical trial.[8] It is quite effective, but agranulocytosis has been reported following its use.

IODIDES

Although a daily intake of about 150 μg of iodide is essential for normal thyroxine synthesis and although low intakes of iodide lead to goiter and cretinism, in large doses iodides can decrease the functional activity of the thyroid in Graves' disease.

Iodides represent the oldest form of antithyroid medication.[19] When as much as 6 mg. of iodide in the form of potassium or sodium iodide is administered daily to a patient with Graves' disease, there is rapid and progressive reduction of metabolic rate, the improvement reaching a maximum in about 10 days. Doses larger than 6 mg./day do not increase the effectiveness of the treatment.

Although iodides can block the synthesis of thyroxine, their actions on the thyroid gland as to size, vascularity, and composition of colloid are quite different from what is seen following medication with an antithyroid drug of the thiouracil type.

Recent evidence suggests that iodide administered to thyrotoxic patients causes an abrupt inhibition of the release of thyroxine, an effect that may be causally related to its beneficial therapeutic action.[24]

Regardless of the mechanism of action of the iodides, they are extremely useful in preparation of patients for thyroidectomy. Generally the antithyroid drugs such as propylthiouracil are used first. These drugs inhibit thyroxine production and produce a euthyroid state, but the gland remains large and highly vascularized, an undesirable state of affairs for the surgeon. It is customary to add iodide therapy during the last 10 days prior to operation in order to produce involution of the thyroid gland.

Iodides are usually administered in the form of a saturated solution of potassium or sodium iodide or as Lugol's solution, which contains 5% elemental iodine and 10% potassium iodide in water. The usual doses of iodides are 100 to 300 mg. one to three times a day. The disadvantages of using iodides are the occurrence of iodism and the possibility that thyroid storm may be elicited when iodides are discontinued during chronic management. It has also been shown that iodides delay the response to therapy from antithyroid drugs of the thiouracil type.

RADIOACTIVE IODINE

Radioactive iodine (^{131}I) emits gamma and beta radiation and has a half-life of 8 days. Since it is handled by the body in the same manner as ordinary iodine, it has become extremely useful in the diagnosis of thyroid disease and in the treatment of hyperthyroidism and carcinoma of the thyroid.

The destructive effect of ^{131}I on thyroid tissue is due to the beta radiation. The gamma rays are useful for estimating the quantity of the radioactive material in the gland by placing suitable counting equipment in front of the neck.

The isotope is available as sodium radioiodide. It is generally taken orally, but intravenous preparations are available. For diagnostic purposes the drug is given in doses of about 30 microcuries (μc), whereas in the treatment of hyperthyroidism about a thousand times as much radioactivity is administered, in other words, 15 to 30 millicuries (mc). The purpose of the treatment is the same as that of subtotal thyroidectomy.

There are several risks involved in the use of radioiodine. Its use in rats has produced malignant tumors of the thyroid gland, but the likelihood of this complication cannot be great on the basis of existing experience in human beings. Other minor risks consist of transient inflammation of the thyroid and adjacent structures and temporary exacerbation of thyrotoxicosis in a few cases.

^{131}I is contraindicated in pregnancy. It is customarily used in patients over 30 years of age. Thyroidectomy is preferred in younger hyperthyroid patients unless surgery represents an unusual hazard, for example, in the presence of heart disease. The most important complication following the use of radioiodine is hypothyroidism.

The usefulness of ^{131}I in the treatment of carcinoma of the thyroid gland with metastasis is limited by the fact that many of these tumors have little concentrating ability. The uptake of the isotope by the tumor may be increased if the normal thyroid tissue is excised or destroyed, if thyrotropic hormone is administered, or if hypothyroidism is induced by means of the antithyroid drugs.

References

1 Astwood, E. B.: Mechanism of action of various antithyroid compounds, Ann. N. Y. Acad. Sci. **50**:419, 1949.

2 Astwood, E. B., Sullivan, J., Bissell, A., and Tyslowitz, R.: Action of certain sulfonamides and of thiourea upon the function of the thyroid gland of the rat, Endocrinology **32**:210, 1943.

3 Barker, S. B.: Peripheral actions of thyroid hormones, Fed. Proc. **21**:635, 1962.

4 Beall, G. N., and Solomon, D. H.: Inhibition of long-acting thyroid stimulator by thyroid particulate fractions, J. Clin. Invest. **45**:552, 1966.

5 Buccino, R. A., Spann, J. F., Jr., Pool, P. E., Sonnenblick, E. H., and Braunwald, E.: Influence of the thyroid state on the intrinsic contractile properties and energy stores of the myocardium, J. Clin. Invest. **46**:1669, 1967.

6 Cairoli, V. J., and Crout, J. R.: Role of the autonomic nervous system in the resting tachycardia of experimental hyperthyroidism, J. Pharmacol. Exp. Ther. **158**:55, 1967.

7 Canary, J. J., Schaaf, M., Duffy, B. J., Jr., and Kyle, L. H.: Effects of oral and intramuscular administration of reserpine in thyrotoxicosis, New Eng. J. Med. **257**:435, 1957.

8 Crooks, J., and Wayne, E. J.: A comparison of potassium perchlorate, methylthiouracil, and carbimazole in the treatment of thyrotoxicosis, Lancet **1**:401, 1960.

9 Gaffney, T. E., Braunwald, E., and Kahler, R. L.: Effects of guanethidine on tri-iodothyronine-induced hyperthyroidism in man, New Eng. J. Med. **265**:16, 1961.

10 Greer, M. A., Meihoff, W. C., and Studer, H.: Treatment of hyperthyroidism with a single daily dose of propylthiouracil, New Eng. J. Med. **272**:888, 1965.

11 Gross, J., and Pitt-Rivers, R.: The identification of 3:5:3'-1-triiodothyronine in human plasma, Lancet **1**:439, 1952.

12 Gross, J., and Pitt-Rivers, R.: Tri-iodothyronine: isolation from thyroid gland and synthesis, Biochem. J. **53**:645, 1953.

13 Harrington, C. R., and Barger, G.: Thyroxine: constitution and synthesis of thyroxine, Biochem. J. 21:169, 1927.

14 Hershman, J. M., Guiens, J., Cassidy, C. E., and Astwood, E. B.: Long term outcome of hyperthyroidism treated with antithyroid drugs, J. Clin. Endocr. 26:803, 1966.

15 Kendall, E. C.: The isolation in crystalline form of the compound containing iodine which occurs in the thyroid: its chemical nature and physiological activity, Trans. Ass. Amer. Physicians 30:420, 1915.

16 Lehninger, A. L.: Thyroxine and the swelling and contraction cycle in mitochondria, Ann. N. Y. Acad. Sci. 89:484, 1960.

17 MacGregor, A. G.: Why does anybody use thyroid B. P.? Lancet 1:329, 1961.

18 MacKenzie, J. B., MacKenzie, C. G., and McCollum, E. V.: Effect of sulfanilylguanidine on thyroid of rat, Science 94:518, 1941.

19 Plummer, H. S.: Results of administering iodine to patients having exophthalmic goiter, J.A.M.A. 80:1955, 1923.

20 Rawson, R. W., Graham, R. M., and Riddell, C. B.: Physiological reactions of the thyroid-stimulating hormone of the pituitary: the effect of normal and pathological thyroid tissue on the activity of the thyroid-stimulating hormone, Ann. Intern. Med. 19:405, 1943.

21 Selenkow, H. A., Garcia, A. M., and Bradley, E. B.: An autoregulatory effect of iodide in diverse thyroid disorders, Ann. Intern. Med. 62:714, 1965.

22 Taurog, A., Tong, W., and Chaikoff, I. L.: Effects of hypophysectomy on organic iodine formation in rat thyroids. In Wolstenholme, G. E. W., and Millar, E. C. P., editors: Regulation and mode of action of thyroid hormones, Ciba Foundation Colloquia On Endocrinology, Boston, 1957, Little, Brown & Co.

23 Taurog, A., Wheat, J. D., and Chaikoff, I. L.: Nature of the I^{131} compounds appearing in the thyroid vein after injection of iodide I^{131}, Endocrinology 58:121, 1956.

24 Wartofsky, L., Ransil, B. J., and Ingbar, S. H.: Inhibition by iodine of the release of thyroxine from the thyroid glands of patients with thyrotoxicosis, J. Clin. Invest. 49:78, 1970.

25 Webster, B., and Chesney, A. M.: Endemic goiter in rabbits: effect of administration of iodine, Bull. Hopkins Hosp. 43:291, 1928.

26 Weiss, W. P., and Sokoloff, L.: Reversal of thyroxine-induced hypermetabolism by puromycin, Science 140:1324, 1963.

27 Williams, R. H., Kay, G. A., and Jandorf, B. J.: Thiouracil: its absorption, distribution and excretion, J. Clin. Invest. 23:613, 1944.

28 Wilson, I. C., Prange, A. J., McClane, T. K., Rabon, A. M., and Lipton, M. A.: Thyroid-hormone enhancement of imipramine in non-retarded depressions, New Eng. J. Med. 282:1063, 1970.

29 Wilson, W. R., Theilen, E. O., and Fletcher, F. W.: Pharmacodynamic effects of beta-adrenergic receptor blockage in patients with hyperthyroidism, J. Clin. Invest. 43:1697, 1964.

30 Witebsky, E., and Rose, N. R.: Studies in organ specificity, J. Immun. 76:408, 1956.

Recent reviews

31 Astwood, E. B.: Management of thyroid disorders, J.A.M.A. 186:585, 1963.

32 DeGroot, L. J.: Current views on formation of thyroid hormones, New Eng. J. Med. 272:243, 297, 1965.

33 Harrison, M. J.: The prevention and treatment of thyroid storm, Pharmacol. Physicians 2(1):1, 1968.

34 Hoch, F. L.: The pharmacologic basis for the clinical use of thyroid hormones, Pharmacol. Physicians 4(4):1, 1970.

35 Ingbar, S. H.: Management of emergencies. IX. Thyroid storm, New Eng. J. Med. 274:1252, 1966.

36 Levy, G. S.: Catecholamine sensitivity, thyroid hormone and the heart, Amer. J. Med. 50:413, 1971.

37 Liberti, P., and Stanbury, J. B.: The pharmacology of substances affecting the thyroid gland, Ann. Rev. Pharmacol. 11:113, 1971.

38 Maloof, F., and Soodak, M.: Intermediary metabolism of thyroid tissue and the action of drugs, Pharmacol. Rev. 15:43, 1963.

39 McKenzie, J. M.: Review: pathogenesis of Graves' disease: role of the long-acting thyroid stimulator, J. Clin. Endocr. 25:424, 1965.

40 Ochi, Y., and DeGroot, L. J.: Long acting thyroid stimulator of Graves' disease, New Eng. J. Med. 278:718, 1968.

41 Oppenheimer, J. H.: Role of plasma proteins in the binding, distribution and metabolism of the thyroid hormones, New Eng. J. Med. 278:1153, 1968.

42 Rosenberg, I. N.: Evaluation of thyroid function, New Eng. J. Med. 286:924, 1972.

43 Senior, R. M., and Birge, S. J.: The recognition and management of myxedema coma, J.A.M.A. 217:61, 1971.

44 Volpe, R.: The immunologic basis of Graves's disease, New Eng. J. Med. 287:463, 1972.

45 Waldstein, S. S.: Thyroid-catecholamine interrelations, Ann. Rev. Med. 17:123, 1966.

46 Werner, S. C., and Nauman, J. A.: The thyroid, Ann. Rev. Physiol. 30:213, 1968.

40 Parathyroid extract and vitamin D

GENERAL CONCEPT

The normal calcium concentration of plasma is about 10 mg./100 ml. About half of this is protein bound, whereas most of the remainder is ionized. These two fractions are in equilibrium, influenced by the plasma protein concentration.[15]

The two major determinants of plasma calcium level are the hormonal activity of the parathyroid glands and the intake of various forms of vitamin D. The parathyroid hormone or hormones regulate the equilibrium between calcium salts in the blood and the bones. They mobilize calcium from bone and influence phosphate excretion in the kidney. Vitamin D primarily promotes absorption of calcium and phosphate from the intestine.

Important new developments have taken place in relation to the parathyroid hormones and vitamin D. It appears that there may be more than one parathyroid hormone. Immunoassay studies indicate that plasma parathyroid hormone is immunochemically different from extracts of parathyroid glands. Striking new developments have taken place also in relation to vitamin D metabolism. It appears that vitamins D_2 and D_3 are metabolically activated in the liver and the kidney.[24]

PARATHYROID EXTRACT

Extract of parathyroid glands was found to improve the tetany that develops in parathyroidectomized dogs and to increase blood calcium.[7] Parathyroid injection is biologically assayed and contains 100 USP units/ml. The definition of a unit states that 100 units represents the subcutaneous dose able to raise blood calcium of dogs by 1 mg./100 ml.

The parathyroid hormone is a highly active polypeptide obtained from parathyroid extract.[16] The bovine hormone consists of 84 amino acids.

There is increasing evidence for the existence of more than one parathyroid hormone. Immunoassay and gel-filtration studies indicate that there are three different parathyroid hormones having different molecular weights and amino acid compositions.[24]

A major disadvantage of the parathyroid injection is that its prolonged use often induces resistance to its action. This is probably due to the development of antibodies.

Mode of action

Patients with hypoparathyroidism show markedly elevated serum phosphorus levels and hypocalcemia. When the calcium level falls to 7 mg./100 ml., tetany may ensue. It can be demonstrated in experimental animals that these blood chemical changes occur within a few hours following parathyroidectomy. This indicates that hormonal output is required continuously in order to maintain normal levels of cal-

499

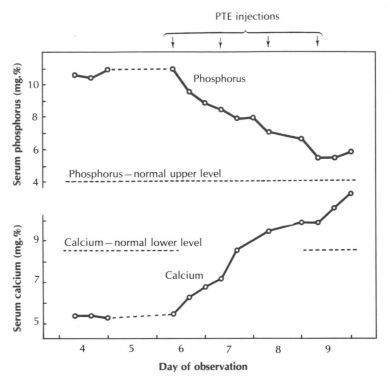

Fig. 40-1. Effect of parathyroid extract **(PTE)** on serum inorganic phosphorus and calcium in patient with idiopathic hypoparathyroidism. (From Munson, P. L.: Fed. Proc. **19:**593, 1960.)

cium and phosphate in the blood and tissues. It is believed that the output of parathyroid hormones is regulated by the level of serum calcium acting through a feedback mechanism.

As shown in Fig. 40-1, the injection of parathyroid extract in patients having idiopathic hypoparathyroidism results in phosphaturia, lowering of serum phosphorus, and gradual elevation of serum calcium. This sequence of events has been interpreted by Albright and Ellsworth[1] as indicative of a primary action of the parathyroid extract on phosphate excretion.

Although parathyroid extract does promote renal excretion of phosphate, there is much experimental evidence to indicate that the most important action of the parathyroid hormones is direct mobilization of calcium from bones. The action of parathyroid extract on serum calcium has been demonstrated in nephrectomized animals.[11] In addition, it has been shown that parathyroid transplants exert a local resorptive effect on bone.[4,6] This effect has also been demonstrated in tissue cultures.

According to more recent views, the parathyroid hormone has important effects on the translocation of phosphate, calcium, and other ions across biologic membranes.[18] It stimulates the uptake of phosphate into mitochondria, promotes the release of calcium and hydrogen ions, and stimulates mitochondrial respiration. It is likely that the actions of the hormone on both bone and kidney primarily involve membrane effects on the movement of ions.

500

Calcium homeostasis and parathyroid extract

A variety of factors contribute to the maintenance of extracellular calcium within narrow limits. The daily diet contributes about 1 Gm. of calcium, the absorption of which is influenced by vitamin D and to some extent by parathyroid hormone. Also, the phosphate, oxalate, and phytate content of the diet will decrease calcium absorption. Antacids containing $Al(OH)_3$ promote calcium absorption by binding phosphate in the intestine.

Extracellular calcium is in equilibrium with the exchangeable calcium of bone. When extracellular calcium falls, the exchangeable portion of bone calcium aids in returning it toward normal. In addition, renal reabsorption of calcium, renal excretion of phosphate, and resorption of nonexchangeable bone are important in opposing decreases in extracellular calcium levels. Bone resorption is promoted by the parathyroid hormone and by some steroids related to vitamin D. The release of parathyroid hormone is under the influence of the level of extracellular calcium.[9]

Although bone resorption is considered to be an active process, the mechanism of the deposition of calcium in the bone is not as well understood. It is believed by some workers that the extracellular fluid is actually supersaturated with calcium *with respect to bone*.[27] When femurs were incubated in plasma at normal calcium and phosphate levels, these ions actually deposited on the bone.[27] According to this view, the deposition of the ions may then be a consequence of supersaturation, whereas the supersaturation itself is maintained by continuous activity of the parathyroids.

Calcitonin, or thyrocalcitonin, is a second hormone involved in calcium homeostasis. Calcitonin is secreted by the parafollicular cells of the thyroid. These cells originate from the ultimobranchial body, a separate organ in some animals. Calcitonin produces hypocalcemia by inhibiting bone resorption. Calcitonin also promotes the urinary excretion of calcium and phosphate.[8,16]

Calcitonin is normally present in the blood, and its concentration increases when calcium salts are administered. Its concentration is greatly increased in patients having medullary carcinoma of the thyroid.[20] The function of calcitonin may be a protective one against hypercalcemia induced by increased calcium intake.

Calcitonin has been used clinically in Paget's disease, hypercalcemia, and osteoporosis. Its usefulness is limited by its short duration of action. In addition, resistance develops to its continued use, perhaps because of compensatory increase in the secretion of parathyroid hormone.[26]

VITAMIN D
Current nomenclature

It was discovered more than 40 years ago that irradiation of plant sterols could yield antirachitic compounds. The active sterol produced by irradiation of ergosterol became known as vitamin D_2 or *ergocalciferol*. What was previously called vitamin D_1 was a mixture of active and inactive products. The vitamin that is produced in the skin by irradiation of 7-dehydrocholesterol was named vitamin D_3 or *cholecalciferol*. Although both vitamins D_2 and D_3 are active and undergo similar metabolic transformations, most of the circulating and stored vitamin D is ergocalciferol. This is a consequence of the high dietary intake of irradiated ergosterol. Vitamin D_3 differs from vitamin D_2 only in lacking a double bond between C22 and C23.

The structural formulas of vitamin D_2 and dihydrotachysterol follow.

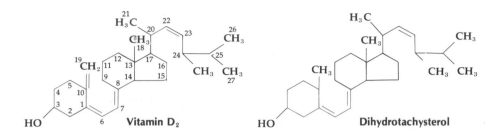

Metabolic activation of vitamin D

Both vitamins D_2 and D_3 must be hydroxylated in the C25 position by the liver to become active. The resulting compounds are referred to as 25-hydroxyergocalciferol and 25-hydroxycholecalciferol, respectively. These compounds are carried in the circulation by a binding protein. Eventually, the microsomal enzymes of the liver convert them to inactive polar metabolites.

A further activating step occurs in the kidney for vitamin D_3. The 25-hydroxycholecalciferol is further hydroxylated to 1,25-hydroxycholecalciferol, which may be the final active form of vitamin D_3. On the other hand, dihydrotachysterol does not require further activation in the kidney.

Drug interactions with vitamin D metabolism

Phenobarbital and diphenylhydantoin are known to increase microsomal hydroxylase activity in the liver. It is possible that the great frequency of rickets and osteomalacia in patients on anticonvulsants is a consequence of increased enzymatic transformation of vitamin D_2 and D_3 to inactive metabolites.[24]

The main function of vitamin D is to promote absorption of calcium and phosphorus from the intestine.[17] Deficiency of the vitamin in children leads to rickets, which may be prevented by the daily requirement of 800 units. Very rarely, osteomalacia can occur in adults following vitamin D deficiency.

In large doses, vitamin D has effects similar to those of parathyroid extract on bone resorption and phosphate excretion. Dihydrotachysterol may be looked upon as having intermediate effects between those of vitamin D and parathyroid hormone: less effect than vitamin D on calcium absorption but much greater effect on phosphate excretion and bone resorption.

In the treatment of hypoparathyroidism, vitamin D_2 may be administered in large doses (400,000 IU) initially, and maintenance doses may vary from 100,000 to 200,000 IU/day. Dihydrotachysterol may be administered initially in doses of 3 to 8 mg. (compared with 10 mg. or more of vitamin D_2), and for maintenance a dose of about 1 mg./day is usually sufficient.

TOXIC EFFECTS OF PARATHYROID EXTRACT AND VITAMIN D

Toxic effects of parathyroid injection and of vitamin D are manifest as (1) hypercalcemia with numerous clinical consequences, (2) demineralization of bones, and (3) renal calculi and metastatic calcifications in soft tissues.

Hypercalcemia is associated with a number of clinical manifestations such as weakness, vomiting, diarrhea, and lack of muscle tone. The electrocardiographic changes that may occur at various levels of serum calcium are shown in Fig. 40-2.

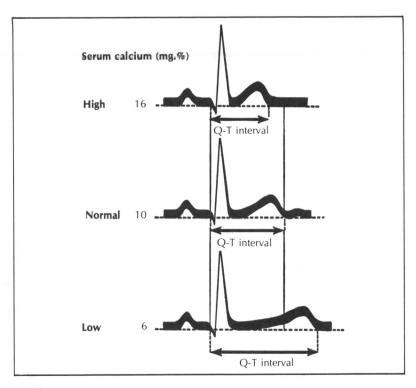

Fig. 40-2. Effect of varying calcium levels on electrocardiogram. (From Burch, G. E., and Winsor, T.: A primer of electrocardiography, Philadelphia, 1960, Lea & Febiger.)

Serious toxic manifestations may be seen at calcium blood levels of 15 mg./100 ml. Signs of hypocalcemia are tetany, cataracts, and mental lethargy.

Toxicity of very large doses of vitamin D is probably due to the parathyroid-like effect of this vitamin. The marked hypercalcemia is more likely due to bone resorption than to increased absorption of calcium from the intestine, since the latter is not greatly increased above what may be expected from therapeutic doses of the vitamin.

OTHER DRUGS INFLUENCING SERUM CALCIUM CONCENTRATIONS

Phosphates, sodium sulfate, sodium citrate, and **disodium edetate** (Endrate), when given by intravenous infusion, can lower calcium levels in the blood. Their administration should not be undertaken without considering their adverse effects. Sodium sulfate may be the most useful drug in this group.

Glucocorticoids are effective in reducing the hypercalcemia caused by sarcoidosis and that caused by vitamin D. **Calcitonin**, commented on before, lowers serum calcium, but its action is of short duration. **Thiazide diuretics** increase calcium excretion at first but may have the opposite effect on long-continued administration. The thiazides have been used in the treatment of idiopathic hypercalciuria for the prevention of stone formation. **Mithramycin**, an inhibitor of RNA synthesis introduced for cancer chemotherapy, was found to produce hypocalcemia in patients with cancer. Its use is strictly experimental.

For the initial treatment of *hypocalcemia*, the intravenous injection of a 10% solution of **calcium gluconate** is highly effective. **Calcium gluceptate** may also be given intravenously or intramuscularly. Calcium salts used orally include calcium gluconate, calcium phosphate dibasic, calcium phosphate tribasic, calcium lactate, and calcium carbonate precipitated. Vitamin D and parathyroid injection have been discussed previously.

References

1 Albright, F., and Ellsworth, R.: Studies on the physiology of the parathyroid glands: calcium and phosphorus studies in a case of idiopathic hypoparathyroidism, J. Clin. Invest. 7:183, 1929.

2 Arnaud, C. D., Sizemore, G. W., Oldham, S. B., Fischer, J. A., Tsao, H. S., and Littledike, E. T.: Human parathyroid hormone: glandular and secreted molecular species, Amer. J. Med. 50: 630, 1971.

3 Aurbach, G. D., and Potts, J. T.: Parathyroid hormone, Amer. J. Med. 42:1, 1967.

4 Barnicot, N. A.: The local action of the parathyroid and other tissues on bone in intracerebral grafts, J. Anat. 82:233, 1948.

5 Bijvoet, O. L. M., Veer, J. V., De Vries, H. R., and Van Koppen, A. T. J.: Natriuretic effect of calcitonin in man, New Eng. J. Med. 284:681, 1971.

6 Chang, H. Y.: Grafts of parathyroid and other tissues to bone, Anat. Rec. 111:23, 1951.

7 Collip, J. B.: The parathyroid glands, Harvey Lect. 21:113, 1925–1926.

8 Copp, D. H.: Parathyroids, calcitonin, and control of plasma calcium, Recent Progr. Hormone Res. 20:59, 1964.

9 Copp, D. H., Moghadam, H., Mensen, E. D., and McPherson, G. D.: The parathyroids and calcium homeostasis. In Greep, R. O., and Talmage, R. V., editors: The parathyroids, Springfield, Ill., 1961, Charles C Thomas, Publisher.

10 DeLuca, H. F.: 25-Hydroxycholecalciferol, Arch. Intern. Med. 124:442, 1969.

11 Grollman, A.: The role of the kidney in the parathyroid control of the blood calcium as determined by studies on the nephrectomized dog, Endocrinology 55:166, 1954.

12 Haddad, J. G., Birge, S. J., and Avioli, L. V.: Effects of prolonged thyrocalcitonin administration on Paget's disease of bone, New Eng. J. Med. 283:549, 1970.

13 Harrison, H. E., Lifshitz, F., and Blizzard, R. M.: Comparison between crystalline dihydrotachysterol and calciferol in patients requiring pharmacologic vitamin D therapy, New Eng. J. Med. 276:894, 1967.

14 Kenny, A. D., Draskóczy, P. R., and Goldhaber, P.: Citric acid production by resorbing bone tissue culture, Amer. J. Physiol. 197:502, 1959.

15 McLean, F. C., and Hastings, A. B.: The state of calcium in the fluids of the body: the conditions affecting the ionization of calcium, J. Biol. Chem. 108:285, 1935.

16 Munson, P. L.: Recent advances in parathyroid hormone research, Fed. Proc. 19:593, 1960.

17 Nicolaysen, R., Eeg-Larsen, N., and Malm, O. J.: Physiology of calcium metabolism, Physiol. Rev. 33:424, 1953.

18 Rasmussen, H., DeLuca, H. F., Sallis, J. D., and Engstrom, G. W.: The relationship between vitamin D and parathyroid hormone, J. Clin. Invest. 42:967, 1963.

Recent reviews

19 DeLuca, H. F., and Suttie, J. W.: The fat-soluble vitamins, Madison, 1970, University of Wisconsin Press.

20 Foster, G. V.: Calcitonin (thyrocalcitonin), New Eng. J. Med. 279:349, 1968.

21 Hirsch, P. F., and Munson, P. L.: Thyrocalcitonin, Physiol. Rev. 49:548, 1969.

22 Kimberg, D. V.: Effects of vitamin D and steroid hormones on the active transport of calcium by the intestine, New Eng. J. Med. 280:1396, 1969.

23 Munson, P. L., Hirsch, P. F., and Tashijan, A. H., Jr.: Parathyroid gland, Ann. Rev. Physiol. 25: 325, 1963.

24 Raisz, L. G.: A confusion of Vitamin D's, New Eng. J. Med. 287:926, 1972.

25 Raisz, L. G.: Parathyroid gland metabolism, Arch. Intern. Med. 124:389, 1969.

26 Raisz, L. G.: The pharmacology of bone, Rational Drug Therapy 5:1, June, 1971.

27 Rasmussen, H., and Reifenstein, E. C.: The parathyroid glands. In Williams, R. H., editor: Textbook of endocrinology, Philadelphia, 1962, W. B. Saunders Co.

28 Talmage, R. V., and Toft, R. J.: The problem of the control of parathyroid secretion. In Greep, R. O., and Talmage, R. V., editors: The parathyroids, Springfield, Ill., 1961, Charles C Thomas, Publisher.

29 Tashjian, A. H.: Soft bones, hard facts and calcitonin therapy, New Eng. J. Med. 283:593, 1970.

30 Tenenhouse, A., Rasmussen, H., Hawker, C. D., and Arnaud, C. D.: Thyrocalcitonin, Ann. Rev. Pharmacol. 8:319, 1968.

41 Posterior pituitary hormones — vasopressin and oxytocin

The posterior lobe of the pituitary body, the neurohypophysis, contains hormones having vasoactive, antidiuretic, and oxytocic properties. The original material was separated into two fractions.[9] One contained most of the vasoactive and antidiuretic portion, whereas the other was predominantly oxytocic. Both active fractions, vasopressin and oxytocin, have been synthesized.[6,7]

Chemistry and preparations

Both vasopressin and oxytocin are polypeptides containing eight amino acids. Vasopressin (in several species) contains the following amino acids: tyrosine, cystine, aspartic acid, glutamic acid, glycine, proline, arginine, and phenylalanine. In vasopressin obtained from hog pituitary, arginine is replaced by lysine.

Oxytocin resembles vasopressin in having six identical amino acids but contains leucine and isoleucine instead of arginine and phenylalanine.

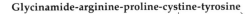

Glycinamide-arginine-proline-cystine-tyrosine

Phenylalanine

Asparagine-glutamine

Vasopressin (beef)

Glycinamide-leucine-proline-cystine-tyrosine

Isoleucine

Asparagine-glutamine

Oxytocin

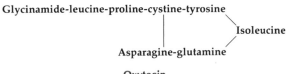

Preparations of these hormones are standardized by bioassay. Vasopressin preparations are standardized on the basis of the action of such preparations on the blood pressure of the dog. One USP unit is the activity present in 0.5 mg. of standard powder of posterior pituitary. Oxytocic potency is determined by the depressor effect of oxytocin preparations on the blood pressure of the chicken.

VASOPRESSIN

The most significant effect of vasopressin is exerted on the kidney. In addition, the hormone can constrict various blood vessels, including the coronary vessels. The only clearly established physiologic function of vasopressin is its antidiuretic action.

The antidiuretic potency of vasopressin is very great. The infusion of less than 0.1 μg of vasopressin per hour produces maximal antidiuresis in man.[11] It is believed that the antidiuretic action of vasopressin is exerted on water reabsorption by the distal tubule and also by the collecting ducts. In physiologic doses the hormone does not influence electrolyte absorption. Larger doses in some experiments have shown increased output of sodium and chloride, probably an indirect effect.

The antidiuretic hormone is elaborated by certain hypothalamic structures such as the supraoptic nuclei and is then transported to the neurohypophysis, where it is stored. The release of the antidiuretic hormone is influenced by the osmolarity of the extracellular fluid and by many drugs. Endogenous neurohumoral agents also may play an important role in the release of antidiuretic hormone since pain and emotions have important influences. It is generally accepted that some hypothalamic structures are sensitive to changes in the osmolarity of the extracellular fluid and act as osmoreceptors.[15] Thus the ingestion of water and dilution of the extracellular fluid lead to inhibition of antidiuretic hormone secretion, whereas hypertonic solutions promote this process.

Diabetes insipidus, occurring spontaneously in man or produced experimentally by pituitary stalk section, is characterized by failure of distal tubular water reabsorption. As a consequence, persons with diabetes insipidus excrete large amounts of dilute urine and drink large quantities of water.

The mode of action of the antidiuretic hormone is now generally attributed to an increase in the size of pores or channels for the flow of water along osmotic gradients.[3] There is evidence for this action on isolated systems such as the skin of toads and frogs.[1]

In regard to the basic mechanism of action of the antidiuretic hormone, three theories have been presented in recent years. The first of these, no longer accepted, suggests that vasopressin promotes secretion of hyaluronidase by tubular cells. The second postulates interactions between the disulfide bridge in the vasopressin molecule and free sulfhydryl groups in the cell membrane. According to the third hypothesis, based on much experimental evidence, vasopressin directly increases the concentration of adenosine-3'-5'-monophosphate, which then alters permeability.[21]

Drug effects on antidiuretic hormone release

In addition to changes in osmolarity of the extracellular fluid, release of the antidiuretic hormone is influenced by a variety of drugs. The existence of a cholinergic mechanism for this process has been suggested on the basis of experiments which showed that injections of *acetylcholine* or diisopropyl fluorophosphate into the supraoptic nuclei caused release of antidiuretic hormone.[12] *Nicotine* has been shown to inhibit water diuresis in man, probably through the release of antidiuretic hormone. *Alcohol* inhibits the release of antidiuretic hormone in response to dehydration and produces inappropriate water diuresis in a dehydrated individual.[10] Alcohol does not block the action of nicotine on the release of the hormone.[10]

Antidiuresis that occurs during general anesthesia[2] and following the injection of histamine, morphine, and barbiturates (but not thiopental[2]) has also been attributed to the release of antidiuretic hormone. Since muscular exercise, pain, and emotional excitement also cause inhibition of water diuresis, it is likely that some central control mechanism of antidiuretic hormone release is very susceptible to neural or neurohumoral influences. Of the large variety of drugs that can influence antidiuretic hormone release, many are known to alter neural activity or to act as stressful stimuli.

Certain hyponatremic syndromes are associated with "inappropriate" secretion of the antidiuretic hormone. They are characterized by primary water retention unassociated with sodium retention and edema. Some of the underlying diseases are broncho-genic carcinoma, head injury, and tuberculous meningitis.[4,5]

Extrarenal effects

Although the main therapeutic advantage of vasopressin is its antidiuretic action, the hormone has a stimulant effect on the smooth muscles of the blood vessels, intestine, and uterus. This action appears to be a direct musculotropic effect, not mediated by nerves or neurohumoral agents. When posterior pituitary preparations are used in the treatment of diabetes insipidus, the smooth muscle effects are undesirable side effects and usually indicate overdosage.

Preparations containing vasopressin constrict the coronary arteries and are therefore dangerous in persons who suffer from coronary disease. Although intravenous injection of posterior pituitary extract into animals causes marked peripheral vasoconstriction, blood pressure often increases only moderately. This is attributed to the fact that the coronary arteries are also constricted. Tachyphylaxis develops to the pressor action of vasopressin.

Antidiuretic preparations

Posterior pituitary USP is available as a powder for topical application, administered by inhalation or directly to the nasal mucosa. It may cause mucosal irritation. The duration of its antidiuretic effect is such that the drug must be used several times a day. Contraindicated in pregnancy, posterior pituitary should be used with caution in patients with coronary artery disease. The dose is 40 to 60 mg. topically three or four times daily.

Posterior pituitary injection is obsolete, being replaced by vasopressin injection.

Vasopressin injection (Pitressin) produces an antidiuretic effect lasting two to eight hours when administered by subcutaneous or intramuscular injection. The solution may also be used topically. Vasopressin may cause fluid retention, hypertension, myocardial ischemia, gastrointestinal and uterine contractions, and allergic reactions. The available solution for injection contains 10 pressor units/ml.

Vasopressin tannate injection (Pitressin tannate) is a suspension in peanut oil of the insoluble tannate of the hormone, suitable for intramuscular administration. The duration of action is two to three days. Vasopressin tannate injection is available in oil, 5 pressor units/ml.

OXYTOCIN

Oxytocin is a polypeptide amide that consists of eight amino acids and ammonia. Its molecular weight is 1,007. Although the physiologic functions of the hormone seem to be related to reproductive function in the female, its presence in the male suggests that it must have other functions also.[16]

The separation of posterior pituitary extracts into the oxytocic and vasopressor-antidiuretic fractions was accomplished as early as 1928. More recently, oxytocin has been purified, chemically identified, and synthesized.[7]

Oxytocin differs from vasopressin in the following respects:
1. It contains leucine and isoleucine instead of phenylalanine and arginine; the other six amino acids are identical in the two hormones.

2. It has no effect on water diuresis.
3. It is a potent stimulant of the gravid uterus at term and postpartum.
4. It does not produce vasoconstriction and may even lower blood pressure in certain species.
5. It may produce milk let-down during the postpartum period.
6. It has little effect on intestinal smooth muscle and coronary arteries.

Bioassay

Oxytocin preparations are bioassayed on the basis of the vasodepressor activity in chickens. The oxytocic activity associated with vasopressin preparations is assayed on the guinea pig uterus.

Oxytocin preparations

Oxytocin injection, synthetic (Pitocin; Syntocinon; Uteracon) is a synthetic preparation used for induction of labor. It is also used to control postpartum uterine atony, but for the latter indication, ergonovine is often preferred. The drug is available in solutions containing 5 units/0.5 ml. or 10 units/ml. Dosage varies according to the indication. To control postpartum bleeding, oxytocin may be administered intramuscularly, 3 to 10 units. When given by intravenous injection for the same indication, its dosage should be reduced to 0.6 to 1.8 units. For intravenous infusion by the drip method, oxytocin, 2 units, is added to 500 ml. of normal saline.

Adverse effects

Adverse effects include overstimulation of the uterus with tetany, water intoxication, hypertensive episodes, and allergic reactions. The fetus may manifest bradycardia or other cardiac arrhythmias.

References

1 Anderson, B., and Ussing, H. H.: Solvent drag on non-electrolytes during osmotic flow through isolated toad skin and its response to antidiuretic hormone, Acta Physiol. Scand. 39:228, 1957.

2 Aprahamian, H. A., Vanderveen, J. L., Bunker, J. P., Murphy, A. J., and Crawford, J. D.: The influence of general anesthetics on water and solute excretion in man, Ann. Surg. 150:122, 1959.

3 Berliner, R. W., Levinsky, N. G., Davidson, D. G., and Eden, M.: Dilution and concentration of the urine and the action of antidiuretic hormone, Amer. J. Med. 24:730, 1958.

4 Carter, N. W., Rector, F. C., Jr., and Seldin, D. W.: Hyponatremia in cerebral disease resulting from the inappropriate secretion of antidiuretic hormone, New Eng. J. Med. 264:67, 1961.

5 Clift, G. V., Schletter, F. E., Moses, A. M., and Streeten, D. H. P.: Syndrome of inappropriate vasopressin secretion, Arch. Intern. Med. 118:453, 1966.

6 du Vigneaud, V.: The isolation and proof of structure of the vasopressins and the synthesis of octapeptide amides with pressor-antidiuretic activity. In Liébecq, C., editor: Proceedings of the Third International Congress on Biochemistry, New York, 1956, Academic Press, Inc.

7 du Vigneaud, V., Ressler, C., Swan, J. M., Roberts, C. W., Katsoyannis, P. G., and Gordon, S.: The synthesis of an octapeptide amide with the hormonal activity of oxytocin: enzymatic cleavage of glycinamide from vasopressin and a proposed structure for this pressor-antidiuretic hormone of the posterior pituitary, J. Amer. Chem. Soc. 75:4879, 1953.

8 Earley, L. E., and Orloff, J.: The mechanism of antidiuresis associated with the administration of hydrochlorothiazide to patients with vasopressin-resistant diabetes insipidus, J. Clin. Invest. 41:1988, 1962.

9 Kamm, O. H., Aldrich, T. B., Grottee, I. W., Rowe, L. W., and Bugbee, E. P.: The active principles of the posterior lobe of the pituitary gland, J. Amer. Chem. Soc. 50:573, 1928.

10 Kleeman, C. R., Rubini, M. E., Lamdin, E., and Epstein, F. H.: Studies on alcohol diuresis. II. The evaluation of ethyl alcohol as an inhibitor of the neurohypophysis, J. Clin. Invest. **34**:448, 1955.

11 Lauson, H. D.: The problem of estimating the rate of secretion of antidiuretic hormone in man, Amer. J. Med. **11**:135, 1951.

12 Pickford, M.: Antidiuretic substances, Pharmacol. Rev. **4**:254, 1952.

13 Poisner, A. M., and Douglas, W. W.: A possible mechanism of release of posterior pituitary hormones involving adenosine triphosphate and an adenosine triphosphatase in the neurosecretory granules, Molec. Pharmacol. **4**:531, 1968.

14 Silva, Y. J., Moffat, R. C., and Walt, A. J.: Vasopressin effect on portal and systemic hemodynamics, J.A.M.A. **210**:1065, 1969.

15 Verney, E. B.: The antidiuretic hormone and the factors which determine its release, Proc. Roy. Soc. [Biol.] **135**:25, 1947.

Recent reviews

16 Berde, B.: Recent progress in oxytocin research, Springfield, Ill., 1959, Charles C Thomas, Publisher.

17 Farrell, G., Fabre, L. F., and Rauschkolb, E. W.: The neurohypophysis, Ann. Rev. Physiol. **30**: 557, 1968.

18 Guillemin, R.: Hypothalamic polypeptides stimulating the secretion of pituitary hormones. In Proceedings of the Twenty-Third International Congress of Physiological Sciences, International Congress Series No. 87, Amsterdam, 1965, Excerpta Medica Foundation.

19 Leaf, A.: Membrane effects of antidiuretic hormone, Amer. J. Med. **42**:745, 1967.

20 Milne, M. D.: Renal pharmacology, Ann. Rev. Pharmacol. **5**:119, 1965.

21 Orloff, J., and Handler, J. S.: The cellular mode of action of antidiuretic hormone, Amer. J. Med. **36**:686, 1964.

22 Reichlin, S.: Functions of the median-eminence gland, New Eng. J. Med. **275**:600, 1966.

23 Wakim, K. G.: Reassessment of the source, mode and locus of action of antidiuretic hormone, Amer. J. Med. **42**:394, 1967.

42 Anterior pituitary gonadotropins and sex hormones

GENERAL CONCEPT

The anterior pituitary is made up of six or seven different secretory types of cells that can function independently in producing their characteristic hormones.[31] These hormones are the thyroid-stimulating hormone (TSH), adrenocorticotropic hormone (ACTH), luteinizing hormone (LH), follicle-stimulating hormone (FSH), melanocyte-stimulating hormone (MSH), prolactin (PL), and growth hormone (GH).

The secretion of these hormones is stimulated by hypothalamic releasing factors also known as hypophysiotropic hormones such as TSH-releasing hormone (TRH), ACTH-releasing factor (CRF), LH-releasing factor (LRF), FSH-releasing factor (FRF), MSH-releasing and -inhibiting factors (MRF and MIF), prolactin-inhibiting and -releasing factors (PIF and PRF), and growth hormone-releasing and -inhibiting factors (GRF and GIF). The general scheme of the anterior pituitary hormones and their releasing factors is shown in Fig. 42-1.

Since there is great interest in the interaction between neuropharmacologic agents and the releasing factors, this subject will be summarized before discussing the pharmacology of gonadotropins and sex hormones.

NEUROPHARMACOLOGIC AGENTS AND HYPOTHALAMIC RELEASING FACTORS

Several neuropharmacologic agents alter anterior pituitary secretions by acting on the elaboration of hypothalamic releasing factors. It is believed that the neurons that secrete the releasing factors are located in the ventral hypothalamus,[23] and various neurotransmitters regulate their functional activities. Among the possible transmitters, dopamine, norepinephrine, and serotonin have received the most consideration. Many drugs influence the elaboration of various releasing factors by interactions with their neurotransmitters. A brief summary based on a more extensive review[23] will be attempted, classifying these drug effects according to the individual releasing factors.

TSH-releasing factor. Although TRH has been well characterized and synthesized, little is known about drug effects on its secretion. It has been hypothesized that serotonin might be involved in the elaboration of TRH,[23] but this is not clearly established.

Corticotropin-releasing factor. Dextroamphetamine stimulates the release of CRF, which is blocked by an alpha adrenergic blocking agent. Reserpine causes a transient increase in basal secretion. The phenothiazines such as chlorpromazine reduce the responses of CRF secretion to hypoglycemia, metyrapone, and pyrogens. These actions could be due to an antiadrenergic, antidopaminergic, or antiserotoninergic effect of the phenothiazines.

LH- and FSH-releasing factors. Experimental studies indicate that dopamine is a stimulatory and serotonin is an inhibitory neurotransmitter involved in the release

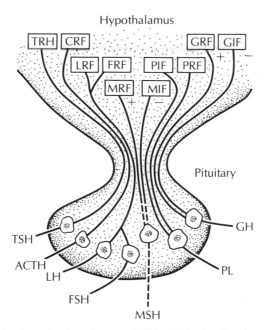

Fig. 42-1. Hypothalamic releasing factors. **TRH,** TSH-releasing hormone; **CRF,** ACTH-releasing factor; **LRF,** LH-releasing factor; **FRF,** FSH-releasing factor; **MRF** and **MIF,** MSH-releasing and -inhibiting factors; **PIF** and **PRF,** prolactin-inhibiting and -releasing factors; **GRF** and **GIF,** GH-releasing and -inhibiting factors; **TSH,** thyroid-stimulating hormone; **ACTH,** adrenocorticotropic hormone; **LH,** luteinizing hormone; **FSH,** follicle-stimulating hormone; **MSH,** melanocyte-stimulating hormone; **PL,** prolactin; **GH,** growth hormone. (From Frohman, L. A.: New. Eng. J. Med. **286**:1391, 1972.)

of LRF and FRF. The administration of L-dopa leads to a rise in plasma FSH and a more variable rise in plasma LH. The phenothiazines have been claimed to inhibit LRF secretion, whereas FRF was unaffected or even stimulated.

Prolactin-inhibiting factor. Galactorrhea is produced by a variety of psychotropic drugs, such as the phenothiazine reserpine, methyldopa, and imipramine. It is believed that dopamine promotes the secretion of a prolactin-inhibiting factor. The problem is complicated, however, and the previously mentioned effect of imipramine could not be explained on the basis of such a simple hypothesis. On the other hand, a prolactin-lowering effect of L-dopa has been reported, an observation that would favor the basic hypothesis of a dopaminergic control.

Growth hormone–releasing factor. There is a strong suspicion of an adrenergic control of GRF secretion. Dextroamphetamine stimulates GRF, the effect being enhanced by propranolol. GRF appears to be stimulated by alpha adrenergic and inhibited by beta adrenergic mechanisms. Reserpine and chlorpromazine reduce the GRF hypoglycemia. In an acromegalic patient, chlorpromazine caused a decrease in growth hormone levels.

It should be emphasized that the field of hypothalamic releasing factors is a relatively new one, and many of the statements in the previous discussion may have to be modified in the light of new evidence. Nevertheless, this is an area of great interest and it is satisfying to find that some of the unusual effects of commonly used psychotropic agents, such as galactorrhea, can be explained on the basis of this new information.

GONADOTROPINS AND SEX HORMONES

Gonadotropin secretion is regulated by hypothalamic centers that communicate with the anterior pituitary by means of releasing factors. Dopamine plays an important role in these central regulations.[15] FSH promotes the growth of the folliculus and the secretion of estrogens. LH, which is identical to the interstitial cell–stimulating hormone (ICSH), produces ovulation and promotes secretion of progesterone from the corpus luteum. Estrogens and progesterone exert a negative feedback on the secretion of gonadotropins.

Estrogens promote the growth of the reproductive organs in the female. They promote growth and cornification of the vaginal epithelium and stimulate cervical mucous secretion. Progesterone contributes to the differentiation in the female reproductive organs and is responsible for the secretions of the endometrium during the luteal phase of the menstrual cycle.

In the male, testosterone is secreted by the interstitial cells of Leydig. The anterior pituitary stimulates the activities of the Leydig cell by means of the interstitial cell–stimulating hormone (ICSH; LH).

OVULATORY CYCLE

The traditional schema of the hormonal control of menstruation is shown in Fig. 42-2, whereas the actual measurements of the serum concentrations of various hormones in normal women are depicted in Fig. 42-3.

The rise of serum follicle-stimulating hormone (FSH) and luteinizing hormone (LH) concentrations in the early phase of the cycle is probably responsible for the initial growth and development of the follicles. FSH and LH act synergistically with regard to follicular maturation.

Ovulation is preceded by a surge of LH and also FSH. The LH surge is of primary importance in causing rupture of the follicle.[18] Progesterone secretion follows the LH surge.

ESTROGENS, PROGESTERONE, AND MENSTRUATION

The administration of estrogen to a woman without ovarian function can lead to withdrawal bleeding, breakthrough bleeding, or no bleeding, depending on dose and timing. Withdrawal bleeding occurs when the estrogen is employed in low doses for weeks and is suddenly stopped. Bleeding is like normal menstruation except that it is painless and more prolonged. Withdrawal bleeding can also be produced by administration of a single dose of estrogen.

Breakthrough bleeding occurs during the continued administration of a dose of estrogen that is *larger* than the amount necessary to induce withdrawal bleeding. Breakthrough bleeding is unpredictable in onset or amount. If the dose of estrogen is further increased, breakthrough bleeding will cease.

If progesterone is added to the continued administration of estrogen for a few days

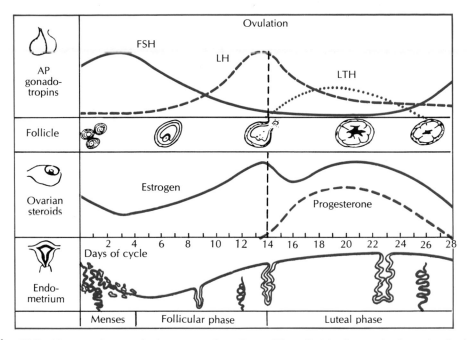

Fig. 42-2. Hormonal control of menstruation. (From Riley, G. M.: Gynecologic endocrinology, New York, 1959, Hoeber Medical Division, Harper & Row, Publishers, Inc.)

and then is stopped, menstruation that resembles normal menses will occur. Bleeding is predictable and painful and occurs 3 days after progesterone administration is stopped.

CHORIONIC GONADOTROPIN

Human chorionic gonadotropin, obtained from the urine of pregnant women, is a glycoprotein having LH or ICSH activity. It may produce ovulation in anovulatory women (p. 518). Human chorionic gonadotropin (HCG) is used in cryptorchidism and for other purposes when stimulation of Leydig cells is desired. Menotropins (Pergonal) are gonadotropins extracted from the urine of postmenopausal women. They have both FSH and LH activity, in contrast with HCG. The main usefulness of menotropins is in the promotion of ovulation in anovulatory women (p. 518).

The gonadotropin obtained from *pregnant mare serum* differs from human chorionic gonadotropin in several respects. It has marked follicle-stimulating activity, whereas the human pregnancy hormone behaves as an ICSH. The main disadvantage of the animal hormone is its antigenicity. Allergic reactions and the development of antihormones have been described following its use.

BIOSYNTHESIS OF STEROIDS

The gonadotropins are believed to promote the synthesis of enzymes, which in turn catalyze the various steps in steroidal biosynthesis. These steps in the formation

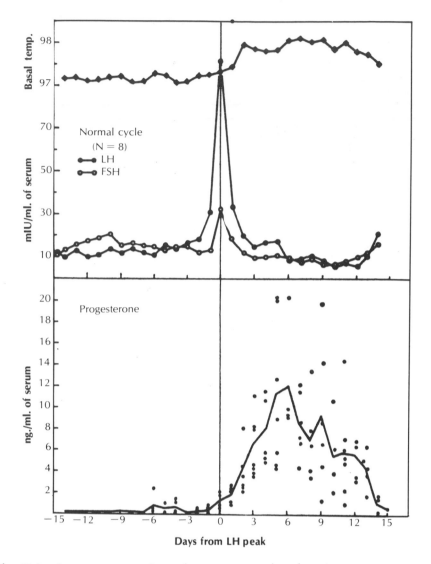

Fig. 42-3. Serum concentrations of progesterone plotted against mean concentrations of FSH and LH determined in normal women. Centered according to day of LH peak (day 0). (From Yen, S. S. C., Vela, P., Rankin, J., and Littell, A. S.: J.A.M.A. **211:**1513, 1970.)

of androstenedione are the same in testis, ovary, and adrenal cortex and may be summarized in the following manner:

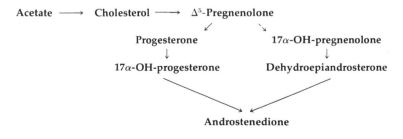

Androstenedione either may be converted directly to estrone or may form testosterone, which in turn is converted to estradiol.

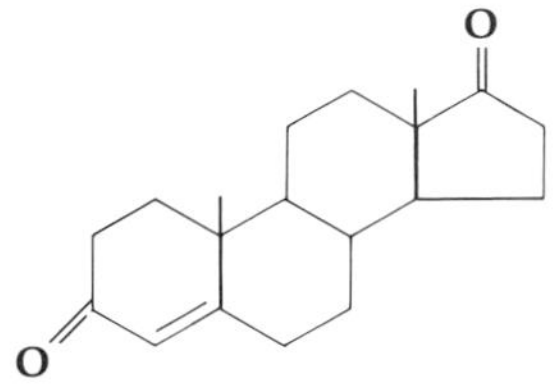

Androstenedione

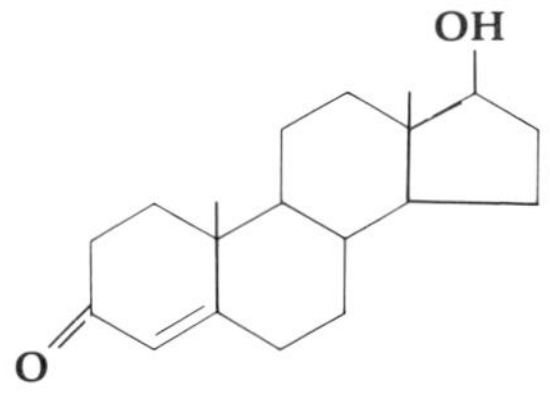

Testosterone

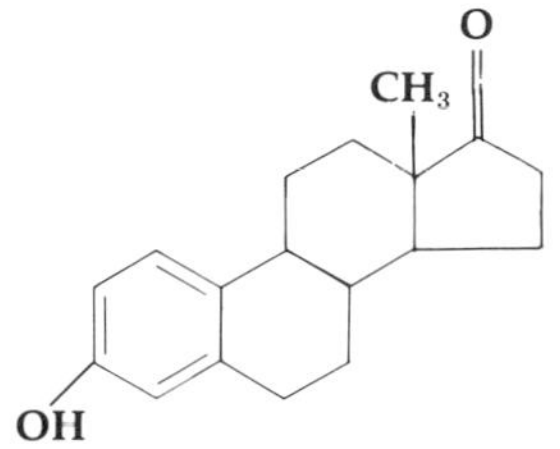

Estrone

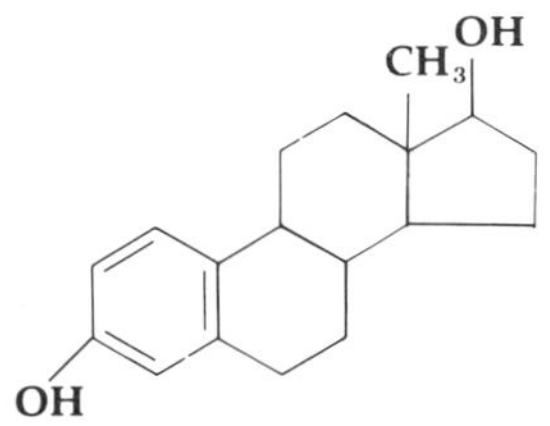

Estradiol

Testosterone may be formed not only in the testis but also in the ovary and the adrenal cortex. Testosterone in women originates from these nontesticular sources. Plasma testosterone levels are about ten times higher in males than in females.[26]

ESTROGENS

The estrogens have important effects on uterine development and cyclic endometrial changes associated with ovulation. They are also responsible for secondary sex characteristics in the female. Study of the estrogens has been greatly facilitated by the early development of a bioassay method[1] based on changes the estrogens produce in the vaginal smear of the rat. The first estrogen isolated and synthesized was estrone, originally called *Theelin*.

Types

The available estrogens are of two types: the natural and semisynthetic compounds and the synthetic estrogens. The members of the first group either occur naturally or represent slight chemical modifications of such natural compounds.

The synthetic drugs such as diethylstilbestrol appear to be quite different chemically.

Natural and semisynthetic estrogens. Estradiol, also known as α-estradiol or 17β-estradiol, is the most potent estrogen produced by the ovary. It is used in doses of 0.1 to 0.5 mg. three times a day in the form of tablets. It is also available in pellets of 0.4 mg. for vaginal suppositories. Oily preparations can also be obtained for intramuscular injection.

Estradiol benzoate, estradiol cyclopentylpropionate, and estradiol dipropionate are available in solution in oil for intramuscular injection.

Estrone is used for intramuscular injection and vaginal suppositories.

Estrogenic substances, conjugated, contain a mixture of estrogens obtained from the urine of pregnant mares. The estrogens are in a conjugated form and are water soluble, whereas the previously mentioned preparations have low water solubility. This mixture is commonly used in the form of tablets, but solutions for parenteral administration are also available. These preparations contain sodium estrone sulfonate and equine estrogens. Their activity is expressed in terms of an equivalent amount of sodium estrone sulfonate. An example of this type of preparation is Premarin. Tablets of this preparation contain amounts varying from 0.3 to 2.5 mg. A synthetic conjugated estrogen is piperazine estrone sulfate.

Ethinyl estradiol is a semisynthetic estrogen of high potency. It is available in tablets and is administered in doses of 0.02 to 0.05 mg. one to three times a day. The 3-methyl ether of ethinyl estradiol, known as *mestranol,* is commonly used in contraceptive progestin-estrogen combinations.

Estriol may be a conversion product of estradiol. It is available in tablet form and is administered in doses of 0.06 to 0.12 mg. one to four times a day.

The structural formulas of these naturally occurring and semisynthetic estrogens are shown below.

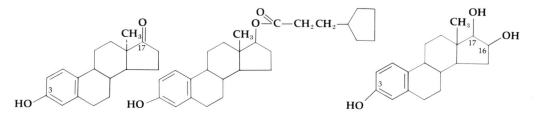

Estrone   Estradiol cyclopentylpropionate   Estriol

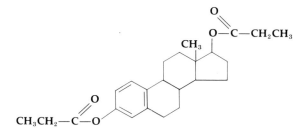

Estradiol dipropionate

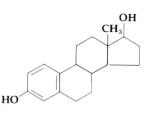

Estradiol

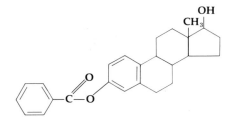
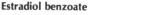

Estradiol benzoate

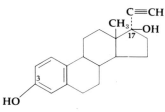

Ethinyl estradiol

516

Synthetic (nonsteroidal) estrogens. The synthesis of diethylstilbestrol[4] led to recognition of the fact that simple derivatives of stilbene can produce all the effects of naturally occurring estrogens in the body. In addition, they are highly effective when administered by mouth. Many of the synthetic estrogens can be visualized as having basic structural similarities to estradiol. Others, termed proestrogens, must undergo metabolic alteration before they become active in the body. A prime example of a proestrogen is chlorotrianisene.

Diethylstilbestrol is used in tablet form, in ointments and suppositories, and in oily solutions for intramuscular injection. The usual dose is 0.5 to 1 mg./day.

Other synthetic estrogens are dienestrol, hexestrol, benzestrol, and promethestrol dipropionate. The doses of these are of the same order of magnitude as those of diethylstilbestrol.

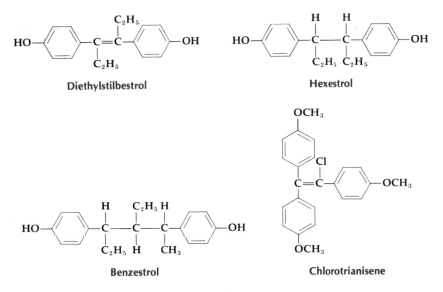

Diethylstilbestrol

Hexestrol

Benzestrol

Chlorotrianisene

Chlorotrianisene (Tace) has a very long duration of action, probably as a consequence of its storage in body fat. It is believed to be converted to an active compound in the body. It is available in capsules containing 12 mg. in corn oil.

Clomiphene (Clomid), a drug structurally related to chlorotrianisene, appears to stimulate pituitary gonadotropin output in women, although it inhibits the pituitary in the rat. It is being tried with some success in treatment of some types of infertility.[5] Clomiphene has been termed an *antiestrogen*. Its stimulant effect on gonadotropin output in women may be a consequence of removal of inhibition exerted by estrogens.

Clomiphene, available in 50 mg. tablets, is used for promoting ovulation. Administered in courses of several days, the drug is highly effective. It can also have adverse effects, causing menopausal symptoms (hot flashes), enlargement of the ovaries, and multiple pregnancies that are more common than in normally ovulating women. This incidence has been estimated as 5 to 10%.

Other fertility drugs. It is of considerable investigational interest that extracts of human pituitary or of menopausal urine (human menopausal gonadotropins) are highly effective in promoting ovulation. Given by injection, these investigational drugs cause considerable enlargement of the ovary and an abnormally high incidence of multiple pregnancies.

The preparation of **human menopausal gonadotropins (menotropins)** contains large amounts of FSH and LH. Its mode of action involves the ovary directly, whereas clomiphene acts indirectly as an antiestrogen on the production of the gonadotropins. Enlargement of the ovary occurs within two weeks after the administration of menotropins and may lead to ascites, bleeding, and rupture of ovarian cysts. Multiple births may occur in 20% of women who become pregnant after the use of menotropins.

The preparation is injected intramuscularly and is administered daily for ten days. Menotropins (Pergonal) are available as a powder containing 75 IU of FSH and 75 IU of LH to make a solution for intramuscular injection.

Effects

The estrogens are responsible for the proliferative changes of the endometrium during the ovulatory cycle. In rodents their effect is recognizable by the appearance of the vaginal smear, since induction of estrus is associated with cornification of the vaginal epithelium. The international unit for the estrogens is the activity of 0.1 μg of estrone. This small quantity is sufficient to produce changes in the vaginal smear of a castrated mouse. It may be estimated that the quantity of estrogen necessary for replacing normal ovarian activity in the human female over a period of weeks may be as much as 1 million units. This apparently large quantity is equivalent to 100 mg. of estrone and considerably less of the more potent estrogens.

The activity of the various estrogens in the human female may be estimated on the basis of withdrawal bleeding that takes place when the estrogen is administered to amenorrheic women for about 2 weeks and is then suddenly discontinued. When assayed in this manner on ovariectomized women, the various estrogens could be placed in the following order according to their potency[2]: ethinyl estradiol (oral), estradiol dipropionate (intramuscular), diethylstilbestrol (oral), estrone (intramuscular), hexestrol (oral), estradiol (oral), and estrone (oral).

The high activity of oral ethinyl estradiol may be attributed to the protection that this chemical modification of estradiol confers against gastrointestinal and hepatic inactivation of the ingested hormone.

Several extrauterine actions of the estrogens have also received attention. These compounds depress the secretion of FSH. The urinary excretion of FSH is increased in ovariectomized women, but this elevation is abolished by the administration of estrogens. The ability of estrogens to inhibit ovulation on chronic administration is probably due to this interaction with FSH.

Estrogens can also cause salt and water retention and an increase in transcortin and thyroxine-binding proteins in the serum and can exert complex effects on plasma lipoproteins. Plasma cortisol and protein-bound iodine levels become elevated.

Metabolism

There is much experimental evidence to indicate that the natural estrogens are inactivated in the body, the liver being considered the most important organ affecting this biotransformation. Persons with liver damage, as in cirrhosis, may excrete a much higher percentage of an estrogen than do normal persons. This hepatic inactivation is also the probable reason for the greater effectiveness of the natural estrogens when administered parenterally. Estrone, for example, may be ten times as effective by the intramuscular route as by mouth. On the other hand, the synthetic estrogens are highly effective by mouth. This and other evidence indicate that synthetic estrogens are not degraded as rapidly or as completely as are the natural forms. Chlorotrianisene has a prolonged action because it is stored in body fat.

Toxicity

The only adverse effects of the estrogens observed in a significant number of patients are anorexia, nausea, and vomiting. These symptoms are more likely to develop following the use of the synthetic compounds, diethylstilbestrol being the worst offender in this respect. It is likely, however, that some women become nauseated following the use of any of the estrogens.

There is increasing suspicion of an association between maternal intake of diethylstilbestrol during pregnancy and the appearance of vaginal carcinoma years later in the offspring.[8] Because of this, appropriate warnings on the labels of estrogens are now required by the Food and Drug Administration.

Therapeutic applications

Estrogens are used widely for menopausal disturbances, atrophic vaginitis, inhibition of lactation, menstrual disturbances, osteoporosis, and some types of prostatic and mammary carcinoma.

Commonly used estrogens and their daily doses for the menopausal syndrome are as follows: esterified or conjugated equine estrogens, 1.25 mg.; ethinyl estradiol, 0.05 mg.; dienestrol, 0.50 mg.; methallenestril (Vallestril), 3 mg.; diethylstilbestrol, 0.20 mg.

The use of estrogens in osteoporosis is based on the belief that in postmenopausal patients there is an osteoblastic defect attributable to estrogen deficiency. More recent studies indicate that osteoporosis results from excessive bone resorption. Furthermore, estrogens or high calcium intake may slow down the progress of the disease but will not bring bone density back to normal, even in postmenopausal patients. The importance of high calcium intake in slowing progression of osteoporosis is increasingly emphasized.

PROGESTERONE

Progesterone is produced by the corpus luteum and has also been prepared synthetically. Its structural formula is shown below along with that of **ethisterone**.

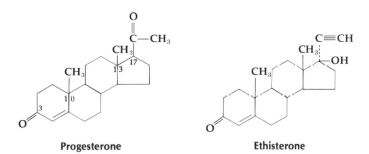

Progesterone   Ethisterone

Progesterone is responsible for the secretory phase of endometrial development. Its effects on the vaginal epithelium and on cervical mucous secretions are the opposite of those of the estrogens. Withdrawal of progesterone results in menstruation. Progesterone is metabolically degraded to pregnanediol, which appears in the urine.

Pharmacologic effects of large doses of progesterone include suppression of ovulation, inhibition of the contractility of the uterus, increased sodium excretion, and negative nitrogen balance.

The hormone is assayed in the rabbit on the basis of its progestational effect on the endometrium; the international unit is 1 mg. of purified progesterone.

Metabolism

Progesterone is not well absorbed from the gastrointestinal tract following oral administration. It is much more effective when injected by the intramuscular route or administered sublingually. The intramuscular dose is 10 mg. Similar or even larger doses are used sublingually. Progesterone is metabolically altered in the body, the liver playing an important role in this respect. The urinary excretory products of progesterone are pregnanediol and pregnanolone.

Clinical uses

Progesterone and particularly the *progestogens* find applications in numerous clinical situations. The progestogens are synthetic derivatives of 19-nortestosterone or progesterone. In contrast with progesterone, they are effective when given orally. They differ also in that some preparations are androgenic, but others have estrogenic activity.

Progesterone and the progestogens are used for the cyclic treatment of amenorrhea and dysmenorrhea besides antifertility effects. In addition, these hormones may be useful in the treatment of threatened abortions and as replacement therapy in infertile women.

Progesterone itself is available in the form of parenteral preparations in water or oil for intramuscular injection. The drug is ineffective when given by mouth.

The following progestogens are used for purposes other than contraception.

Hydroxyprogesterone caproate (Delalutin) is a progesterone derivative without estrogenic activity and without masculinizing effect on the fetus. It is available as an injectable solution in oil, 125 mg./ml., administered intramuscularly.

Dydrogesterone (Duphaston; Gynorest) is a progesterone derivative that is active by oral administration. The drug has no estrogenic or androgenic activity. It is available in tablets containing 5 and 10 mg.

Norethindrone (Norlutin) and **norethindrone acetate** (Norlutate) are derivatives of 19-nortestosterone, having some androgenic activity. They should not be used in threatened abortion because of masculinizing effect on the fetus. Both drugs are available in tablets containing 5 mg.

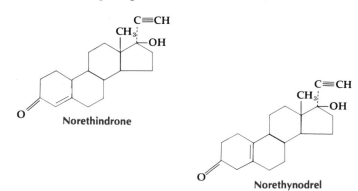

Norethindrone

Norethynodrel

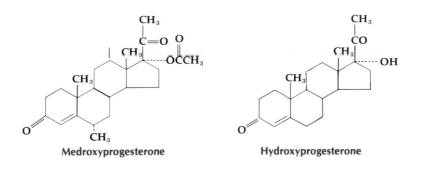

Medroxyprogesterone   Hydroxyprogesterone

ORAL CONTRACEPTIVES

The first report on the successful inhibition of ovulation by orally administered norethynodrel-mestranol appeared in 1956. Just 10 years later more than seven million women were taking oral contraceptives. Results indicate that such drugs are the most effective means of controlling fertility, although all the ultimate consequences of such a mass medication are not completely known.

The contraceptive medications are of three types: (1) progestogen-estrogen combinations, (2) sequential estrogen-progestogen contraceptives, and (3) low-dosage progestogens.

Progestogen-estrogen combinations. The mode of action of the combined administration of progestogens and estrogens involves the inhibition of ovulation by an interference with hypothalamic-pituitary mechanisms. They may also have additional sites of action. There is good evidence for an alteration of the characteristics of cervical mucus by the combined treatment. It is possible also that the changes in the endometrium or the secretions of the fallopian tubes are such as to interfere with fertilization.

The progestogen-estrogen combinations are used in the following manner. A single dose a day is taken from the fifth through the twenty-fourth day of the cycle, counting from the first day of menstruation. Withdrawal bleeding occurs within 3 to 4 days after the last dose.

Sequential estrogen-progestogen contraceptives. Estrogen alone is administered from the fifth through the nineteenth or twentieth day of the cycle. After that, progestogen is added to the estrogen for 4 to 5 days. The estrogen in the first part of the cycle probably inhibits ovulation, although ovulations do occur on occasion. Progestogen is added for the purpose of promoting complete maturation and subsequent prompt shedding of the endometrium during the withdrawal bleeding. Withdrawal bleeding usually occurs 2 to 5 days after discontinuing the medication.

Low-dosage progestogens. Continued low-dosage progestogen is also being tried as an approach to the contol of fertility. Chlormadinone, an analog of medroxyprogesterone, has antifertility effects in very small doses. This form of treatment does not prevent ovulation. The mode of action of low-dosage progestogen is not clear. It may put the endometrium out of phase with ovulation or it may alter cervical mucus or tubal physiology. These explanations are purely speculative.

Adverse effects

A number of adverse effects may occur during the administration of the oral contraceptives. Breakthrough bleeding is not uncommon and may call for an increase in dosage or discontinuation of medication to allow withdrawal bleeding to take place. Enlargement of the breast and mastalgia are common. Increases in transcortin and thyroxine-binding protein interfere with tests for thyroid and adrenal function. Disturbances in liver function and glucose tolerance have been observed, but sodium retention has not been found. Headache and cerebral and visual disturbances may be seen occasionally.

Other adverse effects of oral contraceptives are nausea and vomiting, elevation of blood pressure, skin reactions, and a drug interaction with the coumarin drugs, requiring an increase in dosage of the anticoagulants.

The possible relationship between oral contraceptives and thromboembolic disorders is receiving increasing attention. The British Committee on the Safety of Drugs recommended to all practicing physicians (December, 1969) that the lower-dose estrogen products be used instead of the high-dose products. It is believed by competent authorities in the United States that oral contraceptives and estrogens per se increase the risk of thromboembolic disorders. It is also believed that a higher estrogen dose is correlated with increased risk and therefore the lowest estrogen dose is preferable. While the risk of thromboembolic disorders is not as great in women who take oral contraceptives as in those who become pregnant, it nevertheless does exist and should be taken into consideration by the physician in making his therapeutic decision.

ANDROGENS
TESTOSTERONE

The principal testicular hormone is testosterone. Its isolation and synthesis from testicular extracts were preceded by the isolation of one of its metabolic products, androsterone.

Esterification of testosterone results in compounds with certain advantages. For example, methyltestosterone is effective when given in tablet form by mouth, whereas testosterone is destroyed rapidly when given by the same route. Testosterone propionate is available in buccal tablets for absorption from the oral cavity.

The most widely used androgens are testosterone, methyltestosterone propionate, and testosterone cyclopentylpropionate. The structural formulas of these compounds are shown below.

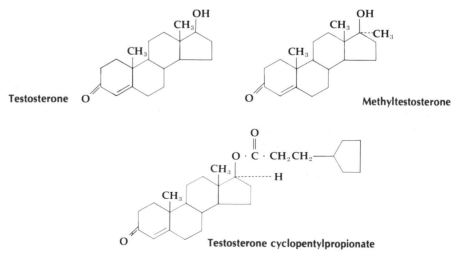

Testosterone

Methyltestosterone

Testosterone cyclopentylpropionate

Effects

The male sex hormone is responsible for the development and maintenance of male secondary sex characteristics, the male sex organs, and related structures.

The physiologic effects of testosterone can be reproduced when the hormone is administered as replacement therapy in males with gonadal deficiency due to prepuberal or postpuberal castration. Testosterone also has many other actions that may be looked upon as pharmacologic.

In the female, testosterone produces masculinization, with hirsutism, growth of the clitoris, change in the voice, and acne. It is of great importance to realize that clinical use of the hormone in the female can cause personality changes and marked increase in libido.

The androgens, just as the estrogens, not only can accelerate the growth of epiphyseal cartilage but also can promote closure of the epiphysis.

Testosterone is generally said to have a protein anabolic effect; that is, it can produce a positive balance of nitrogen and also of potassium, phosphorus, and sodium.

The protein anabolic effect of testosterone is exerted mainly on secondary sex tissue, although increased protein deposition has also been demonstrated at other sites. The stimulation of protein synthesis by testosterone is not caused by an influence on amino acid transport but is a specific action on microsomal ribonucleic acid fraction.[17] The conversion of testosterone to dihydrotestosterone in the body has been demonstrated.[18]

METABOLISM OF ANDROGENS

The various androgens are well absorbed from the gastrointestinal tract but are rapidly metabolized by the liver. Methyltestosterone is absorbed effectively when swallowed or held in the mouth and is not destroyed as rapidly by the liver. Testosterone propionate and testosterone cyclopentylpropionate are available in oil for intramuscular injection. Because of the slow absorption from the intramuscular site, the duration of action of these preparations is prolonged. Thus a single injection may produce effects for 1 or 2 days. Subcutaneous implantation of pellets or the use of aqueous suspensions of testosterone propionate can have greatly prolonged effects.

Testosterone is metabolized in the body to several steroidal compounds. Androsterone and isoandrosterone retain some androgenic activity, whereas etiocholanolone is inactive. The androgens appear in the urine in the conjugated form. Most of them are 17-ketosteroids that originate from the testis or from the adrenal cortex. Conversion to dihydrotestosterone may be of great interest.[18]

ANABOLIC STEROIDS

After the anabolic effects of testosterone were demonstrated, efforts were made to dissociate them from the androgenic effects. This research has resulted in a group of drugs known as *anabolic steroids*. Although these steroids have a greater effect on nitrogen retention than their virilizing action would predict, the separation of these effects is not complete. As a consequence, they should be used with great caution in children with growth problems.

The anabolic steroids are used sometimes in the treatment of osteoporosis and various conditions in which a negative nitrogen balance exists.

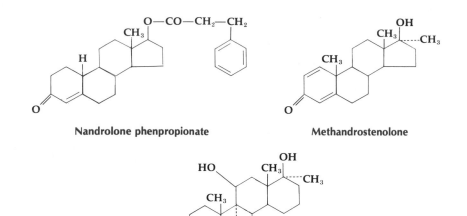

Nandrolone phenpropionate

Methandrostenolone

Fluoxymesterone

The anabolic steroids available for oral administration are ethylesternol (Maxibolin), methandrostenolone (Dianabol), norethandrolone (Nilevar), oxandrolone (Anavar), oxymetholone (Adroyd; Anadrol), and stanozolol (Winstrol). Anabolic steroids for intramuscular use include nandrolone phenpropionate (Durabolin), nandrolone decanoate (Deca-Durabolin), and norethandrolone injection (Nilevar). Fluoxymesterone (Halotestin; Ora-Testryl; Ultandren) is used not only as an anabolic steroid but also for androgen deficiency.

The anabolic steroids have numerous disadvantages. They may cause sodium retention, masculinization of the fetus if used in pregnant women (a definite contraindication), and aggravation of carcinoma of the prostate. Their use is hazardous in children because of their virilizing effect. In addition, androgens or estrogens may actually lead to premature epiphyseal closure when used in children to stimulate their growth. Another adverse effect caused by anabolic steroids that resemble methyltestosterone (17-alkyl-substituted steroids) is cholestatic jaundice.

References

1 Allen, E., and Doisy, E. A.: An ovarian hormone: preliminary report on its localization, extraction and partial purification, and action in test animals, J.A.M.A. 81:819, 1923.

2 Allen, W. M.: The biological activity of various estrogens, Southern Med. J. 37:270, 1944.

3 DeCosta, E. J.: Those deceptive contraceptives, J.A.M.A. 181:122, 1962.

4 Dodds, E. C., Goldberg, L., Lawson, W., and Robinson, R.: Oestrogenic activity of alkylated stilboestrols, Nature 142:34, 1938.

5 Greenblatt, R. B., Rey, S., Mahesh, V. B., Barfield, W. E., and Jungck, E. C.: Induction of ovulation, Amer. J. Obstet. Gynec. 84:900, 1962.

6 Greep, R. O.: Physiology of the anterior hypophysis in relation to reproduction. In Young, I. W. C., editor: Sex and internal secretions,

vol. 1, Baltimore, 1961, The Williams & Wilkins Co.

7 Hazzard, W. R., Spiger, M. J., Bagdade, J. D., and Bierman, E. L.: Studies on the mechanism of increased plasma triglyceride levels induced by oral contraceptives, New Eng. J. Med. 280: 471, 1969.

8 Herbst, A. L., Ulfelder, H., and Proskanzer, D. C.: Adenocarcinoma of the vagina: association of maternal stilbestrol therapy with tumor appearance in young women, New Eng. J. Med. 284:878, 1971.

9 Kamberi, I. A., Mical, R. S., and Porter, J. C.: Luteinizing hormone-releasing activity in hypophysial stalk blood and elevation by dopamine, Science 166:388, 1969.

10 Kobayashi, Y. Kupelian, J., and Maudsley, D. V.: Ornithine decarboxylase stimulation in rat

ovary by luteinizing hormone, Science **172**:379, 1971.

11 Lin, T. J., Durkin, J. W., Jr., and Kim, Y. J.: The control of reproduction and of the functions of certain endocrine organs as reflected by biochemical and biological assays, Curr. Ther. Res. **6**:225, 1964.

12 Masi, A. T., and Dugdale, M.: Cerebrovascular diseases associated with the use of oral contraceptives, Ann. Intern. Med. **72**:65, 1970.

13 Pincus, G.: The physiology of ovarian hormones. In Pincus, G., and Thimann, K. V., editors: The hormones: physiology, chemistry and applications, vol. 2, New York, 1950, Academic Press, Inc.

14 Saruta, T., Saade, G. A., and Kaplan, N.: A possible mechanism for hypertension induced by oral contraceptives, Arch. Intern. Med. **126**: 621, 1970.

15 Schneider, H. P. G., and McCann, S. M.: Release of LH-releasing factor (LRF) into the peripheral circulation of hypophysectomized rats by dopamine and its blockade by estradiol, Endocrinology **87**:249, 1970.

16 Tyler, E. T.: Treatment of anovulation with menotropins, J.A.M.A. **205**:16, 1968.

17 Wilson, J. D.: Localization of the biochemical site of action of testosterone on protein synthesis in the seminal vesicle of the rat, J. Clin. Invest. **41**:153, 1962.

18 Yen, S. S. C., Vela, P., Rankin, J., and Littel, A. S.: Hormonal relationships during the menstrual cycle, J.A.M.A. **211**:1513, 1970.

Recent reviews

19 Berczeller, P. H., Young, I. S., and Kupperman, H. S.: The therapeutic use of progestational steroids, Clin. Pharmacol. Ther. **5**:216, 1964.

20 Bogdanove, E. M.: Hypothalamic-hypophysial interrelationships: basic aspects. In Balin and Glasser, eds., Reproductive biology, Amsterdam, 1972, Excerpta Medica Foundation.

21 Clinical aspects of oral gestogens, No. 326, WHO Technical Report Series, 1966.

22 Evaluation of oral contraceptives, J.A.M.A. **199**:650, 1967.

23 Frohman, L. A.: Clinical neuropharmacology of hypothalamic releasing factors, New Eng. J. Med. **286**:1391, 1972.

24 Kellie, A. E.: The pharmacology of the estrogens, Ann. Rev. Pharmacol. **11**:97, 1971.

25 Lednicer, D.: Contraception: the chemical control of fertility, New York, 1969, Marcel Dekker, Inc.

26 Lipsett, M. B., and Korenman, S. G.: Androgen metabolism, J.A.M.A. **190**:757, 1964.

27 Lloyd, C. W., and Weisz, J.: Some aspects of reproductive physiology, Ann. Rev. Physiol. **28**:267, 1966.

28 McCann, S. M., and Porter, J. C.: Hypothalamic pituitary stimulating and inhibiting hormones, Physiol. Rev. **49**:240, 1969.

29 Nalbandov, A. V., and Cook, B.: Reproduction, Ann. Rev. Physiol. **30**:245, 1968.

30 Pincus, G., and Bialy, G.: Drugs used in control of reproduction, Advances Pharmacol. **3**:285, 1964.

31 Reichlin, S.: Anterior pituitary — six glands and one, New Eng. J. Med. **287**:1351, 1972.

32 Rogers, J.: Estrogens in the menopause and postmenopause, New Eng. J. Med. **280**:364, 1969.

33 Rudel, H. W.: Mechanisms of action of hormonal antifertility agents, Pharmacol. Physicians **2**(2):1, 1968.

34 Turkington, R. W.: Prolactin secretion in patients treated with various drugs, Arch. Intern. Med. **130**:349, 1972.

35 Tyler, E. T.: Antifertility agents, Ann. Rev. Pharmacol. **7**:381, 1967.

36 Wilson, J. D.: Recent studies on the mechanism of action of testosterone, New Eng. J. Med. **287**: 1284, 1972.

43 Pharmacologic approaches to gout

Gout is a disease characterized by hyperuricemia, history of arthritis, presence of urate crystals in the synovial fluid, and clinical response to colchicine within 24 hours. The disease may be of the primary familial type or may be secondary to renal disease, to drugs that block urate excretion, or to metabolic overproduction of urates.

The uric acid concentration in the serum of normal persons is 2 to 5 mg./100 ml. In gouty individuals the mean uric acid level may be 8.8 mg./100 ml.[4] Interestingly, however, the metabolic abnormality may exist in members of the families of gouty patients without these persons' having the disease. This fact, together with the lesser incidence of the disease in women, suggests that gout may depend on multiple factors, only one of which is the metabolic error related to uric acid.

Not only is the uric acid level in the serum elevated in the gouty patient, but the miscible pool of uric acid as determined with ^{15}N-labeled compound is increased also.[19] It is believed by many investigators that the metabolic error consists of an increased production of uric acid, not just as an end product of the breakdown of purines from exogenous and endogenous sources, but by a pathway through which glycine may be converted to uric acid.[10, 11] A disturbance in urinary ammonia production and glutamine metabolism may also contribute to the increased uric acid production.[13]

The pharmacologic approach to an acute attack is different from the management of the chronic disease. The acute attack is a form of acute arthritis that responds best to *colchicine,* although *phenylbutazone, oxyphenbutazone, indomethacin,* or *adrenal corticoids* may also be effective. The aim of management of the chronic form of the disease is to reduce the uric acid content of the body with uricosuric drugs such as *probenecid* or *sulfinpyrazone.* The use of *allopurinol,* a xanthine oxidase inhibitor, may have advantages over the uricosuric drugs in some cases.

[handwritten: Rela to salicylates]

COLCHICINE

Colchicine is an alkaloid obtained from *Colchicum autumnale,* or meadow saffron, a plant belonging to the lily family. Colchicum has been used for centuries for arthralgia that is presumably of gouty origin. Its effect in acute gout is quite remarkable, although its mode of action is still completely obscure.

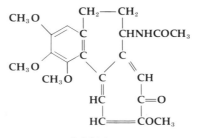

Colchicine

526

When colchicine is given in doses of 0.5 to 1 mg. every hour to a patient having an attack of acute gouty arthritis, relief occurs in 2 to 3 hours, but in severe attacks a somewhat longer period is required. It is quite common for gastrointestinal disturbances such as anorexia, nausea, vomiting, diarrhea, and abdominal pain to appear with about the same dosage as the one required for relief. As a consequence, colchicine is administered every hour until relief is obtained or significant gastrointestinal symptoms develop. In addition to gastrointestinal side effects, colchicine may also cause, though rarely, fever, alopecia, liver damage, and neural and hematopoietic complications.[6]

The mode of action of colchicine is quite mysterious. The drug is not an analgesic and does not benefit arthritis, except that seen in gout. It does not promote excretion of uric acid and fails to alter the concentration of uric acid in the serum or the miscible pool of the compound in the body.

Colchicine can arrest cell division in the metaphase, and it is an interesting tool in the study of chromosomes. Its basic morphologic effect is on microtubules in cells, which become destroyed or disorganized.

An interesting suggestion has been advanced concerning acute gouty inflammation and the action of colchicine.[17] The injection of sharp urate crystals into the knee joint was followed by a typical gouty attack, whereas the effect of amorphous urate was much less. The inflammatory action of the crystals is associated with phagocytosis by leukocytes. It is suggested that colchicine may block the inflammatory response or the phagocytosis of the urate crystals.

In chronic gout the administration of colchicine appears to have prophylactic value with regard to the incidence of acute exacerbations. In addition, it is generally believed that the promotion of uric acid excretion through the use of the uricosuric drugs is beneficial in the gouty patient. The most effective uricosuric agents are the salicylates, probenecid, and sulfinpyrazone.

PROBENECID

Probenecid (Benemid) was developed for the purpose of inhibiting tubular secretion of penicillin.[1] Although effective, it is seldom used for this purpose because it is simpler to increase the dosage of penicillin rather than to use two drugs to achieve a higher blood level of the antibiotic. Whereas the original purpose in the development of probenecid appears unimportant now, the drug was found to be a potent uricosuric agent.

The structural formula of probenecid is as follows:

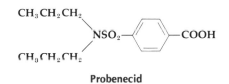

Probenecid

Probenecid causes marked increase in excretion of uric acid in gouty patients. The drug has been given in doses of 0.5 Gm. three or four times daily for years to gouty patients and has produced significant lowering of serum uric acid. In fact, increased urinary concentration of uric acid may lead to development of urate stones, and therefore alkalinization of the urine may be desirable in the early stages of therapy.

The uricosuric effect of probenecid is exerted on the renal tubules and is generally attributed to inhibition of uric acid reabsorption. Interestingly, the simultaneous administration of salicylates appears to nullify the uricosuric action of probenecid.

Renal handling of uric acid apparently involves glomerular filtration, tubular reabsorption, and tubular secretion.[2] Organic anions such as salicylates and probenecid cause retention of uric acid at low doses but are uricosuric at high doses.[21] It is likely that in small doses they compete with uric acid for secretion.

The ability of thiazide diuretics and pyrazinamide to cause uric acid retention may be explained also by an interference with uric acid secretion.[8]

Problem 43-1. Since pyrazinamide blocks uric acid secretion, what would be its effect on the uricosuric action of probenecid? This problem has been investigated in man.[18] Assuming that pyrazinamide selectively inhibits the tubular secretion of urate whereas probenecid acts by increasing the excretion of filtered urate, then the uricosuric response (the increment in urate excretion) should have been unaffected by pyrazinamide. The results of the studies show, however, that the uricosuric responses to probenecid were significantly depressed by pyrazinamide. This finding suggests that probenecid facilitates the excretion of both filtered and secreted urate.

In addition to its uricosuric effect, probenecid inhibits tubular secretion of penicillin, iodopyracet (Diodrast), and p-aminohippurate. It also blocks conjugation of benzoic acid with glycine and increases the blood levels of p-aminosalicylate by some unknown mechanism.

Probenecid is rapidly absorbed from the gastrointestinal tract. It is conjugated with glycuronic acid and is excreted largely in this form.[3]

During the use of probenecid for chronic gout, adverse effects may occur in a small percentage of patients. The figure generally given is less than 2%, but in some series adverse reactions or side effects have occurred in 8% of patients.[5] Nausea and vomiting, skin rash, and drug fever may occur. Urate stones may cause renal colic.

SULFINPYRAZONE

Sulfinpyrazone (Anturan), structurally related to phenylbutazone, is an effective uricosuric agent. This drug prevents tubular reabsorption of uric acid. Its action is antagonized by salicylates but not by probenecid. The marked increase in urate excretion may predispose to urolithiasis. An acute gouty attack may occur at the beginning of treatment, and epigastric distress has been seen. The similarity in structure between sulfinpyrazone and phenylbutazone suggests caution with regard to hematologic disturbances. The usual dose is 50 mg. four times daily initially, which may be gradually increased until as much as 400 mg. is given daily.

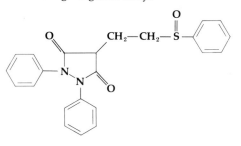

Sulfinpyrazone

ALLOPURINOL

An interesting approach to the treatment of gout is the use of an inhibitor of xanthine oxidase. Allopurinol (Zyloprim) was developed originally for the purpose of protecting 6-mercaptopurine against rapid inactivation in the body. The drug causes a marked decrease in plasma uric acid concentration and in urinary uric acid excretion. Although the oxypurines xanthine and hypoxanthine replace uric acid under these circumstances, renal clearance of the oxypurines is much greater than that of uric acid.

Allopurinol is rapidly oxidized in the body to alloxanthine, and 90 to 95% of allopurinol administered is excreted as alloxanthine, the remainder as the original allopurinol. The renal clearance of allopurinol is rapid, while that of alloxanthine is slow — only two or three times the clearance of uric acid. Probenecid promotes the excretion of alloxanthine.

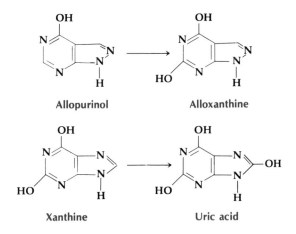

Allopurinol   Alloxanthine

Xanthine   Uric acid

In a series of gouty subjects who showed an intolerance to uricosuric agents or failed to respond to them, normal serum urate levels were achieved with doses of 200 to 600 mg./day of allopurinol.[16]

A summary of the present position of allopurinol in the treatment of gout is as follows. While uricosuric agents are effective in controlling hyperuricemia in most gouty patients, allopurinol may prove to be more useful for a number of reasons. Gouty nephropathy and the formation of urate stones are less likely with allopurinol therapy because the drug *reduces* the amount of uric acid excreted. Colchicine is still the treatment of choice in acute gout and is helpful in the prevention of acute attacks. In severe cases associated with impaired renal function and urate stones, allopurinol appears to be the agent of choice. In addition, the anti-inflammatory drugs phenylbutazone and indomethacin may be very useful in the treatment of acute gout.

Reactions to allopurinol have been mild or moderate, although about 3% of patients taking the drug may develop skin eruptions, fever, hepatomegaly, and leukopenia.

References

1 Beyer, K. H.: Functional characteristics of renal transport mechanisms, Pharmacol. Rev. 2:227, 1950.

2 Beyer, K. H., and Baer, J. E.: Physiological basis for the action of newer diuretic agents, Pharmacol. Rev. 13:517, 1961.

3 Beyer, K. H., et al.: "Benemid," *p*-(di-*n*-propyl-sulfamyl)-benzoic acid: its renal affinity and its elimination, Amer. J. Physiol. 166:625, 1951.

4 Bishop, C., and Talbott, J. H.: Uric acid: its role in biological processes and the influence upon it of physiological, pathological, and pharmacological agents, Pharmacol. Rev. 5:231, 1953.

5 Boger, W. P., and Strickland, S. C.: Probenecid (Benemid): its uses and side effects in 2502 patients, Arch. Intern. Med. 95:83, 1955.

6 Carr, A. A.: Colchicine toxicity, Arch. Intern. Med. 115:29, 1965.

7 DeConti, R. C., and Calabresi, P.: Use of allopurinol for the prevention and control of hyperuricemia in patients with neoplastic disease, New Eng. J. Med. **274**:481, 1966.

8 Demartini, F. E., Wheaton, E. A., Healey, L. A., and Laragh, J. A.: Effect of chlorothiazide on the renal excretion of uric acid, Amer. J. Med. **32**:572, 1962.

9 Goldfinger, S., Klinenberg, J., and Seegmiller, J. E.: The renal excretion of oxypurines, J. Clin. Invest. **44**:623, 1965.

10 Gutman, A. B.: Uric acid metabolism and gout, Amer. J. Med. **9**:799, 1950.

11 Gutman, A. B.: Primary and secondary gout, Ann. Intern. Med. **39**:1062, 1953.

12 Gutman, A. B., Yu, T.-F., and Berger, L.: Tubular secretion of urate in man, J. Clin. Invest. **38**:1778, 1959.

13 Gutman, A. B., and Yu, T.-F.: Urinary ammonia excretion in primary gout, J. Clin. Invest. **44**:1474, 1965.

14 Klinenberg, J. R., Goldfinger, S. E., and Seegmiller, J. E.: The effectiveness of the xanthine oxidase inhibitor allopurinol in the treatment of gout, Ann. Intern Med. **62**:639, 1965.

15 Pagliara, A. S., and Goodman, D.: Elevation of plasma glutamate in gout; its possible role in the pathogenesis of hyperuricemia, New Eng. J. Med. **281**:767, 1969.

16 Rundles, R. W., Metz, E. N., and Silberman, H. R.: Allopurinol in the treatment of gout, Ann. Intern. Med. **64**:229, 1966.

17 Seegmiller, J. E., Howel, R. R., and Malawista, S. E.: The inflammatory reaction to sodium urate: its possible relationship to the genesis of acute gouty arthritis, J.A.M.A. **180**:469, 1962.

18 Steele, T. H., and Boner, G.: Origins of the uricosuric response, J. Clin. Invest. **52**:1368, 1973.

19 Stetten, DeW., Jr.: On the metabolic defect in gout, Bull. N. Y. Acad. Med. **28**:664, 1952.

20 Wallace, S. L., Omokoku, B., and Ertel, N. H.: Colchicine plasma levels, Amer. J. Med. **48**:443, 1970.

21 Yu, T.-F., and Gutman, A. B.: Study of the paradoxical effects of salicylate in low, intermediate and high dosage on the renal mechanisms for excretion of urate in man, J. Clin. Invest. **38**:1298, 1959.

Recent reviews

22 Calkins, E.: The treatment of gout, Rational Drug Therapy **5**:1, Feb., 1971.

23 Goldfinger, S. E.: Treatment of gout, New Eng. J. Med. **285**:1303, 1971.

24 Gutman, A. B., and Yu, T.-F.: Uric acid metabolism in normal man and in primary gout, New Eng. J. Med. **273**:252, 1965.

25 Krakoff, I. H.: Clinical pharmacology of drugs which influence uric acid production and excretion, Clin. Pharmacol. Ther. **8**:124, 1967.

26 Rundles, R. W., and Wyngaarden, J. B. L.: Drugs and uric acid, Ann. Rev. Pharmacol. **9**:345, 1969.

27 Steele, T. H.: Control of uric acid secretion, New Eng. J. Med. **284**:1193, 1971.

28 Sorensen, L. B., and Pepe, P.: Hypoxanthine-guanine phosphoribosyltransferase deficiency, Bull. Rheum. Dis. **21**:621, 1970.

44 Antianemic drugs

The maintenance of normal red cell mass and the synthesis of hemoglobin are normally adjusted to take care of the physiologic loss of the blood elements. Anemia results when there is excessive loss or diminished replacement of red cells.

Most anemias are deficiency diseases resulting from inadequate tissue concentrations of *iron, vitamin B_{12},* or *folic acid.* Correction of the deficiency is highly successful provided an accurate diagnosis is made. In addition to the use of iron, vitamin B_{12}, and folic acid for correction of deficiencies, other drugs such as *anabolic steroids* and *pyridoxine* may be useful in some forms of anemia. *Erythropoietin* may be of great importance but is currently only of research interest.

IRON
Metabolism and effects

Iron is contained in the body in various forms, principally as hemoglobin. Normal blood contains about 15 grams of hemoglobin/100 ml., and each gram of hemoglobin contains 3.4 mg. of iron. It may be calculated then that the total normal blood volume contains about 2.6 grams of iron, and each milliliter of blood contains 0.5 mg.

In addition to hemoglobin, iron is contained in ferritin, the storage form for iron in the tissues, and in the serum attached to the carrier substance, the globulin transferrin. Minute quantities are also present in the cytochrome enzymes and myoglobin of muscle. Quantitatively, hemoglobin and ferritin contain the bulk of the iron in the body, amounting to a total of about 4 to 5 grams.

Under normal circumstances red cells are broken down at a steady rate, their lifespan being on the order of 120 days. Most of the iron released from the breakdown of hemoglobin is reutilized. As a consequence, the daily iron requirement in a normal adult is quite low, about 1 mg. Growth, menstruation, and pregnancy increase the iron requirement.

Absorption and excretion

Perhaps the most remarkable fact about the metabolism of iron is the inability of the body to get rid of significant quantities of this element. Only minute quantities are excreted into the feces, and the urinary loss of iron is even less. This is the reason for the very low iron requirement of normal persons.

Since the body does not readily eliminate iron, there must be a mechanism that limits its absorption. Otherwise the iron content of the body would steadily increase and hemochromatosis would develop. The mechanism that limits the absorption of iron from the intestine is often referred to as the mucosal block.

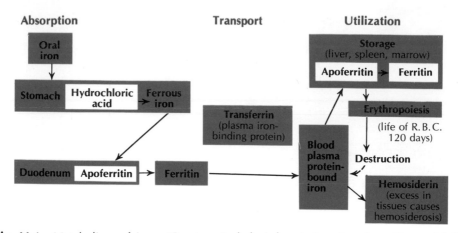

Fig. 44-1. Metabolism of iron. (Courtesy Lederle Laboratories, American Cyanamid Co., Pearl River, N. Y.)

Mucosal block

The mucosal cells of the small intestine contain a large-molecule compound known as *apoferritin*. Iron is absorbed in the ferrous state (Fe^{++}) and is changed to ferric iron (Fe^{+++}), which then combines with apoferritin to form ferritin. The latter dissociates again into apoferritin and iron. The Fe^{+++} is reduced to the ferrous form and finds its way to the blood, where it eventually attaches itself to the iron-binding globulin known as transferrin, again in the ferric form.[9, 10]

The mucosal block is attributed to the fact that if apoferritin is saturated with iron, it hinders the further absorption of ferrous iron. These relationships are shown schematically in Fig. 44-1. Mucosal block is not sufficient to account for all known facts concerning iron absorption. It is nevertheless a useful concept to explain the adjustment of absorption to the needs of the body for iron. The capacity of the mucosal block may be exceeded when very large, unphysiologic doses of iron are ingested. In such instances perhaps a second transport system becomes operative.

The iron-binding globulin transferrin, or siderophilin, is present in normal blood at such a concentration that when fully saturated it can carry 300 μg of iron/100 ml. of blood. Since the normal serum iron level is about 100 μg/100 ml., this means that transferrin is only one-third saturated. The globulin combines with two molecules of iron per protein molecule.

The normal daily diet contains approximately 20 mg. of iron. Of this, only about 10% is absorbed, but this quantity is adequate for taking care of the very small daily losses of iron. In iron-deficiency anemia, however, the dietary iron is quite insufficient for reasonably rapid correction of the hemoglobin deficit, even though the mucosal block is greatly diminished.

The degree of the mucosal block reflects the state of iron stores in the body. Experiments utilizing isotopically labeled iron have shown that iron-deficient persons absorb more iron than do normal persons.[7] On the other hand, there must be an additional absorptive mechanism, since large doses of orally administered iron preparations may lead to iron accumulation in normal persons. Increased absorption of iron from the intestines occurs in a variety of hematologic disorders in which red cell formation is increased. Thus patients with chronic hemolytic anemia may develop hemochromatosis when they are treated unnecessarily with oral iron. In hemochromatosis, iron absorption continues despite the large excess of the metal in the body.[16]

In addition to the mucosal block, other factors influence the absorption of iron. It is generally believed that ferrous iron is more effectively absorbed than the ferric form.[11] On the other hand, a diet rich in phytate, phosphate (milk), or alkalinizing agents such as used for patients with peptic ulcer tends to decrease absorption of iron.

Therapeutic preparations

Dosages of therapeutic iron preparations should be calculated on the basis of their elemental iron content. For the treatment of iron deficiency anemias in adults a dose of 50 to 100 mg. of elemental iron three times daily is recommended.

Iron preparations can be administered both orally and parenterally.

Oral. There are many iron preparations, both organic and inorganic, that may be utilized in treatment of hypochromic anemias. These drugs differ in absorption from the gastrointestinal tract. It is customary to administer a large excess because not more than 15% of an oral dose is absorbed of even the most effective preparation, ferrous sulfate. The percentage of absorption is considerably less when certain other preparations such as reduced iron are administered. The recommended dosages of the various preparations are such that they may be expected to provide absorption of 15 to 25 mg. of iron a day in an individual suffering from hypochromic anemia. The following doses are often used:

Ferrous sulfate tablets	0.3 Gm. three times a day
Ferric ammonium citrate	1.0 Gm. three times a day
Reduced iron	0.5 Gm. three times a day
Ferrous gluconate	0.6 Gm. three times a day
Ferrous fumarate	0.5 Gm. three times a day
Ferrocholinate	0.5 Gm. three times a day

Parenteral. Because of the low degree of efficiency of gastrointestinal absorption of iron, several injectable forms of iron have been introduced.

Iron dextran complex (Imferon) is a useful preparation when parenteral administration of iron is mandatory. It was temporarily withdrawn when carcinogenicity in rats and mice and one questionable case in a human being were reported. The preparation contains 50 mg. of iron/ml. The dose is 1 to 4 ml. daily intramuscularly. Occasional anaphylactoid and allergic reactions have been reported following its use. Nevertheless, it is less likely to produce severe shocklike states and phlebitis, which may follow the use of the intravenous preparations of iron.

Iron sorbitex (Jectofer) is another intramuscular preparation with characteristics similar to iron dextran.

Dextriferron (Astrafer) is an iron-dextrin complex containing 20 mg./ml. of iron. It is replacing saccharated iron oxide (Proferrin) as an intravenous dosage form. The intravenous iron preparations should be used only with the realization of their dangers. They may cause hypotension, vascular collapse, headache, nausea, and anaphylactoid reactions.

Adverse effects

The oral iron preparations tend to produce nausea and vomiting through a local irritant effect on the stomach. For this reason the preparations are generally administered immediately after meals. Large doses of ferrous sulfate and of ferrous gluconate have produced poisoning in children. If large amounts of iron are absorbed, it seems that symptoms resembling those of heavy metal poisoning may result.[5]

Increasing attention is being paid to the danger of producing hemochromatosis in patients who receive iron medication for a long time. In some of these instances the patient may absorb a greater percentage of the administered iron than would a normal individual, the mucosal block apparently not operating efficiently.

CHELATING AGENTS IN TREATMENT OF IRON POISONING

Acute iron poisoning is an important cause of accidental death in small children. The metal chelating agent edathamil calcium disodium has been used to lessen the toxic effects of iron. More recently, the potent and specific iron chelating agent deferoxamine (Desferal) has been used with apparent benefit both in treatment of acute toxic reactions to ferrous gluconate[13] and for removal of iron in patients with overload.[18]

Deferoxamine, also known as desferrioxamine B, is a water-soluble substance of three molecules of trihydroxamic acid. Its molecular weight is 597, and one molecule chelates one molecule of Fe^{+++} ions. The drug is derived from the microbial product ferrioxamine B by removal of iron.

Deferoxamine removes iron from ferritin and transferrin but not from hemoglobin.[18] It is not itself absorbed from the intestine and blocks the absorption of iron. When administered by the intravenous or intramuscular route, deferoxamine promotes renal excretion of iron at a rate of 1 to 3 mg./day in a normal person and up to 50 mg. in hemochromatosis.

In acute iron poisoning, deferoxamine, 8 to 12 Gm., is administered by gastric tube. In addition, 1 to 2 Gm. of the drug may be injected intramuscularly or intravenously. In a small child, repeated doses of deferoxamine (92 mg./kg.) have been used with apparent benefit. Smaller doses, 400 to 600 mg. daily, are sufficient for promotion of iron excretion in hemochromatosis.

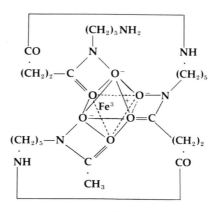

Deferoxamine (in combination with iron)

USE OF IRON IN ANEMIAS

Iron is effective in the treatment of iron-deficiency anemias.[23] In these states the mean corpuscular volume is below 80 μ^3, and the mean corpuscular hemoglobin concentration is below 30%. These anemic states are generally caused by chronic blood loss or a deficient dietary supply of iron. The latter is more likely to occur in a growing child.

In most instances ferrous sulfate is quite adequate for the treatment of iron deficiency. Its main disadvantages are gastric irritation, diarrhea, and constipation. It may be advisable to use small doses at first and to increase the dose gradually over a period of 1 or 2 weeks. In general there is no advantage in the addition of cobalt, other metals, or folic acid to preparations whose purpose is to supply iron. Ferrous fumarate may be better tolerated than other iron preparations by some patients. The danger of overdosage should be kept in mind, particularly in children.

METALS OTHER THAN IRON IN TREATMENT OF ANEMIAS

The effect of cobalt on hemoglobin synthesis has received particular attention. This metal in the form of its various salts can produce polycythemia regularly in experimental animals. The therapeutic usefulness of cobalt in the treatment of anemias is still in an experimental stage. A number of adverse reactions such as nausea and diarrhea have been reported from its premature clinical use. An unusual effect is enlargement of the thyroid gland.

Although vitamin B_{12} contains cobalt, there is no relationship between the polycythemic effect of cobalt salts and the vitamin. It has been postulated that cobalt may exert the same effect on the bone marrow as anoxia, perhaps by tying up sulfhydryl groups.

VITAMIN B_{12}

Vitamin B_{12} (cyanocobalamin) is a cobalt-containing compound having a molecular weight of 1,400. Its isolation from liver[25] brought to a successful conclusion more than 20 years of investigation aimed at finding the cause of *pernicious anemia.*

Until 1926 pernicious anemia was entirely incurable. At that time the key observation was made that large amounts of liver had a beneficial effect in the treatment of the disease.[17] Subsequent work was aimed at purification of the liver factor responsible for the curative effect. Soon injectable purified liver extracts of great potency were available.

The problem of pernicious anemia appeared more complex, however, than a simple deficiency of a liver factor. Clinical experiments showed that normal gastric juice contained an intrinsic factor which had to interact with a dietary extrinsic factor in order for the erythrocyte maturation factor present in liver to be obtained.[4]

When folic acid was isolated in 1943, it was felt at first that the compound was in some way related to the etiology of pernicious anemia. It was soon found, however, that whereas folic acid could remedy the hematologic manifestations of the disease, it either had no effect or aggravated the neurologic symptoms. Since liver extract was effective against both these aspects of pernicious anemia, it was clear that folic acid could not represent the liver factor.

The picture became clarified when vitamin B_{12} was isolated in 1948. It appears that the absorption of vitamin B_{12} requires the presence of the intrinsic factor of Castle. This is lacking in true addisonian pernicious anemia. Furthermore, injected vitamin B_{12} remedies both hematologic and neurologic disturbances in pernicious anemia. When reasonable doses of the vitamin are administered by mouth to patients with pernicious anemia, they are ineffective unless some normal gastric juice is given simultaneously. Thus there is little doubt at present that vitamin B_{12} represents both the extrinsic factor and the erythrocyte maturation factor. The function of the intrinsic factor has to do with the absorption of vitamin B_{12}.

Chemistry

The structural formula of vitamin B_{12} is as follows:

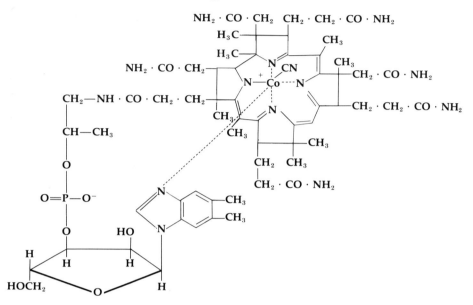

Vitamin B_{12}

The vitamin has been called cyanocobalamin and is only one member of several cobalamins, all of which have vitamin B_{12} activity. The compound has been isolated not only from liver but also from fermentation liquors of *Streptomyces griseus,* the organism that produces streptomycin.

Unlike many other vitamins, vitamin B_{12} is not present in higher plants but can be synthesized by certain microorganisms. Human liver contains at least 400 μg of the vitamin/kg., and beef liver may contain up to 100 μg/kg. Cow's milk contains more than human milk, up to 4 μg/L.[18]

Indication for use

The vitamin is indicated in treatment of megaloblastic states due to a deficient supply or absorption of vitamin B_{12}. In the majority of cases the deficiency is in the absorption. This is certainly the case in pernicious anemia and following gastrectomy. In *Diphyllobothrium latum* (fish tapeworm) infestation the worm itself may concentrate much of the vitamin supplied in the diet.

There are other megaloblastic states in which a deficiency of folic acid exists, and treatment should be based on correction of the deficiency rather than on administration of vitamin B_{12}. Some of these megaloblastic states are nutritional macrocytic anemia, certain cases of sprue, megaloblastic anemia of pregnancy, megaloblastic anemia of infants, and certain cases of adult scurvy.

Absorption and fate

Much has been learned about the absorption and excretion of the vitamin as a result of the availability of ^{60}Co-labeled vitamin B_{12}.

When 0.5 μg of labeled vitamin B_{12} was administered orally to normal persons, about 31% was excreted in the feces. In patients with pernicious anemia the fecal excretion averaged 88%.[3] When an intrinsic factor preparation was administered simultaneously, the excretion of the vitamin in patients with pernicious anemia decreased to normal levels. Fecal excretion of the labeled vitamin was also very high in patients following gastrectomy. On the other hand, in megaloblastic anemia of pregnancy there is no deficiency in the absorption of vitamin B_{12}.

Vitamin B_{12} does not appear in urine under normal circumstances, probably because the compound is bound to plasma proteins. However, if a large dose of nonlabeled vitamin B_{12} (1,000 μg) is injected intramuscularly following oral administration of the labeled compound, normal individuals excrete as much as 30% of the radioactivity in the urine within 24 hours. Apparently the nonradioactive material displaces the labeled compound from its binding sites. This observation has been adapted to the diagnosis of pernicious anemia, since under similar circumstances a patient suffering from the disease will excrete only insignificant quantities in the urine, usually less than 2.5% of the administered dose.

Following intramuscular injection of large doses, much of vitamin B_{12} is excreted in the urine, both in normal individuals and in patients with pernicious anemia. The percentage of the dose excreted increases with the quantity administered. Thus when 40 μg is injected, 7.5% appears in the urine, whereas 60% of the dose may be similarly excreted when 1,000 μg of the vitamin is injected.[19]

Oral administration of very large doses of vitamin B_{12} (such as 3,000 μg) may result in some absorption, even in patients with pernicious anemia. This may indicate that the deficiency of intrinsic factor is not absolute or that there is some other mechanism of absorption.

Basic mode of action

Vitamin B_{12} and folic acid correct megaloblastosis by influencing DNA synthesis. The characteristic delayed nuclear maturation in megaloblastosis results from inadequate DNA synthesis, a consequence of deficiencies of Vitamin B_{12} and/or folic acid.

The pathway affected by vitamin B_{12} and folic acid is that leading to the synthesis of DNA thymine from deoxyuridylate (dUMP) through the following steps:

Deoxyuridine $\rightarrow$ **Deoxyuridylate** $\rightarrow$ **Thymidylate** $\rightarrow$ **DNA thymine**

The methylation of deoxyuridylate to thymidylate requires 5,10-methylene-tetrahydrofolic acid. This requirement explains the role of folic acid in DNA synthesis.

The role of vitamin B_{12} is in the regeneration of tetrahydrofolic acid from 5-methyltetrahydrofolic acid by homocysteine transmethylation:

5-Methyltetrahydrofolic acid $\Longrightarrow$ **Tetrahydrofolic acid**
Vitamin B_{12}
Homocysteine   **Methionine**

These relationships and the possible role of pyridoxal phosphate are shown in Fig. 44-2.

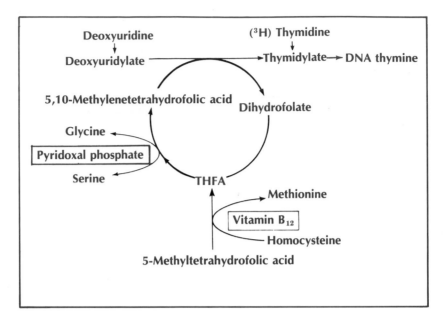

Fig. 44-2. Pathways for DNA thymine synthesis. (From Waxman, S., Corcino, J., and Herbert, V.: J.A.M.A. **214**:101, 1970, copyright 1970, American Medical Association.)

Preparations and clinical uses

Vitamin B_{12} contains 10 or 15 μg of the vitamin/ml. Injectable liver extracts are now standardized on the basis of their vitamin B_{12} content rather than in terms of USP units, which were based on the hematologic response of patients in relapse with pernicious anemia.

In a severely anemic patient, vitamin B_{12} is injected intramuscularly in a dosage of 15 μg. The injection may be repeated every 2 hours for three or four doses. Following this initial treatment, injections of 30 μg of vitamin B_{12} are usually given once a week. In megaloblastic anemias due to vitamin B_{12} deficiency, a characteristic reticulocyte response appears within 10 days. Some signs of improvement in the general condition of the patient may develop within 48 hours.

FOLIC ACID
Chemistry and nomenclature

Folic acid is pteroylglutamic acid and has the following structural formula:

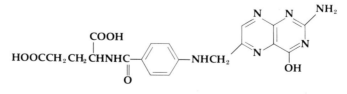

Folic acid

The compound may be looked upon as a combination of pteridine, *p*-aminobenzoic acid, and glutamic acid. In natural materials such as green vegetables the compound occurs in a conjugated form, being attached to six additional glutamic acid residues.

Folic acid is a growth factor for certain microorganisms such as *Streptococcus faecalis* R. Its deficiency causes anemia and leukopenia in monkeys and in man. Folic acid has been synthesized.[1]

Folinic acid (citrovorum factor; Leucovorin) is closely related to folic acid.

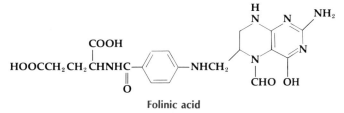

Folinic acid

Folic acid is converted in the body to folinic acid. It has been shown that rats fed folic acid excrete some folinic acid in the urine. It has also been demonstrated that rat liver can convert folic acid to folinic acid in vitro,[21] a conversion accelerated by ascorbic acid.

Functions

The reactions in which folic acid participates are important in the synthesis of DNA (Fig. 44-2). As a consequence, deficiency of folic acid, whether induced by dietary means or by administration of the folic acid antagonists such as aminopterin, leads to damage in those tissues in which DNA synthesis and turnover are rapid. These include the hematopoietic tissues, the mucosa of the gastrointestinal tract, and the developing embryo.

Preparations and clinical uses

Folic acid is available in capsules and tablets containing 5 mg. The vitamin is well absorbed from the gastrointestinal tract, and injectable preparations, although available, are generally unnecessary.

The main use for folic acid is in nutritional macrocytic anemia, certain cases of sprue, megaloblastic anemia of pregnancy, certain cases of megaloblastic anemia in infancy, and scurvy.

It is contraindicated in pernicious anemia. It should not be used in multiple vitamin preparations because it would obscure the diagnosis of unrecognized pernicious anemia. Although it improves the megaloblastic anemia in this instance, it does not protect against the nervous system manifestations of the disease and may even aggravate them.

Folinic acid has no advantages over folic acid in megaloblastic or deficiency states. It may be advantageous, however, in counteracting the toxic manifestations of the folic acid antagonists. This use, along with the folic acid antagonists, is discussed more fully in Chapter 54, which deals with drugs used in chemotherapy of neoplastic diseases.

ERYTHROPOIETIN

There is evidence for the existence of a circulating erythropoiesis-stimulating factor. This factor, called erythropoietin or hemopoietin, has been detected in the plasma of animals made anemic, exposed to lowered pressures, or treated with cobalt. Such a factor has also been demonstrated in the plasma and urine of anemic human beings. Although this factor is of no therapeutic importance at present, it is of great experimental interest and may eventually become important in treatment of certain anemias.[8]

The kidney has been suggested as the site of erythropoietin formation, on the basis of experiments on nephrectomized rats whose response to severe anemia and hypoxia was strikingly reduced.[15] In man, however, there must be extrarenal sources of erythropoietin, since nephrectomy reduces but does not abolish erythropoiesis.[20] It has also been suggested that the kidney elaborates an erythropoietic factor (REF), the release of which is stimulated by anoxia.[33] This REF acts on a plasma globulin to form erythropoietin.

References

1 Angier, R. B., et al.: Structure and synthesis of liver L. casei factor, Science 103:667, 1946.
2 Barker, H. A., Weissbach, H., and Smyth, R. D.: A coenzyme containing pseudovitamin B_{12}, Proc. Nat. Acad. Sci. 44:1093, 1958.
3 Callender, S. T., Turnbull, A., and Wakisaka, G.: Estimation of intrinsic factor of Castle by use of radioactive vitamin B_{12}, Brit. Med. J. 1:10, 1954.
4 Castle, W. B.: Etiology of pernicious anemia and related macrocytic anemias, Ann. Intern. Med. 7:2, 1933.
5 Charney, E.: A fatal case of ferrous sulfate poisoning, J.A.M.A. 178:326, 1961.
6 Desforges, J. F.: Anemia in uremia, Arch Intern. Med. 126:808, 1970.
7 Dubach, R., Callender, S. T., and Moore, C. V.: Studies in iron transportation and metabolism: absorption of radioactive iron in patients with fever and with anemias of varied etiology, Blood 3:526, 1948.
8 Gordan, A. S.: Hemopoietine, Physiol. Rev. 39:1, 1959.
9 Granick, S.: Ferritin: increase of the protein apoferritin in the gastrointestinal mucosa as a direct response to iron feeding. The function of ferritin in the regulation of iron absorption, J. Biol. Chem. 164:737, 1946.
10 Granick, S.: Ferritin: its properties and significance for iron metabolism, Chem. Rev. 38:379, 1946.
11 Hahn, P. F., Jones, E., Lowe, R. C., Meneely, G. R., and Peacock, W.: The relative absorption and utilization of ferrous and ferric iron in anemia as determined with the radioactive isotope, Amer. J. Physiol. 143:191, 1945.
12 Helleiner, C. W., and Woods, D. D.: Cobalamin and the synthesis of methionine by cell-free extracts of Escherichia coli, Biochem. J. 63:26, 1956.
13 Henderson, F., Vietti, T. J., and Brown, E. B.: Desferrioxamine in the treatment of acute

toxic reaction to ferrous gluconate, J.A.M.A. 186:1139, 1963.
14 Hwang, Y. F., and Brown, E. B.: Evaluation of deferoxamine in iron overload, Arch. Intern. Med. 114:741, 1964.
15 Jacobson, L. O., Goldwasser, E., Fried, W., and Plzak, L.: Role of kidney in erythropoiesis, Nature 179:633, 1957.
16 Mendel, G. A.: Iron metabolism and etiology of iron storage diseases: an interpretive formulation, J.A.M.A. 189:45, 1964.
17 Minot, G. R., and Murphy, W. P.: Treatment of pernicious anemia by special diet, J.A.M.A. 87:470, 1926.
18 Moeschlin, S., and Schnider, U.: Treatment of primary and secondary hemochromatosis and acute iron poisoning with a new, potent iron-eliminating agent (desferrioxamine-b), New Eng. J. Med. 269:57, 1963.
19 Mollin, D. L., and Ross, G. I. M.: Vitamin B_{12} concentrations of serum and urine in the first seventy-two hours after intramuscular injections of the vitamin, J. Clin. Path. 6:54, 1953.
20 Nathan, D. G., Shupak, E., Stohlman, F., Jr., and Merrill, J. P.: Erythropoiesis in anephric man, J. Clin. Invest. 43:2158, 1964.
21 Nichol, C. A., and Welch, A. D.: Synthesis of citrovorum factor from folic acid by liver slices: augmentation by ascorbic acid, Proc. Soc. Exp. Biol. Med. 74:52, 1950.
22 Nieweg, H. O., Faber, J. G., de Vries, J. A., and Kroese, W. F. S.: The relationship of vitamin B_{12} and folic acid in megaloblastic anemias, J. Lab. Clin. Med. 44:118, 1954.
23 Pritchard, J. A., and Mason, R. A.: Iron stores of normal adults and replenishment with oral iron therapy, J.A.M.A. 190:897, 1964.
24 Reissman, K. R., Nomura, T., Gunn, R. W., and Brosius, F.: Erythropoietic response to anemia or erythropoietin injection in uremic rats with or without functioning renal tissue, Blood 16: 1411, 1960.

25 Rickes, E. L., Brink, N. G., Koniuszy, F. R., Wood, T. R., and Folkers, K.: Comparative data on vitamin B_{12} from liver and from a new source, Streptomyces griseus, Science 108:634, 1948.

26 Schade, S. G., Cohen, R. J., and Conrad, M. E.: Effect of hydrochloric acid on iron absorption, New Eng. J. Med. 279:672, 1968.

27 Welch, A. D., and Heinle, R. W.: Hematopoietic agents in macrocytic anemias, Pharmacol. Rev. 3:345, 1951.

Recent reviews

28 Brown, E. B.: Clinical pharmacology of drugs used in the treatment of iron deficiency anemia, Pharmacol. Physicians 2(11):1, 1968.

29 Erslev, A. J.: The search for erythropoietin, New Eng. J. Med. 284:849, 1971.

30 Fisher, J. W.: Erythropoietin: pharmacology, biogenesis and control of production, Pharmacol. Rev. 24:459, 1972.

31 Friend, D. G.: Iron therapy, Clin. Pharmacol. Ther. 4:345, 1951.

32 Glass, G. B. J.: Gastric intrinsic factor and its function in the metabolism of vitamin B_{12}, Physiol. Rev. 43:529, 1963.

33 Gordon, A. S., Cooper, G. W., and Zangani, E. D.: The kidney and erythropoiesis, Seminars Hemat. 4:337, 1967.

34 Hallberg, L., Harwerth, H. G., and Vannotti, A.: Iron deficiency, New York, 1970, Academic Press, Inc.

35 Krantz, S. B., and Jacobson, L. O.: Erythropoietin and the regulation of erythropoiesis, Chicago, 1970, University of Chicago Press.

45 Vitamins

GENERAL CONCEPT

The early discoveries of vitamins followed observations on naturally occurring diseases such as scurvy and beriberi. The improvement noted in these diseases when modifications were made in the diet suggested that a deficiency of some sort was the cause of the pathologic process. Discoveries came much more rapidly when feeding experiments were performed on experimental animals, and soon the essential nature of many vitamins was recognized. More recently, the study of vitamins and their functions was further stimulated by observations on growth factors in microbial metabolism.

Vitamin deficiencies can occur in man as a result of inadequate intake, lack of intestinal absorption, or increased need in relation to intake. The purpose of administering vitamins is to provide daily requirements or to correct an already existing deficiency. In a few instances excessive amounts may be used for a definite therapeutic purpose, such as in the case of vitamin D in parathyroid deficiency or vitamin K for antagonizing the action of the coumarin anticoagulants. In most instances, however, an excess of vitamins performs no useful function and can even produce toxic effects.

WATER-SOLUBLE VITAMINS

Many of the water-soluble vitamins are coenzymes or essential parts of a coenzyme and thus have an essential function in the enzymatic machinery of cells.

THIAMINE

Thiamine in the form of thiamine pyrophosphate or cocarboxylase has been shown to play an important role in the decarboxylation of α-keto acids such as pyruvate. The structural formula is shown below.

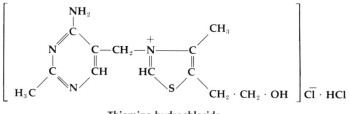

Thiamine hydrochloride

Deficiency

Severe deficiency results in the disease beriberi, characterized by high-output heart failure and peripheral polyneuritis. Other symptoms include anorexia, nausea, intestinal atony, disturbances of peripheral nerves, and mental disorders.

542

Occurrence

Thiamine is present in sufficient quantities in yeast, wheat germ, and pork. One international or USP unit is equal to 3 μg of thiamine hydrochloride.

NICOTINIC ACID

Nicotinic acid (niacin) is an integral part of at least two important coenzymes, nicotinamide adenine dinucleotide (NAD), formerly called diphosphopyridine nucleotide (DPN), and nicotinamide adenine dinucleotide phosphate (NADP), formerly called triphosphopyridine nucleotide (TPN). The structural formulas of NAD, nicotinic acid, and nicotinamide are as follows:

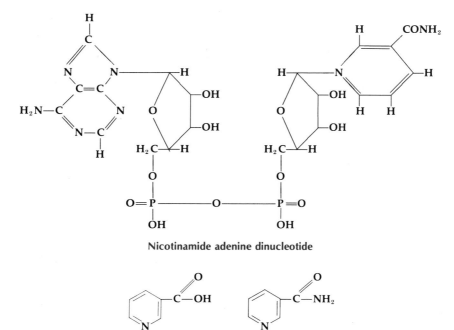

Nicotinamide adenine dinucleotide

Nicotinic acid   Nicotinamide

NAD and NADP can exist in an oxidized or reduced state and can thus act as hydrogen acceptors or donors in many enzymatic reactions of intermediary metabolism. Microsomal enzymes requiring NADP play an important role also in the metabolism of many drugs.

Deficiency

Pellagra is the disease caused by niacin deficiency. It is characterized by skin lesions, _dermatitis_ gastrointestinal mucosal changes with diarrhea, and neurologic symptoms including mental disorders. _dementia_

Occurrence

Nicotinic acid is found in significant amounts in yeast, rice, bran, and liver and other meats. Mammals can synthesize nicotinic acid from tryptophan. Pellagra can occur in patients having carcinoid tumor as a consequence of utilization of tryptophan for serotonin (5-hydroxytryptamine) synthesis.

Pharmacology

Nicotinic acid, but not nicotinamide, produces marked dilatation of small vessels, an effect that is transient but may be severe on parenteral administration. On a purely empirical basis, nicotinic acid is used experimentally for lowering serum cholesterol and as a vasodilator, but it is not definitely useful.

RIBOFLAVIN

Riboflavin is present in flavin adenine dinucleotide (FAD), which is a coenzyme of flavoprotein enzymes. There is also a flavin mononucleotide (FMN). The structural formulas of riboflavin and flavin adenine dinucleotide are shown below.

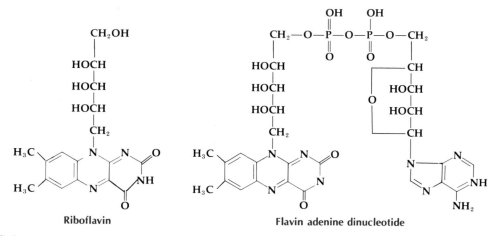

Riboflavin   Flavin adenine dinucleotide

Deficiency

A deficiency of riboflavin will cause cheilosis, stomatitis, and keratitis.

Occurrence

Riboflavin is present in significant quantities in yeast, green vegetables, liver and other meats, eggs, and milk.

PYRIDOXINE

Pyridoxine and also pyridoxal and pyridoxamine are various forms of vitamin B_6. Pyridoxal phosphate functions as a coenzyme in many reactions such as the decarboxylation of amino acids and transamination reactions between amino acids and keto acids. The structural formulas of pyridoxine hydrochloride, pyridoxal, and pyridoxamine dihydrochloride follow:

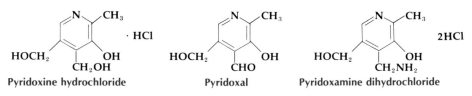

Pyridoxine hydrochloride   Pyridoxal   Pyridoxamine dihydrochloride

Deficiency

A deficiency of pyridoxine results in dermatitis and convulsions. Thiosemicarbazide may act as a convulsant by this mechanism. Isoniazid may also cause pyridoxine deficiency.

Occurrence

Pyridoxine is present in significant amounts in yeast, liver, rice, bran, and wheat germ.

PANTOTHENIC ACID

Pantothenic acid is a part of a very important coenzyme known as coenzyme A, the structural formula of which follows:

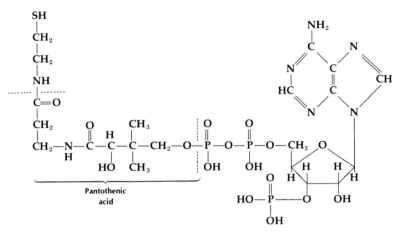

Coenzyme A

Coenzyme A in the form of acetyl coenzyme A is essential for a variety of acetylation reactions such as the formation of acetylcholine from choline and the acetylation of *p*-amino compounds. The coenzyme plays an important role in the Krebs cycle since citric acid is formed from oxaloacetic acid, acetyl coenzyme A, and water, the reaction regenerating coenzyme A. The coenzyme also plays an important role in fatty acid metabolism.

Deficiency

Pantothenic acid deficiency is not well recognized in man. In animals it may cause dermatitis, adrenal degeneration, and central nervous system symptoms.

Occurrence

Pantothenic acid is found particularly in yeast, bran, egg yolk, and liver.

ASCORBIC ACID

Ascorbic acid is a reducing agent whose exact biologic function is not understood. It may be a cofactor for the transformation of folic to folinic acid and may be necessary for adrenal cortical function and maintenance of normal connective tissue. The recent claim for asorbic acid in the prevention of the common cold is not based on convincing evidence, although large-scale, controlled clinical trials are not available for proving or disproving its efficacy.

Deficiency

The classic disease scurvy is characterized by abnormalities in the connective tissue, capillaries and bone being severely affected.

Occurrence

Ascorbic acid is present in large quantities in citrus fruits, green peppers, tomatoes, and fruits and vegetables in general.

OTHER WATER-SOLUBLE VITAMINS

There are several other water-soluble factors essential for experimental animals and presumably for man. These include biotin, folic acid, choline, and inositol.

The exact biochemical functions of the other water-soluble vitamins are not known, although there is much information available on the clinical consequences of their deficiency.

FAT-SOLUBLE VITAMINS
VITAMIN A

Vitamin A performs an important function in connection with dark adaptation, being part of the visual purple of the retina. It also maintains the integrity of various epithelial structures.

Deficiency of vitamin A produces night blindness, keratinization of the conjunctiva (xerophthalmia), and ulcerations of the cornea (keratomalacia). The skin becomes rough because of hyperkeratosis. Respiratory infections occur in animals deficient in vitamin A, perhaps due to changes in the bronchial epithelium, but there is no good evidence to indicate any connection between vitamin A deficiency and respiratory infection in human beings.

The assay for vitamin A is based on saponification of the oil (palmitate or acetate) by potassium hydroxide, extraction with ethyl ether, and the measurement of the absorbance of ultraviolet light through an isopropanol dilution in a quartz cell at wavelengths of 310, 325, and 334 mμ.

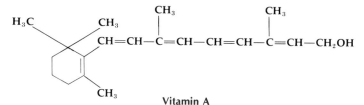

Vitamin A

Occurrence

Vitamin A occurs particularly in eggs, milk, vegetables, and fish liver oils.

Pharmacology and toxicity

Vitamin A is stored in the liver. In large quantities the vitamin may cause toxic effects such as anorexia, hepatomegaly, loss of hair, and periosteal thickening of long bones.

Cod liver oil contains 850 IU of vitamin A per gram, a unit being equal to 0.6 μg of β-carotene. Both percomorph liver oil and a water-miscible vitamin A preparation contain 50,000 IU/Gm. The administration of more than 25,000 IU/day is seldom justified.

VITAMIN D

Vitamin D refers to one of several sterols. Vitamin D_2 (calciferol) is obtained by irradiation of ergosterol. The striking new developments in relation to vitamin D metabolism are discussed on p. 502.

Vitamin D_3 is present in fish liver oils and is produced in the skin by the action of sunlight on 7-dehydrocholesterol. Dihydrotachysterol has actions resembling those of the parathyroid hormone and was discussed in connection with that subject.

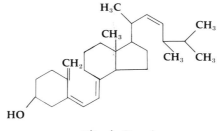

Vitamin D_2

Deficiency of vitamin D brings forth the various manifestations of rickets in growing children and animals. There is a disturbance in calcification of bones and teeth. The bones may become soft. Swollen epiphyses and lack of normal calcification are demonstrable by radiologic examination.

The main function of vitamin D appears to be exerted on the intestinal absorption of calcium and phosphate. In large quantities the vitamin may exert an effect on bone dissolution similar to the action of the parathyroid hormone.

The daily requirement of vitamin D depends on the calcium needs of the individual. Growing children and pregnant or lactating women require more of the vitamin because their daily calcium absorption must be greater.

Vitamin D preparations are standardized by determining their effect of calcification in rats maintained on a diet deficient in vitamin D. The international unit is 0.025 μg of vitamin D_3.

Adults require 100 units of vitamin D in 24 hours. Infants, children, and also pregnant or lactating women may require as much as twice this amount.

It may be administered in the form of fish liver oils, as calciferol (Drisdol), or as synthetic oleovitamin D. Dihydrotachysterol (Hydrocalciferol) is used in hypoparathyroidism to raise the serum calcium level.

Toxicity

Excessive doses of the D vitamins cause hypercalcemia, with anorexia and metastatic calcifications in the kidney.

VITAMIN E

Vitamin E is present in wheat-germ oil and in many foods. Its role in animal reproduction has been well established, and the term *tocopherol* implies its importance in childbearing. There are several tocopherols, but α-tocopherol has the highest activity.

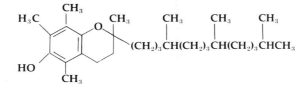

α-**Tocopherol**

Deficiency of vitamin E produces abortion in the female animal and degeneration of the germinal epithelium in the male animal. Muscular dystrophy also develops in animals on a vitamin E–deficient diet. Many other functions have been claimed for α-tocopherol, and many of its therapeutic applications have been suggested largely on the basis of uncritical clinical observations. The exact daily requirements of vitamin E in man are not known, but quantities of 5 to 30 mg. or more have been used in many clinical series.

The feeding of large amounts of unsaturated fats may increase the tocopherol requirements. It has been suggested that tocopherol functions as a biologic antioxidant whose function becomes particularly important when tissues contain peroxidizable lipids.

VITAMIN K

Vitamin K is essential for production of prothrombin by the liver, and in its absence hemorrhagic manifestations occur. Various 1,4-naphthoquinones have vitamin K activity. Vitamin K_1 is 2-methyl-3-phytyl-1,4-naphthoquinone. The structural formulas of vitamin K_1 and of menadione are as follows:

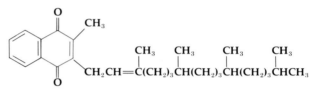

Vitamin K₁

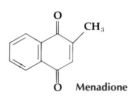

Menadione

These naphthoquinone compounds are very insoluble in water and are suitable primarily for oral administration. Emulsions of vitamin K_1, however, can be injected intravenously in hemorrhagic emergencies due to hypoprothrombinemia.

Water-soluble derivatives of naphthoquinones have also been prepared. The structural formulas of two such compounds, menadiol sodium diphosphate and menadione sodium bisulfite, are shown below:

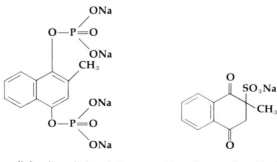

Menadiol sodium diphosphate   **Menadione sodium bisulfite**

Vitamin K preparations are useful in bleeding caused by hypoprothrombinemia. Causes of hypoprothrombinemia are severe liver disease, biliary obstruction, malabsorption syndromes, coumarin and indandione drugs, salicylates in large doses, reduction of intestinal flora by chemotherapeutic agents, and hypoprothrombinemia of small infants.

Commonly used preparations are vitamin K_1 (phytonadione; Mephyton) and various forms of vitamin K_3 (menadione; menadiol sodium diphosphate, water soluble, or Synkayvite; and menadione sodium bisulfite or Hykinone, also water soluble).

The daily requirement for vitamin K cannot be stated because considerable quantities are synthesized by the bacterial flora of the intestine. The dosage varies greatly, depending on the nature and severity of prothrombin deficiency. Doses of 1 to 2 mg. by mouth or injection may suffice. On the other hand, very large doses may have to be administered in emergency situations when prothrombin levels have been depressed by the anticoagulant drugs. As much as 100 mg. or more of vitamin K_1 emulsion has been used in this situation by the intravenous route.

Toxicity

Individuals who are subject to primaquine-sensitive anemia may react with hemolysis to large doses of vitamin K. Such doses can also aggravate liver disease and produce jaundice, particularly in infants.

ANTIVITAMINS

Of great experimental interest are structural analogs of some of the vitamins that can induce experimental vitamin deficiency.

Some of the vitamins and their antagonists are as follows:

Vitamins	Antagonists
Thiamine	Pyrithiamine and oxythiamine
Nicotinic acid	Inhibitor in corn
Pyridoxine	Deoxypyridoxine
Ascorbic acid	Glucoascorbic acid
Vitamin K	Coumarins and indandiones

MEDICAL USES OF VITAMINS

Vitamins are used in medicine for various reasons. A clear-cut deficiency of any of these factors calls for therapeutic measures aimed at its correction. In addition, growing children, pregnant and lactating women, and persons on unusual diets may require multiple vitamins for the prevention of deficiencies. It is also possible that acutely ill persons may need more than the normal daily requirements of vitamins.

There may also be justification for using large amounts of ascorbic acid in debilitated patients who need an operation, to promote healing and mesenchymal integrity.

In most cases, however, vitamins are used by the medical profession and the laity under the mistaken belief that larger amounts than the minimum daily requirement will promote optimal health. This feeling has been further promoted by popular statements concerning the inadequacy of our modern manufactured foods with regard to vitamin and mineral content. It is believed by critical authorities that most of the

Table 45-1. Recommended daily dietary allowances and therapeutic doses of vitamins

Vitamin	Average daily adult requirement	Therapeutic dose
Thiamine	1.5 mg.	2-10 mg.
Nicotinamide	20 mg.	100-300 mg.
Riboflavin	2 mg.	2-10 mg.
Pyridoxine	2 mg.	10 mg.
Ascorbic acid	60 mg.	100-150 mg.
Vitamin A	4,000 units	25,000 units
Vitamin D	400 units	5,000 units or more
Vitamin E	Unknown	30 units

widespread use of vitamins by the population is wasteful and that benefits claimed by many persons must be due to a placebo effect.

ADVERSE EFFECTS OF VITAMINS

Although slight excesses of vitamin intake are more wasteful than dangerous, large doses of several of the vitamins can produce adverse effects.

The water-soluble vitamins are generally harmless except in special circumstances. Thiamine injected intravenously has produced a shocklike state, and an anaphylactic-type sensitization to it has been suspected. Nicotinic acid is a fairly potent vasodilator, and for that reason nicotinamide, which does not affect the blood vessels, is preferred. Folic acid may be dangerous in persons who have pernicious anemia, since it may aggravate the neurologic manifestations of the disease. For this reason the modern tendency is to eliminate folic acid from multiple vitamin preparations. Ascorbic acid is remarkably nontoxic. When administered in large quantities, the vitamin is rapidly cleared by the kidney.

The fat-soluble vitamins are more likely to produce distinct pathologic changes when given in excessive quantities.

Hypervitaminosis A has been described as occurring in children when doses of the order of 100,000 units or more are administered for many days. Changes in skeletal development, hepatomegaly, anemia, loss of hair, and other symptoms have been described in these patients.

When used in large quantities, vitamin D can produce hypercalcemia with metastatic calcification in the kidney and blood vessels. This is not likely to happen in the treatment of rickets, but occasionally large amounts of vitamin D_2 are used in other diseases such as lupus vulgaris in which there is no reason to suspect a deficiency.

Hemolytic anemia and jaundice have been reported following parenteral use of large doses of the various vitamin K preparations.

The occurrence of these adverse reactions is an additional reason for maintaining a rational attitude toward the use of vitamins in cases in which their indications are not clear.

References

1 Almquist, H. J.: Vitamin K, Physiol. Rev. 21:194, 1941.
2 Axelrod, A. E.: Immune processes in vitamin deficiency states, Amer. J. Clin. Nutr. 24:265, 1971.
3 Elvehjem, C. A.: The vitamin B complex: Council on Foods and Nutrition, J.A.M.A. 138: 960, 1948.

4 Finkel, M. J.: Vitamin K_1 and vitamin K analogues, Clin. Pharmacol. Ther. **2**:794, 1961.

5 Gribetz, D., Silverman, S. H., and Sobel, A. E.: Vitamin A poisoning, Pediatrics 7:372, 1951.

6 Sebrell, W. H., and Harris, R. S., editors: The vitamins, New York, 1954, Academic Press, Inc.

7 Streif, R. R., and Little, A. B.: Folic acid deficiency in pregnancy, New Eng. J. Med. **276**: 776, 1967.

8 Suttie, J. W.: Mechanism of action of vitamin K: demonstration of a liver precursor of prothrombin, Science **179**:192, 1973.

9 Symposium on vitamin E, Ann. N. Y. Acad. Sci. **52**:63, 1949.

10 Unglaub, W. G., and Hunter, F. M.: Essential fatty acids, Amer. J. Med. Sci. **233**:90, 1957.

11 Vietti, T. J., Murphy, T. P., James, J. A., and Pritchard, J. A.: Observations on the prophylactic use of vitamin K in the newborn infant, J. Pediat. **56**:343, 1960.

12 Wald, G.: The chemistry of rod vision, Science **113**:287, 1951.

13 Youmans, J. B.: Deficiencies of the water-soluble vitamins, J.A.M.A. **144**:386, 1950.

Recent reviews

14 DeLuca, H. F.: Vitamin D, New Eng. J. Med. **281**:1103, 1969.

15 DeLuca, H. F., and Suttie, J. W.: The fat-soluble vitamins, Madison, 1970, University of Wisconsin Press.

16 Rivlin, R. S.: Riboflavin metabolism, New Eng. J. Med. **283**:463, 1970.

17 Rosenberg, L. E.: Vitamin-dependent genetic disease, Hosp. Practice **5**:59, 1970.

18 Symposium on the detection of nutrition deficiencies in man, Amer. J. Clin. Nutr. **20**:513, 1967.

19 Symposium on recent advances in the appraisal of the nutrient intake and the nutritional status of man, Amer. J. Clin. Nutr. **11**:331, 1962.

20 Symposium on some findings and observations on the nutritional status of residents of the U. S. A., Amer. J. Clin. Nutr. **17**:189, 1965.

SECTION NINE

CHEMOTHERAPY

46 Introduction to chemotherapy; mechanisms of antibiotic action

HISTORICAL DEVELOPMENT

Prior to 1935 systemic bacterial infections could not be effectively treated with drugs. There were many *antiseptics* and *disinfectants* that could eradicate infections when applied topically, but their systemic use was precluded by their unfavorable therapeutic index. Certain parasitic infections such as malaria, amebiasis, and spirochetal infections could be treated effectively. This was an indication that the concept of "chemotherapy" as envisioned by Ehrlich was not unreasonable. Still, systemic bacterial infections, whether seen in patients or produced experimentally in animals, seemed to be hopelessly beyond the reach of existing drugs.

In 1935 a paper appeared in the German medical literature claiming that the red azo dye Prontosil was able to protect mice against a systemic streptococcal infection and was curative in patients suffering from such infections.[4] This was a milestone in the history of chemotherapy. In the test tube, Prontosil was ineffective against the bacteria.

It was soon demonstrated that Prontosil is broken down in the body to *p*-aminobenzenesulfonamide, known later as sulfanilamide.[11] It was also demonstrated that the chemotherapeutic activity of Prontosil was due to the breakdown product sulfanilamide.

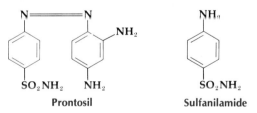

Prontosil   **Sulfanilamide**

These observations initiated a new era in medicine. Numerous derivatives of sulfanilamide were synthesized, and soon a considerable number of systemic infections could be controlled by these drugs. Not only was the treatment of many infectious diseases revolutionized, but study of these drugs led to many great discoveries about bacterial metabolism, opening many new fields in pharmacology. The study of biologic antagonism and the discovery of the carbonic anhydrase inhibitors, antithyroid drugs, and many other agents were greatly influenced by basic studies on the sulfonamides.

The successes obtained with the new sulfonamides revived interest in observations on *antibiotics*, or compounds produced by some microorganisms that inhibit the growth of other microorganisms. There were several isolated observations on the phenomenon of antibiosis. One of the most remarkable of these was Fleming's discovery that a mold of the genus *Penicillium* prevented multiplication of staphylococci and that culture filtrates of this mold had similar properties.[5] A concentrate of this antibacterial factor was eventually prepared, and its remarkable activity and lack of toxicity were demonstrated by a team at Oxford, led by Florey.[1,3]

555

The enormous potency and lack of toxicity of penicillin turned the attention of many investigators in the direction of the antibiotics as potential sources of useful chemotherapeutic agents. Soon hundreds of antibiotics were discovered. The great majority of these were too toxic for clinical use, but a few represented welcome additions to therapeutics. Streptomycin, the tetracyclines, chloramphenicol, polymyxin, bacitracin, neomycin, and several newer antibiotics have greatly increased the range of effectiveness of antibacterial chemotherapy.

The end result of these exciting discoveries is the susceptibility of the majority of systemic infections to drug therapy. With the exception of certain infections caused by fungi, gram-negative bacilli, and viruses, generalized infections today can be treated quite effectively. New problems have arisen, however. Certain microorganisms such as staphylococci and gram-negative bacilli have acquired great resistance to many of the antibacterial agents. The widespread use of the antibiotics has also produced new problems such as superinfection. However, on the whole, the chemotherapy of bacterial infection represents perhaps the most brilliant chapter in pharmacology. It is a good example of what can be achieved by *selective action* of drugs within the body.

GENERAL CONCEPTS

A number of important concepts have been derived from the extensive studies on antibacterial chemotherapy.[12]

Antibacterial spectrum refers to the range of activity of a compound. A broad-spectrum antibacterial agent is one capable of inhibiting a wide variety of microorganisms, including usually both gram-positive and gram-negative bacteria.

Potency, or activity per milligram, of a chemotherapeutic agent is usually expressed on the basis of the lowest concentration at which a chemotherapeutic agent is capable of inhibiting the multiplication of one of the susceptible microorganisms. Although potency varies greatly, depending on the test organism, the activity per milligram of some of the antibiotics against their most susceptible microorganisms is far greater than the activity of the sulfonamides against the agents that are most susceptible to them. The differences in potency are reflected in the dosage of the various chemotherapeutic agents.

Bacteriostatic activity refers to the ability of a compound to inhibit multiplication of microorganisms. *Bactericidal activity* means an actual killing effect, which can only be demonstrated by techniques that are more complex than the usual plate or tube-dilution methods used for the demonstration of bacteriostatic activity. It is an interesting generalization that those antibacterial substances that disturb the synthesis or function of the microbial cell wall or the cell membrane are usually the ones that are bactericidal.

The necessity of maintaining *blood levels* varies greatly. This is important in the case of the sulfonamides, but it may be less so in the case of some of the antibiotics such as penicillin. Blood levels in a given situation can generally be predicted from the dose and the weight of the patient. Determinations of blood levels are important only in some condition such as renal failure that makes it impossible to predict blood levels on the basis of the dose administered.

The terms *antibiotic synergism* and *antibiotic antagonism* usually refer to the magnitude of *bactericidal* activity when combinations of chemotherapeutic agents are used. The *bacteriostatic* activities of such drug combinations are usually additive. For example, if two antibiotics such as penicillin and streptomycin exert greater bactericidal activity when given together rather than singly, a phenomenon of *antibiotic synergism* is said to exist. If a bacteriostatic antibiotic interferes with the killing effect of a bactericidal antibiotic, the phenomenon is referred to as *antibiotic antagonism*. These concepts are discussed in greater detail in connection with penicillin.

Indications for the combined use of antibiotics are to increase the effectiveness of therapy against a resistant organism and to take advantage of a possible synergistic killing effect, to delay the development of resistance, and to broaden the antibacterial spectrum in mixed infections or in cases in which reliable bacteriologic diagnosis is unavailable.

There are many disadvantages to the combined use of antibiotics, which may be entirely unnecessary and wasteful. Combinations expose the patient to the adverse effects of the various members, superinfection may develop, and in rare instances, antibiotic antagonism may be promoted.

RESISTANCE

Resistance to antibiotics makes it necessary to periodically revise the drugs of choice for various infections. Tetracycline has generally been considered a satisfactory alternative to penicillin in the treatment of pneumococcal and streptococcal infections when some contraindication to the use of penicillin exists. But several cases of tetracycline-resistant Group A streptococci have been isolated, which would seem to leave erythromycin as a logical alternative.[9] At the same time, however, resistance to erythromycin can be induced rather easily in the laboratory, raising doubt as to how long this antibiotic will remain consistently effective. To minimize the development of resistance, antibiotics should not be used promiscuously or in inadequate dosage.

Resistance to chemotherapeutic agents may be of several types. Microorganisms may destroy the antibiotic by adaptative development of enzymes. The *penicillinase* present in resistant strains of staphylococci is an example.

In most instances the resistant bacteria do not destroy the antibiotic, but rather have learned to live with it. Just how this is achieved is often not clear, although several mechanisms have been postulated. If the antibacterial drug is an antimetabolite, bacteria may have learned to synthesize the growth factor, such as *p*-aminobenzoic acid in the case of the sulfonamides. In other instances the bacteria may have developed new enzymes and new metabolic pathways or may have learned not to take up or bind the antibiotic.

Bacterial resistance is usually based on genetic changes. Mutations occur spontaneously, and the more resistant cells have a selective advantage for survival in the presence of an antibacterial drug. With many successive generations, the bacterial population will become more and more resistant to the therapeutic agent employed. In addition to this mechanism, resistance may depend on other factors.

Nonmultiplying or metabolically inactive bacteria are often resistant to the killing effect of some antibiotics. Thus penicillin is much more bactericidal at 37° C. than at refrigerator temperatures, at which the organisms become metabolically inactive. The resting or "persisting" bacteria may survive in the body and start multiplying when treatment is discontinued. This is not true bacterial resistance, however, since the multiplying organisms are still susceptible and will be killed when treatment is reinstituted.

A novel mechanism of resistance was revealed by studies on the resistance transfer factor (RTF) and infectious drug resistance.

INFECTIOUS DRUG RESISTANCE

It was recognized in Japan in 1959 that bacterial resistance to several unrelated anti-biotics can be transferred to susceptible organisms by cell-to-cell contact or conjugation.[19]

Bacteria contain extrachromosomal genetic elements called R factors that are made up of DNA and act like viruses without coats. Transfer of resistance by RTF, a portion of the R factor, can occur among *Shigella, Salmonella, Klebsiella, Vibrio, Pasturella,* and *Escherichia coli.* The last-named may be a great reservoir for the transmission of bacterial resistance.

In addition to the gram-negative organisms, staphylococci may also contain extra-chromosomal particles called *plasmids,* which may be transferred from cell to cell by phages, a form of *transduction.*

The ultimate importance of infectious drug resistance cannot be stated. Resistance of gram-negative bacteria is becoming the most important problem in antibiotic therapy. It is likely that the widespread use of antibiotics not only in medicine but also in live-stock feed contributes to this problem by promoting the survival of bacteria that can spread infectious drug resistance.

MECHANISM OF ACTION OF ANTIBACTERIAL CHEMOTHERAPEUTIC AGENTS

Most of the commonly used antibacterial chemotherapeutic agents act by one of the following basic mechanisms: competitive antagonism of some metabolite, inhibition of bacterial cell wall synthesis, action on cell membranes, inhibition of protein synthesis, or inhibition of nucleic acid synthesis.

Competitive antagonism. There are a few examples in which antibacterial sub-stances act as antimetabolites. The sulfonamides compete with *p*-aminobenzoic acid for the synthesis of folic acid in bacteria. This concept of competitive antagonism arose from studies on substrates that tended to inhibit the activity of the sulfonamides in vitro. It was shown that the antagonistic effect of yeast extract was probably due to the presence of *p*-aminobenzoic acid.[16] The structural similarity between this compound and sulfanilamide and the competitive nature of their interaction suggested the pos-sibility that *p*-aminobenzoic acid may be an essential growth factor for certain micro-organisms. It was postulated that sulfanilamide, because of its structural similarity, would compete with the utilization of this growth factor.

It has subsequently been shown that folic acid, a noncompetitive inhibitor of the sulfonamides, contains *p*-aminobenzoic acid. It now appears that certain bacteria re-quire *p*-aminobenzoic acid for the synthesis of folic acid and that the sulfonamides prevent this synthesis by substrate competition. The structural formulas of *p*-amino-benzoic acid, sulfanilamide, and folic acid are as follows:

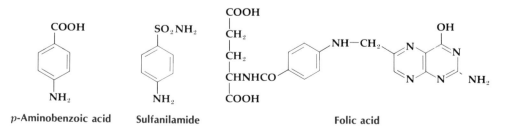

p-Aminobenzoic acid   Sulfanilamide   Folic acid

Since mammalian organisms do not synthesize folic acid but require it as a vitamin, the sulfonamides are not expected to interfere with the metabolism of mammalian cells. This difference between microorganisms and mammals explains the favorable therapeutic index of the sulfonamides in the treatment of various infections.

There are other examples of competitive antagonism in antibacterial chemotherapy. p-Aminosalicylate also competes with p-aminobenzoic acid. Interestingly, p-amino-salicylate is ineffective against bacteria other than the tubercle bacillus, although these bacteria may require p-aminobenzoic acid and are inhibited by the sulfonamides. A reasonable explanation for this invokes a difference in the receptive mechanisms in the two types of microorganisms.

Inhibition of bacterial cell wall synthesis. Several antibiotics including penicillin, the cephalosporins, cycloserine, and bacitracin act by inhibiting the synthesis of the rigid bacterial cell wall. This cell wall, in contrast with mammalian cell membranes, is rigid, making it possible for bacteria to maintain a very high internal osmotic pressure. If the synthesis of the cell wall is blocked, the high osmotic pressure leads to an extrusion of bacterial protoplasm through defects in the supporting structure and eventually to lysis of the cell when exposed to the isosmotic environment present in mammalian tissues.

The structural element of the bacterial cell wall is known as *murein*. The synthesis of murein is divided into three phases[15]: (1) synthesis of nucleotide intermediates, UDP-N-acetylglucosamine and UDP-N-acetylmuramyl-pentapeptide, terminating in D-alanyl-D-alanine; (2) assembly of the disaccharide intermediate and its incorporation into murein; and (3) the cross-linking of the peptides by transpeptidation with release of D-alanine.

It was known for many years that penicillin is particularly effective against rapidly multiplying bacteria. It was also known that the antibiotic produced morphologic changes in bacteria, such as swelling, large body formation, and lysis. Subsequently it was shown by Lederberg[8] that *Escherichia coli* cells were converted to protoplasts in the presence of penicillin and sucrose. Protoplasts are believed to represent cellular units deprived of their rigid cell wall.

Problem 46-1. Since both penicillin G and ampicillin act on a transpeptidase to block cell wall synthesis, why is ampicillin so much more potent against gram-negative bacilli, such as *E. coli?* It has been shown[15] that in cell-free systems both antibiotics were nearly equally active against the transpeptidase. On the other hand, in the case of penicillin G about ten times as much was required for growth inhibition of *E. coli* as for transpeptidase inhibition in cell-free systems. This finding suggests permeability as the explanation for the different antibacterial spectrum of the two antibiotics.

Action on cell membranes. Some antibiotics act on cell membranes, altering their permeability. This mode of action is sometimes referred to as a detergent-like action. The best examples of this mechanism are provided by the polymyxins and the antifungal polyene antibiotics.

Although antibiotics acting on cell membranes have some selective toxicity for microorganisms, they may be quite toxic for mammalian cells also. For example, the polymyxins cause renal tubular damage when administered in doses somewhat larger than therapeutic. They can also cause histamine release from mast cells both in vitro and in vivo (p. 188).

The polyene antibiotics such as amphotericin B complex have sterols in the cell wall. Fungi, but not bacteria, possess such sterols in their cell membranes and this explains the selective toxicity of the polyenes for fungi. On the other hand, mammalian cells also possess sterols in their cell membranes and the polyenes can lyse red cells and cause numerous toxic effects.

Streptomycin has an effect on the bacterial cell membrane, but it also inhibits protein synthesis.

Inhibition of protein synthesis. Most of the commonly used antibiotics inhibit protein synthesis. The list includes the tetracyclines, chloramphenicol, streptomycin, erythromycin, and lincomycin. In addition, the highly toxic experimental tools puromycin and cycloheximide (Actidione) are potent inhibitors of protein synthesis both in microorganisms and in mammals.

The selective toxicity of a protein synthesis for microorganisms is understood only in a few instances. Chloramphenicol interferes with the attachment of amino acids to the ribosomes in bacteria. In mammalian organisms, on the other hand, it only prevents the attachment of *new* messenger RNA to ribosomes. As a consequence, chloramphenicol

Table 46-1. Mechanism of action of antibiotics*

Mechanism	Antibiotic	Site of action	Mode of action
Cell wall synthesis	Penicillin and cephalosporins	Phase 3†	Inhibition of a transpeptidase
	Cycloserine	Phase 1	Competitive inhibition of alanine racemase and dipeptide synthetase
	Vancomycin (ristocetin)	Phase 2	Blockade of murein polymerase
	Bacitracin	Phase 2	Inhibition of a lipid pyrophosphatase
Protein synthesis	Tetracyclines	30 S subunit	Blockade of A site that binds tRNA where mRNA attaches
	Chloramphenicol	50 S subunit	Competitive inhibition of binding aminoacyl-tRNA to ribosome
	Aminoglycosides	30 S subunit	Unclear
	Macrolides	50 S subunit	Inhibition of translocation from A to P site
	Puromycin	50 S subunit	Substitution for aminoacyl-tRNA; transfer to peptide causing its release
	Lincomycin	50 S subunit	Inhibition of peptidyl transferase
DNA synthesis	Mitomycins	Double-stranded DNA	Bifunctional alkylation causing cross linkages between DNA strands
RNA synthesis	Rifamycins	DNA-dependent RNA polymerase	Binding to polymerase with inhibition
	Actinomycin	DNA segment	Blockade of transcription by binding to DNA

*Based on data from Hash, J. H.: Ann. Rev. Pharmacol. **12**:35, 1972.
†The three phases in cell wall synthesis are as follows: *Phase 1*—synthesis of the nucleotide intermediates; *Phase 2*—assembly and modification of the disaccharide intermediate; *Phase 3*—the cross-linking of the peptide chains by transpeptidation

exerts an effect on the synthesis of new antibodies in animals without influencing protein synthesis in general.

Streptomycin and probably the other aminoglycoside antibiotics inhibit protein synthesis. They also act on the bacterial cell membrane, and it is impossible to tell which of these actions is more important or how they may be related.

Inhibition of nucleic acid synthesis. Some highly toxic antibiotics such as actinomycin complex with DNA at the deoxyguanosine level. As a consequence, messenger RNA formation is blocked. The drug is highly toxic and is used only experimentally and rarely against some forms of malignancies (Wilms' tumor).

Griseofulvin has been considered a possible inhibitor of nucleic acid synthesis, but the evidence for this is incomplete. Idoxuridine (5-iodo-2'-deoxyuridine) blocks the synthesis of DNA and is used by topical application in the treatment of herpes keratitis. Rifampin blocks RNA synthesis in susceptible organisms. (See Table 46-1.)

References

1 Abraham, E. P., et al.: Further observations on penicillin, Lancet **2**:177, 1941.

2 Anderson, E. S., and Lewis, M. J.: Drug resistance and its transfer in Salmonella typhimurium, Nature **206**:579, 1965.

3 Chain, E. B.: The development of bacterial chemotherapy, Antibiot. Chemother. (Basel) **4**:215, 1954.

4 Domagk, G.: Ein Beitrag zur Chemotherapie der bakteriellen Infektionen, Deutsch. Med. Wschr. **61**:250, 1935.

5 Fleming, A., editor: Penicillin: its practical application, Philadelphia, 1946, The Blakiston Co.

6 Izaki, K., and Strominger, J. L.: Biosynthesis of the peptidoglycan of bacterial cell walls. VIII. Peptidoglycan transpeptidase and D-alanine carboxypeptidase: penicillin-sensitive enzymatic reaction in strains of *Escherichia coli*, J. Biol. Chem. **243**:3180, 1968.

7 Jawetz, E., and Gunnison, J. B.: Antibiotic synergism and antagonism: an assessment of the problem, Pharmacol. Rev. **5**:175, 1953.

8 Lederberg, J.: Bacterial protoplasts induced by penicillin, Proc. Nat. Acad. Sci. **42**:574, 1956.

9 McCormack, R. C., Kaye, D., and Hook, E. W.: Resistance of Group A streptococci to tetracycline, New Eng. J. Med. **267**:323, 1962.

10 Park, J. T., and Strominger, J. L.: Mode of action of penicillin: biochemical basis for the mechanism of action of penicillin and for its toxicity, Science **125**:99, 1957.

11 Trefouel, J., Trefouel, Mme. J., Nitti, F., and Bovet, D.: Activité du p-aminophénylsulfamide sur les infections streptococciques expérimentales de la souris et du lapin, C. R. Soc. Biol. **120**:756, 1942.

12 Welch, H., and Lewis, C. N.: Antibiotic therapy, Washington, D. C., 1951, The Arundel Press, Inc.

Recent reviews

13 Burchall, J. J., Ferone, R., and Hitchings, G. H.: Antibacterial chemotherapy, Ann. Rev. Pharmacol. **5**:53, 1965.

14 Feingold, D. S.: Antimicrobial chemotherapeutic agents: the nature of their action and selective toxicity, New Eng. J. Med. **269**:900, 957, 1963.

15 Hash, J. H.: Antibiotic mechanisms, Ann. Rev. Pharmacol. **12**:35, 1972.

16 Hayes, W.: Conjugation in Escherichia coli, Brit. Med. Bull. **18**:36, 1962.

17 Lorian, V.: The mode of action of antibiotics on gram-negative bacilli, Arch. Intern. Med. **128**:623, 1971.

18 Seneca, H.: Biological basis of chemotherapy of infections and infestations, Philadelphia, 1971, F. A. Davis Co.

19 Watanabe, T.: Infective heredity of multiple drug resistance in bacteria, Bact. Rev. **27**:87, 1963.

20 Weinstein, L., and Dalton, A. C.: Host determinants of response to antimicrobial agents, New Eng. J. Med. **279**:467, 524, 1968.

47 Sulfonamides

GENERAL CONCEPT

Despite the availability of numerous antibiotics, the sulfonamides still have important therapeutic uses, particularly in the treatment of acute urinary tract infections. In addition to a discussion of the pharmacology of the sulfonamides, reference will be made in this chapter to other drugs also that find applications chiefly in infections of the urinary tract. (See Table 47-2.)

SULFONAMIDE DRUGS
Chemistry

The majority of clinically useful sulfonamides may be looked upon as derivatives of sulfanilamide. As a rule, only those sulfonamides that have a free p-amino group show antibacterial activity. Compounds that are substituted in the amino group become active only if the substituent is removed in the body. This was the reason for the lack of activity of Prontosil in vitro, whereas it had considerable effectiveness in vivo.

Substitutions in the amide group have produced some of the most important sulfonamides, whose advantages over sulfanilamide consist of greater potency, wider antibacterial spectrum, and greater therapeutic index. The structural formulas of some of the most important sulfonamides for systemic use and those for local intestinal use are depicted in Table 47-1.

The sulfonamides that are substituted in the amino group may be useful as intestinal antiseptics if the substituent is removed slowly in the intestine and the compound is not absorbed to a great extent. Succinylsulfathiazole and phthalylsulfathiazole are examples of such drugs.

When sulfadiazine was introduced into therapeutics, it soon became obvious that it was superior to such previously used sulfonamides as sulfapyridine and sulfathiazole. The superiority manifested itself particularly in less toxicity than sulfapyridine and less sensitizing effect than sulfathiazole. Still, sulfadiazine has two major disadvantages. It has to be administered rather frequently in order to maintain a therapeutic level in the body, and it is also somewhat insoluble at the usual urinary hydrogen ion concentration—acteylsulfadiazine, its biotransformation product, being even more insoluble. As a consequence, there is always a danger of crystalluria.

The newer sulfonamides such as sulfisoxazole proved to be much more soluble at the usual urinary pH. A further aim in the development of the newer sulfonamides has been the prolongation of the half-life of the drug in the body to decrease the necessity of frequent administration. This objective has been achieved with such sulfonamides as sulfamethoxypyridazine, sulfadimethoxine, and sulfaphenazole.

Combinations of sulfamethoxazole and trimethoprim may increase the usefulness of the sulfonamides.

Antibacterial spectrum

The sulfonamides are effective against many gram-positive organisms, against some gram-negative diplococci and bacilli, and against certain large viruses of the *lymphopathia-psittacosis* group.

Sulfonamides are highly effective in the treatment of *nocardiosis, chancroid, trachoma,* and *inclusion conjunctivitis.* They are also quite effective in the treatment of *meningococcal meningitis,* although they are not the drugs of choice because of the appearance of resistant strains of meningococci. Sulfonamides are useful in the treatment of urinary tract infections, especially those caused by *Escherichia coli* or *Proteus mirabilis.* Other indications include prophylaxis of rheumatic fever and the treatment of chloroquine-resistant malaria caused by *Plasmodium falciparum.* Some former indications have become obsolete because of the development of bacterial resistance or the availability

Table 47-1. Structures of sulfonamides

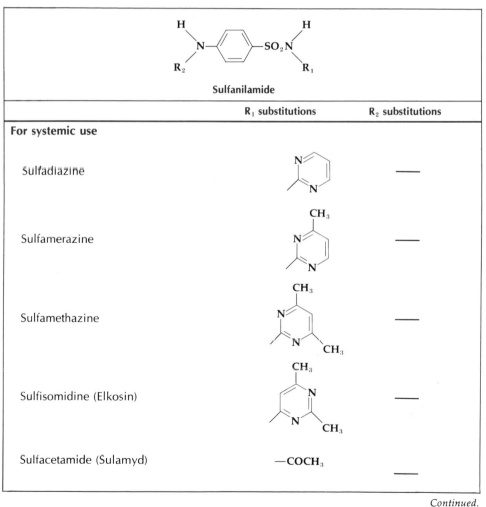

	R_1 substitutions	R_2 substitutions
For systemic use		
Sulfadiazine		—
Sulfamerazine		—
Sulfamethazine		—
Sulfisomidine (Elkosin)		—
Sulfacetamide (Sulamyd)	—$COCH_3$	—

Continued.

Table 47-1. Structures of sulfonamides—cont'd

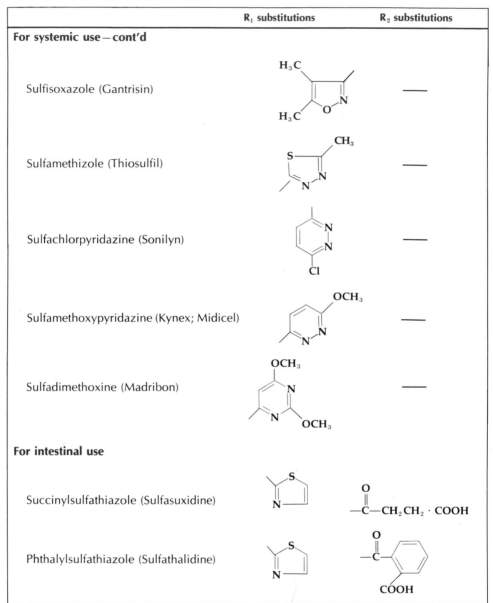

	R₁ substitutions	R₂ substitutions
For systemic use—cont'd		
Sulfisoxazole (Gantrisin)		—
Sulfamethizole (Thiosulfil)		—
Sulfachlorpyridazine (Sonilyn)		—
Sulfamethoxypyridazine (Kynex; Midicel)		—
Sulfadimethoxine (Madribon)		—
For intestinal use		
Succinylsulfathiazole (Sulfasuxidine)		—C—CH₂CH₂ · COOH
Phthalylsulfathiazole (Sulfathalidine)		

of more effective antibacterial agents. Thus *Shigella* dysentery and infections caused by Group A streptococci are no longer considered indications for sulfonamide therapy.

The *potency* of these drugs is such that growth inhibition may be achieved in simple media at a concentration of about 0.1 to 1 mg./ml. and at blood levels of the order of 10 mg./100 ml. The potency of these drugs in the test tube is greatly influenced by the nature of the culture medium. Thus enrichment with yeast extract, pus, or *p*-aminobenzoic acid causes marked decrease in the effectiveness of these drugs. Even in a simple synthetic medium the potency or activity per milligram of the sulfonamides is very much smaller than that of the most clinically useful antibiotics. For this reason, when compared with most antibiotics, relatively large doses of the sulfonamides must be administered.

Mode of action

The sulfonamides compete with *p*-aminobenzoic acid for incorporation into folic acid in susceptible bacteria (p. 558).

A study of the in vitro activity of various sulfonamides and the ionization and electron density of their SO_2 group led to the concept that a definite relationship exists between this physical property and activity in the test tube. Activity appeared maximal at around pK_a 6.5 and was less either below or above this figure.[1] Since the pK_a of sulfadiazine was close to the optimal figure, it was thought unlikely that any sulfonamide acting by competition with *p*-aminobenzoic acid would have greater activity than sulfadiazine. This means that newer sulfonamides are more likely to offer advantages on the basis of solubility, metabolism, renal handling, or lack of sensitizing properties than by having a significantly greater antibacterial potency.

SULFADIAZINE AS PROTOTYPE OF SULFONAMIDES

The pharmacology of sulfadiazine will be discussed in some detail. The other sulfonamides will be described by contrasting their pharmacology with that of sulfadiazine.

Metabolism

Sulfadiazine is absorbed rapidly from the gastrointestinal tract, mostly from the small intestine. If a single dose of 4 Gm. is administered, the blood level of the free drug is about 2 mg./100 ml. in 1 hour, reaching a peak of 8 mg./100 ml. in 4 hours. After 4 hours, the blood level gradually declines as a result of renal clearance. In 24 hours, more than half of the administered drug has been eliminated, and blood levels are generally less than 3 mg./100 ml.

If 6 Gm. of sulfadiazine is administered daily in divided doses, maintenance blood levels of 10 to 15 mg./100 ml. may be achieved.

About 80 to 90% of the drug in the body is in its original free form. The remainder is acetylsulfadiazine, which is formed in the liver by conjugation of the *p*-amino group.

A significant fraction of the drug is bound to plasma proteins.[3] In the case of sulfadiazine this bound fraction is about 25%. The bound fraction is not active against bacteria and does not penetrate into the spinal fluid under normal circumstances. As the free and acetylated drugs are excreted, the bound fraction undergoes equilibrium resorption and eventually is also excreted.

The volume of distribution of sulfadiazine, calculated on the basis of sulfadiazine concentration in the plasma filtrate (nonprotein-bound fraction), approaches the volume of total body water. This and other evidence indicate that the drug penetrates into various cells of the body.

Renal handling of sulfadiazine is similar to that of urea. The free drug is filtered through the glomeruli and is then partially reabsorbed. The acetylsulfadiazine is also filtered but is apparently not reabsorbed. As a consequence, renal clearance of acetylsulfadiazine is greater than that of sulfadiazine, and its concentration in the urine may be greater in relation to the free drug than in the plasma.

Just as in the case of urea, urinary concentrations of sulfadiazine are much greater than simultaneous blood levels. In fact, it may be as much as twenty-five times greater, so that in the presence of a blood level of 10 mg./100 ml. the urinary concentration of sulfadiazine may be 250 mg./100 ml. The high concentrations of sulfadiazine and acetylsulfadiazine in the urine predispose to precipitation of these compounds in the urinary tract. This is one of the few serious disadvantages of sulfadiazine.

The solubility of sulfadiazine in the urine is a function of the hydrogen ion concentration. At a neutral pH the urine can dissolve as much as 200 mg./100 ml. of sulfadiazine and even more of acetylsulfadiazine. On the other hand, the solubility of these compounds declines markedly as the urinary pH decreases. Thus at pH 5.5 only about 20 mg./100 ml. of these compounds can be dissolved in the urine, and crystalluria becomes inevitable at the usual doses of sulfadiazine.

The relationship between the pH and the solubility of the various sulfonamides is due to the fact that these compounds behave as weak acids because of the dissociation of the sulfamyl group ($-SO_2NH-$). Substitutions of the sulfamyl nitrogen can produce considerably stronger acids than sulfanilamide. The salts (ions) of the sulfonamides are much more soluble than the molecular form; thus the solubility of these drugs increases greatly when the pH is above the pK_a of the drug.

Sulfanilamide is such a weak acid that its solubility in the urine cannot be increased significantly by alkalinization. On the other hand, it has been shown that the solubility of sulfadiazine in urine at pH 7.4 is thirty-five times greater than in unbuffered water. Many of the newer sulfonamides are more soluble at the usual pH of the urine because they are stronger acids.

The implications of these findings are obvious. The urinary volume must be adequate. Alkalinization with sodium bicarbonate may be necessary. Another approach consists of using mixtures of sulfonamides.

It has been shown that when several sulfonamides are dissolved in water or urine, the presence of one does not influence the solubility of the others.[7,8] Since the antibacterial effects of such mixtures are additive, whereas their tendency to precipitate does not increase, this discovery provides a sound basis for simultaneous use of several sulfonamides. Such a therapeutic procedure can produce a higher total sulfonamide concentration in the urine, with diminished tendency for crystal formation.

Toxicity and hypersensitivity

Most of the adverse reactions to sulfadiazine are not due to direct toxicity but to acquired hypersensitivity. Experimental animals and most normal persons can tolerate enormous amounts of the sulfonamide without demonstrable changes in various physiologic functions or pathologic changes in various organs. On the other hand, some adverse reactions can be seen in about 6% of patients taking the drug. Most of these reactions such as dermatitis, leukopenia, hemolytic anemia, and drug fever may be related to acquired hypersensitivity or drug allergy. The renal lesions may be due to precipitation of sulfadiazine and its acetyl derivative in the urinary tract, but some renal damage has been attributed to a direct toxic effect on the kidney tubules. The latter is quite uncommon.

Many other toxic and hypersensitivity reactions to the sulfonamide drugs have been described, including hepatic damage, peripheral neuritis, and a condition resembling periartheritis nodosa.

Drug interactions

Sulfonamides and methenamine should not be administered simultaneously for the treatment of urinary tract infections, since formaldehyde liberated from methenamine in acid urine forms a precipitate with some of the sulfonamides. The binding of sulfonamides by plasma proteins leads to displacement of other drugs and may cause increased drug effects. Thus the actions of tolbutamide may be intensified, and kernicterus may be caused by the sulfonamides. The action of coumarins may also be intensified.

Clinical uses

Sulfadiazine is usually administered in the form of 0.5 Gm. tablets. The daily adult dose is 4 to 6 Gm. The soluble sodium salt of sulfadiazine is available for intravenous injection.

Indications for the use of sulfonamides have been changing as a consequence of the availability of numerous antibiotics. The Food and Drug Administration has concluded that the short-acting systemic sulfonamides, including sulfadiazine, are indicated only in the following conditions:

1. Chancroid
2. Trachoma
3. Inclusion conjunctivitis
4. Nocardiosis
5. Uncomplicated urinary tract infections caused by susceptible organisms such as *Escherichia coli, Klebsiella-Enterobacter, Staphylococcus aureus, Proteus mirabilis,* and less frequently, *Proteus vulgaris*
6. Toxoplasmosis—as adjunctive therapy with pyrimethamine
7. Malaria caused by chloroquine-resistant strains of *Plasmodium falciparum*—as adjunctive therapy
8. Meningococcal meningitis in which susceptible organisms have been demonstrated
9. *Haemophilus influenzae* meningitis—as adjunctive therapy with parenteral streptomycin
10. Prophylaxis of rheumatic fever—as an alternative to penicillin (only sulfadiazine has been demonstrated to have substantial effectiveness)*

Bacteria can develop resistance to the sulfonamides. The mechanism of resistance may be related to the ability of the bacteria to produce antagonists to the drug. In some cases increased production of *p*-aminobenzoic acid by the resistant organism has been demonstrated.

Comparison of other sulfonamides with sulfadiazine

The earlier sulfonamides, **sulfapyridine** and **sulfathiazole**, have been largely eliminated from clinical use because of greater toxicity and much greater incidence of hypersensitivity reactions.

Sulfamerazine and **sulfamethazine** resemble sulfadiazine in most respects, except for the fact that they are excreted more slowly by the kidney and are bound to plasma proteins to a much greater extent. The main usefulness of these methylated sulfadiazines is their inclusion in the **triple-sulfonamide mixtures.**

Since it was recognized that the low solubility of sulfadiazine and acetylsulfadiazine in acid urine is a major drawback, many efforts have been made to prevent the

---

* Quoted, with slight modifications, from FDA circular letter, Sept. 12, 1969.

precipitation of sulfonamides in the urine. Alkalinization and forcing fluids to maintain adequate urinary volume are helpful but generally do not completely solve the problem. Since the various sulfonamides can exist in solution without influencing their respective solubilities, it has been proposed that mixtures of three or more of these drugs would allow maintenance of higher blood levels and higher urinary concentrations of total sulfonamide without the danger of crystalluria.[7]

The usual dose of a triple-sulfonamide mixture is 2 to 4 Gm. initially, followed by 1 Gm. every 6 hours in adults. Children receive 60 to 100 mg./kg. initially, followed by one fourth of this dose every 6 hours.

In minimizing the renal complications due to insolubility of the drugs, the physician has a choice between using the triple-sulfonamide mixtures and using some of the newer sulfonamides that are more soluble.

Sulfisoxazole (Gantrisin) has similar antibacterial properties to those of sulfadiazine. Its solubility at pH 6 is much greater than that of sulfadiazine. In fact, it is more than ten times as soluble. At pH 5.5 its solubility in human urine is only about 120 mg./100 ml., which is still four times as great as the solubility of sulfadiazine but is no guarantee against crystal formation. Sulfisoxazole is cleared rather rapidly from the blood and produces high urinary levels. A comparison of sulfisoxazole and sulfadiazine with regard to blood levels and urinary excretion is shown in Fig. 47-1.

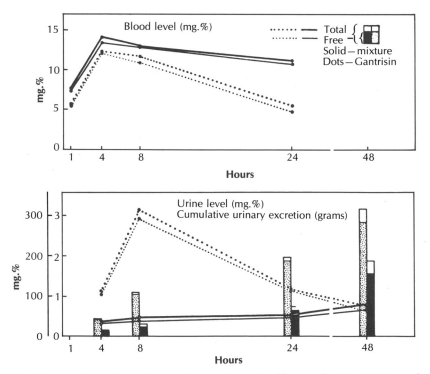

Fig. 47-1. Comparative absorption and excretion of sulfisoxazole (Gantrisin) and triple mixture of sulfadiazine-sulfamerazine-sulfamethazine in a group of three human subjects. Single oral dose of 4 Gm.; crossed experiment, sulfisoxazole first, mixture 6 days later. (From Lehr, D.: Antibiot. Chemother. [Basel] **3:**71, 1953.)

Acetyl sulfisoxazole (Gantrisin acetyl) differs from sulfisoxazole mainly in being tasteless and suitable for liquid oral preparations. The drug is deacetylated in the intestine, and the active drug is absorbed. Sulfisoxazole diolamine (Gantrisin diolamine) is less irritating and is thus suitable for topical use. Sulfamethoxazole (Gantanol), a congener of sulfisoxazole, is more slowly absorbed and excreted than the parent drug. It may cause crystalluria.

Other soluble sulfonamides that are used primarily for urinary tract infections are sulfamethizole (Thiosulfil), sulfisomidine (Elkosin), and sulfachlorpyridazine (Sonilyn). Sulfacetamide (Sulamyd) is quite soluble also but is useful primarily as a topical drug in ophthalmic infections, being less effective for the treatment of urinary tract infections.

More recent developments in sulfonamide therapy have to do with the introduction of drugs that have very low renal clearance. As a consequence, relatively small doses given infrequently ensure sustained blood levels. Sulfamethoxypyridazine (Kynex; Midicel) is excreted so slowly that 24 hours after administration of 1 Gm. of the drug the blood levels of 5 to 10 mg./100 ml. are still maintained. As a consequence, an initial priming dose of 2 Gm. followed by 1 Gm. once a day is sufficient to maintain therapeutic blood levels. Another sulfonamide that is cleared very slowly is sulfadimethoxine (Madribon).

The slowly excreted sulfonamides such as sulfamethoxypyridazine or sulfadimethoxine have been associated with the development of serious, even fatal, Stevens-Johnson syndrome (erythema multiforme exudativum). For this reason the short-acting sulfonamides are much preferred.

Co-trimoxazole (Bactrim, Septrin) is a synergistic combination of sulfamethoxazole and trimethoprim, the latter being a methotrexate analog. The combination is truly synergistic because the sulfonamide inhibits the conversion of para-aminobenzoic acid to dihydrofolic acid, and trimethoprim interferes with the synthesis of tetrahydrofolic acid by bacteria. This combination extends greatly the usefulness of the sulfonamides in the treatment of urinary infections, gonorrhea, bronchitis, and typhoid fever caused by strains of Salmonella typhi resistant to ampicillin and chloramphenicol. On the other hand, adverse reactions to the drug combination, including hematologic complications, are significant and may limit its use in many of its possible applications.

TOPICAL SULFONAMIDES

The topical application of sulfonamides is generally undesirable because the effectiveness of the drugs is antagonized by pus and sensitization is common. An exception to this statement is mafenide (Sulfamylon).

Mafenide acetate (Sulfamylon acetate) and mafenide hydrochloride (Sulfamylon hydrochloride) are useful when applied topically to infected wounds and for the treatment of burns. These drugs are not inactivated by pus or p-aminobenzoic acid. The acetate is available as a cream, and the hydrochloride as a topical solution. Structurally mafenide differs from all other useful sulfonamides in that it is α-amino-p-toluenesulfonamide rather than a benzenesulfonamide.

Problem 47-1. Ten burned patients were treated with topical mafenide acetate cream. The urine became persistently alkaline in 9 of the 10 patients. What was the probable mechanism? Mafenide is absorbed in part and acts as a carbonic anhydrase inhibitor.[12]

Table 47-2. Antibacterial agents used principally for urinary tract infections*

Drug	Activity spectrum and characteristics	Dosage	Route	Side effects
Sulfonamides	Short-acting sulfonamides are best because of high urinary concentration and good solubility at acid pH; more active in alkaline urine; especially effective against *E. coli* and *Pr. mirabilis*; many strains of *Klebsiella, Aerobacter, Proteus,* and *Pseudomonas* are resistant Sulfisoxazole (Gantrisin) Sulfamethizole (Thiosulfil) Sulfisomidine (Elkosin) Sulfachlorpyridazine (Sonilyn) Sulfamethoxazole (Gantanol)	Varies with drug	P.O.	Allergic reactions; skin rash, drug fever, pruritus, photosensitization; periarteritis nodosa, S.L.E., Stevens-Johnson syndrome, serum sickness syndrome, myocarditis; neurotoxicity (psychosis, neuritis); hepatotoxicity; blood dyscrasias, usually agranulocytosis; crystalluria; nausea and vomiting, headache, dizziness, lassitude, mental depression, acidosis, sulfhemoglobin; hemolytic anemia in G6PD-deficient individuals; possible teratogenic effects; should not be used in newborn infants or in women near term.
Cephaloglycin (Kafocin)	Many gram-positive (including enterococci) and gram-negative organisms; as relates to urinary tract, cephaloglycin is effective against likely pathogens except *Pseudomonas*	0.25-0.5 Gm. q.6h.	P.O.	G.I. (22%), hypersensitivity, eosinophilia, fever, dizziness, possible balanitis
Nitrofurantoin (Furadantin)	Many gram-positive and gram-negative organisms; as relates to urinary tract, nitrofurantoin is effective against likely pathogens except *Pseudomonas* and some *Klebsiella-Enterobacter* and *Proteus* species; high urinary concentration (ineffective in renal failure); increased activity in acid urine; action much reduced at pH 8 or over	100 mg. q.6h. (5-7 mg./kg.)	P.O. I.V.	Nausea and vomiting, hypersensitivity, peripheral neuropathy, pulmonary infiltrate, intrahepatic cholestasis, hemolytic anemia in G6PD deficiency; contraindicated in renal failure; should not be used in infants less than 1 month of age

Methenamine mandelate (Mancelamine)	Combination effect against most organisms in vitro; methenamine has no action per se but in acid medium is slowly decomposed with liberation of formaldehyde; mandelic acid also requires acid pH; effective only when acid urine (preferably about pH 5) can be maintained; limited place in therapy; should not be used in tissue infection (pyelonephritis)	1 Gm. q.6h.	P.O.	Nausea and vomiting; contraindicated in renal failure because it leads to acidosis
Nalidixic acid (NegGram)	Gram-negative urinary tract pathogens (*Enterobacteriaceae*) except *Pseudomonas*; high degree of resistance may develop rapidly during therapy	1 Gm. q.6h.	P.O.	G.I. hypersensitivity, fever, eosinophilia, photosensitivity, neurologic disturbances (H.A., malaise, drowsiness, dizziness, visual disturbances); convulsions, pseudotumor; cerebri (?); mild leukopenia, thrombocytopenia, hemolytic anemia; can produce false elevations of 17-ketosteroids and 17-ketogenic steroids in urine

*Courtesy Dr. Jay P. Sanford, Dallas.

SULFONAMIDES AS INTESTINAL ANTISEPTICS

Sulfonamides that are poorly absorbed from the intestine may be used for decreasing intestinal bacterial flora. **Sulfaguanidine** was the first sulfonamide introduced for this purpose. However, about one third of the administered dose was absorbed. As a consequence, it was soon replaced for this specialized purpose by drugs whose absorption was much less.

Succinylsulfathiazole (Sulfasuxidine) and **phthalylsulfathiazole** (Sulfathalidine) are substituted in the *p*-amino portion of the sulfathiazole molecule. As a consequence, they have no antibacterial activity in the test tube. However, when they are swallowed and reach the large intestine, they are hydrolyzed, and the free sulfathiazole reaches high local concentrations. This sulfathiazole is not well absorbed from the large intestine. Either drug is administered in large doses prior to bowel operation and for treatment of certain intestinal infections. Not more than 3 to 5% of the administered dose is absorbed, and adverse reactions to this medication are infrequent.

The coliform and clostridia organisms are markedly decreased in the intestine and the volume and character of the feces change when these intestinal antiseptic sulfonamides are administered for several days. Certain organisms such as *Proteus, Pseudomonas, Salmonella,* and enterococci may be resistant to the action of these drugs.

The usual daily doses for adults are 0.125 to 0.25 Gm./kg. The antibiotic neomycin, given orally, has largely replaced the sulfonamides in intestinal antisepsis.

ANTIBACTERIAL AGENTS USED PRINCIPALLY FOR URINARY TRACT INFECTIONS

In addition to the sulfonamides, a number of antibacterial agents are used almost exclusively in the treatment of urinary tract infections. Their major characteristics are summarized in Table 47-2.

Nitrofurantoin (Furadantin) is one of a series of nitrofurans that have been introduced as antibacterial agents.

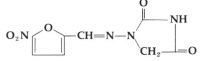

Nitrofurantoin

The drug is absorbed rapidly, and much of it is excreted unchanged in the urine. It has a wide antibacterial spectrum, and both gram-positive and gram-negative bacteria can be inhibited at levels that are obtainable in the urine following the daily oral administration of 5 to 10 mg./kg. It may cause a variety of sensitivity reactions: nausea and vomiting, skin sensitization, peripheral neuritis, and cholestatic jaundice. A macrocrystalline preparation (Macrodantin) may be less nauseating. The sodium salt of nitrofurantoin may be administered intravenously.

Preparations of **nitrofurantoin** as Furadantin include tablets containing 50 and 100 mg. and a suspension, 25 mg./5 ml.; and as Macrodantin, capsules containing 50 and 100 mg. **Nitrofurantoin sodium.** (Furadantin sodium is available for intravenous injection as a powder, 180 mg. in 20 ml. containers.)

No bacteriostatic blood levels are produced following oral administration of nitrofurantoin. Its use in systemic infections is not supported by the available evidence.[11]

Drugs related to nitrofurantoin are available for special applications. **Nitrofurazone** (Furacin) is used topically for infections of the skin, but it may cause sensitization. **Furazolidone** is used orally for bacterial and giardial intestinal infections. Furazolidone is an inhibitor of monoamine oxidase, and foods rich in tyramine should be avoided when the drug is used. It may also cause disulfiram-like reactions when alcohol is ingested. **Furazolidone** (Furoxone) is available in tablets containing 100 mg.

Methenamine mandelate (Mandelamine) is a combination of two fairly old urinary antiseptics, methenamine (Urotropin) and mandelic acid.

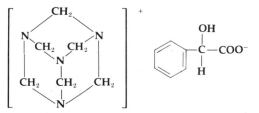

Methenamine mandelate

Methenamine, or hexamethylenetetramine, liberates *formaldehyde* in acid urine. Mandelic acid is bactericidal also if the pH of the urine is low. If the pH of the urine is higher than 6, it is necessary to administer ammonium chloride in amounts of 0.5 to 1 Gm. three or four times daily.

Methenamine mandelate is relatively nontoxic, but gastric irritation may occur following its use. This is probably related to production of some formaldehyde in the acid gastric juice. For the same reason urinary frequency may also occur. The usual dose of methenamine mandelate is 0.5 to 1 Gm. three times a day.

Methenamine mandelate has the advantage of being well tolerated and is suitable for long-continued administration without the development of tolerance. Although much more potent drugs are available, the drug is useful in the treatment of urinary tract infections caused by gram-negative bacteria such as *E. coli.*

In addition to methenamine mandelate (Mandelamine), the hippurate salt of methenamine (Hiprex) is also available.

Nalidixic acid (NegGram), a relatively new drug, is chemically unrelated to other urinary antiseptics.[2] It is well absorbed from the gastrointestinal tract and is largely excreted in the urine, in part as glucuronide.

Nalidixic acid is effective *only* against gram-negative bacteria such as *E. coli, Proteus* and some strains of *Pseudomonas, Enterobacter,* and *Klebsiella.* Resistance to the drug develops readily. Nalidixic acid is ineffective against systemic infections because its activity is greatly reduced in the presence of proteins.

Nausea, vomiting, diarrhea, allergic reactions, and neurological disturbances may occur as a consequence of the administration of nalidixic acid.

Preparations of **Nalidixic acid** (NegGram) include tablets of 250 and 500 mg.

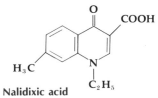

Nalidixic acid

References

1 Bell, P. H., and Roblin, R. O., Jr.: Studies in chemotherapy: a theory of the relation of structure to activity of sulfanilamide type compounds, J. Amer. Chem. Soc. **64**:2905, 1942.

2 Carroll, G.: NegGram (nalidixic acid), a new antimicrobial chemotherapeutic agent, J. Urol. **90**:476, 1963.

3 Davis, B. D.: The binding of sulfonamide drugs by plasma proteins: a factor in determining the distribution of drugs in the body, J. Clin. Invest. **22**:753, 1943.

4 Goldstein, A.: Antibacterial chemotherapy, New Eng. J. Med. **240**:98, 137, 180, 1949.

5 Kass, E. H.: Chemotherapeutic and antibiotic drugs in the management of infection of the urinary tract, Amer. J. Med. **18**:764, 1955.

6 Knight, V., Draper, J. W., Brady, E. A., and Attmore, C. A.: Methenamine mandelate: antimicrobial activity, absorption and excretion, Antibiot. Chemother. (Basel) **2**:615, 1952.

7 Lehr, D.: Inhibition of drug precipitation in the urinary tract by the use of sulfonamide mixtures; sulfathiazole-sulfadiazine mixture, Proc. Soc. Exp. Biol. Med. **58**:11, 1945.

8 Lehr, D.: Comparative merits of 3,4-dimethyl-5-sulfanilamido-isoxazole (Gantrisin) and a sulfapyrimidine triple mixture (an evaluation of properties important at the bedside), Antibiot. Chemother. (Basel) **3**:71, 1953.

9 Poth, E. J., and Ross, C. A.: The clinical use of phthalylsulfathiazole, J. Lab. Clin. Med. **29**:785, 1944.

10 Richards, W. A., Riss, E., Kass, E. H., and Finland, M.: Nitrofurantoin: clinical and laboratory studies in urinary tract infections, Arch. Intern. Med. **96**:437, 1955.

11 Sanford, J. P.: Nitrofurantoin in extragenito-urinary infections? Curr. Ther. Res. **2**:476, 1960.

12 White, M. G., and Asch, M. J.: Acid-base effects of topical mafenide acetate in the burned patient, New Eng. J. Med. **284**:1281, 1971.

13 Woods, D. D.: Relation of *p*-aminobenzoic acid to mechanism of action of sulphanilamide, Brit. J. Exp. Path. **21**:74, 1940.

14 Work, T. S., and Work, E.: The basis of chemotherapy, New York, 1948, Interscience Publishers, Inc.

Recent reviews

15 Draper, J. W.: Development of sulfonamides: historical account, Curr. Med. Digest **23**:855, 1965.

16 Struller, T.: Long-acting and short-acting sulfonamides; recent developments, Antibiot. Chemother. (Basel) **14**:179, 1968.

17 Weinstein, I., Madoff, M. A., and Samet, C. A.: The sulfonamides, New Eng. J. Med. **263**:793, 842, 1960.

48 Antibiotic drugs

Among the hundreds of compounds produced by microorganisms that have inhibitory action on other microorganisms, only a relatively small number have a favorable therapeutic index. These are the clinically useful antibiotics. In the present discussion, particular attention will be paid to the potency, antibacterial spectrum, metabolism, and mode of action of these various antibiotic drugs.

ANTIBIOTIC SYNERGISM AND ANTAGONISM

It has been assumed for years that the actions of various chemotherapeutic agents are simply additive. Certain studies have shown, however, that other antibiotics may enhance or interfere with the killing effect of penicillin.[29] Although this concept is important only in a few clinical situations, its application in these cases may make the difference between success and failure.

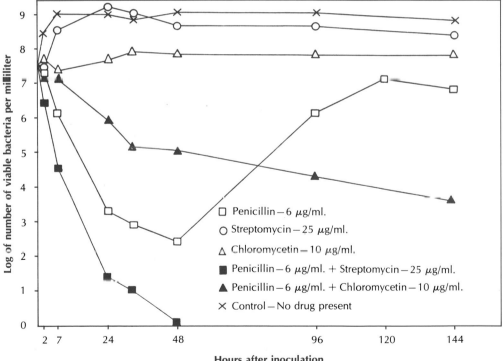

Fig. 48-1. Effect of penicillin, streptomycin, and chloramphenicol (Chloromycetin) on enterococci in vitro. (From Jawetz, E., Gunnison, J. B., and Coleman, V. R.: Science **111:**254, 1950.)

575

On the basis of these studies the antibiotics have been divided into two groups:

Group I: Penicillin, streptomycin, bacitracin, neomycin, and polymyxins

Group II: Chloramphenicol, the tetracyclines, erythromycin, novobiocin, and also the sulfonamides

Members of Group I have additive effects and may be synergistic with regard to bactericidal effect. Members of Group II may have additive bacteriostatic effects, but they are never truly synergistic in a bactericidal sense and may antagonize the killing effect of penicillin and other members of Group I.

The current view is that the general guidelines for antibiotic synergism and antagonism, as outlined, may not apply in a given case unless special tests are performed on the causative organism. Nevertheless, penicillin and streptomycin are used together in enterococcus infections, while the simultaneous use of chlortetracycline and penicillin is frowned upon in pneumococcus meningitis. These are illustrations of the practical importance of antibiotic synergism and antagonism.

Experimental demonstration of antibiotic synergism and antagonism is shown in Fig. 48-1.

It is important to emphasize that the concepts of antibiotic synergism and antagonism may be relatively unimportant if the defense mechanisms of the body are operating efficiently. These concepts may be of vital importance in the absence of such favorable conditions. In any case, the mere existence of antibiotic antagonism, rare as it may be, should be a warning against shotgun therapy with antibiotic drugs.

PENICILLIN

When Florey and co-workers reported in 1941 on the remarkable effectiveness of penicillin, attention was immediately directed toward producing this antibiotic in quantity and determining its structure. Both of these problems have been solved. It now appears that penicillin is one of several closely related compounds having similar antibacterial spectrums but differing in ease of manufacture and degree of protein binding in the body.

Other problems are finding injectable forms with delayed absorption and preparation of semisynthetic penicillins, which may have advantages over naturally occurring compounds. Much effort is being expended at present in the hope that oral absorption may be improved by certain chemical manipulations of the penicillin molecule and that the antibacterial spectrum may also be modified.

The greatest recent advance in the preparation of new semisynthetic penicillins resulted from isolation of 6-aminopenicillanic acid from fermentation media and synthetic attachment of various chemical groups to this basic structure. The discovery of penicillins that are resistant to penicillinase has considerably broadened the useful spectrum of this antibiotic. It may be anticipated that many important new penicillins will be introduced in the future.

Penicillin is an organic acid. Its sodium, potassium, and procaine salts are commonly used. There are several other naturally occurring penicillins that differ from penicillin G in having a side chain other than benzyl. Some of these are penicillin F, dihydro F (amylpenicillin), and also K and X. None of these naturally occurring compounds have a significant advantage over penicillin G, and some, such as K, may be much less effective in vivo because of a high degree of plasma protein binding.

Although several biosynthetic penicillins have been prepared by adding various precursors of the side chain to the *Penicillium* culture medium, more recently a new procedure has opened up a field for the preparation of new penicillins. A key intermediate, 6-aminopenicillanic acid, is produced by fermentation, and new penicillins are prepared by adding various groups to this intermediate. One of the first of these new "synthetic" penicillins, phenethicillin (Syncillin), is the N-acylation product of 6-amino-

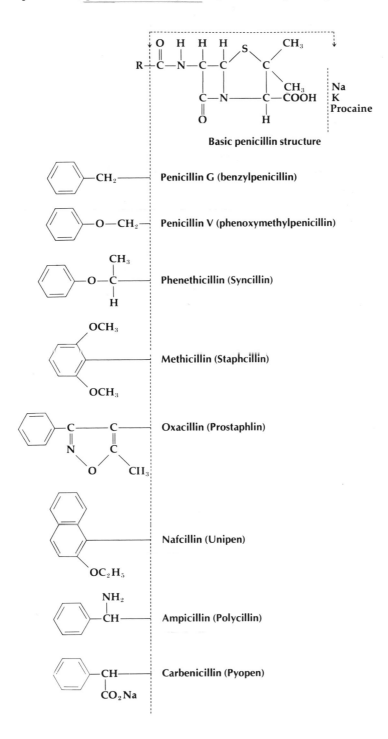

Basic penicillin structure

Penicillin G (benzylpenicillin)

Penicillin V (phenoxymethylpenicillin)

Phenethicillin (Syncillin)

Methicillin (Staphcillin)

Oxacillin (Prostaphlin)

Nafcillin (Unipen)

Ampicillin (Polycillin)

Carbenicillin (Pyopen)

penicillanic acid and α-phenoxypropionic acid. Its structural formula is similar to that of penicillin V (phenoxymethylpenicillin). It is quite stable in acid, as is penicillin V. It occurs as a mixture of the L isomer and the D isomer.

Penicillin has been completely synthesized through cooperative efforts of several groups of workers. Total synthesis is much too difficult for commercial production.

Penicillin is very soluble in water. It is labile in solution, particularly in an acid medium. In the powder form it is quite stable. The greater resistance of penicillin V and phenethicillin to acid decomposition has been noted previously.

Potency and antibacterial spectrum

Penicillin preparations are standardized on the basis of their growth-inhibition potency against test organisms such as *Bacillus subtilis* or staphylococci. Activity is expressed in units and is measured in comparison with a standard preparation by determining the zone of inhibition of bacterial growth on an inoculated agar plate. The amount of activity represented by 1 unit is sufficient to prevent multiplication of a susceptible organism such as *Bacillus subtilis* or certain staphylococci in as much as 20 to 50 ml. of broth. One milligram of penicillin G represents 1,667 units. This means that 1 unit is equivalent to 0.6 μg of penicillin G.

The enormous activity of penicillin may be appreciated from the fact that, if 1 mg. of the antibiotic were placed in about 5 gallons of broth, the growth of several susceptible organisms would be prevented by the resulting minute concentration of the antibiotic. By contrast, it would be necessary to add 2 to 20 Gm. of a sulfonamide to this volume of culture medium in order to obtain similar growth inhibition. The majority of the clinically useful antibiotics have a much greater potency than do the sulfonamides but not as great as that of penicillin. These differences in potency are reflected in the recommended dosages of these various drugs.

Microorganisms inhibited by less than 1 unit of penicillin/ml. may be considered moderately susceptible. The highly susceptible infective agents are usually inhibited by less than 0.1 unit/ml. Blood levels of 0.1 to 1.0 unit/ml. can be achieved without difficulty in clinical practice. Representative microorganisms that are readily inhibited by such penicillin concentrations are *Streptococcus (Diplococcus) pneumoniae, Neisseria gonorrhoeae, Neisseria meningitidis, Streptococcus pyogenes,* some strains of *Micrococcus pyogenes (Staphylococcus), Bacillus anthracis, Treponema pallidum,* and *Actinomyces bovis.* Clostridia and the causative agents of leptospirosis and diphtheria also are susceptible to penicillin. On the other hand, most gram-negative bacilli such as *Escherichia coli, Salmonella* organisms, *Klebsiella, Shigella, Proteus,* and *Pseudomonas* are highly resistant. The same is true for *Streptococcus faecalis,* many strains of *Micrococcus pyogenes (Staphylococcus),* mycobacteria, yeast, and fungi. As a consequence, penicillin must be considered an antibiotic having a relatively narrow antibacterial spectrum when compared with tetracyclines and other broad-spectrum antibiotics.

Mode of action

Penicillin is both bacteriostatic and bactericidal. Even with very low concentrations of penicillin present, susceptible bacteria may not multiply. If they do, they may acquire abnormal morphologic characteristics and may undergo lysis.

The bactericidal activity of penicillin is quite different from that of the common disinfectants. Penicillin does not kill bacteria rapidly on contact. It apparently produces some alteration in the bacteria that makes them more susceptible to death and disruption. It has been established that rapidly multiplying bacteria are most susceptible to the killing effect of penicillin.

Metabolism

The absorption of penicillin G from the gastrointestinal tract is incomplete and variable. In order to obtain comparable blood levels it is usually necessary to administer five times as much of the antibiotic by the oral route as by intramuscular injection. The reasons for this incomplete absorption are inactivation of the drug by the gastric juice and, once it reaches the large intestine, by bacteria as well. Some of the newer penicillin preparations such as penicillin V or phenethicillin are fairly resistant to the acid of an acid environment. Oral administration of these newer penicillins produces higher blood levels, particularly when large doses are administered.

The absorption of penicillin following oral administration is greatly influenced by the presence of food in the stomach and the rate of gastric emptying. More predictable results are obtained if the drug is taken on an empty stomach.

Blood levels obtained following administration of 100,000 units of penicillin G sodium by various routes are shown in Fig. 48-2. It is clear that very transient high levels reaching 2 to 4 units/ml. can be obtained by either the intravenous or intramuscular route. The same dose given orally produces a blood level of only about 0.4 unit/ml., but demonstrable activity remains for a longer time.

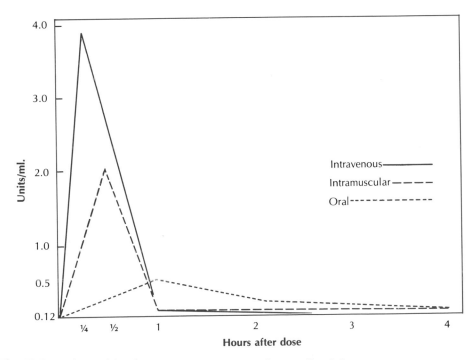

Fig. 48-2. Relative blood serum concentrations of penicillin following intravenous, intramuscular, and oral administration of 100,000 units of crystalline sodium penicillin G. (From Welch, H., et. al.: Principles and practice of antibiotic therapy, New York, 1954, Medical Encyclopedia, Inc.)

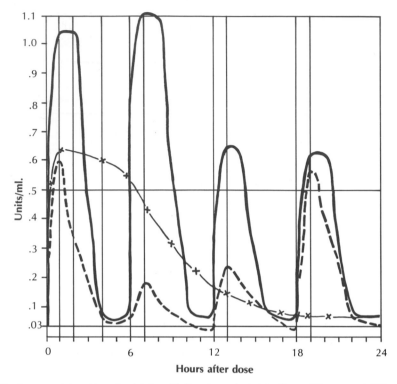

Fig. 48-3. Average blood levels obtained following administration of three penicillin prepara-tions: ——, oral penicillin V, 400,000 μg every 6 hours; ----, oral penicillin G, 400,000 μg; —×—×—×—, intramuscular aqueous procaine penicillin G, 400,000 μg. (From Symon, W. E.: In Antibiotics annual, 1955–1956, New York, 1956, Medical Encyclopedia, Inc.)

A comparison of blood levels following oral administration of 400,000 units of peni-cillin G and the same dose of penicillin V is shown in Fig. 48-3. It also shows the blood levels obtained following intramuscular injection of the same dose of aqueous procaine penicillin G. Penicillin V gave blood levels up to 1 unit/ml., which fell to less than 0.1 unit/ml. in about 4 hours. Penicillin G was not quite as effective and gave more variable results. Aqueous procaine penicillin G injected intramuscularly produced levels in the blood of about 0.6 unit/ml., and significant levels persisted for a much longer time, even up to 24 hours. It should be recalled that most highly susceptible microorganisms are inhibited by penicillin concentrations of 0.1 unit/ml. or less.

The rapid decline of penicillin blood levels is due to rapid renal clearance of the antibiotic. It has been well established that penicillin is actively secreted by the renal tubules, apparently by the same mechanism as *p*-aminohippurate or iodopyracet (Diodrast). Drugs have been developed that can block this tubular secretory mechanism. One of these is probenecid (Benemid), which is quite effective. It is of little use in penicillin therapy, however, since it is just as easy to use larger doses of penicillin as to administer a second drug for the purpose of preventing its excretion. Probenecid, on the other hand, has an important clinical application as a uricosuric drug.

A number of repository preparations of penicillin are available for the purpose of producing sustained blood levels. Procaine penicillin G and benzathine penicillin G

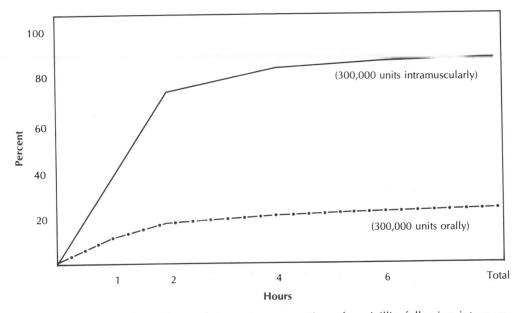

Fig. 48-4. Comparison of cumulative urinary excretion of penicillin following intramuscular and oral administration of crystalline sodium penicillin G. (From Welch, H., et al.: Principles and practice of antibiotic therapy, New York, 1954, Medical Encyclopedia, Inc.)

are two such preparations. With the latter preparation, demonstrable penicillin blood levels can be maintained for as long as 20 days. It is important to keep in mind, however, that demonstrable blood levels are often defined as 0.03 unit/ml. or more. This low concentration of the antibiotic may not suffice in many infections although it may be beneficial in prevention of streptococcal infections and prophylaxis of rheumatic fever.

Distribution of penicillin in the body is far from uniform. First, the antibiotic is partially bound to plasma proteins. Under normal circumstances it penetrates poorly into the cerebrospinal fluid, aqueous humor, and joint fluids. On the other hand, inflammation at these various sites greatly increases the permeability to penicillin.

The cumulative urinary excretion of sodium penicillin G following its oral and intramuscular administration is shown in Fig. 48-4. As much as 80% of the intramuscularly administered dose may be recovered in the urine in less than 4 hours. Only about 20% is usually recovered following the oral administration of the antibiotic. With oral administration, this difference is due to lack of absorption of much of the administered dose.

Toxicity and hypersensitivity

The inherent toxicity of penicillin as determined in animal experiments is extremely low. In several animal species the acute toxicity of penicillin is so low that death from overdosage has been attributed to the cation rather than to penicillin itself.

Unfortunately, however, a significant percentage of the human population show hypersensitivity reactions to penicillin. These reactions are of many different types, ranging from immediate anaphylactic reactions to late manifestations of the serum sickness type. It is believed that several hundred severe anaphylactic reactions have occurred following penicillin injections, many terminating fatally.

Hypersensitivity reactions are seen most often following topical use of penicillin and most rarely after oral administration. The incidence of such reactions has been estimated to vary from 1 to 8% in the general population.

Skin tests for the determination of penicillin allergy are unreliable and dangerous when penicillin G itself is injected in small quantities intracutaneously. On the other hand, preparations are available, at least for experimental purposes, in which penicilloylpolylysine (PPL) is suitable for testing allergy to the major determinant. Also, a mixture of penicillin, penicilloate, and other products are suitable for testing allergy to the minor determinants. Despite these refinements in diagnosing penicillin allergy, tests are not completely reliable. As a consequence, the history of previous reactions is very important, and even in the presence of a negative intradermal test, it is best to be prepared for the possibility of anaphylactic reaction whenever the antibiotic is injected.

In addition to the hypersensitivity reactions, penicillin is capable of producing other adverse effects. Neural tissue may be susceptible to penicillin, particularly when the drug is injected intrathecally or applied directly to the surface of the brain. Convulsive phenomena have been noted following such procedures. There is seldom any reason for injecting penicillin intrathecally.

Therapeutic uses

Despite the development of many new antibiotics, penicillin remains one of the most important anti-infective agents. A special advantage of this antibiotic is its killing effect on bacteria, which allows it to eradicate infections even in clinical situations in which the defense mechanisms of the body are not functioning in an efficient manner. In subacute bacterial endocarditis, certain forms of meningitis, and infections complicating agranulocytosis, this is a special advantage of penicillin when compared with the merely bacteriostatic antibiotics or the sulfonamides.

Such repository types of penicillin preparations as aqueous procaine penicillin G, procaine penicillin G in oily vehicles, or benzathine penicillin G (N,N-dibenzylethylenediamine dipenicillin) have been designed for the purpose of achieving sustained blood levels. In many instances the susceptibility of the infective agents may be such that sustained low blood levels will not suffice for obtaining the desired therapeutic effect, and additional quantities of aqueous penicillin must be given by the intramuscular or intravenous route. As much as 100 million units have been injected daily in some cases of subacute bacterial endocarditis. With these enormous doses, the adverse effects of the cation of the penicillin salt may become a problem.

Disadvantages

The major disadvantage of penicillin is its sensitizing capacity. A significant percentage of the general population is allergic to penicillin, and alarming, even fatal, anaphylactic reactions may occur following its use.

NEWER PENICILLINS AND CEPHALOSPORINS

The discovery of semisynthetic penicillins that are resistant to staphylococcal penicillinase was a milestone in penicillin therapy. Oxacillin (Prostaphlin), cloxacillin, nafcillin, and methicillin (Staphcillin) belong to this group.[38] A broad-spectrum penicillin introduced recently is ampicillin (Polycillin). It is quite active against many

Table 48-1. Newer penicillins and cephalothin

Drug	Properties		
	Acid stability	Penicillinase resistance	Broad spectrum
Penicillin G	0	0	0
Methicillin	0	+	0
Oxacillin	+	+	0
Nafcillin	+	+	0
Ampicillin	+	0	+
Cephalothin	0	+	+

gram-negative bacilli but not against many strains of *Proteus, Enterobacter,* and *Pseudomonas.* It is susceptible to penicillinase. Carbenicillin (Pyopen) differs from other penicillins in its activity against *Pseudomonas aeruginosa.* It inhibits most strains in vitro at a concentration of 25 to 200 μg/ml. It is not effective against penicillinase-producing staphylococci or *Klebsiella.*[9, 10]

It is of great importance to put the advantages and disadvantages of the newer penicillins in their proper perspective in relation to penicillin G (Tables 48-1 and 48-2).

Penicillin G is much more active per unit weight against many microorganisms than are oxacillin, methicillin, and ampicillin. It remains the drug of choice for infections caused by gram-positive cocci, including nonpenicillinase-producing staphylococci, and for syphilis, gonorrhea, and meningococcal meningitis. The advantages of oxacillin and methicillin are in regard to penicillinase-producing staphylococci. Methicillin should be used only parenterally. Oxacillin may be used by oral administration, but the oral use of any penicillin in a severe infection is questionable.

Ampicillin has no advantages over penicillin G in most infections and is much more costly. Its advantage is in relation to certain gram-negative organisms such as *Proteus mirabilis, Haemophilus influenzae, Escherichia coli,* and some strains of *Klebsiella* and *Salmonella.*

The penicillinase-resistant drugs oxacillin and nafcillin should not be used routinely as substitutes for penicillin G. They are less active against most microorganisms. Furthermore, staphylococci can develop resistance to these newer penicillins, and the resistance thus developed extends to penicillin G. Several instances of methicillin-resistant staphylococci have been reported recently.

The dose of oxacillin is 2 to 3 Gm./day taken in divided doses on an empty stomach. About 60% of the drug is absorbed. Oxacillin is generally as active as nafcillin, but both are less active than penicillin G, except against penicillinase-producing staphylococci. Methicillin is administered in doses of 1 Gm. by either the intramuscular or intravenous route, but because of its low potency, it is being replaced by nafcillin or oxacillin. Oxacillin and nafcillin are very similar in clinical characteristics, except that oxacillin is better absorbed from the gastrointestinal tract whereas nafcillin is more active against pneumococci and Group A streptococci.

The recently introduced semisynthetic cloxacillin resembles oxacillin both structurally and in regard to its pharmacology.

Important new antibiotics, structurally related to penicillin, are produced by a *Cephalosporium* mold. Cephalosporins differ in their basic nucleus from the penicillins by having a *six-membered* ring containing sulfur. The greatest advantages of the cephalo-

Table 48-2. Summary of current usage of penicillins and cephalosporins*

Agent Generic name (Trade name)	Spectrum of activity	Usual adult dosage (G.I. absorption)	Route	Mode of action (cidal or static)	Side effects
Ampicillin	Gram-positive (*not* resistant staph), gram-negative (especially *H. influenzae*)	0.25-0.5 Gm. q.6h. 150-200 mg./kg./day	P.O. I.M. I.V.	cidal	G.I., skin rash (especially in patients with infectious mono), fever, rare ↑ SGOT, anaphylactoid reactions, convulsions (with excessively rapid I.V.)
Carbenicillin (Pyopen, Geopen)	Gram-positive (*not* resistant staph), gram-negative (especially *Pseudomonas, Proteus, E. coli, Enterobacter, H. influenzae,* not *Klebsiella*)	5.0 Gm. q.4h. given over 2 hr. period (nonabsorbed)	I.V.	cidal	Similar to other penicillins, ↑ SGOT, nausea, neutropenia, hemolytic anemia, convulsions (high dose in patients with renal failure), possible abnormalities in coagulation tests (high dose in patients with uremia) [Note: 4.7 mEq. (108 mg.) Na$^+$/ Gm.], possible hypokalemia
Cephalothin (Keflin)	Gram-positive, gram-negative (especially *E. coli, Pr. mirabilis*)	0.5-3.0 Gm. q.6h. (nonabsorbed)	I.M. I.V.	cidal	Rash, fever, eosinophilia, ↑ SGOT, neutropenia, anaphylactoid reactions, convulsions (high dose in patients with renal failure), positive Coombs test, thrombocytopenia, false positive "Clinitest"
Cephaloridine (Loridine)	Gram-positive (variable against resistant staph), gram-negative (especially *E. coli, Pr. mirabilis*)	0.5-1.0 Gm. q.6-8h. (nonabsorbed)	I.M. I.V.	cidal	Rash, eosinophilia, acute tubular necrosis, ↑ SGOT, neutropenia, anaphylactoid reactions, rare nausea and vomiting
Cephaloglycin (Kafocin)	Use limited to urinary tract infections				
Cephalexin (Keflex)	Gram-positive (*not* enterococci, variable against resistant staph and *Neisseriae*), gram-	0.25-0.5 Gm. q.6h.	P.O.	cidal	Similar to the other cephalosporins

Drug	Spectrum	Dose	Route	cidal/static	Toxicity and reactions
	negative (urinary infections due to most *E. coli*, *Pr. mirabilis*, and some *Klebsiella*; variable against *Salmonella* and *Shigella*)				
Methicillin (Staphcillin, Dimocillin)	Gram-positive, especially staph	1.0-2.0 Gm. q.6h. (nonabsorbed)	I.M. or I.V.	cidal	Similar to penicillin G plus eosinophilia, leukopenia, nephrotoxicity, Coombs positive hemolytic anemia
Oxacillin (Prostaphlin or Resistopen)	Gram-positive, especially staph	0.5-1.0 Gm q.4-6h.	P.O., I.M., or I.V.	cidal	Occasional G.I., fever, skin rash, asymptomatic ↑ SGOT, ↓ hemoglobin, neutropenia; transient hematuria (infants)
Dicloxacillin (Dynapen, Pathocil, Veracillin)	Gram-positive, especially staph	0.125-0.5 Gm. q.6h. ac	P.O.	cidal	Similar to cloxacillin
Nafcillin (Unipen)	Gram-positive, especially staph	0.25-1.0 Gm. q.6h. ac / 0.5-1.0 Gm. q.4-6h.	P.O. / I.M. or I.V.	cidal	G.I., fever, skin rash, asymptomatic ↑ SGOT
Hetacillin	Same as ampicillin	0.225 Gm. q.6h.	P.O.	cidal	Same as ampicillin
Penicillin G	Gram-positive, gram-negative, *E. coli*, *Pr. mirabilis*, *H. influenzae*; *Shigella* and *Salmonella* in high concentration	Usual dose 600,000 to 1,200,000 u.	I.M.	cidal	Anaphylactoid reactions, drug fever, skin rashes, Coombs positive hemolytic anemia
		Large dose 10-12,000,000 u.	I.V.	cidal	Skin rashes, convulsions (high dose, especially in renal failure)
Benzathine penicillin G (Bicillin)		Usual dose 1,600,000 u. (1.0 Gm.) before meals	P.O.	cidal	G.I.–uncommon
		600,000 to 1,200,000 u.	I.M.	cidal	As above, plus local reactions

*Courtesy Dr. Jay P. Sanford, Dallas.

sporins are their relative resistance to staphylococcal penicillinase and their somewhat broad antibacterial spectrum, being active against not only gram-positive organisms but also against *Proteus mirabilis, Escherichia coli, Klebsiella,* and *Enterobacter.*

Several cephalosporins have become of clinical importance, particularly cephalothin (Keflin) and cephalexin monohydrate (Keflex). Cephaloridine (Keflordin) and cephalexin (Keforal) have also had some applications.

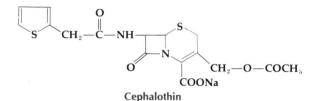

Cephalothin

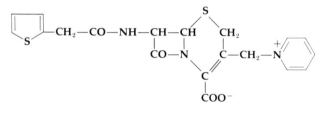

Cephaloridine

Cephalothin (Keflin) and **cephaloridine** (Keflordin) are derivatives of the naturally occurring antibiotic cephalosporin C, and they may be looked upon as semisynthetic cephalosporins. They are obtained by attaching various groups to the 7-aminocephalosporanic acid nucleus, which is analogous to the 6-aminopenicillanic acid nucleus. Cephaloridine produces higher and more sustained blood levels and is better tolerated than cephalothin after intramuscular injection.[50] Cephaloridine in large doses may cause renal damage.

Both cephalothin and cephaloridine are administered intramuscularly in doses of 0.5 to 1 Gm. every 4 to 6 hours.

Cephalexin (Keforal) is a new cephalosporin antibiotic that is much better absorbed following oral administration than related cephalosporins. Cephalexin is acid stable. The suggested dose is 250 mg. four times a day.

Cephalexin monohydrate (Keflex) is another new cephalosporin antibiotic that is effective after oral administration. It is rapidly excreted unchanged in the urine and is particularly useful in urinary tract infections caused by susceptible organisms. The drug is rapidly replacing cephalexin. Occasional gastrointestinal disturbances and allergic reactions may result from its use.

AMINOGLYCOSIDES: STREPTOMYCIN, NEOMYCIN, KANAMYCIN, AND GENTAMICIN

The aminoglycoside antibiotics are inhibitors of protein synthesis in microorganisms. Although they are bactericidal and have a broad antibacterial spectrum, they also

Table 48-3. Summary of characteristics of aminoglycosides*

Agent Generic name (Trade name)	Spectrum of activity	Usual adult dosage (G.I. absorption)	Route	Mode of action (cidal or static)	Side effects
Streptomycin	Gram-positive, gram-negative, TBC	0.5-2.0 Gm./day (nonabsorbed)	I.M.	cidal	Vestibular damage, auditory damage, drug fever, neuromuscular blockade, skin rash, circumoral paresthesias with flushing
Neomycin	Similar to kanamycin				
Kanamycin (Kantrex)	Gram-positive, gram-negative, TBC; especially staph-resistant	15 mg./kg./day divided q.6h. (nonabsorbed)	I.M. I.V.	cidal	Ototoxicity (auditory), nephrotoxicity, neuromuscular blockade, skin rash (rare)
Gentamicin (Garamycin)	Gram-positive, gram-negative (both *Proteus* and *Pseudomonas)*	0.8-5.0 mg./kg./day divided q.8h. (nonabsorbed)	I.M. I.V.	cidal	Nephrotoxicity (protein, ↑ BUN), vestibular toxicity, fever, skin rash. Avoid concurrent use with ethacrynic acid.

*Courtesy Dr. Jay P. Sanford, Dallas.

demonstrate certain characteristic toxic effects in man. Their essential features are shown in Table 48-3.

STREPTOMYCIN

Streptomycin, discovered in 1944,[46] differs from penicillin in being an organic base rather than an acid. It is not absorbed from the gastrointestinal tract, has a much broader antibacterial spectrum although a generally lower potency, and has direct toxic effects in the mammal. At present the main usefulness of this antibiotic is in the treatment of tuberculosis and in combination with penicillin, in which the synergism between the two drugs may be of great importance in selected cases.

The structural formula of streptomycin follows.

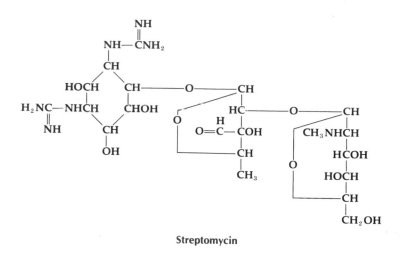

Streptomycin

Bacterial resistance

A unique disadvantage of streptomycin is the extraordinary tendency of bacteria to develop resistance to it. The development of resistance has been demonstrated with a variety of microorganisms, both in the test tube and in vivo. While resistance to most other chemotherapeutic agents develops slowly and gradually, it happens very rapidly when streptomycin is used. For example, when this antibiotic is given by mouth, intestinal flora are inhibited and bacterial counts of the feces decline. In just a few days, however, the bacterial counts return to essentially their previous value despite continued streptomycin therapy. The same phenomenon has been observed in urinary infections. The tubercle bacillus may also show considerable resistance.

Not only can resistance to streptomycin develop, but in patients being treated with streptomycin, microorganisms have been isolated that have become dependent on the drug and will not grow in its absence.

Metabolism

Streptomycin is not significantly absorbed following oral administration. The drug is generally injected by the intramuscular route at intervals of 6 to 12 hours in a total dosage of 1 to 2 Gm./day. Under these conditions blood levels of the drug reach 10 to 15 μg/ml. Since most susceptible organisms are inhibited by concentrations of 1μg/ml., the usual blood levels appear to be quite adequate.

The distribution of streptomycin in the body is largely extracellular. The drug does not penetrate well into the cerebrospinal fluid. In meningitis, however, this is not the case.

Most of the streptomycin is excreted in the kidney. It appears that the antibiotic is filtered through the glomeruli and is not reabsorbed. Renal clearance of streptomycin is lower than that of inulin, probably as a consequence of partial protein binding in the plasma. In renal insufficiency, plasma levels of streptomycin may rise to dangerous heights.

Toxicity

Streptomycin is directly toxic to the eighth cranial nerve and can lead to vestibular and auditory disturbances in both man and experimental animals.

If more than 1 Gm. of streptomycin is administered daily for more than a month, disturbances in equilibration and vertigo will appear in most persons. Larger doses or intrathecal administration accelerates development of these disturbances. In addition to vestibular damage, streptomycin can cause significant impairment of hearing and even complete deafness, which may be permanent. The greater tendency of dihydro-streptomycin to cause auditory impairment has caused it to fall in disfavor.

Other adverse effects resulting from the use of streptomycin are unimportant when compared with its effect on the eighth nerve. Still, various allergic reactions and eosinophilia have been described.

AMINOGLYCOSIDES — NEOMYCIN, KANAMYCIN, AND GENTAMICIN

Neomycin is a nephrotoxic and ototoxic antibiotic that is quite valuable for intestinal chemotherapy and for topical application. This drug was isolated from cultures of the soil organism *Streptomyces fradiae*.[51] It has a much broader antibacterial spectrum than bacitracin or polymyxin, inhibiting both gram-positive and gram-negative bacteria and having an effect even on the tubercle bacillus. Fungi, however, are resistant to it. Chemically, neomycin along with streptomycin and kanamycin belong to the aminoglycoside group of antibiotics.

Neomycin is a potent intestinal antiseptic. It is available in 0.5 Gm. tablets. Several grams may be administered prior to bowel surgery because the drug is poorly absorbed from the intestine. A combination of neomycin with phthalylsulfathiazole (Sulfathalidine) may be advantageous. Neomycin reduces the number of coliform organisms in the intestinal contents, and phthalylsulfathiazole aids in the reduction of clostridial organisms.[44]

Neomycin has been valuable for the topical treatment of skin infections. For this purpose it is often combined with other antibiotics and even the anti-inflammatory steroids. A few cases of skin sensitization have occurred following its topical use.

The systemic use of neomycin is quite hazardous because of its nephrotoxicity and neurotoxicity. The latter is characterized by deafness caused by damage to the eighth cranial (auditory) nerve. This damage is similar to that caused by dihydrostreptomycin and is often irreversible. As a consequence, the systemic use of neomycin carries the same risk as the combined use of polymyxin B and dihydrostreptomycin. For this reason parenteral use of the drug is very seldom justified. Although neomycin is poorly absorbed, its prolonged oral administration may cause deafness.

Continued intestinal use of neomycin may lead to steatorrhea, malabsorption, and damage to the intestinal villi.

Kanamycin (Kantrex), along with neomycin, belongs structurally to the streptomycin group of antibiotics. It differs from streptomycin in the slower development of resistance to it by bacteria. It also can cause hearing damage. Despite this disadvantage and the necessity of intramuscular injection, kanamycin is quite useful in infections caused by such gram-negative organisms as *Proteus* that may be resistant to all other antibiotics. Its prophylactic use prior to prostatectomy has been recommended by some investigators, who found that it decreases the chance of urinary infections. Kanamycin is administered intramuscularly in doses of 0.5 Gm. every 6 hours. The drug is quite dangerous and should not be used for more than a week.

Gentamicin (Garamycin) is an aminoglycoside antibiotic that is becoming the drug of choice for many serious infections caused by gram-negative bacilli. Administered along with carbenicillin, it is effective even in *Pseudomonas* infections. The two anti-

Table 48-4. Summary of characteristics of tetracyclines*

Agent Generic name (Trade name)	Spectrum of activity	Usual adult dosage (G.I. absorption)	Route	Mode of action (cidal or static)	Side effects
Tetracycline, chlortetracycline, oxytetracycline	Gram-positive, gram-negative, including *Bacteroides*, *Chlamydiae* (LGV), *M. pneumoniae*, *Rickettsiae*. Oxytetracycline—TBC	0.25-0.5 Gm. q.6h. 0.2-0.6 Gm./day 0.5-1.0 Gm. q.12h.	P.O. I.M. I.V.	static	G.I., skin rash, anaphylactoid reactions (rare), deposition in teeth, negative N balance, hepatotoxicity, enamel agenesis, benign ↑ CSF pressure, possible hematotoxicity, (outdated drug—Fanconi syndrome), neuromuscular blockade
Demeclocycline (Declomycin)	Gram-positive, gram-negative, *Mycoplasma pneumoniae*, *Chlamydiae*	0.15-0.3 Gm. q.6h.	P.O.	static	G.I., skin rash, deposition in teeth, negative N balance, *phototoxicity*, hepatotoxicity, benign ↑ CSF pressure, *onycholysis*, anaphylactoid reactions
Minocycline (Minocin)	Gram-positive, gram-negative, *Chlamydiae*	100 mg. q.12h.	P.O.	static	Similar to other tetracyclines
Doxycycline (Vibramycin)	Gram-positive, gram-negative, *M. pneumoniae*, *Chlamydiae*	0.1 Gm. q.12h. on 1st day, then 0.1 Gm./day	P.O.	static	Similar to other tetracyclines, phototoxicity less than demethylchlortetracycline, probably greater than tetracycline
Methacycline (Rondomycin)	Gram-positive, gram-negative, *Chlamydiae*	0.15 Gm. q.6h.	P.O.	static	Similar to other tetracyclines

*Courtesy Dr. Jay P. Sanford, Dallas.

biotics should not be mixed in the same intravenous solution because inactivation of gentamicin occurs. Just as the other aminoglycosides, gentamicin is nephrotoxic and ototoxic. Since the antibiotic is excreted largely by the kidney, its dosage should be carefully adjusted in cases of renal impairment. In patients with normal renal function gentamicin is administered in doses of 1 to 2 mg./kg. intramuscularly every 8 to 12 hours. The serum half-life of the antibiotic in such patients is between 2 and 4 hours, and the interval between doses is three to four half-lives. In patients with renal impairment the gentamicin half-life has been estimated as 3 to 4 times the serum creatinine concentration (in mg./100 ml.). The interval between doses in such patients should be extended correspondingly.[15]

Neuromuscular effect of aminoglycosides

Neomycin and probably other aminoglycosides are capable of depressing neuromuscular transmission.[78] This blocking effect may be reversed by calcium administration,[1] and it may involve transmitter release from motor nerves.

Problem 48-1. In an anesthetized patient, respiratory arrest occurred when neomycin was instilled into the peritoneal cavity. What is the probable mechanism? This is probably related to the neuromuscular blocking effect of neomycin.[78]

TETRACYCLINES

The three tetracycline antibiotics, **chlortetracycline** (Aureomycin), **oxytetracycline** (Terramycin), and **tetracycline** were discovered as a result of extensive screening experiments on antibiotics produced by soil organisms. These drugs are characterized by a wide antibacterial spectrum, effectiveness of oral administration, and a very favorable therapeutic index. They are essentially bacteriostatic drugs, except in very high concentrations. Their use may in some cases modify the infection rather than eradicate it completely. Their characteristics are summarized in Table 48-4.

The structural formulas of these well-known tetracycline antibiotics accompany this discussion. They are very similar from the standpoint of potency, antibacterial spectrum, and metabolism. Tetracycline has become most widely used because it is less likely to cause gastrointestinal disturbances in patients.

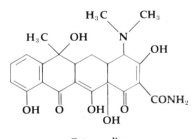

Tetracycline

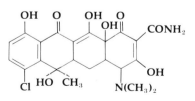

Chlortetracycline

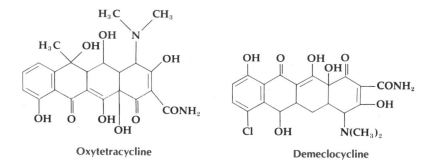

Oxytetracycline   Demeclocycline

In addition to the three well-known tetracycline antibiotics, other derivatives have been introduced. **Demeclocycline** (Declomycin) was introduced a few years ago. Although certain advantages have been claimed for this drug, some cases of photosensitization have been reported following its use. Its ultimate status in relation to the other tetracyclines cannot be stated at present. **Methacycline** (Rondomycin) resembles demeclocycline in its pharmacology. **Doxycycline monohydrate** (Vibramycin monohydrate) differs from other tetracyclines in that less frequent administration is effective because the drug is less readily excreted. It may cause phototoxicity. **Rolitetracycline** (Syntetrin) is a very soluble derivative of tetracycline and is suitable for parenteral administration. It may be injected intravenously or intramuscularly.

Problem 48-2. The causative agent in a stubborn urinary tract infection was found to be most susceptible to the tetracyclines. The physician selected doxycycline because of the convenience of twice-daily administration. Was this a good choice? No, because doxycycline is not excreted in the urine to the same extent as some other tetracyclines.[39]

Metabolism

All these drugs are absorbed rapidly but incompletely from the gastrointestinal tract. Calcium salts prevent their absorption. Variable amounts may remain in the large intestine, and the bacterial flora of the intestinal contents may be altered considerably. The development of serious staphylococcal gastroenteritis during therapy with one of the tetracyclines has been attributed to the phenomenon of *superinfection*, with micrococci producing exotoxin.

Oral administration of 250 mg. of tetracycline will produce a serum level of about 0.7 μg/ml. in less than 2 hours (Fig. 48-5). This level will decline very gradually to about one half this value in approximately 12 hours. This slow decline may be explained by the low renal clearance of the drug. During the first 12 hours only about 10 to 20% of the dose appears in the urine.

The drug is widely distributed in the various tissues and probably penetrates into cells, but its level in the cerebrospinal fluid is less than in plasma. Probably as a consequence of its chelating properties, tetracycline tends to localize in bones and teeth, where it may be detected by its fluorescence.[41] Tetracycline fluorescence is widespread but tends to disappear from normal tissues, except from bones and teeth, in about 24 hours. It tends to remain in inflammatory tissue somewhat longer, while it clings to neoplastic tissue for a surprisingly long time. Fluorescence of the gastric sediment induced by demethylchlortetracycline has been used as a diagnostic procedure for differentiating malignant from benign gastric lesions.[8]

The absorption of the tetracyclines from the gastrointestinal tract has received much

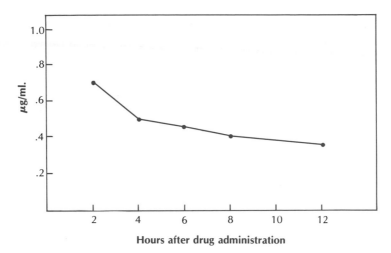

Fig. 48-5. Average serum concentration following oral administration of 0.25 Gm. of tetracycline. (From Welch, H., et al.: Principles and practice of antibiotic therapy, New York, 1954, Medical Encyclopedia, Inc.)

attention. It has been observed that antacids of the aluminum hydroxide type decrease absorption of the antibiotic. Later it was realized that calcium salts also tend to diminish absorption of these drugs.

Problem 48-3. Inhibition of gastrointestinal absorption of tetracycline by gastric antacids is generally attributed to chelation. Would sodium bicarbonate interfere with the absorption of the antibiotic, and if so, by what mechanism? In an experimental study of this problem[7] it was found that sodium bicarbonate interferes with the dissolution of tetracycline contained in capsules, and thus interferes with absorption.

Toxicity and other adverse effects

Adverse effects caused by tetracyclines include nausea, vomiting, enterocolitis, stomatitis, and superinfections. Phototoxicity may occur after the administration of demeclocycline (Declomycin).

Administration of the tetracyclines in large doses has produced liver damage in patients, as proved by liver biopsy. Recent evidence suggests that tetracycline in large doses produces a negative nitrogen balance and probably exerts an antianabolic action. Interference with protein synthesis may be the basis of these effects. A similar action may explain the mechanism of its action against bacteria.[61]

CHLORAMPHENICOL

Chloramphenicol (Chloromycetin) is a broad-spectrum antibiotic having an antibacterial spectrum and potency very similar to those of the tetracyclines. It is not effective, however, against *Entamoeba histolytica* but is more effective than the tetracyclines in the treatment of typhoid fever.

It may be seen from the structural formula of chloramphenicol that this antibiotic is a derivative of nitrobenzene.

$$NO_2\text{—}\left\langle\bigcirc\right\rangle\text{—}\overset{\overset{\displaystyle OH}{|}}{CH}\text{—}\overset{\overset{\displaystyle CH_2OH}{|}}{CH}\text{—}NH\text{—}\overset{\overset{\displaystyle O}{\|}}{C}\text{—}CHCl_2$$

Chloramphenicol

The drug is well absorbed from the gastrointestinal tract. It is largely metabolized in the body, so that only about 10% of an administered dose appears in the urine in the unchanged form.

The mode of action of chloramphenicol is not completely understood. The drug is largely bacteriostatic. Considerable evidence indicates that it interferes with protein synthesis in bacteria and also in human protein-synthesizing systems, at least as demonstrated with human bone marrow cells in tissue culture.[61]

Toxicity

The acute toxicity of chloramphenicol in experimental animals is about the same as that of the tetracyclines. In clinical usage many minor side effects such as gastrointestinal disturbances, glossitis, skin rash, and superinfection may occur. These are similar to the effects produced by the tetracyclines. On the other hand, it is generally recognized that chloramphenicol has a much greater tendency than have commonly used antibiotics to produce blood dyscrasias such as aplastic anemia. Although the incidence of this serious toxic effect is small, it is sufficient to make physicians very cautious in the use of chloramphenicol. Chloramphenicol is particularly dangerous in infants, in whom it can lead to a symptom complex often referred to as the "gray syndrome."

The gray syndrome occurs in premature and newborn infants when chloramphenicol is administered during the first few days of life. Symptoms consist of cyanosis, vascular collapse, and elevated chloramphenicol levels in the blood. The syndrome results from lack of development of glucuronyl transferase in the liver, which normally detoxifies the antibiotic by changing it to the glucuronide.[55]

Chloramphenicol sodium succinate, a water-soluble derivative, is available for parenteral administration.

POLYPEPTIDE ANTIBIOTICS

Bacitracin, polymyxin, and colistin are discussed as a group for two reasons. First, all three are nephrotoxic when administered systemically in large enough doses. Second, they are used mostly for special purposes and only rarely as systemic chemotherapeutic agents.

BACITRACIN

Bacitracin, a mixture of polypeptides, was first isolated from cultures of a gram-positive bacillus.[40] Its name was derived from Tracy, the name of the patient from whom the bacillus was isolated.

The antibacterial spectrum of bacitracin is remarkably similar to that of penicillin. It is particularly effective against gram-positive organisms, those of the *Neisseria* group, and spirochetes.

The main usefulness of bacitracin is in treating infections of the skin and mucous membranes, where it can be applied topically. When used by intramuscular injection, renal tubular damage regularly occurs in patients or experimental animals if large enough doses are used.

The activity of bacitracin is expressed in a unit that represents 26 μg of a standard preparation. For topical use, ointments containing 500 units/Gm. of base are available.

Bacitracin is valuable for topical application and, compared to penicillin, has the great advantage of seldom causing sensitivity reactions. The drug is not absorbed from the gastrointestinal tract.

POLYMYXINS, INCLUDING COLISTIN

Polymyxin B is one of a series of polypeptide antibiotics produced by *Bacillus polymyxa*, a soil bacillus. This antibiotic has a potent bactericidal effect on gram-negative bacilli. Unfortunately, when administered to patients in daily doses exceeding 4 mg./kg., it is likely to cause renal tubular damage. This appears to be a direct toxic effect, readily demonstrable in experimental animals.

The main usefulness of polymyxin is for topical application. Many preparations are available for this purpose, and the drug is generally combined with either bacitracin or neomycin in order to widen the antibacterial spectrum. The polymyxins are useful also in the treatment of severe urinary tract infections.

The systemic use of polymyxin is hazardous, and the daily dose should not exceed 3 to 4 mg./kg. in adults.

In addition to the nephrotoxic action, systemic use of polymyxin can produce central nervous system effects such as vertigo and paresthesia.

An interesting feature of the chemistry of polymyxin is the fact that it contains α,γ-diaminobutyric acid. This amino acid analog is being used experimentally for blocking amino acid transport into cells.

Polymyxin B is not absorbed significantly from the gastrointestinal tract and may occasionally be used by mouth for intestinal chemotherapy. When the drug is applied to open wounds, absorption may take place and the total quantity applied in a day should not exceed 3 to 4 mg./kg.

Colistin is a polypeptide antibiotic very similar in antibacterial spectrum and toxicity to polymyxin B. Although some investigators believe that the drug is less neurotoxic and is not as likely to produce paresthesia, others question the superiority of this drug over polymyxin B.[43] It is available as sodium colistimethate (Coly-Mycin), used in daily doses of 2 to 5 mg./kg. by intramuscular injection.

ERYTHROMYCIN AND NEWER ANTIBIOTICS AGAINST GRAM-POSITIVE ORGANISMS

Since penicillin and the broad-spectrum antibiotics became available, several important additional discoveries have been made in the fight against gram-positive organisms, such as the introduction of erythromycin, the discovery of newer antibiotics effective against resistant micrococci (staphylococci), and the development of the newer penicillins.

Erythromycin (Ilotycin) was isolated from a strain of *Streptomyces*. It is an organic base having a molecular weight of about 700. This antibiotic is particularly effective against gram-positive microorganisms, although gonococci, *Haemophilus* organisms, and the large viruses of the lymphogranuloma venereum group are somewhat affected by it. Its antibacterial spectrum is between that of penicillin and of the tetracyclines, but the gram-negative bacilli such as *Escherichia coli* and *Salmonella* organisms are not inhibited by it. Its mode of action appears to be largely bacteriostatic, since it has a true killing effect only at very high concentrations. Erythromycins are among the safest antibiotics commonly used for respiratory infections, particularly in patients that are allergic to penicillin. Erythromycins should not be used in serious staphylococcal infections or in the treatment of gonococcal infections because better drugs are available.

Gastric juice tends to destroy erythromycin, but enteric-coated preparations and the erythromycin stearate are well absorbed. It is given in doses of 0.5 Gm. every 6 hours, and blood levels of 2 μg/ml. or more can be obtained. Many gram-positive organisms are inhibited by levels below this amount.

Erythromycin estolate (Ilosone) is claimed to be stable in acid, is well absorbed, and is excreted in lesser amounts in bile. Thus, when taken with food, it gives faster, higher, and longer lasting blood levels than comparable doses of erythromycin. Cholestatic jaundice has been reported following the use of this drug and other esters of erythromycin. Although this occurs rarely, caution is necessary in its use.

Vancomycin (Vancocin) has been introduced largely for the purpose of treating staphylococcal infections and endocarditis when the causative agent appears to be highly resistant to the usual antibiotics. It is administered by the intravenous route because it is inadequately absorbed from the gastrointestinal tract. Vancomycin can produce nerve deafness when it is given in large doses or when it is not cleared efficiently by the kidney. It also causes thrombophlebitis.

Novobiocin (Albamycin; Cathomycin) is also obtained from *Streptomyces*. The antibiotic is effective in the treatment of infections due to gram-positive organisms, particularly when they are resistant to penicillin. It can be administered by the oral, intramuscular, and intravenous routes. The main disadvantage of this antibiotic is the not infrequent development of skin rash, drug fever, hepatic damage, and blood dyscrasias. Because of these effects, the drug is not recommended.

Lincomycin (Lincocin) is structurally unrelated to previously discussed antibiotics. Its antibacterial spectrum resembles that of erythromycin. It is effective against gram-positive organisms, *Neisseriae,* and *Bacteroides*. It is administered by mouth, intramuscularly, or intravenously. Its usual adult dose is 0.5 Gm. every 6 to 8 hours. Side effects from lincomycin include gastrointestinal manifestations, skin rashes, and anaphylactoid reactions.

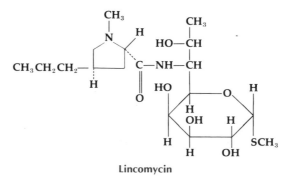

Lincomycin

Clindamycin (Cleocin) is closely related to lincomycin structurally. In fact, it differs only in a chloro substitution of the 7-hydroxyl group. The spectrum of activity of the drug includes gram-positive organisms (not *Neisseriae* or enterococci), *Actinomyces*, and *Bacteroides fragilis*. The drug is administered by mouth in a usual adult dose of 150 to 450 mg. every 6 hours. The drug may be either bactericidal or bacteriostatic and acts by inhibiting protein synthesis in the 50 S subunit of the ribosome. Adverse effects caused by clindamycin include gastrointestinal manifestations, neutropenia, eosinophilia, rashes, and elevated SGOT levels.

Clindamycin phosphate (Cleocin phosphate) is a parenteral form of the drug available for intramuscular or intravenous use. The usual adult dose is 600 to 1,200 mg./day in 2 to 4 equal doses.

ANTIFUNGAL ANTIBIOTICS

Fungal infections have generally been highly resistant to chemotherapy. In fact, alteration of the normal bacterial flora by antibiotic treatment tends to contribute to superinfection with fungi, particularly *Candida albicans (Monilia)*. Some success has been achieved in recent years in developing antifungal antibiotics. One of the first of these, **cycloheximide** (Actidione), showed a remarkable selective effect on *Torula* organisms. Unfortunately the drug is quite toxic, being a potent inhibitor of protein synthesis and resembling emetine in its basic action.[22]

Nystatin (Mycostatin) and **amphotericin B** (Fungizone) are also called *polyene* antibiotics. This name refers to the fact that these antibiotics contain a large ring with a conjugated double-bond system. There is evidence to indicate that the polyene antibiotics injure the membrane of the fungi, perhaps by complexing with sterols that occur in these membranes. Because of this interaction, sterols protect yeasts against the action of these antibiotics. Bacterial membranes are not injured by the polyenes. On the other hand, the hemolytic anemia sometimes caused by the polyene antibiotics may be a consequence of injury of the red cell membrane, which is known to contain cholesterol.[61]

Nystatin is effective against *Candida albicans* and some other fungi. It appears to be useful against those monilial infections that can be reached by topical application. The drug is inactivated by gastric juice, and no systemic effects can be expected when it is administered orally, although it has been incorporated in tetracycline preparations.

Amphotericin B appears to be the most effective antibiotic against deep-seated mycotic infections.[45] The usefulness of the antibiotic has been demonstrated against histoplasmosis, cryptococcosis, blastomycosis, and coccidioidomycosis. It has also proved to be effective in systemic infections due to *Candida albicans*.[35]

The drug is administered intravenously but can cause thrombophlebitis at the site of injection and may also produce some renal damage, skin rash, and gastrointestinal upset. Test doses of 1 to 5 mg. are injected first. If there is no untoward reaction, these may be followed by daily doses of 20 to 50 mg. Although amphotericin B is obviously a dangerous drug, its use may be justified in severe systemic fungus infections. Its intravenous LD_{50} in mice is of the order of 5 mg./kg.

The drug is poorly absorbed from the intestine.

Griseofulvin represents an interesting development in the treatment of certain dermatomycoses. The antibiotic is produced by a *Penicillium* mold. When given orally for long periods of time, it is apparently incorporated into the skin, hair, and nails and exerts a fungistatic activity against various species of *Microsporum*, *Trichophyton*, and *Epidermophyton*. Prolonged administration is necessary because ringworm of the skin may require several weeks for improvement. In fungal infections of the nails,

Table 48-5. Summary of antifungal drugs and their side effects*

Type of infecting fungi	Site of infection	Antifungal agent	Route of administration	Dosage	Side effects and comments
Candida species	Superficial	Amphotericin B or nystatin	Topical	Not applicable	Apply 3 or 4 times daily for 7 to 14 days; with vaginitis, daily or twice daily for 14 days Side effects: essentially none
	Intestinal	Nystatin (Mycostatin)	P.O.	500,000 u. 3 times daily for 7 to 14 days	Side effects: essentially none; large doses, occasionally G.I. distress and diarrhea
	Systemic — not endocarditis	Amphotericin B (Fungizone)	I.V.	Initial dose 0.25 mg./kg. I.V. over 6 hr. (suspend in 5% glucose solution, NOT saline), then increase stepwise to 1.0 mg./kg./administration daily or 3 times/wk; total dose 0.5 to 1.0 Gm.	If administered rapidly, convulsions, anaphylaxis, hypotension, ventricular fibrillation or cardiac arrest; phlebitis, fever, nausea, vomiting, anorexia, metallic taste, abdominal pain, nephrotoxicity, anemia, hypokalemia, ↓ urinary 170H corticoids
		or flucytosine (Ancobon)	P.O.	50-150 mg./kg./day	G.I. distress (nausea, vomiting, diarrhea), leukopenia
	Systemic — endocarditis	Amphotericin B	I.V.	As above	Removal of prosthesis or primary surgery usually required
Dermatophytes	Intradermal and hair	Griseofulvin (Fulvicin, Grifulvin, Grisactin)	P.O.	12.5 mg./kg. or 500 mg./day in adults	Photosensitivity, urticaria, G.I. upset, fatigue, leukopenia (rare); interferes with coumarin drugs; increases blood and urine porphyrins, therefore should not be used in patients with porphyria Adjunct treatment: tolnaftate (Tinactin) or "Desenex" 2 to 3 times daily
	Onychomycosis	Griseofulvin	P.O.	12.5 mg./kg. or 500 mg./day in adults for 6 to 12 mo.	

Fungi causing deep mycoses: Actinomycosis		Penicillin G or ampicillin or tetracycline		10,000 to 20,000 u./kg. 50 mg./kg. 25 mg./kg.	See Tables 48-2 and 48-4
Nocardia		Sulfonamide— rapid-acting, and/or cycloserine (Seromycin) Sulfamethoxazole-tri-methoprim	P.O.	1.0 Gm. q.4h. 15 mg./kg.	See Table 47-2 See Table 49-1
Sporotrichosis	Cutaneous anc lymphatic	Potassium iodide, saturated solution			
Histoplasmosis, coccidioidomycosis, systemic sporotrichosis, aspergillosis, mucormycosis, chromablastomycosis	Systemic	Amphotericin B		See Candida, systemic, not endocarditis	Total dosage variable, but usually 2 5 Gm. or more
Blastomycosis	Systemic	Amphotericin B or 2-hydroxy-stilbamidine		See Candida, systemic, not endocarditis	
Cryptococcosis	Systemic	Amphotericin B or flucytosine		See Candida, systemic, not endocarditis	

*Courtesy Dr. Jay P. Sanford, Dallas.

treatment may have to be continued for several months. The most common side effects consist of gastric discomfort, diarrhea, and headache. Urticaria and skin rash may also occur. The antibiotic is available in 250 mg. tablets. The dose for adults is one tablet four times a day.[37] Phenobarbital accelerates the metabolism of griseofulvin.[13,14]

The structural formula of griseofulvin is as follows:

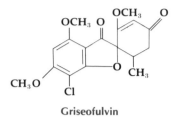

Griseofulvin

ANTIVIRAL AGENTS

Until recently chemotherapy of true viral diseases has been essentially nonexistent. The larger viruses such as the causative agents of trachoma and lymphogranuloma venereum responded quite well to tetracycline and other antibiotics. In other viral diseases such as measles, poliomyelitis, and influenza, considerable success has been achieved in recent years with vaccines but not with chemotherapeutic agents.

Several developments have taken place in this field during the last few years (Table 48-6). The inhibitor of nucleic acid synthesis, idoxuridine, has produced spectacular results by topical application in herpetic keratitis, and the new drug amantadine has provided a new approach to the prevention of influenza A_2 infections. Amantadine blocks the penetration of the virus into the host cell.[64] In addition to these approaches, there is great interest in the stimulation of interferon production by synthetic polyanions of defined composition such as pyran copolymer.[66]

Idoxuridine (5-iodo-2'-deoxyuridine; IDU; Stoxil) is a pyrimidine analog that blocks the synthesis of nucleic acids. It is applied topically in a 0.1% solution to the conjunctiva every 1 to 2 hours in the treatment of herpetic keratitis caused by the herpes simplex virus. This is an important therapeutic advance because herpetic keratitis can lead to blindness. No effective treatment existed prior to the introduction of idoxuridine. Unfortunately the drug is ineffective by systemic administration, probably because of rapid destruction. Nevertheless, the drug has been used systemically in the treatment of herpes simplex encephalitis and varicella-zoster infections. Some of the toxic effects of idoxuridine are bone marrow depression, alopecia, gastric ulcers, loss of fingernails, and hepatotoxicity.

Amantadine (Symmetrel) is a new synthetic drug of unusual structure that inhibits the penetration of certain viruses into the host cell. In vitro it is effective against influenza and rubella viruses. In man its effectiveness as a chemoprophylactic measure against influenza A_2 (Asian) virus has been demonstrated. Amantadine reduced the number of clinical illnesses and also diminished the serologic response to influenza infection. Mice could be protected against several strains of influenza A_2 virus even when treatment was delayed as much as 72 hours after inoculation.[68]

Amantadine is available in capsules containing 100 mg. of the drug and also as a syrup. The adult daily dose is 200 mg.

While amantadine appears to be quite nontoxic on the basis of animal experiments, it can produce central nervous system stimulation and even convulsions when given

Table 48-6. Summary of currently used antiviral drugs*

Drug	Indication	Usual adult dosage	Route	Side effects	Comments
Amantadine (Symmetrel)	Prophylaxis of influenza A; possible therapy of influenza A in elderly or chronically ill patients if seen less than 20 hr. after onset of illness	100 mg. B.I.D.	P.O.	Jitteriness, inability to concentrate, insomnia, tremors, confusion, depression, and hallucinations; incidence generally at a low level and is dose-related	Primary reliance on prevention of influenza A infections remains with immunization
5-iodo-2'-deoxyuridine, idoxuridine (IDUR) (Stoxil)	Severe herpes simplex virus infections (encephalitis, generalized diseases of newborn)	Total dose 430 mg./kg. given over a 5-day period (always less than 30 Gm.)	I.V.	Leukopenia, thrombocytopenia, stomatitis, alopecia, fingernail loss, and occasionally jaundice; nausea and vomiting can occur during infusion	IDUR poorly soluble and pH must be adjusted to 8.2-8.6 before drug goes into solution (3 to 8 Gm./1000 ml. D5W); filter sterilize before use
	Herpes simplex keratitis		Topical		
Cytosine arabinoside (Ara-C) (Cytosar)	Progressive varicella-zoster virus infections in compromised host; primary varicella pneumonia in adult	100 mg./M²/day for 3 to 5 days; ≤4 hr. infusion	I.V.	Leukopenia, thrombocytopenia, anemia with reticulocytopenia, and megaloblastoid changes; chromosomal changes acutely; anorexia, nausea, and vomiting occur	
	Severe herpes simplex virus infections (encephalitis, generalized diseases of newborn); progressive cytomegalovirus pneumonia in compromised host		As above		Current information insufficient to determine whether IDUR or Ara-C is first drug of choice
Methisazone	Progressive vaccinia (vaccinia necrosum)	Initial dose 200 mg./kg. followed by 8 doses of 50 mg./kg. at 6 hourly intervals	P.O.	Anorexia, nausea, and vomiting; hepatotoxicity	

*Courtesy Dr. Jay P. Sanford, Dallas.

Table 48-7. Drugs of choice for various infections

Causative agent	Drugs
Gram-positive	
Streptococcus pyogenes	Penicillin; erythromycin; a cephalosporin
*Streptococcus viridans**	Penicillin with streptomycin; ampicillin; vancomycin
Enterococcus*	Penicillin with streptomycin; vancomycin with streptomycin
Pneumococcus	Penicillin; erythromycin; tetracycline
Staphylococcus aureus	
Penicillinase-producing	Oxacillin; nafcillin; cloxacillin; others based on susceptibility such as a cephalosporin, erythromycin, lincomycin, vancomycin
Nonpenicillinase-producing	Penicillin; erythromycin; a cephalosporin; lincomycin
Clostridium	Penicillin; erythromycin; tetracycline
Corynebacterium diphtheriae	Penicillin; erythromycin; tetracycline
Actinomyces	Penicillin with tetracycline; sulfonamides
Gram-negative	
Neisseria meningitidis	Penicillin; sulfonamides; tetracycline
Neisseria gonorrhoeae	Penicillin; tetracycline; erythromycin
Salmonella	Chloramphenicol; ampicillin
Shigella	Tetracycline; ampicillin
*Escherichia coli**	Ampicillin; kanamycin; tetracycline
*Enterobacter**	Kanamycin; tetracycline
*Klebsiella**	A cephalosporin; kanamycin; chloramphenicol; polymyxin B; colistimethate
Brucella	Tetracycline; chloramphenicol
Haemophilus influenzae	Ampicillin; chloramphenicol
Haemophilus ducreyi	Tetracycline; sulfonamides
Bordetella pertussis	Ampicillin; tetracycline
*Pseudomonas**	Polymyxin B; colistimethate; gentamicin
*Proteus**	Kanamycin; neomycin; chloramphenicol (penicillin for *Proteus mirabilis*)
Bacteroides	Clindamycin; chloramphenicol; tetracycline
Miscellaneous	
Fusobacterium (Vincent's angina)	Penicillin; erythromycin; tetracycline
Treponema pallidum	Penicillin; erythromycin; tetracycline
Leptospira	Penicillin; tetracycline
Rickettsia	Tetracycline; chloramphenicol
Psittacosis-lymphogranuloma group	Tetracycline; chloramphenicol
Histoplasma capsulatum	Amphotericin B
Candida	Amphotericin B; nystatin
Cryptococcus	Amphotericin B
Coccidioides	Amphotericin B
Blastomyces	Amphotericin B
Microsporum and *Trichophyton*	Griseofulvin

* Susceptibility tests may be essential.

in large doses. Nervousness, dizziness, hallucinations, and even grand mal convulsions have been associated with the use of the drug in man. These adverse reactions are not common, however, and are more likely to occur following the administration of large doses.

Amantadine is a new approach to viral diseases. Its ultimate place in chemoprophylaxis in comparison with immunization procedures is a matter of debate.[64] Amantadine has some therapeutic effect in parkinsonism (p. 132).

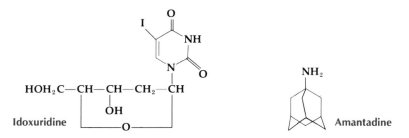

Idoxuridine   Amantadine

Methisazone, or *n*-methylisatin-beta-thiosemicarbazone, shows some therapeutic promise against the poxviruses such as smallpox and complications of vaccination.

Cytarabine (Cytosar), or cytosine arabinoside, is an inhibitor of DNA synthesis. It is used largely as an antineoplastic agent, although it may become useful in varicella-zoster infections in patients with lymphomas.

Interferon inducers represent a novel approach to antiviral chemotherapy. Interferon is an antiviral protein produced by cells as a consequence of virus infections.[25] Not only viruses but also bacteria and their products are capable of inducing the formation of interferon by the cells of the host.[66] More recently, it has been shown that chemically defined substances such as a polyanionic pyran copolymer or double-stranded RNA from a synthetic source can also act as interferon inducers. Early trials in man and animals indicate that these synthetic materials may induce demonstrable serum interferon levels.[66]

CLINICAL PHARMACOLOGY OF ANTIBACTERIAL AGENTS
SELECTION OF A CHEMOTHERAPEUTIC AGENT

Clinical experience with chemotherapeutic agents in a wide variety of infections allows certain generalizations regarding the best choice. These will be summarized, based on a more extensive report.[38] There may be exceptions to these recommendations in individual cases in which susceptibility tests reveal resistance of the causative agent to a drug that ordinarily would be a good choice (Table 48-7).

CAUSES OF FAILURE OF ANTIBACTERIAL THERAPY

With the availability of effective weapons against infection, it is inexcusable not to cure an infection that would be curable with optimal treatment. Some of the causes of failure of anti-infective therapy are unavoidable. Others, however, may be iatrogenic.

Some of the causes of failure are as follows:

Incorrect clinical or bacteriologic diagnosis
Improper selection of drugs
Improper method of administration or inadequate dose
Futile prophylaxis

>Alteration in bacterial flora and superinfection
>Inaccessible lesion
>Drug resistance
>Deficiency in host defenses
>Drug toxicity and hypersensitivity

GASTROINTESTINAL EFFECTS OF ANTIBIOTICS

The possible effects of antibiotics on the gastrointestinal tract are of two types. They may alter the bacterial flora or they may have direct toxic effects unrelated to the bacterial flora.[76]

Alteration of the bacterial flora is deliberately sought when antibiotics are used prior to bowel surgery. The nonabsorbable antibiotics such as neomycin, kanamycin, and certain sulfonamides have often been employed for this purpose. Despite some enthusiastic proponents of such a prophylactic measure, many investigators feel that it has no advantages over the preoperative cleansing of the bowel.

Staphylococcal enterocolitis has occurred in patients who received oxytetracycline, neomycin, multiple antibiotics, or preoperative bowel antisepsis.

Candidiasis is commonly seen in patients who receive long-term treatment with broad-spectrum antibiotics. The number of yeasts in the stools can be diminished by the simultaneous use of nystatin, but it is not certain that the gastrointestinal symptoms are caused by the yeasts. The condition improves if the antibiotic is discontinued.

Prophylaxis of hepatic coma is an indication for the use of neomycin, kanamycin, or paromomycin, a closely related drug. The mode of action of these antibiotics in the prevention of hepatic coma is explained by their inhibitory effect on ammonia production in the intestine.

Malabsorption syndrome may result from the continued oral administration of neomycin. Changes in the jejunal mucosa and interference with the absorption of fat, glucose, D-xylose, iron, and vitamin B_{12} have been demonstrated.

Liver disease may be induced by some antibiotics. Large doses of intravenously administered tetracycline are quite hepatotoxic. Erythromycin estolate and triacetyl-oleandomycin can produce an obstructive type of hepatitis. Novobiocin can increase serum bilirubin in newborn infants by inhibiting the enzyme glucuronyl transferase.

HOST FACTORS IN ANTIBIOTIC THERAPY

Effectiveness and safety of antibiotic therapy depend on several host factors that will be summarized briefly.

Defense mechanisms of the host have much to do with the success or failure of treatment. Debilitating diseases or the administration of large doses of corticosteroids or immunosuppressant drugs may interfere with antibiotic therapy.

The age of the patient influences both the effectiveness and safety of antibiotic therapy. Infants in the first month of life excrete penicillin more slowly, presumably because of a less developed tubular secretory mechanism. Older infants and children require larger doses of penicillin than adults. Tetracycline may be deposited in tooth enamel and dentin and perhaps also in the bones of children. Chloramphenicol can cause the "gray syndrome" when given to infants during the first month of their life (p. 594).

Undeveloped glucuronide conjugation by the liver makes chloramphenicol more hazardous.

Pregnancy is a contraindication to the use of many drugs. Tetracyclines can cause dental defects in the fetus.

Liver disease may be aggravated by chloramphenicol, the tetracyclines, novobiocin, and erythromycin. *Defective renal function* would cause the accumulation of sulfonamides, tetracycline, and other antibiotics that are largely cleared by the kidney. *Urinary obstructions* in any part of the urinary tract are a most important host factor in making the eradication of the infection very difficult.

Pharmacogenetic defects such as glucose-6-phosphate dehydrogenase deficiency may predispose an individual to hemolytic anemia from various antimicrobial drugs such as sulfamethoxypyridazine, sulfadimethoxine, sulfisoxazole, nitrofurantoin, and chloramphenicol.

References

1 Adams, H. R.: Neuromuscular blocking effect of aminoglycoside antibiotics in non-human primates, J. Amer. Vet. Med. Assoc. **163**:613, 1973.

2 Ambrose, C. T., and Coons, A. H.: Studies on antibody production. VIII. Inhibitory effect of chloramphenicol on synthesis of antibody in tissue culture, J. Exp. Med. **117**:1075, 1963.

3 Anand, N., and Davis, B. D.: Effect of streptomycin on Escherichia coli, Nature **185**:22, 1960.

4 Anand, N., Davis, B. D., and Armitage, A. K.: Uptake of streptomycin by Escherichia coli, Nature **185**:23, 1960.

5 Andriole, V. T., and Kravetz, H. M.: The use of amphotericin B in man, J.A.M.A. **180**:269, 1962.

6 Baldwin, D. S., Levine, B. B., McCluskey, R. T., and Gallo, G. R.: Renal failure and interstitial nephritis due to penicillin and methicillin, New Eng. J. Med. **279**:1245, 1968.

7 Barr, W. H., Adir, J., and Garrettson, L.: Decrease of tetracycline absorption in man by sodium bicarbonate, Clin. Pharmacol. Ther. **12**:779, 1971.

8 Berk, J. E., and Kantor, S. M.: Demethylchlortetracycline-induced fluorescence of gastric sediment: use to differentiate benign and malignant gastric lesions, J.A.M.A. **179**:998, 1962.

9 Bodey, G. P., Rodriquez, V., and Stewart, D.: Clinical pharmacological studies of carbenicillin, Amer. J. Med. Sci. **257**:185, 1969.

10 Bodey, G. P., and Terrell, L. M.: In vitro activity of carbenicillin against gram-negative bacilli, J. Bact. **95**:1587, 1968.

11 Brown, B. C., Price, E. V., and Moore, M. B.: Penicilloyl-polylysine as an intradermal test of penicillin sensitivity, J.A.M.A. **189**:599, 1964.

12 Bryson, V., and Demerec, M.: Bacterial resistance, Amer. J. Med. **18**:723, 1955.

13 Busfield, D., Child, K. J., Atkinson, R. M., and Tomich, E. G.: An effect of phenobarbitone on blood-levels of griseofulvin in man, Lancet **2**:1042, 1963.

14 Busfield, D., Child, K. J., and Tomich, E. G.: An effect of phenobarbitone on griseofulvin metabolism in the rat, Brit. J. Pharmacol. **22**:137, 1964.

15 Cutler, R. E., Gyselynck, A. M., Fleet, W. P., and Forrey, A. W.: Correlation of serum creatinine concentration and gentamicin half-life, J.A.M.A. **219**:1037, 1972.

16 Deal, W. B., and Sanders, E.: Efficacy of rifampin in treatment of meningococcal carriers, New Eng. J. Med. **281**:641, 1969.

17 Dubos, R. J.: Studies on a bactericidal agent extracted from a soil bacillus: preparation of the agent. Its activity in vitro, J. Exp. Med. **70**:1, 1939.

18 Eagle, H.: The binding of penicillin in relation to its cytotoxic action. I. Correlation between the penicillin sensitivity and combining activity of intact bacteria and cell-free extracts, J. Exp. Med. **99**:207, 1954; II. The reactivity with penicillin of resistant variants of streptococci, pneumococci, and staphylococci, J. Exp. Med. **100**:103, 1954; III. The binding of penicillin by mammalian cells in tissue culture (HeLa and L strains), J. Exp. Med. **100**:117, 1954.

19 Eagle, H., Fleischman, R., and Levy, M.: On the duration of penicillin action in relation to its concentration in the serum, J. Lab. Clin. Med. **41**:122, 1953.

20 Frimpter, G. W., Timpanelli, A. E., Eisenmenger, W. J., Stein, H. S., and Ehrlich, L. I.: Reversible "Fanconi syndrome" caused by degraded tetracycline, J.A.M.A. **184**:111, 1963.

21 Grieco, M. H.: Cross-allergenicity of the penicillins and cephalosporins, Arch. Intern. Med. **119**:141, 1967.

22 Grollman, A. P.: Structural basis for inhibition

of protein synthesis by emetine and cyclohexi-mide based on an analogy between ipecac alkaloids and glutarimide antibiotics, Proc. Nat. Acad. Sci. 56:1867, 1966.

23 Grüneberg, R. N., and Kolbe, R.: Trimethoprim in the treatment of urinary infections in hospital, Brit. Med. J. 1:545, 1969.

24 Hahn, F. E., and Ciak, J.: Penicillin-induced lysis of Escherichia coli, Science 125:119, 1957.

25 Hartmann, G., Honikel, K. O., Knüsel, F., and Nuesch, J.: The specific inhibition of DNA-directed RNA synthesis by rifamycin, Biochem. Biophys. Acta 145:843, 1967.

26 Hinman, A. R., and Wolinsky, E.: Nephrotoxicity associated with the use of cephaloridine, J.A.M.A. 200:724, 1967.

27 Isaacs, A., and Lindenmann, J.: Virus interference. I. Interferon, Proc. Roy. Soc. London [Biol.] 147:258, 1957.

28 Jao, R. L., and Jackson, G. G.: Gentamicin sulfate: a new antibiotic against gram-negative bacilli, J.A.M.A. 189:817, 1964.

29 Jawetz, E., and Gunnison, J. B.: Antibiotic synergism and antagonism: an assessment of the problem, Pharmacol. Rev. 5:175, 1953.

30 Koch-Weser, J., and Gilmore, E. B.: Benign intracranial hypertension in an adult after tetracycline therapy, J.A.M.A. 200:345, 1967.

31 Lederberg, J.: Bacterial protoplasts induced by penicillin, Proc. Nat. Acad. Sci. 42:574, 1956.

32 Levison, M. E., Johnson, W. D., Thornhill, T. S., and Kaye, D.: Clinical and in vitro evaluation of cephalexin, J.A.M.A. 209:1331, 1969.

33 Lewis, C. N., Putnam, L. E., Hendricks, F. D., Kerlan, I., and Welch, H.: Chloramphenicol (Chloromycetin) in relation to blood dyscrasias, with observations on other drugs, Antibiotics Chemother. 2:601, 1952.

34 Long, P. H., editor: Symposium: antibiotics derived from Bacillus polymyxa, Ann. N. Y. Acad. Sci. 51:853, 1949.

35 Louria, D. B., and Dineen, P.: Amphotericin B in treatment of disseminated moniliasis, J.A.M.A. 174:273, 1960.

36 McCormack, R. C., Kaye, D., and Hook, E. W.: Resistance of Group A streptococci to tetracycline, New Eng. J. Med. 267:323, 1962.

37 McCuistion, C. H., Jr., Lawlis, M. G., and Gonzalez, B. B.: Toxicological studies and effectiveness of griseofulvin in dermatomycosis, J.A.M.A. 171:2174, 1959.

38 Medical Letter 5:17, 1963.

39 Medical Letter 14:4, 1972.

40 Meleney, F. L., Longacre, A. B., Altemeier, W. A., Reisner, E. H., Pulaski, E. J., and Zintel, H. A.: The efficacy and the safety of the intramuscular administration of bacitracin in various types of surgical and certain medical infections, with analysis of 270 cases, Surg. Gynec. Obstet. 89:657, 1949.

41 Owen, L. N.: Fluorescence of tetracyclines in bone tumours, normal bone, and teeth, Nature 190:500, 1961.

42 Park, J. T., and Strominger, J. L.: Mode of action of penicillin: biochemical basis for the mechanism of action of penicillin and for its toxicity, Science 125:99, 1957.

43 Petersdorf, R. G.: Colistin—a reappraisal, J.A.M.A. 183:123, 1963.

44 Poth, E. J.: Intestinal antisepsis in surgery, J.A.M.A. 153:1516, 1953.

45 Procknow, J. J., and Loosli, C. G.: Treatment of deep mycoses, Arch. Intern. Med. 101:765, 1958.

46 Schatz, A., Bugie, E., and Waksman, S. A.: Streptomycin, a substance exhibiting antibiotic activity against gram-positive and gram-negative bacteria, Proc. Soc. Exp. Biol. Med. 55:66, 1944.

47 Schimpff, S., Satterlee, W., Young, V. M., and Serpick, A.: Empiric therapy with carbenicillin and gentamycin for febrile patients with cancer and granulocytopenia, New Eng. J. Med. 284:1061, 1971.

48 Sidell, S., Burdick, R. E., Brodie, J., Bulger, R. J., and Kirby, W. M. M.: New antistaphylococcal antibiotics, Arch. Intern. Med. 112:21, 1963.

49 Steer, P. L., Marks, M. I., Klite, P. D., and Eickhoff, T. C.: 5-Fluorocytosine: an oral antifungal compound, Arch. Intern. Med. 76:15, 1972.

50 Turk, M., Belcher, D. W., Ronald, A., Smith, R. H., and Wallace, J. F.: New cephalosporin antibiotic—cephaloridine, Arch. Intern. Med. 119:50, 1967.

51 Waksman, S. A.: Neomycin: nature, formation, isolation, and practical application, New Brunswick, N. J., 1953, Rutgers University Press.

52 Walters, E. W., Romansky, M. J., and Johnson, A. C.: Lincomycin. In Laboratory and clinical studies: antimicrobial agents and chemotherapy, Ann Arbor, Mich., 1963, American Society for Microbiology.

53 Weinstein, L., Kaplan, K., and Chang, T.: Treatment of infections in man with cephalothin, J.A.M.A. 189:829, 1964.

54 Weinstein, M. J., Luedemann, G. M., Oden, E. M., Wagman, G. H., Rosselet, J. P., Marquez, J. A., Coniglio, C. T., Charney, W., Herzog, H. L., and Black, J.: Gentamycin, a new antibiotic complex from Micromonospora, J. Med. Chem. 6:463, 1963.

55 Weiss, C. F., Glazko, A. J., and Weston, J. K.: Chloramphenicol in the newborn infant. A

physiological explanation of its toxicity when given in excessive doses, New Eng. J. Med. **262**:787, 1960.

56 Wisseman, C. L., Jr., Smadel, J. E., Hahn, F. E., and Hopps, H. E.: Mode of action of chloramphenicol: action of chloramphenicol on assimilation of ammonia and on synthesis of proteins and nucleic acids in Escherichia coli, J. Bact. **67**:662, 1954.

57 Wright, W. A., Boyer, D. D., and Strode, J. W.: Genetic aspects of antimicrobial therapy. In Antibiotics annual, 1955–1956, New York, 1956, Medical Encyclopedia, Inc.

Recent reviews

58 Abraham, E. P.: The cephalosporins, Pharmacol. Rev. **14**:473, 1962.

59 Abraham, E. P.: The chemistry of new antibiotics, Amer. J. Med. **39**:692, 1965.

60 Bennett, J. E.: The treatment of systemic mycoses, Rational Drug Ther. **4**:1, Apr. 1973.

61 Burchall, J. J., Ferone, R., and Hitchings, G. H.: Antibacterial chemotherapy, Ann. Rev. Pharmacol. **5**:53, 1965.

62 Butler, W. T.: Pharmacology, toxicity and therapeutic usefulness of amphotericin B, J.A.M.A. **195**:371, 1966.

63 Caldwell, J. R., and Cluff, L. E.: The real and present danger of antibiotics, Rational Drug Ther. **7**:1, Jan. 1973.

64 Council on Drugs: The amantadine controversy, J.A.M.A. **201**:372, 1967.

65 Dowling, H. F.: Present status of therapy with combinations of antibiotics, Amer. J. Med. **39**:796, 1965.

66 Editorial: Interferon induction, New Eng. J. Med. **277**:1316, 1967.

67 Editorial: Rifampin—a major new chemotherapeutic agent for the treatment of tuberculosis, New Eng. J. Med. **280**:615, 1969.

68 Eggers, H. J., and Tamm, I.: Antiviral chemotherapy, Ann. Rev. Pharmacol. **6**:231, 1966.

69 Feingold, D. S.: Antimicrobial chemotherapeutic agents: the nature of their action and selective toxicity, New Eng. J. Med. **269**:900, 957, 1963.

70 Gale, E. F.: Mechanisms of antibiotic action, Pharmacol. Rev. **15**:481, 1963.

71 Gill, A. F., and Hook, E. W.: Changing patterns of bacterial resistance to antimicrobial drugs, Amer. J. Med. **39**:780, 1965.

72 Goldberg, I. H.: Mode of action of antibiotics. II. Drugs affecting nucleic acid and protein synthesis, Amer. J. Med. **39**:722, 1965.

73 International symposium on gentamicin, a new aminoglycoside antibiotic, J. Infect. Dis. **119**: 341, 1969.

74 Kunin, C. M.: Clinical pharmacology of the new penicillins. I. The importance of serum protein binding in determining antimicrobial activity and concentration in serum, Clin. Pharmacol. Ther. **7**:166, 1966.

75 Kunin, C. M.: Clinical pharmacology of the new penicillins. II. Effect of drugs which interfere with the binding to serum proteins, Clin. Pharmacol. Ther. **7**:180, 1966.

76 Kunin, C. M.: Effects of antibiotics on the gastrointestinal tract, Clin. Pharmacol. Ther. **8**:495, 1967.

77 Kunin, C. M., and Finland, M.: Clinical pharmacology of the tetracycline antibiotics, Clin. Pharmacol. Ther. **2**:51, 1961.

78 Pittinger, C. B., and Adamson, R.: Antibiotic blockade of neuromuscular function, Ann. Rev. Pharmacol. **12**:169, 1972.

79 Rollo, I. M.: Antibacterial chemotherapy, Ann. Rev. Pharmacol. **6**:209, 1966.

80 Sabath, L. D., Elder, H. A., McCall, C. E., and Finland, M.: Synergistic combinations of penicillins in the treatment of bacteriuria, New Eng. J. Med. **277**:232, 1967.

81 Schoenfield, L. J.: Biliary excretion of antibiotics, New Eng. J. Med. **284**:1213, 1971.

82 Seneca, H.: Biological basis of chemotherapy of infections and infestations, Philadelphia, 1971, F. A. Davis Co.

83 Smith, D. H.: The current status of R factors, Ann. Intern. Med. **67**:1337, 1967.

84 Strominger, J. L., and Tipper, D. J.: Bacterial cell wall synthesis and structure in relation to the mechanism of action of penicillins and other antibacterial agents, Amer. J. Med. **39**:708, 1965.

85 Utz, J. P.: Chemotherapeutic agents for the systemic mycoses, New Eng. J. Med. **268**:938, 1963.

86 Utz, J. P.: Antimicrobial therapy in systemic fungal infections, Amer. J. Med. **39**:826, 1965.

87 VanArsdel, P. P., Jr.: Allergic reactions to penicillin, J.A.M.A. **191**:240, 1965.

88 Yaffe, S. J.: Antibiotic dosage in newborn and premature infants, J.A.M.A. **193**:818, 1965.

49 Drugs used in treatment of tuberculosis

The *primary* drugs in the treatment of tuberculosis are *isoniazid, streptomycin,* and *p-aminosalicylic acid.* The *secondary* group of drugs includes *ethambutol, cycloserine, ethionamide, pyrazinamide, viomycin,* and *rifampin.*

Isoniazid is the most effective drug, and it would be almost ideal if it were not for the emergence of resistance in the tubercle bacillus. The same difficulty is encountered with streptomycin. *p*-Aminosalicylic acid, although much less effective than the other two primary drugs, is very useful in delaying resistance to them. The secondary drugs are generally more toxic than the members of the primary group but may have important applications in selected cases (Table 49-1).

Tuberculosis represents one of the few examples in which combinations of drugs are highly recommended. The purpose of these combinations is to prevent the appearance of resistant strains of tubercle bacilli.

STREPTOMYCIN

Streptomycin was the first antibiotic that, even at concentrations as low as 1 μg/ml., could prevent multiplication of mycobacteria and cure experimental infections due to *Mycobacterium tuberculosis.* It was also the first drug that was clinically effective and could actually elicit a cure of tuberculous meningitis in man.

Streptomycin is injected intramuscularly in doses of 1 Gm./day. Many different dosage schedules are used in treatment of pulmonary tuberculosis. Since resistance usually develops to its action when as much as 60 Gm. has been given, many investi-

Table 49-1. Current antituberculous agents and side effects*

Primary agents	Usual dosage†	Route	Side effects, toxicity, and precautions
Isoniazid (INH)	3-5 mg./kg./day, usually 300 mg./day	P.O. (I.M. available)	Peripheral neuropathy (less than 1%); pyridoxine 50 to 100 mg. daily will reduce this incidence; other neurologic sequelae include convulsions, optic neuritis, toxic encephalopathy, psychosis, muscle twitching, dizziness, and alterations of sensorium (all rare); allergic skin rashes, fever, hepatitis (less than 1%); blood dyscrasias (rare)

*Courtesy Dr. Jay P. Sanford, Dallas.
†Adult dosages only.

Table 49-1. Current antituberculous agents and side effects—cont'd

Primary agents	Usual dosage	Route	Side effects, toxicity, and precautions
Para-aminosalicyclic acid (PAS) (Na⁺ or K⁺ salt)	10-12 Gm./day (200 mg./kg./day)	P.O.	Gastrointestinal irritation (10 to 15%); goitrogenic action (rare); depressed prothrombin activity (rare); G6PD-mediated anemia (rare); drug fever, rashes, hepatitis, myalgia, arthralgia; Na⁺ or K⁺ must be taken into account in those with heart failure or renal insufficiency; give medication with meals or antacids
Streptomycin	1.0 Gm./day initially for 60 to 90 days, then 1.0 Gm. 2 or 3 times/wk. (15 mg./kg./day)	I.M.	Vestibular dysfunction (vertigo); paresthesias; dizziness and nausea (all less in patients receiving 2 or 3 doses/wk.); tinnitus and high frequency loss (1%); nephrotoxicity (rare); peripheral neuropathy (rare); allergic skin rashes (4 to 5%); drug fever, lymphadenopathy, blood dyscrasias and anaphylactoid reactions (rare); audiogram, estimation of renal function in older patients or when otherwise indicated
Ethambutol	25 mg./kg./day for 2 mo., then 15 mg./kg./day	P.O. (I.V. available)	Optic neuritis with decreased visual acuity, central scotomata, and loss of green and red perception; peripheral neuropathy and headache (rare), rashes (rare); monthly evaluation of visual acuity, with greater than 10% loss considered significant, usually reversible if drug is discontinued
Rifampin	600 mg./day (single dose)	P.O.	Although toxicity is uncommon, the following have been reported: gastrointestinal irritation, drug fever, skin rash, mental confusion, thrombocytopenia, leukopenia, transient abnormalities in liver function (SGOT, alkaline phosphatase). Interferes with some chemical determinations of bilirubin (false elevation); eosinophilia (rare); avoid in first trimester of pregnancy; discolors urine a brownish color. Increases requirement for coumarin-type anticoagulants.

Continued.

Table 49-1. Current antituberculous agents and side effects—cont'd

Secondary agents	Usual dosage	Route	Side effects, toxicity, and precautions
Etionamide	500-750 mg./day (10-15 mg./kg./day)	P.O.	Gastrointestinal irritation (up to 50% on large dose); goiter; peripheral neuropathy (rare); convulsions (rare); changes in affect (rare); difficulty in diabetes control; rashes, hepatitis; purpura; stomatitis; give drug with meals or antacids; 50 to 100 mg. pyridoxine/day concomitantly; SGOT monthly
Pyrazinamide (PZA)	25 mg./kg./day (maximum 2.5 Gm./day)	P.O.	Hyperuricemia (with or without symptoms); hepatitis (not over 2% if recommended dose not exceeded); gastric irritation; photosensitivity (rare); SGOT monthly; serum uric acid periodically, or if symptomatic gouty attack occurs
Cycloserine	750-1000 mg./day (15 mg./kg./day)	P.O.	Convulsions, psychoses (5 to 10% of those receiving 1.0 Gm./day); headache; somnolence; hyperreflexia; increased CSF protein and pressure; contraindicated in epileptics; 100 mg. pyridoxine (or more) daily should be given concomitantly
Kanamycin	1.0 Gm. 3 or 4 times/wk. (or 0.5 Gm. daily)	I.M.	Ototoxicity (largely hearing loss); vertigo less common; nephrotoxicity; neuromuscular blockade; paresthesias; eosinophilia; drug fever; rashes; anaphylactoid reactions (rare); periodic renal functional assessments; audiograms when indicated
Viomycin	1.0 Gm. 3 or 4 times/wk. (or 0.5 Gm. daily)	I.M.	Similar to kanamycin; hypocalcemia and hypokalemia; edema
Experimental agent	**Usual dosage**	**Route**	**Side effects, toxicity, and precautions**
Capreomycin (experimental)	1.0 Gm./day (15 mg./kg./day)	I.M.	Similar to kanamycin and viomycin

gators find it advantageous to administer streptomycin only twice weekly and to combine it with some other agent such as *p*-aminosalicylic acid, which helps in delaying the development of resistance.

Vestibular damage and resistance are the main limitations in the use of streptomycin. For these reasons isoniazid is now considered the most important drug in the treatment of tuberculosis.

PARA-AMINOSALICYLIC ACID

The discovery of the usefulness of *p*-aminosalicylic acid (PAS) in the treatment of tuberculosis[3] was a consequence of fundamental studies on the effect of various substances, including salicylic acid, on the oxygen uptake of the tubercle bacillus.[1] Salicylic acid was found to increase the oxygen consumption of virulent tubercle bacilli, and it became of interest to study the effect of related drugs.

p-Aminosalicylic acid inhibits growth of virulent tubercle bacilli at concentrations as low as 1 μg/ml. It has no effect on virulent saprophytic mycobacteria. In patients the drug is less effective than streptomycin and must be administered in very large doses, even up to 15 to 20 Gm./day. The great value of the drug results from the fact that it delays development of resistance to other tuberculostatic drugs.[6]

The structural formulas of salicylic acid and *p*-aminosalicylic acid are shown below:

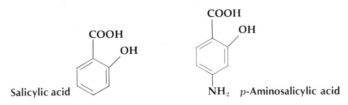

Salicylic acid   NH₂ *p*-Aminosalicylic acid

The adverse effects of *p*-aminosalicylic acid consist of gastrointestinal disturbances, occasional skin rash, and, rarely, hepatic damage and interference with thyroid function.

The inhibitory effect of *p*-aminosalicylic acid on the tubercle bacillus is antagonized by *p*-aminobenzoic acid, a finding that suggests that its mode of action may be related to antagonism to this growth factor.

p-Aminosalicylic acid is an important drug in the treatment of tuberculosis. It is well absorbed and is excreted after being partially acetylated in the body. Its only disadvantage is gastric irritation. Various salts of the acid may be less irritating.

ISONIAZID

The potent effect of isoniazid on the tubercle bacillus was discovered somewhat by accident as the result of routine screening of chemical intermediates in the synthesis of thiosemicarbazones.

Isoniazid is remarkably potent against the tubercle bacillus. It inhibits growth in the test tube at concentrations of less than 1 μg/ml. Its mechanism of action is not known, but it is of interest that pyridoxal antagonizes its neurotoxic effect without preventing its antibacterial action. It is also possible that the drug is incorporated into nicotinamide-containing coenzymes in mycobacteria. Some of the central nervous system effects of isoniazid have been attributed to interference with enzymes that require pyridoxal.

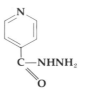

Isoniazid

Although isoniazid can form a complex in vitro with pyridoxal phosphate, it is not likely that this is the mechanism of its killing effect on mycobacteria. Loss of acid fastness of tubercle bacilli on isoniazid treatment suggests interference with synthesis of the lipid-rich envelope as an important factor in the lethal effect of the drug.[14]

Isoniazid is rapidly absorbed from the gastrointestinal tract. It is widely distributed in the body and penetrates efficiently into the cerebrospinal fluid. Its metabolism is not completely known, but acetylation is one of the important processes of biotransformation. The acetyl derivative and some of the original drug are cleared by the kidney.

Genetically conditioned differences in the ability to acetylate isoniazid are good examples of pharmacogenetics. Persons who show low acetylating ability maintain higher blood levels and may be more subject to the toxic effects of the drug.[14]

Isoniazid is administered in doses of 3 to 4 mg./kg. once a day. Larger doses have been used in tuberculous meningitis. Oral administration is preferred, but parenteral routes of administration can also be used.

Among the toxic manifestations, neurotoxicity appears to be the most important. From 1 to 5% of patients taking isoniazid may develop *headache, vertigo,* and *peripheral neuropathy.* It has been suggested that pyridoxine is effective in the prevention of these manifestations without interference with chemotherapeutic activity. Depression of bone marrow, liver damage, and skin rash have also been observed.

Resistance to isoniazid can develop fairly rapidly, and simultaneous use of *p*-aminosalicylic acid delays this undersirable development.

Although the administration of vitamin B_6 may prevent neurotoxicity of isoniazid, there is no reason to believe that the effect of the drug on mycobacteria involves interference with this vitamin, as mycobacteria can synthesize B_6. Furthermore, pyridoxal phosphate does not prevent the effect of isoniazid on the tubercle bacillus.[14]

ETHIONAMIDE

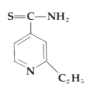

Ethionamide

Ethionamide (Trecator) is a pyridine derivative, as is isoniazid. It is used in the treatment of tuberculosis in doses of 0.5 to 1 Gm./day. It is less effective than isoniazid.

OTHER DRUGS

A number of drugs are looked upon as alternatives to the previously discussed agents or secondary agents in the treatment of tuberculosis. Because of their frequent and serious side effects, this use should be limited to severe infections in which the less hazardous drugs may be ineffective.

Cycloserine (Oxamycin; Seromycin) has been somewhat effective in treatment of tuberculosis in combination with other drugs. Unfortunately it is neurotoxic. It is administered by mouth in doses of 250 mg. daily. Frequent side effects such as nausea, vomiting, hypotension, and peripheral neuritis limit the usefulness of cycloserine.

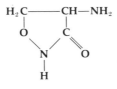

Cycloserine

The mechanism of action of cycloserine involves competition for D-alanine as a precursor of some cell wall component.[2] As a consequence, the drug induces protoplast formation. Despite its neurotoxicity, cycloserine has some usefulness as a second-line drug in the treatment of tuberculosis and also in some urinary infections.

Cycloserine is well absorbed from the gastrointestinal tract, is widely distributed in the body, and penetrates well into the spinal fluid. It is excreted mostly unchanged into the urine, although part is metabolized.

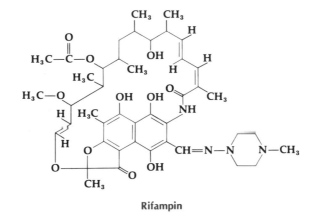

Rifampin

Rifampin is a semisynthetic derivative of rifamycin B produced by *Streptomyces mediterranei*. The drug is highly effective in the treatment of tuberculosis.[7,8,11] The antibacterial spectrum of rifampin is broad, since it includes both gram-positive and gram-negative organisms. Its therapeutic efficacy in the elimination of meningococcal carriers has been demonstrated.[10] Rifampin inhibits DNA-dependent RNA polymerase,[12] the bacterial enzyme being more susceptible than its mammalian counterpart. After oral administration of 600 mg. of rifampin, blood levels of 8 μg/ml. are attained in less than 2 hours.[10] Serum antibacterial activity is often present in 12 hours.[7] Combinations of isoniazid and rifampin are highly effective in the treatment of tuberculosis.[7]

The development of rifampin may be considered a major advance in antituberculosis chemotherapy. It is of great value in patients with drug-resistant infections. Since resistance develops to rifampin, it is imperative to use it in combination with another antituberculous agent. In some clinical studies,[7] no toxicity attributable to rifampin was found.

Viomycin, a polypeptide antibiotic, is also somewhat effective against the tubercle bacillus but causes renal and auditory damage.

Pyrazinamide (pyrazinoic acid amine) is an analog of nicotinamide. It is inhibitory to the tubercle bacillus when administered in large doses, 3 Gm./day. It can cause hepatic damage and retention of uric acid.

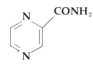

Pyrazinamide

Ethambutol (Myambutol) is a new drug for the treatment of tuberculosis. It is available in 100 and 400 mg. tablets. The drug seems promising, although it may cause visual disturbances.[13] Ethambutol may replace PAS as a primary antituberculosis drug.

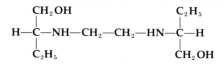

Ethambutol

References

1 Bernheim, F.: The effect of various substances on the oxygen uptake of the tubercle bacillus, J. Bact. **41**:387, 1941.

2 Hoeprich, P. D.: Alanine: cycloserine antagonism, Arch. Intern. Med. **112**:405, 1963.

3 Lehmann, J.: Determination of pathogenicity of tubercle bacilli by their intermediate metabolism, Lancet **1**:14, 1946.

4 Raleigh, J. W., and Steele, J. D.: Recent developments in the treatment of tuberculosis in man, J.A.M.A. **166**:921, 1958.

5 Ruiz, R. C.: D-Cycloserine in the treatment of tuberculosis resistant to standard drugs. A study of 116 cases, Dis. Chest **45**:181, 1964.

6 Thoren, M., and Hinshaw, H. C.: Therapy of pulmonary tuberculosis with isoniazid alone and in combination with streptomycin and with para-aminosalicylic acid, Stanford Med. Bull. **10**:316, 1952.

7 Vall-Spinosa, A., Lester, W., Moulding, T., Davidson, P. T., and McClatchy, J. K.: Rifampin in the treatment of drug-resistant *Mycobacterium tuberculosis* infections, New Eng. J. Med. **283**:616, 1970.

8 Verbist, L., and Gyselen, A.: Antituberculous activity of rifampin in vitro and in vivo and the concentrations obtained in human blood, Amer. Rev. Resp. Dis. **98**:923, 1968.

9 Walker, A. M.: Chemotherapy of tuberculosis in man, J.A.M.A. **147**:253, 1951.

Recent reviews

10 Deal, W. B., and Sanders, E.: Efficacy of rifampin in treatment of meningococcal carriers, New Eng. J. Med. **281**:641, 1969.

11 Editorial: Rifampin — a major new chemotherapeutic agent for the treatment of tuberculosis, New Eng. J. Med. **280**:615, 1969.

12 Hartmann, G., Honikel, K. O., Knüsel, F., and Nuesch, J.: The specific inhibition of DNA-directed RNA synthesis by rifamycin, Biochim. Biophys. Acta **145**:843, 1967.

13 Mitchell, R. S.: Control of tuberculosis, New Eng. J. Med. **276**:842, 905, 1967.

14 Robson, J. M., and Sullivan, F. M.: Antituberculosis drugs, Pharmacol. Rev. **15**:169, 1963.

50 Drugs used in treatment of leprosy

The most effective drugs in the treatment of leprosy are certain sulfones. Shortly after the introduction of the sulfonamides, diaminodiphenylsulfone and related drugs received attention because of their greater effectiveness against the tubercle bacillus. They proved somewhat toxic in clinical trials and not as useful in human tuberculosis as did streptomycin and the other tuberculostatic compounds. It was found, however, that some of the sulfones are quite useful in the treatment of leprosy.

The structural formulas of 4,4'-diaminodiphenylsulfone (DDS; dapsone; Avlosulfon) and 2-amino-5-sulfanilylthiazole (Promizole) are shown below.

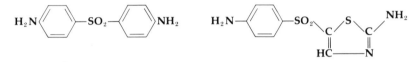

4,4'-Diaminodiphenylsulfone   **2-Amino-5-sulfanilylthiazole**

It is believed that the mode of action of these sulfones is similar to that of the sulfonamides, since p-aminobenzoic acid tends to antagonize their bacteriostatic activities. It is not known why these compounds have greater effectiveness than do the sulfonamides against leprosy.

Chaulmoogra oil (hydnocarpus oil) has been used for many years in the treatment of leprosy. Despite the fairly extensive use of this oil, usually by intramuscular injection, there is no unanimity among the experts concerning its effectiveness. Some even believe that it has no effect at all.

Sulfone therapy is still the treatment of choice in leprosy. In addition to 4,4'-diaminodiphenylsulfone, which is most often prescribed, other sulfones such as sulfoxone (Diasone) and solapsone (Sulphetrone) are also recommended. Initial dosage of the sulfones should be small, since the patient's condition may become much worse when treatment with full doses is initiated in certain phases of the disease.[3]

With sulfone treatment, greatest improvement is noted in the ulcerative lesions. Nasal obstruction improves in 3 to 6 months. Bacteria disappear very slowly, and even after 5 years of treatment one half of lepromatous patients continue to have positive smears.[2] Ethambutol and rifampin may be effective in the treatment of leprosy.

References

1 Bushby, S. R. M.: The chemotherapy of leprosy, Pharmacol. Rev. **10**:1, 1958.
2 Smith, J. W.: Leprosy, Texas Med. **67**:58, 1971.

3 Trautman, J. R.: The management of leprosy and its complications, New Eng. J. Med. **273**: 756, 1965.

51 Antiseptics and disinfectants

GENERAL CONCEPT

There are many drugs that are useful in decreasing the bacterial flora when applied directly to the skin, infected wounds, instruments, or excreta. These locally effective drugs have a low enough therapeutic index to make them unsuited as systemic chemotherapeutic agents.

Antiseptics are drugs that are applied to living tissues for the purpose of killing bacteria or inhibiting their growth. *Disinfectants* are bactericidal drugs that are applied to nonliving materials. Other terms related to antiseptics and disinfectants that are commonly misused are as follows:

germicide anything that destroys bacteria but not necessarily spores.
fungicide anything that destroys fungi.
sporicide anything that destroys spores.
sanitizer an agent that reduces the number of bacterial contaminants to a safe level, as may be judged by public health requirements.
preservative an agent or process that prevents decomposition by either chemical or physical means.

BRIEF HISTORY

Disinfectants were used long before the discovery of bacteria. The first germicides used were deodorants, since foul odors were associated with disease. Chlorinated soda was used on infected wounds as early as 1825 (Labarraque) and its use was recommended at about the same time for the purification of drinking water.

Phenol was used also as a deodorant and later as an antiseptic for infected wounds. Lister (1867) is usually credited with the introduction of phenol into surgery, but it was actually used long before the nature of infections was understood.

The use of alcohol was delayed for many years because Koch (1881) had reported that it did not kill anthrax spores. The superior germicidal properties of 70% alcohol were established by Beyer (1912).

Tincture of iodine was introduced into the *United States Pharmacopeia* in 1830, but it was not used extensively until the Civil War.

The importance of cleansing the hands with chlorine-containing solutions for the prevention of puerperal fever was clearly demonstrated by Semmelweis. This clinician, while working as an assistant at the Lying-in Hospital in Vienna, made some shrewd observations on the cause of puerperal fever. The ward where he worked was used for the training of medical students. Semmelweis noted that the mortality on the ward was lower when the medical students were on vacation. This observation by itself could have had many different explanations. He also noted, however, the odor from the autopsy room whenever the students were present. He suspected that the students were carrying "decomposing organic matter" from the autopsy room to the delivery room. He proved his hypothesis when cleansing of the students' hands with a solution of chloride and lime resulted in a marked reduction in mortality from puerperal sepsis. (For a detailed history see Reddish.[8])

POTENCY OF ANTISEPTICS

Prior to the discovery of chemotherapeutic agents there was much preoccupation with the development of more and more potent antiseptics. Much effort was expended in synthesizing new compounds that could kill bacteria rapidly at high dilutions. The new antiseptics were generally compared with phenol, and the ratio of the dilutions necessary for killing test organisms in vitro was called the *phenol coefficient*. These efforts were so successful that antiseptics were synthesized that were hundreds of times more potent than phenol in killing bacteria in less than 10 minutes.

In retrospect, much of this effort was misdirected. Any drug that can kill bacteria in a few minutes is bound to have toxic effects on mammalian tissues. It is not surprising that even the most potent antiseptics were completely incapable of curing a systemic bacterial infection because the testing method used for their development was designed for *potency* and not for a favorable *therapeutic index*. The discoverers of Prontosil decided to test every compound against a systemic infection in mice. The sulfonamides and penicillin would never have been discovered by testing methods such as the use of the phenol coefficient. Not only the phenol coefficient but all tools for the evaluation of antiseptics are poor. It is not surprising that the field is dominated by empiricism and is greatly influenced by fashion.

COMMONLY USED ANTISEPTICS AND DISINFECTANTS
PHENOLS

Phenol is a caustic substance that precipitates proteins. In a 1:90 dilution it can kill many bacteria in less than 10 minutes. Phenol has considerable systemic toxicity and is absorbed from denuded surfaces or burned areas. It can cause convulsions and renal damage.

Many derivatives of phenol find some application as antiseptics or disinfectants. Saponated solutions of cresol (Lysol), resorcinol, and thymol have some medicinal uses, but the most widely used phenol derivative is hexachlorophene. The latter is incorporated into soaps and creams. In a 3% solution, hexachlorophene causes a marked reduction of bacterial counts on the skin without being irritating. Soaps containing hexachlorophene are generally used for preoperative scrubbing of the surgeon's hands and for the antisepsis of the patient's skin.

The safety of hexachlorophene preparations, particularly for bathing newborn infants, has been seriously questioned. Such infants absorb some of the drug through the skin when the bath contains 3% of the antiseptic. Although no obvious toxicity has been demonstrated in human infants, newborn monkeys washed daily for 90 days with 3% solutions of hexachlorophene showed mean plasma levels of 2.3 μg/ml. and developed brain lesions.[2] The Food and Drug Administration now advises against the use of 3% hexachlorophene for total body bathing. Such a product is still considered effective as a bacteriostatic skin cleanser and possibly effective in the treatment of staphylococcal skin infection. Evidence is lacking for the effectiveness and safety of hexachlorophene as an "aid to personal hygiene."

HALOGEN COMPOUNDS

Tincture of iodine containing 2% iodine is often used for the preoperative preparation of the skin. The tincture stains the skin and is irritating to some individuals.

Povidone-iodine is a complex of polyvinylpyrrolidone and iodine. It releases iodine slowly and is claimed to be less irritating than tincture of iodine.

SODIUM HYPOCHLORITE AND CHLORAMINE T

Sodium hypochlorite and chloramine T release chlorine. They were popular at one time for the cleansing of infected wounds.

Halazone, tetraglycine hydroperiodide (Globaline), and aluminum hexaurea sulfate triiodide (Hexadine S) are among the compounds that are used for water disinfection by means of halogen release.

OXIDIZING AGENTS

Hydrogen peroxide, 3%, releases "nascent" oxygen in the presence of catalase in the tissues. Probably its only value lies in its ability to remove foreign material by means of the oxygen bubbles it forms. Other oxidizing antiseptics are potassium permanganate, zinc peroxide, and sodium perborate.

ALCOHOLS AND ALDEHYDES

Ethyl alcohol is most bactericidal at 70% concentration by weight (78% by volume). It is commonly used as a skin antiseptic.

Isopropyl alcohol is at least as good an antiseptic as ethyl alcohol. It may be used as a 50% solution, but it is quite active when concentrated.

Formaldehyde in 40% concentration in formalin is used for the disinfection of instruments and excreta. It probably kills bacteria by combining with their proteins.

SURFACE-ACTIVE COMPOUNDS

Surface-active compounds have both hydrophilic and hydrophobic groups. They tend to accumulate in interfaces and probably disturb bacterial cell membranes that contain lipids. The surface-active antiseptics are of two types: anionic and cationic.

Anionic antiseptics. The various soaps and detergents such as sodium lauryl sulfate and sodium ethasulfate are antibacterial largely against gram-positive organisms. They are not nearly as important as the cationic antiseptics.

Cationic antiseptics. The hydrophilic group is usually a quaternary ammonium. Common representatives are benzalkonium (Zephiran), cetylpyridinium (Ceepryn), and benzethonium (Phemerol).

The cationic surface-active antiseptics are more potent at a higher pH. Their activity is decreased by soaps. In general they kill both gram-positive and gram-negative organisms, with some exceptions in the latter category.

The cationic antiseptics such as benzalkonium are commonly used for antisepsis of the skin and disinfection of instruments. The phenol coefficient of these compounds is very high, up to 500, but is reduced in the presence of pus and organic matter in general.

METAL-CONTAINING ANTISEPTICS

Mercuric chloride in a 1:1,000 solution has been used widely as a skin antiseptic. It undoubtedly combines with SH groups in bacteria. Yellow mercuric oxide ointment, 1%, is used in the treatment of conjunctivitis.

The organic derivatives of mercury have been widely used as skin antiseptics. Some popular preparations are thimerosal (Merthiolate), nitromersol (Metaphen), and merbromin (Mercurochrome). These antiseptics are largely bacteriostatic.

Silver nitrate in a 1% solution has been traditionally applied to the eyes of newborn infants to prevent ophthalmia neonatorum caused by gonococci. This practice is being replaced by the application of penicillin in the conjunctival sac of the newborn infant.

Zinc salts are mild antiseptics and also astringents. Zinc sulfate ointment is used in some types of conjunctivitis, while zinc oxide ointment is a traditional remedy in the treatment of a variety of skin diseases. Calamine lotion USP contains mostly zinc oxide, with a small amount of ferric oxide. Phenolated calamine lotion USP also contains 1% phenol.

NITROFURANS

Nitrofurazone (Furacin) has been used in the form of ointments and solutions at a concentration of 0.2%. Although quite effective against both gram-positive and gram-negative organisms, it can cause skin sensitization in a large percentage of patients.

ACIDS

Benzoic acid and salicylic acid have been used for many years as fungistatic agents. Whitfield's ointment is a mixture of 6% benzoic acid and 3% salicylic acid. It is commonly used for the treatment of fungal infections of the feet. Undecylenic acid (Desenex) is widely used in the treatment of "athlete's foot" and other fungal infections of the skin.

Mandelic acid and methenamine, used as urinary antiseptics, were discussed on p. 573.

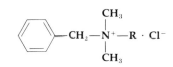

Phenol   Hexachlorophene   Benzalkonium chloride

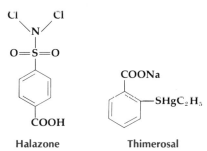

Halazone   Thimerosal

INDICATIONS AND USES OF ANTISEPTICS

With the development of powerful chemotherapeutic agents, the indications for the use of antiseptics have declined. They are unquestionably useful for reducing the bacterial counts on the skin, both on the surgeon's hands and on the patient. They generally have no place in the treatment of fresh wounds or infected wounds, where cleansing with saline is most important. Deeply infected wounds call for systemic chemotherapy.

Preoperative uses. Regular soap, alcohol up to 95%, and 3% hexachlorophene are the only antiseptics used for reducing the bacterial counts on the surgeon's hands and forearms. It is customary to scrub with soap with or without hexachlorophene for 7 minutes. This is followed by washing in 70% alcohol for 3 minutes. A final brushing with soap containing 3% hexachlorophene is used by some surgeons.

Experimental studies indicate that alcohol is an excellent rapidly acting skin antiseptic. Hexachlorophene does not kill bacteria as rapidly. Much of the benefit of hexachlorophene is attributed to the film it leaves on the skin after repeated applications.

The skin cannot be completely sterilized. Cleansing, facilitated by surface-active agents such as the anionic or cationic surfactants, removes the superficial bacterial flora, which probably contains most of the pathogenic organisms. In addition, alcohol is excellent for preoperative preparations of the skin, but mild tincture of iodine and organic mercurials still have some advocates.

References

1 Dineen, P.: The choice of a local antiseptic. In Modell, W., editor: Drugs of choice 1972-1973, St. Louis, 1972, The C. V. Mosby Co.

2 FDA Drug Bulletin, Dec., 1971.

3 Reddish, G. F., editor: Antiseptics, disinfectants, fungicides and chemical and physical sterilization, Philadelphia, 1957, Lea & Febiger.

52 Drugs used in treatment of amebiasis

Amebiasis is caused by the protozoon _Entamoeba histolytica_. It occurs sporadically or in epidemics, the latter often following contamination of a water supply with sewage.

Entamoeba histolytica has two principal phases in its life cycle, the _trophozoite_ and the _cystic_. The trophozoite is motile and can penetrate into the intestine, eventually reaching the liver. Ingested cysts liberate trophozoites in the intestine and cause the intestinal and extraintestinal forms of amebiasis.

From a chemical standpoint the antiamebic drugs can be classified into five general groups: alkaloids of ipecac (emetine), halogenated quinolines (iodoquinolines), arsenical preparations, aminoquinolines (chloroquine), and antibiotics.

Table 52-1. Antiamebic and some other antiprotozoal drugs of choice

Infecting organism	Drug of choice	Usual dosage	Route	Side effects and alternative agents
Entamoeba histolytica Intestinal (nondys-enteric)	Diiodohydroxyquin (Diodoquin) or	650 mg. t.i.d. — 21 days	P.O.	Nausea, abdominal cramps, rash
	Bismuth glycolylar-sanilate (Milibis)	500 mg. t.i.d. — 7 days	P.O.	
Intestinal (dysen-teric	Tetracycline plus emetine hydro-chloride	500 mg. q.i.d. — 10 days	P.O.	
		1 mg./kg. (not more than 65 mg./day)	I.M.	Local pain, electro-cardiographic changes, arrhyth-mias, peripheral neuropathy
Extraintestinal	Metronidazole (Flagyl)	800 mg. t.i.d. — 10 days	P.O.	Nausea, headache, diarrhea; alterna-tives: emetine or chloroquine
Giardia lamblia	Quinacrine hydro-chloride	100 mg. t.i.d. — 5 days		CNS effects, yellow staining of skin and sclerae, urticaria, blood dyscrasias
Balantidium coli	Tetracycline	500 mg. t.i.d. — 7 days		
Trichomonas vaginalis	Metronidazole (Flagyl)	250 mg. t.i.d. — 10 days	P.O.	Nausea, headache, diarrhea, rash, paresthesias

621

From a therapeutic standpoint the amebicides can be divided into intestinal and extraintestinal drugs. The former are often poorly absorbed from the intestine and are used primarily for eradicating the infection at that site. Most antiamebic drugs belong to this category and cannot be relied on for eradication of the trophozoites in the liver or lungs. On the other hand, metronidazole, emetine, and chloroquine are effective in the extraintestinal forms of the disease.

Some of the amebicides such as glycobiarsol, carbarsone, and iodochlorhydroxyquin are effective also in topical treatment of infections caused by *Trichomonas vaginalis*. In addition, the relatively new drug metronidazole is effective in trichomoniasis, even with oral administration (Table 52-1).

ALKALOIDS OF IPECAC — EMETINE

Emetine is obtained from the dried root of *Cephaelis ipecacuanha*, or ipecac. The crude preparation has been used for centuries in treatment of dysentery, although it is only effective against amebic and not bacillary enteric infections. As early as 1912, emetine was used by intramuscular injection in treatment of amebiasis. The drug is still useful in efforts at eradication of the extraintestinal trophozoites. Emetine is useful also in controlling symptoms in acute amebiasis but is not curative.

The structural formula of emetine is shown below. The alkaloid is directly amebicidal at high dilutions in vitro.[1] It exerts similar effects on trophozoites localized in tissues.

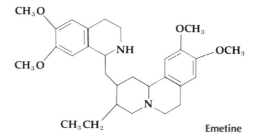

Emetine

It has a marked symptomatic effect in acute amebic dysentery but cannot be relied on for eradication of *Entamoeba histolytica* within the intestinal contents. As a consequence, if used alone, it would convert the acute form of the disease into the chronic or carrier phase.

The only valid uses of emetine hydrochloride are in the treatment of amebic dysentery and in the extraintestinal forms of the disease. For the latter indication, chloroquine may also be used. Ipecac is an emetic (p. 668).

Emetine is a toxic drug. Its main toxic action is manifest on cardiac and skeletal muscle. A dosage schedule of 65 mg./day for 10 days can be tolerated by most adults, but even on this dosage there may occur electrocardiographic changes such as T-wave inversion. Emetine is a cumulative drug, and its administration should not be continued beyond 10 days.

HALOGENATED QUINOLINES — IODOQUINOLINES

The iodinated quinolines such as chiniofon (yatren), iodochlorhydroxyquin (Vioform), and diiodohydroxyquin (Diodoquin) are effective and fairly safe antiamebic compounds that are considered quite useful for intestinal forms of the disease.

In some series a cure rate of 80 to 95% has been reported following oral administration of the iodoquinolines. Diiodohydroxyquin is being widely used because it has less tendency than chiniofon to produce nausea and diarrhea.

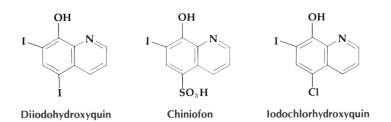

Diiodohydroxyquin   Chiniofon   Iodochlorhydroxyquin

The activity of these compounds in the intestine may be due to liberation of iodine. These compounds are partially absorbed from the intestine and can produce marked elevations in the blood iodine level, which can interfere with tests for thyroid function.

ARSENICAL PREPARATIONS

Certain organic arsenicals are effective for treatment of intestinal amebiasis. As with the iodoquinolines, however, they cannot be expected to eradicate *Entamoeba histolytica* from its extraintestinal localizations.

Carbarsone, or *p*-ureidobenzenearsonic acid, is a pentavalent arsenical that has been used in the treatment of amebiasis for many years. Its effectiveness is comparable to that of the iodoquinolines. Since the drug is absorbed from the gastrointestinal tract, arsenical poisoning may occur, and most experts advise against its use in the presence of liver damage.

Another arsenical, **glycobiarsol** (Milibis), contains both arsenic and bismuth. It is not well absorbed from the gastrointestinal tract and is very effective against the intestinal ameba, although no action can be expected against trophozoites in the tissues. Thus, in hepatic amebiasis, additional amebicides such as chloroquine or emetine are necessary.

The structural formulas of carbarsone and glycobiarsol are as follows:

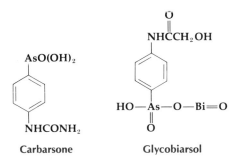

Carbarsone   Glycobiarsol

The dosage of glycobiarsol is 0.5 Gm. three times a day for 7 days. Although the drug is quite nontoxic because of its lack of absorption, it should not be employed if liver damage is present or known intolerance to arsenicals exists.[3] The drug may produce arsenical sensitivity.

AMINOQUINOLINES – CHLOROQUINE

Chloroquine (Aralen) is a well-known antimalarial compound that is highly concentrated in the liver[4] and is highly effective in treatment of amebic hepatitis and amebic abscess of the liver. Its introduction as an extraintestinal amebicide was a most important therapeutic development in view of the many side effects and cardiotoxicity encountered with emetine, the only other effective extraintestinal antiamebic compound.

Chloroquine cannot be expected to eradicate the intestinal form of *Entamoeba histolytica*, and concomitant medication with an intestinal amebicide such as glycobiarsol is mandatory.

The recommended dosage of chloroquine is 0.25 Gm. four times daily for 2 days, followed by 0.25 Gm. twice daily for 2 weeks. Other dosage schedules have also been recommended. Additional information on chloroquine is included in Chapter 54.

ANTIBIOTICS

Early work with the antibacterial drugs has shown that patients with intestinal amebiasis improve more rapidly when these drugs are added to the usual antiamebic regimen. Later the tetracyclines, erythromycin, bacitracin, and paromomycin were found to be quite effective against intestinal forms of the disease.

There has been considerable controversy concerning the mode of action of these antibiotics in amebiasis. Many authorities believe that their beneficial effect is due to alteration of the bacterial flora, which is in itself deleterious to the survival of the ameba. Some work indicates, however, that these antibiotics can exert a direct amebicidal effect. In any case, the antibiotics are effective largely against the intestinal form of the disease, and other amebicides are generally recommended for concomitant use against extraintestinal infestation.[6]

DRUGS USED IN TREATMENT OF TRICHOMONIASIS

Many amebicidal drugs have a killing effect on *Trichomonas vaginalis* also. Most of them such as carbarsone, glycobiarsol, and iodochlorhydroxyquin are effective only when applied topically. In contrast, the relatively new drug **metronidazole** (Flagyl) is highly effective in the treatment of *Trichomonas* infections when given orally. The drug is administered in 250 mg. doses two or three times a day by mouth, usually for 10 days. Metronidazole may cause gastrointestinal symptoms, ataxia, vertigo, hematologic complications such as leukopenia, and secondary monilial infection. Metronidazole may cause a disulfiram-like reaction when alcohol is ingested. The drug is contraindicated in pregnant women.

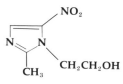

Metronidazole

References

1 Anderson, H. H., and Hansen, E. L.: The chemotherapy of amebiasis, Pharmacol. Rev. 2:399, 1950.

2 Balamuth, W., and Lasslo, A.: Comparative amoebicidal activity of some compounds related to emetine, Proc. Soc. Exp. Biol. Med. 80:705, 1952.

3 Berberian, D. A., Dennis, E. W., and Pipkin, C. A.: The effectiveness of bismuthoxy *p*-N-glycolylarsanilate (Milibis) in the treatment of the intestinal amebiasis, Amer. J. Trop. Med. 30:613, 1950.

4 Conan, N. J., Jr.: The treatment of hepatic amebiasis with chloroquine, Amer. J. Med. 6:309, 1949.

5 Killough, J. H., Magill, G. B., and Smith, R. C.: The treatment of amebiasis with fumagillin, Science 115:71, 1952.

6 Most, H., and Van Assendelft, F.: Laboratory and clinical observations of the effect of terramycin in treatment of amebiasis, Ann. N. Y. Acad. Sci. 53:427, 1950.

7 Sikat, P., Heemstra, J., Brooks, R., and Yankton, S. D.: Metronidazole chemotherapy for Trichomonas vaginalis infections, J.A.M.A. 182:904, 1962.

Recent reviews

8 Anderson, H. H.: Newer drugs in amebiasis, Clin. Pharmacol. Ther. 1:78, 1960.

9 Clark, D., Solomons, E., and Siegal, S.: Drugs for vaginal trichomoniasis, Obstet. Gynec. 20:615, 1962.

10 Most, H.: Treatment of common parasitic infections of man encountered in the United States (second of two parts), New Eng. J. Med. 287:698, 1972.

11 Schnitzer, R. J., and Hawking, F., editors: Experimental chemotherapy, vol. 1, New York, 1963, Academic Press, Inc.

53 Anthelmintic drugs

Worm infections represent the most common parasitic diseases of man. It has been estimated that in various parts of the world more than 800 million persons are infected with helminths.

A number of drugs have been used in the treatment of helminthiasis, largely on an empirical basis. Some of the early anthelmintics were highly toxic, whereas in recent years much more attention is being paid to the safety of such medications.

The drugs of choice for various helminthiases are shown in Table 53-1.

INDIVIDUAL ANTHELMINTICS
PIPERAZINE SALTS

Piperazine citrate anhydrous (Antepar), a close equivalent to piperazine hexahydrate, is highly effective in the treatment of ascariasis and other worm infestations. This simple drug causes paralysis of the musculature of the worm, by a curare-like action. Expelled worms are still alive, although relaxed.

$$HN \begin{array}{c} CH_2 - CH_2 \\ \diagup \qquad \diagdown \\ \diagdown \qquad \diagup \\ CH_2 - CH_2 \end{array} NH \cdot 6H_2O$$

Piperazine hexahydrate

Studies on the mode of action of piperazine indicate that it causes paralysis of susceptible worms by a selective effect on the myoneural junction. The curare-like action is very weak on mammalian muscles, but worms appear to be much more susceptible.

HEXYLRESORCINOL

Hexylresorcinol was perhaps the first anthelmintic developed by a systematic in vitro screening method.[8] It is still valuable in the treatment of *Trichuris* infections.

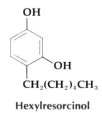

Hexylresorcinol

The drug exerts a paralyzing effect on the worms. It is only partially absorbed from the gastrointestinal tract. Since food interferes with the effectiveness of hexylresorcinol,

Text continued on p. 632.

Table 53-1. Summary of anthelmintic drugs*

Infecting organism	Drug of choice	Usual dosage	Route	Side effects and comments
Nematodes — intestinal				
Trichuris trichiura (whipworm infection)	Thiabendazole (Mintezol)	25 mg./kg. b.i.d. — 3 days	P.O.	Epigastric distress, diarrhea, nausea, vomiting, weakness, "light-headedness," disturbed sleep, "asparagus-like" odor to urine, rash (urticarial or maculopapular), ↑ SGOT; rare: tinnitus, shock
	or			
	Hexylresorcinol	Up to 500 ml. of 0.2% solution	Retention enema for 30 min.	
Enterobius vermicularis (pinworm)	Pyrvinium pamoate (Povan)	5 mg./kg. single dose (maximum 250 mg.); repeat after 2 wk.	P.O.	Red discoloration of stool, nausea, vomiting, occasional diarrhea; rare: photosensitivity
	or			
	Piperazine citrate (Antepar)	75 mg./kg. (maximum 2 Gm.) once daily for 7 days	P.O.	Nausea, vomiting, dizziness, urticaria; rare: reversible asymmetric paralysis, exacerbation of seizure disorder, visual disturbances *Alternative:* pyrantel pamoate, 10 mg./kg. single dose
Ascaris lumbricoides (ascariasis)	Piperazine citrate (Antepar)	75 mg./kg. (maximum 3.5 Gm.) daily for 2 days; may be repeated in 1 wk.	P.O.	See *Enterobius vermicularis*
Necator americanus (hookworm, American or New World)	Tetrachlorethylene	0.12 ml./kg. (maximum 5.0 ml. in single dose)	P.O.	Nausea, vomiting, headache, vertigo; occasional: hepatotoxicity, diarrhea; rare: loss of consciousness. Comment: Usually only available in soft gelatin capsules as a veterinary drug
	or			
	Bephenium hydroxy-naphthoate (Alcopar)	5.0 Cm. (2.5 Gm. of base) b.i.d. for 3 days	P.O.	Nausea, vomiting, diarrhea

*Courtesy Dr. Jay P. Sanford, Dallas.

Continued.

Table 53-1. Summary of anthelmintic drugs—cont'd

Infecting organism	Drug of choice	Usual dosage	Route	Side effects and comments
Nematodes—intestinal— cont'd				
Ancylostoma duodenale	Bephenium hydroxy-naphthoate (Alcopar)	5.0 Gm. (2.5 Gm. of base) b.i.d. for 3 days	P.O.	See *Necator americanus*
Trichostrongylus orientalis	Piperazine citrate or Thiabendazole or Bephenium hydroxy-naphthoate	See *Ascaris lumbricoides* See *Trichuris trichiura* See *Ancylostoma duode-nale*		
Strongyloides stercoralis (strongyloidiasis)	Thiabendazole	25 mg./kg. b.i.d.—2 days	P.O.	Side effects: see *Trichuris trichiura* Alternative: pyrvinium pamoate (see *Enterobius vermicularis* for dosage)
Nematodes—extraintestinal				
Wuchereria bancrofti or *Wuchereria (Brugia) malayi* (filariasis)	Diethylcarbamazine (Hetrazan, Notezine, Banocide)	2 mg./kg. t.i.d.—21 days	P.O. after meals	Fever, malaise, vertigo, urticaria, headache, nausea, vomiting, inflammatory reactions of lymph nodes
Onchocerca volvulus (Onchocerciasis)	Suramin (Naphuride, Bayer 205, Antrypol, Germanin) +	Initial dose of 0.2 Gm. to test for idiosyncrasy, then 1.0 Gm. at weekly intervals for 5 wk.	I.V.	See *Trypanosoma rhodesiense*: also fever, headache, muscle and joint pains; when possible all tumors should be excised
	Diethylcarbamazine (Hetrazan, Notezine, Banocide)	25 mg. daily for 3 days, then 50 mg. daily for 3 days, then 100 mg. daily for 3 days, then 150 mg. daily for 12 days	P.O.	See *Wuchereria*; severe allergic reactions often require antihistamines or corticosteroids
Loa loa (eyeworm disease)	Diethylcarbamazine	2 mg./kg. t.i.d.—21 days	P.O.	See *Wuchereria*: also calabar swellings may appear; pruritus, arthralgia; allergic reactions often require antihistamines or corticosteroids

Organism (Disease)	Drug	Dose	Route	Side effects
Acanthocheilonema perstans (Acanthocheilonemiasis, dipetalonemiasis)	Diethylcarbamazine	See Wuchereria		
Dracunculus medinensis (Dracunculiasis, guinea worm)	Niridazole (Ambilhar)	25 mg./kg. daily—7 days	P.O.	Vomiting, headache, dizziness and ECG changes; rare instances of loss of consciousness, convulsions, psychosis
Trichinella spiralis (Trichinosis)	Thiabendazole (Mintezol)	25 mg./kg. b.i.d.—5 to 7 days	P.O.	Side effects: see Trichuris trichiura; palliative measures include corticosteroids
Cutaneous Larva migrans (creeping eruption, Ancylostoma braziliense, dog and cat hookworm)	Thiabendazole (Mintezol)	25 mg./kg. b.i.d.—2 days, repeat in 3 to 7 days if active lesions persist	P.O.	Side effects: see Trichuris trichiura
Visceral Larva migrans (Toxocara canis, toxocariasis)	Thiabendazole (Mintezol)	25 mg./kg. b.i.d. until symptoms subside or toxicity precludes further treatment	P.O.	Side effects: see Trichuris trichiura
Trematodes Schistosoma haematobium (genitourinary bilharziasis)	Niridazole (Ambilhar)	25 mg./kg. daily—7 days	P.O.	Side effects: see Dracunculus. Alternative: Stibophen (Fuadin); in 50-75 kg. person—1.5 ml. I.M. 1st day; 3.5 ml. 2nd day; 5.0 ml. 3rd day; then 5.0 ml. on alternate days for 18 injections—total of 100 ml. Side effects include nausea, vomiting, arthralgia. Or alternative: Lucanthone hydrochloride (Miracil D, Nilodin), 10 to 20 mg./kg. for 8 to 20 days. Some use it only in children less than 16 years. Side effects: nausea, vomiting, yellow skin, vertigo, restlessness, headache, confusion, and tremor
Schistosoma mansoni (intestinal bilharziasis)	Niridazole (Ambilhar)	25 mg./kg.—7 days	P.O.	Side effects: see Dracunculus. Alternatives: see S. haematobium

Continued.

Table 53-1. Summary of anthelmintic drugs—cont'd

Infecting organism	Drug of choice	Usual dosage	Route	Side effects and comments
Trematodes—cont'd				
Schistosoma japonicum (Oriental schistosomiasis)	Antimony potassium tartrate—0.5% solution	Total dose 360 ml.; 8, 12, 16, 20, 24, 28 ml. on alternate days, then 28 ml. on alternate days to total dose	I.V.	Nausea, vomiting, epigastric distress, conjunctivitis, peripheral neuritis, dizziness, faintness, precordial distress, ST-T wave changes on ECG; arthralgia and myalgia; paroxysmal coughing with injection; vascular collapse and death
Clonorchis sinensis (liver fluke)	Chloroquine phosphate (Aralen, Resochin)	0.5 Gm. b.i.d.—3 days, then 0.5 Gm. daily for 30 days	P.O.	Side effects: see Malaria, *Plasmodium vivax*
Fasciola hepatica (sheep liver fluke disease)	Emetine hydrochloride	30 mg. daily—18 days	I.M.	Side effects: see *Entamoeba histolytica*, dysenteric, intestinal
Paragonimus westermani (lung fluke)	Bithional (Actamer, Bitin)	30 to 50 mg./kg. every other day for 10 to 15 doses	P.O.	Diarrhea, abdominal pain, nausea, vomiting, occasional urticaria
Cestodes				
Diphyllobothrium latum (fish tapeworm)	Niclosamide (Cestocide, Yomesan) or	1.0 Gm. then 1 hr. later 1.0 Gm.	P.O.—chewed	Nausea, abdominal pain, diarrhea, pruritus
	Quinacrine hydrochloride (Atabrine)	0.1 Gm. every 10 min. to total of 0.8 Gm.	P.O.	Comment: 2 hr. after last dose, administer saline purge. Side effects: nausea, vomiting, transient dizziness, yellowish discoloration of skin

Organism	Drug	Dosage	Route	Comments
Taenia saginata (beef tapeworm)	Same as *Diphyllobothrium latum*			*Alternative:* Oleoresin of aspidium, 4 to 8 Gm. plus 8 Gm. of acacia in water, one-half early in morning, the rest 1 hr. later. Side effects include headache, vertigo, gastroenteritis, abdominal pain, diarrhea, nausea, vomiting, visual disturbances
Taenia solium (pork tapeworm)	Quinacrine hydrochloride (Atabrine)	See *Diphyllobothrium latum*		*Alternative:* Oleoresin of aspidium—see *Taenia saginata*
Hymenolepis nana (dwarf tapeworm)	Quinacrine hydrochloride (Atabrine)	0.1 Gm every 10 min. to total of 0.5 Gm.	P.O.	See *Diphyllobothrium latum*
	or			
	Niclosamide	1.0 Gm. then 1 hr. later 1.0 Cm.	P.O.—chewed	See *Diphyllobothrium latum*
Echinococcus granulosus (echinococcosis)	None		—	Complete surgical excision of cyst

it should be administered on an empty stomach, and fatty meals should be avoided the night before.

CYANINE DYES—DITHIAZANINE AND PYRVINIUM PAMOATE

The discovery of the anthelmintic cyanine dyes is an important development in therapeutics because these compounds are effective in the treatment of a variety of worm infestations, some of which have had no satisfactory treatment in the past.

Dithiazanine (Delvex)[9] and pyrvinium pamoate (Povan)[1] are two of the cyanine dyes that have been shown to be effective in certain worm infestations. Their structural formulas are as follows:

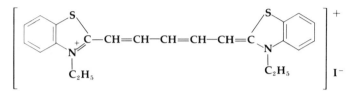

Dithiazanine iodide

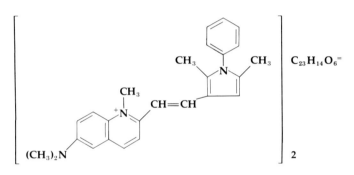

Pyrvinium pamoate

The cyanine dyes may exert an inhibitory effect on the oxidative metabolism of a number of helminths. Respiration and glycolysis of various worms are inhibited by these dyes.

Because of its toxicity, dithiazanine has been withdrawn from the market. Pyrvinium pamoate is administered in a single dose of 5 mg./kg. It is used in the treatment of *Enterobius* infection.

BEPHENIUM HYDROXYNAPHTHOATE

The anthelmintic bephenium hydroxynaphthoate (Alcopar), one of a group of quaternary ammonium compounds, shows considerable promise in the treatment of hookworm infections.[6] It is administered in rather large doses of 5 Gm./day. Very little of the drug is absorbed, and adverse effects so far appear to be limited to nausea and vomiting.

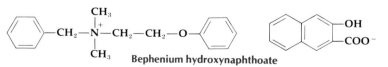

Bephenium hydroxynaphthoate

TETRACHLOROETHYLENE

The use of tetrachloroethylene in the treatment of hookworm infections is an outgrowth of the similar use of carbon tetrachloride. The latter is effective but is markedly toxic to the liver. When fats are avoided in the diet, tetrachloroethylene is absorbed to a much lesser extent from the gastrointestinal tract. It is much less toxic than carbon tetrachloride, probably because of lack of absorption.

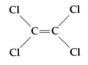

Tetrachloroethylene

QUINACRINE

The well-known antimalarial compound quinacrine (Atabrine) is currently the preferred drug in the treatment of cestodiasis or tapeworm infection.

The drug is sometimes administered by duodenal intubation, which assists in preventing side effects. Administration of sodium bicarbonate with divided doses of quinacrine is favored by some authorities in an effort to counteract the nausea and vomiting commonly associated with large doses.

OLEORESIN OF ASPIDIUM

Oleoresin of aspidium, an ancient medicine, is an extract of the male fern *Dryopteris filix-mas*. It is said to have been used by Galen in treating helminthiasis. Until the effectiveness of quinacrine was demonstrated, this crude preparation was the only effective medication in the treatment of tapeworm infections. It is not available in the United States at present.

The usual dose of the oleoresin for adults is 5 ml., often given in emulsions. The drug is distinctly more toxic than quinacrine, and in addition to abdominal disturbances, it can cause vertigo and impairment of vision, usually temporarily. It has no advantage over quinacrine.

THIABENDAZOLE

Thiabendazole (Mintezol), a benzimidiazole derivative, has the remarkable ability to kill *Trichinella* larvae in muscle. Favorable results have been reported with the drug in treatment of human trichinosis, but results are still not conclusively established[11]

The importance of thiabendazole as an anthelmintic is increasing. In doses of 20 to 25 mg./kg. twice a day for 1 or 2 days, it may be the drug of choice for *Strongyloides* infections. It is the first effective drug for cutaneous larva migrans and is as effective as piperazine in ascariasis. Thiabendazole is also useful in the treatment of hookworm and whipworm infections. Adverse side effects are nausea, vertigo, headache, and weakness in as many as one third of the patients.

DRUGS USED IN TREATMENT OF SCHISTOSOMIASIS
AND FILARIASIS
ANTIMONY COMPOUNDS

Various antimony compounds are effective in the treatment of schistosomiasis.[10] Antimony potassium tartrate (tartar emetic) is quite effective, but it is more toxic than stibophen (Fuadin), which is preferred by many. Stibophen is administered intramuscularly in 5 ml. doses of a 6.3% solution, starting with smaller doses of 1.5 to 3.5 ml. the first 2 days. A course of treatment consists of twenty injections on alternate days. Tartar emetic is still the drug of choice in *Schistosoma japonicum* infections, stibophen having little effect in this species.

The toxic effects of antimony compounds are abdominal disturbance, headache, fainting, skin rash, and electrocardiographic changes. Hepatitis and renal damage have also been observed.

LUCANTHONE

The orally effective drug lucanthone (Miracil D), a thiaxanthone, has the following structural formula:

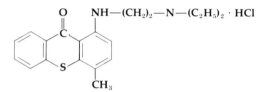

Lucanthone hydrochloride

Its administration in doses of 10 to 20 mg./kg. for 8 to 20 days was found to be effective in the treatment of infestations caused by *Schistosoma haematobium* but less so against *Schistosoma mansoni* or *Schistosoma japonicum*.

Hycanthone mesylate is closely related to lucanthone and is more effective and safe in the treatment of schistosomiasis. The drug is given by intramuscular injection in a dose of 3 to 5 mg./kg. in adults and older children.

DIETHYLCARBAMAZINE

Diethylcarbamazine citrate (Hetrazan), a piperazine derivative, is effective for the treatment of filarial infestations caused by *Wuchereria bancrofti, Onchocerca volvulus,* and *Loa loa.* The usual dose is 2 mg. of the citrate/kg. three times a day for 7 to 21 days. The structural formula of diethylcarbamazine is as follows:

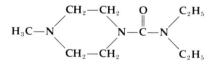

Diethylcarbamazine

The exact mode of action of this drug is not known. Although it contains piperazine, this compound by itself is ineffective in filariasis. The main effect in man consists of disappearance of the microfilariae of *Wuchereria bancrofti* from the circulation. It is believed that the adult worms are killed or sterilized by the drug. The destruction of the microfilariae of *Onchocerca volvulus* by diethylcarbamazine can produce severe allergic manifestations.

NIRIDAZOLE

Niridazole (Ambilhar) is an experimental drug that shows promise in the treatment of infections caused by *Schistosoma haematobium, Schistosoma mansoni,* and *Dracunculus medinensis* and also in amebiasis. Chemically, the drug is 1-(5-nitro-2-thiazolyl)-2-

imidazolidinone. It is effective by the oral route but may cause neurologic and psychiatric side effects rather frequently.

SURAMIN

Suramin (Bayer 205) is effective against the adult worm of onchocerciasis. The drug must be injected intravenously, the usual dose for adults being 20 mg./kg. once a week.

In addition to suramin and diethylcarbamazine, a number of antimonials and arsenicals are also used in treatment of filariasis, with some favorable results. Their unpleasant side effects and the necessity of many injections represent disadvantages in the general use of drugs containing antimony and arsenic.

OLDER AND OBSOLETE ANTHELMINTICS

Some remarkably toxic compounds were used at one time in the treatment of helminthiasis. They will be mentioned only to emphasize the fact that they are dangerous and obsolete. Some of these are carbon tetrachloride, oil of chenopodium, santonin, and pelletierine.

References

1 Beck, J. W., Saavedra, D., Antell, G., and Tejeiro, B.: Treatment of pinworm infections in humans (enterobiasis) with pyrvinium chloride and pyrvinium pamoate, Amer. J. Trop. Med., 8:349, 1959.

2 Brown, H. W.: The actions and uses of anthelmintics, Clin. Pharmacol. Ther. 1:87, 1960.

3 Bueding, E., and Swartzwelder, C.: Anthelmintics, Pharmacol. Rev. 9:329, 1953.

4 Carr, P., Pichardo Sarda, M. E., and Nunez, A.: Anthelmintic treatment of uncinariasis, Amer. J. Trop. Med. 3:495, 1954.

5 Dunn, T. L.: Effect of piperazine derivatives on certain intestinal helminths, Lancet 1:592, 1955.

6 Goodwin, L. G., Jayewardene, L. G., and Standen, O. D.: Clinical trials with bephenium hydroxynaphthoate (Alcopar) against hookworm in Ceylon, Brit. Med. J. 2:1572, 1958.

7 Katz, R., Ziegler, J., and Blank, H.: The natural course of creeping eruption and treatment with thiabendazole, Arch. Derm. 91:420, 1965.

8 Lamson, P. D., Caldwell, E. L., Brown, H. W., and Ward, C. B.: Hexylresorcinol in treatment of human ascariasis, Amer. J. Hyg. 13:568, 1931.

9 McCowen, M. C., Callender, M. E., and Brandt, M. C.: The anthelmintic effect of dithiazanine in experimental animals, Amer. J. Trop. Med. 6:894, 1957.

10 Most, H.: Treatment of schistosomiasis, Amer. J. Trop. Med. 4:455, 1955.

11 Stone, O. J., Stone, C. T., Jr., and Mullins, J. F.: Thiabendazole—probable cure for trichinosis, J.A.M.A. 187:536, 1964.

12 Swartzwelder, J. C.: Intestinal helminthiases and their treatment, J. Louisiana Med. Soc. 111:394, 1959.

13 Swartzwelder, J. C., et. al.: Dithiazanine, an effective broad-spectrum anthelmintic, J.A.M.A. 165:2063, 1957.

Recent reviews

14 Brown, H. W.: The treatment of four common parasitic infections, Pharmacol. Physicians 3(1): 1969.

15 Campbell, W. C., and Cuckler, A. C.: Thiabendazole in the treatment of and control of parasitic infections in man, Texas Rep. Biol. Med. 27 (supp. 2):665, 1969.

16 Desowitz, R. S.: Antiparasite chemotherapy, Ann. Rev. Pharmacol. 11:351, 1971.

17 Elslager, E. F., and Thompson, P. E.: Parasite chemotherapy, Ann. Rev. Pharmacol. 2:193, 1962.

18 Mansour, T. E.: The pharmacology and biochemistry of parasitic helminths, Advances Pharmacol. 3:129, 1964.

19 Most, H.: Treatment of the more common worm infections, J.A.M.A. 185:874, 1963.

20 Most, H.: Treatment of common parasitic infections of man encountered in the United States, New Eng. J. Med. 287:495, 1972.

21 Saz, H. J., and Bueding, E.: Relationships between anthelmintic effects and biochemical and physiological mechanisms, Pharmacol. Rev. 18:871, 1966.

22 Schnitzer, R. J., and Hawking, F., editors: Experimental chemotherapy, vol. 1, New York, 1963, Academic Press, Inc.

23 Thompson, P.: Parasite chemotherapy, Ann. Rev. Pharmacol. 7:77, 1967.

54 Antimalarial drugs

For centuries malaria was treated with cinchona bark, and until fairly recently the cinchona alkaloid, quinine, was the most generally employed antimalarial drug. Since World War II, very important developments have taken place in this field. Much more effective drugs have been developed, and new concepts concerning antimalarial therapy have evolved.

PRESENT CONCEPTS OF MALARIA

The malarial parasite is a protozoan organism of the genus *Plasmodium*. Of the four species of *Plasmodium* that infect man, three are important. These are *Plasmodium falciparum*, *Plasmodium vivax*, and *Plasmodium malariae*. The fourth, *Plasmodium ovale*, is numerically unimportant. Other plasmodia also occur in animals, and some of these have been important in antimalarial screening studies.

The insect vector is the female *Anopheles* mosquito. Public health measures directed at eradication of the mosquito are of great importance. It is unlikely, however, that such efforts will be completely successful. The other approach to the problem of malaria is chemotherapy.

The life cycle of the malarial parasite has been divided into several phases: (1) sporozoite phase, (2) primary tissue phase, (3) asexual blood phase, (4) sexual phase, and (5) secondary tissue phase, which, however, does not occur in *Plasmodium falciparum* infections.

The major new concept of great importance in therapy is recognition of the importance of the primary and secondary tissue phases, which are commonly referred to as the exoerythrocytic cycle of the malarial parasite. The liver is the only organ in which exoerythrocytic stages have been demonstrated.

The *Anopheles* mosquito inoculates *sporozoites* into the bitten person. The various antimalarial agents have no effect on sporozoites, which remain in the bloodstream for a very short time and are localized in various tissues such as the liver.

From this primary tissue localization the parasite penetrates into red cells, where it is first seen as a *trophozoite*, which develops into the mature *schizont*. When the parasitized red cell bursts, it releases *merozoites*, and a malarial chill occurs. Certain modified trophozoites develop into *gametocytes*. These sexual forms represent the link between man and mosquito and are important in the perpetuation of the disease in an area. Fertilization takes place in the mosquito, and sporozoites eventually appear in its salivary glands, ready for the next person who may be bitten.

TREATMENT OF MALARIA

The modern classification of antimalarial drugs is based on the stage of the *Plasmodium* life cycle acted upon. *Primary tissue schizonticides* are primaquine, chlorguanide

636

Table 54-1. Summary of drugs used in the treatment of malaria*

Infecting organism	Drug of choice	Usual dosage	Route	Side effects and comments
Malaria Acute attack due to *Plasmodium vivax, P. malariae, P. ovale,* "chloroquine-sensitive" *P. falciparum*	Chloroquine phosphate (Aralen, Resochin) +	1 Gm. (600 mg. base), then 0.5 Gm. in 6 hr., then 0.5 Gm. daily for 2 days [Total dose 2.5 Gm.]	P.O.	Pruritus, vomiting, headache, skin eruption, depigmentation of hair, partial alopecia, hemolytic anemia, leukopenia, thrombocytopenia, rare deafness, retinal damage
	Primaquine phosphate	26.3 mg. (15 mg. base) daily for 14 days	P.O.	Hemolytic anemia in G6PD defect, neutropenia, G.I., rare CNS symptoms, hypertension, arrhythmias
Acute attack due to *P. falciparum* (chloroquine-resistant strains — S. E. Asia, S. America)	Quinine sulfate +	650 mg. t.i.d. — 10 days	P.O.	Arrhythmias, tinnitus, hypotension, headache, nausea, abdominal pain, visual disturbance, blood dyscrasia
	Pyrimethamine (Daraprim) +	25 mg. every 12 hr. for 3 days	P.O.	Megaloblastic anemia, blood dyscrasia, rare rash, convulsions, shock
	Sulfadiazine	500 mg. q.i.d. — 5 days	P.O.	See Table 47-2 for side effects. *Alternative:* Dapsone (Avlosulfon), 25 mg. daily for 28 days or sulphormethoxine (Fanasil)
Prophylaxis and suppression	Chloroquine phosphate +	500 mg. (300 mg. base) once weekly, continued for 6 wk. after last exposure	P.O.	As above
	Primaquine phosphate	26.3 mg. (15 mg. base) daily for 14 days after last exposure in endemic area	P.O.	As above

*Courtesy Dr. Jay P. Sanford, Dallas.

(Paludrine), and pyrimethamine (Daraprim). *Blood schizonticides* include quinine, quinacrine (Atabrine), chloroquine (Aralen), amodiaquin (Camoquin), chlorguanide (Paludrine), and pyrimethamine (Daraprim).

The primary tissue schizonticides are *causal prophylactic agents,* whereas the blood schizonticides may be termed *suppressive drugs* or *clinical prophylactic agents. Radical cure* means a complete elimination of the plasmodia from the body. This can be achieved by primaquine, a tissue schizonticide against *Plasmodium vivax. Clinical control* may be achieved by the supressive drugs, although they may not eliminate the parasites completely from the body.

Clinical prophylaxis of malaria may be achieved by the administration of 300 mg. of chloroquine once a week in adults.

In addition to the classic antimalarial drugs, the sulfones and sulfonamides have become important adjuncts in the treatment of falciparum malaria caused by strains that have become resistant to other medications (Table 54-1).

CHLOROQUINE

Chloroquine (Aralen), a 4-aminoquinoline derivative, was first synthesized in Germany in 1934. It was considered too toxic on the basis of a few tests in human beings and was discarded. A closely related compound was used by the French in North Africa in World War II and appeared quite effective and well tolerated. Subsequently a large series of related compounds were synthesized in the United States, and extensive studies soon showed that chloroquine was the most satisfactory in the group.

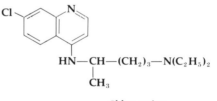

Chloroquine

Antimalarial activity

Chloroquine is highly effective against erythrocytic parasites. It is a suppressive drug that can produce radical cure in susceptible falciparum malaria but will not eliminate the exoerythrocytic forms of *Plasmodium vivax.* Consequently, relapses occur in vivax malaria treated with chloroquine, although the drug can terminate the clinical attacks very efficiently.

Metabolism

Chloroquine is rapidly and almost completely absorbed from the gastrointestinal tract. Its distribution is such that some tissues such as liver may contain more than 500 times as much of the drug as does plasma. This affinity for the liver suggested its use in hepatic amebiasis.

Chloroquine may occasionally be injected by the intramuscular route. However, this is seldom necessary. For intramuscular injection, chloroquine hydrochloride is given in a dose of 250 mg. For other uses see p. 624.

Toxicity

Studies in human volunteers have shown that the toxicity of chloroquine is quite low when suppressive doses are employed.[9] In larger doses dizziness, blurring of vision, headache, diarrhea, and epigastric distress have been reported. These symptoms disappear when the dosage is decreased.[1] Retinopathy and corneal deposits may also occur[11] and may result in blindness.

Resistance to chloroquine

Chloroquine-resistant *Plasmodium falciparum* has been encountered with increasing frequency in South America, Southeast Asia, and Africa.[4,20] Such strains have created a serious problem in South Vietnam since 1965. While combined chloroquine-quinine therapy was usually effective, a very high percentage of patients, more than 40%, had relapses within 2 weeks. Several new drug combinations have been introduced to meet this problem. A long-acting sulfonamide, sulphormethoxine, with pyrimethamine and quinine was successful in reducing the relapse rate. In other treatment schedules the sulfone 4,4'-diaminodiphenylsulfone (dapsone; Avlosulfon), used as a supplement to chloroquine and quinine, reduced the relapse rate to a very low figure.

AMODIAQUIN

Amodiaquin (Camoquin) is similar to chloroquine as an antimalarial. It is given by mouth in doses of 0.6 Gm. daily as a suppressive antimalarial or 1.8 Gm. in divided doses the first day, followed by 0.6 Gm./day for 2 or 3 days for clinical control.

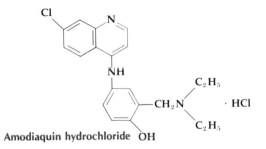

Amodiaquin hydrochloride

PRIMAQUINE

Certain 8-aminoquinolines have the ability to destroy exoerythrocytic malarial parasites. Primaquine is at present considered to be the most effective representative of this group of antimalarial drugs.

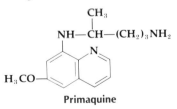

Primaquine

The development of primaquine is a late consequence of studies on the synthetic antimalarial drug pamaquine (Plasmochin). It was shown as early as 1925 that this drug was lethal to gametocytes, although it was not safe enough for complete elimination of the asexual forms from the blood. The drug was tried in some areas in combination with quinine for the purpose of controlling malaria by eliminating the gametocytes. There was an indication during these trials that the relapse rate in vivax malaria was reduced. This finding suggested an important property of the 8-aminoquinolines. Pamaquine was fairly toxic and did not appear promising. On the other hand, when related 8-aminoquinolines were synthesized during World War II, several were found to be safer than pamaquine. Pentaquine was first used as a curative antimalarial drug but was superseded by primaquine because the latter was found to be less toxic.

Antimalarial activity

Primaquine is useful in producing radical cure in *Plasmodium vivax* infections because of its effect on the exoerythrocytic stages. It is also effective against the exoerythrocytic forms of *Plasmodium falciparum*. It has some activity against the asexual forms of these parasites, but this activity is not high enough to make it an efficient suppressive as well as curative drug. For this reason primaquine is usually given in combination with a suppressive antimalarial drug.

Clinical trials in vivax malaria have shown that concomitant administration of chloroquine as a suppressive, coupled with 15 mg. primaquine/day for 14 days, will often achieve a radical cure. In a comparable group receiving chloroquine alone, the relapse rate was 39%.[2]

Metabolism

Primaquine is rapidly absorbed from the gastrointestinal tract. In contrast with chloroquine, however, it is also rapidly metabolized and excreted. Its tissue fixation is very slight, and the drug is altered and excreted in less than 24 hours.

Toxicity

Although primaquine is generally well tolerated at the recommended therapeutic dosages, some patients may complain of anorexia, nausea, abdominal cramps, and other vague symptoms. There may be depression of the activity of the bone marrow, with leukopenia and anemia. The effects on the blood, including some methemoglobinemia, are aggravated by concomitant use of quinacrine.

Hemolytic anemia that follows primaquine therapy is related to an interesting genetic abnormality. It is more likely to occur in dark-skinned races.[12] The red cells of susceptible persons show a defect in the mechanisms that protect hemoglobin against denaturation. The reduced glutathione (GSH) content of such cells was as low as 50 mg./ 100 ml. as compared with 75 mg./100 ml. in normal cells. The metabolic error in primaquine-sensitive red cells appears to be a deficiency of glucose-6-phosphate dehydrogenase.[6] These GSH-deficient red cells are also sensitive to acetanilid, sulfanilamide, phenylhydrazine, sulfoxone, and acetophenetidin[10] (p. 37).

PYRIMETHAMINE

The discovery of the potent antimalarial drug pyrimethamine (Daraprim) was the result of observations on the similarities between the antimalarial drug chlorguanide and certain folic acid antagonists such as the 2,4-diamino-5-substituted pyrimidines. One of these antimetabolites was found to have antimalarial activity in animals, and soon many others were tested. Pyrimethamine is a member of this series.

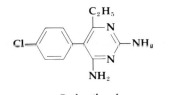

Pyrimethamine

Toxicity

Pyrimethamine appears to be quite safe when administered in doses of 25 to 50 mg. once or twice a week.[8] Megaloblastic anemia of a transient nature has occurred in some persons following the use of pyrimethamine.[13] This action may be related to metabolic antagonism to folic acid or folinic acid. Pyrimethamine blocks the enzyme dihydrofolic acid reductase.

The drug is not recommended for treatment of the acute attack because it is slow-acting. Although it has remarkable gametocidal activity against some strains of *Plasmodium falciparum*, it is ineffective against others. Resistant strains have become common.

TRIMETHOPRIM

Trimethoprim is a synthetic diaminopyrimidine compound related to pyrimethamine. Both inhibit dihydrofolate reductase. Trimethoprim is synergistic with sulfonamides, which is to be expected since it acts sequentially with the latter in blocking the synthesis of folic acid in bacteria. For the same reason pyrimethamine and sulfonamides may be synergistic in the treatment of malaria.[22] Trimethoprim in combination with sulfamethoxazole is being used in the treatment of some bacterial infections (p. 569).

OTHER ANTIMALARIAL DRUGS

Quinine has been the traditional antimalarial remedy that has been gradually replaced by newer drugs. It is a suppressive drug and will not cure vivax malaria. Even as a suppressive, it is not nearly as efficient as chloroquine or other newer antimalarial drugs. The drug has become very important again in the treatment of chloroquine-resistant falciparum malaria.

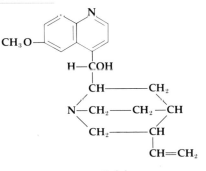

Quinine

The adult dose of quinine sulfate is 1 Gm. three times daily. The drug is rapidly absorbed, and most of it is metabolized, about 10% being excreted unchanged in the urine and the remainder in the form of metabolic products. Metabolism and excretion are both rapid, and no cumulation occurs when quinine sulfate is given daily for long periods of time. In a patient who cannot take or tolerate oral quinine, the drug may be injected as the dihydrochloride by slow intravenous drip. For this purpose 650 mg. of quinine is dissolved in 300 ml. of saline solution.

Quinine can produce a variety of toxic effects, some of which are known by the collective name *cinchonism*. Headache, nausea, tinnitus, and visual disturbances can occur. Allergic skin rashes and asthmatic attacks have also been reported.

Occasionally quinine is used for purposes other than treatment of malaria. The drug can aggravate myasthenia gravis and has been used on occasion as a diagnostic test in this disease. The drug has also been used as a weak antipyretic and analgesic, but it is considered obsolete for these purposes. Quinine salts are also used as sclerosing agents.

Quinacrine (Atabrine) is a yellow acridine derivative. It was at one time an important antimalarial, but chloroquine has so many advantages over quinacrine that the latter is gradually being abandoned in treatment of malaria.

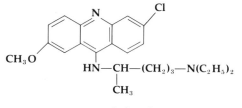

Quinacrine

Quinacrine is probably more valuable at present for purposes other than antimalarial therapy. It is important in the treatment of certain tapeworm infestations.

Chlorguanide (Paludrine) was synthesized in England during World War II. It is a suppressive antimalarial drug. Its action may be related to metabolic antagonism to folic acid, perhaps due to a metabolic product of this compound. The suppressive effect of chlorguanide is somewhat slow in onset.

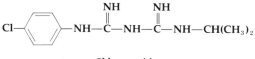

Chlorguanide

Perhaps the greatest disadvantage of this drug has to do with development of resistance by plasmodia. Studies on the chemical relationship between chlorguanide and folic acid antagonists were directly responsible for the development of pyrimethamine. A chlorguanide derivative appears promising as a long-term suppressant when injected as pamoate salt.

Cycloguanide pamoate (Camolar), an insoluble salt of a chlorguanide derivative, is remarkable in that a single intramuscular injection exerts a protective effect for several months.[7] This prolonged effect is a consequence of its extremely slow absorption from muscle. Cycloguanide pamoate may play an important role in eradication of malaria in some parts of the world, provided that its continued use does not reveal serious adverse effects. The drug is not yet generally available.

DRUGS OF CHOICE IN THE TREATMENT OF MALARIA

The selection of the drug of choice in the treatment of malaria depends on the therapeutic objective. For the treatment of uncomplicated attacks caused by any of the plasmodia except resistant strains of *Plasmodium falciparum*, chloroquine is the best drug; an alternative drug is amodiaquin hydrochloride. If the infection is severe, the drug of choice may have to be injected. Chloroquine hydrochloride is available for this purpose.

Malaria caused by resistant strains of *Plasmodium falciparum* is best treated with quinine sulfate plus pyrimethamine and sulfadiazine or dapsone. If oral therapy is not possible, quinine dihydrochloride is available for slow intravenous injection.

Prevention of the disease in an endemic area can be achieved with chloroquine, 500 mg. once a week, but the individual may develop the disease after leaving the area unless he receives primaquine for 14 days thereafter. This is especially necessary for malaria caused by *Plasmodium vivax*, *Plasmodium ovale*, or *Plasmodium malariae*.

References

1 Alving, A. S., et al.: Studies on the chronic toxicity of chloroquine (SN 7618), J. Clin. Invest. 27:60, 1948.

2 Alving, A. S., et al.: Korean vivax malaria: curative treatment with pamaquine and primaquine, Amer. J. Trop. Med. 2:970, 1953.

3 Archibald, H. M.: Preliminary field trials on a new schizonticide, Brit. Med. J. 2:821, 1951.

4 Bartelloni, P. J., Sheehy, T. W., and Tigertt, W. D.: Combined therapy for chloroquine-resistant Plasmodium falciparum infection, J.A.M.A. 109:173, 1967.

5 Beutler, E.: The hemolytic effect of primaquine and related compounds: a review, Blood 14:103, 1959.

6 Carlson, P. E., Flanagan, C. L., Ickes, C. E., and Alving, A. S.: Enzymatic deficiency in primaquine-sensitive erythrocytes, Science 124:484, 1956.

7 Coatney, G. R., Contacos, P. G., and Lunn, J. S.: Further observations on the antimalarial activity of CI-501 (Camolar) against the Chesson strain of vivax malaria, Amer. J. Trop. Med. 13:383, 1964.

8 Coatney, G. R., Myatt, A. V., Hernandez, T., Jeffery, G. M., and Cooper, W. C.: The protective and therapeutic effects of pyrimethamine (Daraprim) against Chesson strain vivax malaria, Amer. J. Trop. Med. 2:777, 1953.

9 Coatney, G. R., Ruhe, D. S., Cooper, W. C., Josephson, E. S., and Young, M. D.: Studies in human malaria: the protective and therapeutic action of chloroquine (SN 7618) against St. Elizabeth strain vivax malaria, Amer. J. Hyg. 49:49, 1949.

10 Dern, R. J., Beutler, E., and Alving, A. S.: The hemolytic effect of primaquine: primaquine sensitivity as a manifestation of a multiple drug sensitivity, J. Lab. Clin. Med. 45:30, 1955.

11 Henkind, P., and Rothfield, N. F.: Ocular abnormalities in patients treated with synthetic antimalarial drugs, New Eng. J. Med. 269:433, 1963.

12 Hockwald, R. S., Arnold, J., Clayman, C. B., and Alving, A. S.: Status of primaquine: toxicity of primaquine in Negroes, J.A.M.A. 149:1568, 1952.

13 Myatt, A. V., Hernandez, T., and Coatney, G. R.: Studies in human malaria: the toxicity of pyrimethamine (Daraprim) in man, Amer. J. Trop. Med. 2:788, 1953.

14 Rieckmann, K. H.: Determination of the drug sensitivity of Plasmodium falciparum, J.A.M.A. 217:573, 1971.

15 Schellenberg, K. A., and Coatney, G. R.: The influence of antimalaria drugs on nucleic acid synthesis in Plasmodium gallinaceum and Plasmodium berghei, Biochem. Pharmacol. 6:143, 1961.

16 Sheehy, T. W., and Dempsey, H.: Methotrexate therapy for Plasmodium vivax malaria, J.A.M.A. 214:109, 1970.

17 Sheehy, T. W., Reba, R. C., Neff, T. A., Gaintner, J. R., and Tigertt, W. D.: Supplemental sulfone (dapsone) therapy: use in treatment of chloroquine-resistant falciparum malaria, Arch. Intern. Med. 119:561, 1967.

18 Van Dyke, K., Lantz, C., and Szustkiewicz, C.: Quinacrine: mechanisms of antimalarial action, Science 169:492, 1970.

Recent reviews

19 Beutler, E.: Drug-induced blood dyscrasias, J.A.M.A. 189:143, 1964.

20 Blount, R. E.: Management of chloroquine-resistant falciparum malaria, Arch. Intern. Med. **119**:557, 1967.

21 Elslager, E. F., and Thompson, P. E.: Parasite chemotherapy, Ann. Rev. Pharmacol. **2**:193, 1962.

22 Hunsicker, L. G.: The pharmacology of anti-malarials, Arch. Intern. Med. **123**:645, 1969.

23 Most, H.: Treatment of common parasitic infections of man encountered in the United States (second of two parts), New Eng. J. Med. **287**:698, 1972.

24 Schnitzer, R. J., and Hawking, F., editors: Experimental chemotherapy, vol. 1, New York, 1963, Academic Press, Inc.

25 Thompson, P. E.: Parasite chemotherapy, Ann. Rev. Pharmacol. **7**:77, 1967.

55 Drugs used in chemotherapy of neoplastic disease

GENERAL CONCEPT

The antineoplastic agents, although not as dramatically successful as the antibacterial drugs, increase the survival of patients with acute leukemia, malignant lymphoma, multiple myeloma, and carcinoma of the colon and breast. They may even produce *cures* in patients with choriocarcinoma and Wilms' tumor.

The majority of drugs used in chemotherapy of neoplastic diseases are highly toxic and also affect rapidly growing cells other than those of the neoplastic process. As a consequence, their therapeutic index is rather low.

Although the results of cancer chemotherapy are not nearly as brilliant as those of antimicrobial therapy, the field can claim some positive achievements. (1) The life expectancy of children with acute leukemia has increased greatly, and some may have been cured. (2) Disseminated choriocarcinoma in young women can be cured with combination chemotherapy. (3) The alkylating agents are as helpful as x-ray therapy in a variety of cases. (4) Hodgkin's disease is being treated effectively with drugs and radiation. (5) Adenocarcinoma of the uterus has responded well to progestational hormones. (6) The discovery of antimetabolites such as 5-fluorouracil has extended the lives of many patients with solid tumors. (7) The discovery of imidazole carboxamide provides a ray of hope in the treatment of malignant melanoma. Other achievements have been made in the treatment of Wilms' tumor, Burkitt's lymphoma, and other tumors.

The current emphasis in cancer chemotherapy centers on the use of synergistic combinations of chemotherapeutic agents linked to an understanding of the portion of the cell cycle on which they act. The cell cycle is divided into several portions. Phase G_1 (18 hours) occurs prior to DNA synthesis. Phase S (20 hours) includes all the processes necessary for DNA synthesis. Phase G_2 (3 hours) consists of protein and RNA synthesis, and the short Phase M represents the process of mitosis. The *alkylating agents* are cell cycle–nonspecific, meaning that they act at any phase of the cycle. On the other hand, the antimetabolites act on Phase S, whereas a few other agents such as the *Vinca alkaloids* have Phases G_2 and M as their points of attack. Based on these concepts, some improvements have occurred in the survival of cancer patients by using synergistic combinations of drugs.

DEVELOPMENT OF ANTINEOPLASTIC CHEMOTHERAPY

The systematic study of agents that are potentially useful for treatment of neoplastic diseases is a fairly recent development.

The antileukemic activity of the nitrogen mustards was discovered during World

645

War II. The discovery was an outgrowth of earlier observations on the leukopenic effect of mustard gas (bis[2-chloroethyl]sulfide). As a result of this discovery, the less toxic nitrogen mustards (bis[chloroethyl]amines) and eventually many other alkylating agents were introduced into chemotherapy of neoplastic diseases.[5]

The development of folic acid antagonists and other antimetabolites as potential antitumor agents originated from observations on the role of folic acid in white cell production. It seemed reasonable that compounds structurally related to folic acid could inhibit white cell production, and this was indeed demonstrated.[4]

These observations stimulated interest in other metabolic antagonists as possible chemotherapeutic agents, and eventually several purine, pyrimidine, and amino acid antagonists were discovered. Nucleic acid biosynthesis has been the chief target of the chemotherapeutic approach.[20]

CLASSIFICATION

The drugs currently employed in the management of malignant diseases fall into the following categories:

Alkylating agents
  Mechlorethamine hydrochloride (nitrogen
    mustard; Mustargen)
  Chlorambucil (Leukeran)
  Cyclophosphamide (Cytoxan)
  TEM (triethylenemelamine)
  Thio-TEPA (triethylenethiophosphoramide)
  Busulfan (Myleran)
  Melphalan (phenylalanine mustard; Alkeran; Sarcolysin)
Antimetabolites
  Methotrexate (amethopterin)
  Mercaptopurine (Purinethol)
  Fluorouracil
  Azaserine
  Azothioprine
  Cytarabine

Hormonal agents
  Adrenal steroids
  Sex hormones
Radioactive isotopes
  Phosphorus (^{32}P)
  Iodine (^{131}I)
  Gold (^{198}Au)
Antibiotics and miscellaneous
  Actinomycin D
  Puromycin
  Daunorubicin and adriamycin
  Bleomycin
  Demecolcin
  Vinblastine (Velban)
  Vincristine (Oncovin)
  Hydroxyurea
  L-Asparaginase
  Procarbazine
  Imidazole carboxamide

ALKYLATING AGENTS

The alkylating agents are highly reactive agents that transfer alkyl groups to important cell constituents by combining with amino, sulfhydryl, carboxyl, and phosphate groups. They are cell cycle–nonspecific, being capable of combining with cells at any phase of their cycle. It is believed that they alkylate DNA and, more specifically, guanine. This basic action may explain the preferential toxicity of these compounds for rapidly mutliplying cells (Table 55-1).

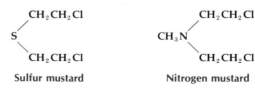

Sulfur mustard   Nitrogen mustard

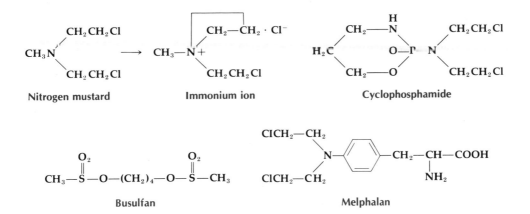

Nitrogen mustard — Immonium ion — Cyclophosphamide — Busulfan — Melphalan

Mechlorethamine hydrochloride (nitrogen mustard; Mustargen) must be injected intravenously because the compound is highly reactive. More recently, attempts have been made to inject the drug intra-arterially in close proximity to the tumor. It is believed that the action of mechlorethamine hydrochloride lasts only a few minutes and that it disappears from the blood very rapidly.

The dose of mechlorethamine hydrochloride is 0.1 to 0.2 mg./kg./day for 4 days, injected intravenously. The drug can cause venous thrombosis, severe vomiting, and delayed depression of the bone marrow. In toxic doses mechlorethamine hydrochloride can cause involution of lymphatic tissues and the thymus, ulcerations of gastrointestinal mucosa, convulsions, and death.

Table 55-1. Dosage and toxicity of alkylating agents

Drug	Route of administration	Usual dose	Toxic effects
Mechlorethamine hydrochloride	Intravenous	0.1 mg./kg./day	Nausea and vomiting; bone marrow depression and bleeding; venous thrombosis
Chlorambucil	Oral	0.1-0.2 mg./kg./day	Bone marrow depression and bleeding
Cyclophosphamide	Intravenous Oral (maintenance)	4 mg./kg./day 1-3 mg./kg./day	Nausea and vomiting; bone marrow depression and bleeding; alopecia may occur
Thio-TEPA	Oral	5-10 mg./day	Bone marrow depression and bleeding
	Intravenous	0.2 mg./kg.	Nausea and vomiting; bone marrow depression and bleeding
Busulfan	Oral	2-8 mg./day	Bone marrow depression and bleeding

The main advantage of the newer alkylating agents is that they are well absorbed when administered orally.

The phenylalanine mustard **melphalan** (Alkeran; Sarcolysin) is particularly effective against multiple myeloma. It is given by mouth, 6 mg. daily.

ANTIMETABOLITES
FOLIC ACID ANTAGONISTS

The folic acid antagonists inhibit nucleic acid synthesis by blocking the enzyme dihydrofolate reductase. **Methotrexate,** formerly known as amethopterin, is effective in the treatment of acute leukemias of children and lymphomas and may be curative in women with choriocarcinoma. In combination with other agents, methotrexate may be useful in the treatment of some solid tumors such as carcinoma of the breast, ovary, and colon. Methotrexate produces many toxic effects such as nausea, vomiting, diarrhea, alopecia, aphthous stomatitis, skin rash, and bone marrow depression. Leucovorin calcium, within a few hours after overdosage, may serve as an antidote. Methotrexate is available in tablets containing 2.5 mg., and methotrexate sodium in a powder for injection, 5 and 50 mg.

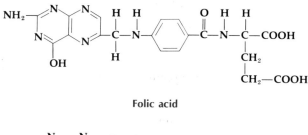

Folic acid

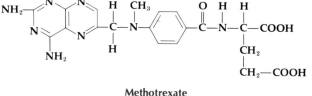

Methotrexate

PURINE ANTAGONISTS

The most important purine antagonist, mercaptopurine, acts by several mechanisms. First, it is converted to the ribonucleotide. As such it competes with enzymes that convert hypoxanthine ribonucleotide (inosinic acid) to adenine and xanthine ribonucleotides. In addition, mercaptopurine is converted into 6-methyl mercaptopurine and its ribonucleotide. This metabolite ties up the enzyme that synthesizes phosphoribosylamine, which is required for RNA and DNA synthesis.

Thioguanine is also metabolized to the ribonucleotide, which enters the pathway of nucleic acid synthesis substituting for guanine. Thus "fraudulent" polynucleotides that block nucleic acid synthesis are produced.

Mercaptopurine is effective in the treatment of acute lymphocytic and chronic myelocytic leukemias. Its toxic manifestations include bone marrow depression, gastrointestinal disturbances, and jaundice. Allopurinol (p. 528) was originally developed for the purpose of blocking the metabolism of mercaptopurine by xanthine oxidase. Mercaptopurine (Purinethol) is obtainable in tablets containing 50 mg.

Thioguanine is an antimetabolite similar to mercaptopurine with essentially the same indications and adverse effects.

Azathioprine, a derivative of mercaptopurine, has become widely used as an immunosuppressive drug in organ transplantation. Bone marrow depression, oral lesions, gastrointestinal disturbances, alopecia, and intercurrent infections are some of the toxic effects of azathioprine. Azathioprine (Imuran) is available in tablets containing 50 mg. Azathioprine is much more useful as an immunosuppressant than in cancer chemotherapy. It splits in the body to 6-mercaptopurine.

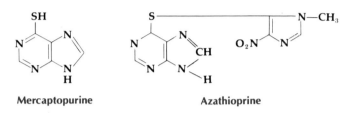

| Mercaptopurine | Azathioprine |

PYRIMIDINE ANTAGONISTS

Fluorouracil is a pyrimidine antimetabolite of some usefulness in the treatment of carcinoma of the colon, breast, ovary, pancreas, and liver. It is a highly toxic drug, producing the same sort of disturbances as mercaptopurine and also hyperpigmentation and photosensitization. The drug is available as a solution, 50 mg./ml., for intravenous injection. Fluorouracil is also available for topical application as Efudex solution or cream. The solution contains 2 or 5% fluorouracil, the cream 5%.

Fluorouracil is converted to the ribonucleotide, which may be reduced to 5-fluoro-2'-deoxyuridine-5'-phosphate (F-dUMP). This enzymatic product inhibits thymidylate synthetase, which is involved in the production of deoxyuridylic acid (dUMP).

Cytarabine (cytosine arabinoside; Cytosar) is a pyrimidine antagonist that differs from deoxycytidine (cytosine deoxyriboside) in containing arabinose rather than deoxyribose. It is converted to the nucleotide, which then blocks the conversion of cytidine nucleotide to deoxycytidine nucleotide. It also prevents the formation of DNA by blocking the incorporation of deoxycytidine triphosphate.

Cytarabine must be injected intravenously, since it is not effective after oral administration. It finds some usefulness in the treatment of acute lymphocytic and acute myelocytic leukemias. It is also of interest as a possible antiviral agent (p. 603).

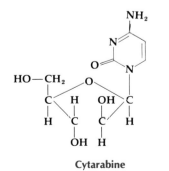

Cytarabine

HORMONAL AGENTS

Steroid hormones such as estrogens, androgens, and corticosteroids are useful in some neoplastic diseases. The estrogens include diethylstilbestrol and ethinyl estradiol. Androgens that are widely used, particularly in the treatment of carcinoma of the breast, include testosterone propionate, fluoxymesterone, and the recently introduced calusterone (Methosarb). The most widely used corticosteroid is prednisone, which is effective in various lymphomas and some other malignancies.

Estrogens, along with castration and other measures, are used in treatment of prostatic carcinoma. Both androgens and estrogens have been employed in management of advanced mammary carcinoma. The choice depends on the age of the patient. Estrogens are used in women well pas' the menopause, whereas androgens may be helpful in patients who are still menstruating. The main benefit obtained from this type of treatment is reduction of pain related to metastatic lesions in the bones.

The *rationale* for the use of the estrogens and androgens is the belief that prostatic and mammary carcinoma are to some extent "hormone dependent."

The adverse effects of the estrogens (diethylstilbestrol) are gastrointestinal symptoms, hypercalcemia, edema, uterine bleeding, and feminization in males. The adverse effects expected from large doses of androgens (testosterone propionate) in the treatment of advanced mammary carcinoma are virilization, edema, and hypercalcemia.

RADIOACTIVE ISOTOPES

Radioactive phosphorus (^{32}P) is used in the treatment of polycythemia vera and also in chronic leukemias. It has a biologic half-life of about 8 days in man. It is handled just like normal phosphorus, being incorporated into nucleic acids and deposited in bone. It emits beta rays that exert a destructive effect on the rapidly multiplying cells in which it is concentrated. ^{32}P is administered in doses of about 1 mc daily for 5 days. Either the oral or intravenous route may be used, and the doses are not greatly different.

Radioactive iodine (^{131}I), radioactive gold (^{198}Au), and other isotopes are not as useful as ^{32}P. Nevertheless, ^{131}I has some limited application in metastatic thyroid carcinoma. Colloidal ^{198}Au has been tried in the treatment of lymphomas and in neoplastic diseases involving serous cavities. Its uses are largely experimental.

ANTIBIOTICS AND MISCELLANEOUS AGENTS

Actinomycin D is a highly toxic antibiotic that combines with DNA and blocks RNA production. It is administered intravenously in doses of 15 to 50 μg/kg. of body weight daily. It can cause nausea, vomiting, bone marrow depression, stomatitis, diarrhea, skin lesions, and alopecia. Its possible usefulness is limited to cases of Wilms' tumor, carcinoma of the testis, and choriocarcinoma.

Mithramycin is a toxic antibiotic that acts in a manner similar to that of actinomycin D. It has an interesting application in treating hypercalcemia that may result from bone metastasis.

Daunorubicin and adriamycin are closely related antibiotics that bind to DNA. Although these drugs may become useful in the treatment of acute leukemias and some carcinomas, they are strictly investigational at present.

Bleomycin, a product of a *Streptomyces,* blocks DNA synthesis and cell division.

Although it is toxic, good results have been claimed for it in the treatment of squamous cell skin carcinomas.

Vinblastine (Velban) is an alkaloid obtained from the periwinkle plant (*Vinca*). It has antineoplastic activity, presumably as a consequence of mitotic arrest. Its toxic effects, commonly seen also with other antimetabolites, include nausea and vomiting, leukopenia, and alopecia. It is administered intravenously in doses of 0.1 to 0.15 mg./kg. daily. Other alkaloids related to vinblastine are also being investigated. It is quite effective in the treatment of Hodgkin's disease and choriocarcinoma.

Vincristine (Oncovin) is a *Vinca* alkaloid that is particularly effective in the treatment of acute leukemia in children and Wilms' tumor. Nausea, vomiting, leukopenia, neurotoxic effects, and alopecia are toxic effects of the *Vinca* alkaloids. Vincristine is a spindle toxin.

Urethan, or ethyl carbamate, is a weak hypnotic that causes leucopenia in man. It has been used in the treatment of leukemias and in multiple myeloma but is now considered obsolete.

L-Asparaginase is an enzyme that is effective in the treatment of human leukemia. Apparently some malignant cells require exogenous asparagine, but normal cells synthesize their own. The discovery of L-asparaginase as an antineoplastic agent resulted from observations[8] on the suppressive effect of guinea pig serum, now known to contain L-asparaginase, on experimental leukemias. The drug is still experimental but is of great interest because it exploits a basic metabolic difference between normal and malignant cells.

Podophyllin, a resin obtained from mandrake or May apple, produces rapid involution of condyloma acuminatum when applied locally as a 25% suspension in mineral oil. Constituents of podophyllin may arrest mitosis by a mechanism similar to that of colchicine. They do not appear promising for systemic use in neoplastic diseases. This resin has been used as a cathartic, but it is now obsolete.

Procarbazine is a hydrazine derivative that is cytotoxic and has numerous adverse effects from monoamine oxidase inhibition to carcinogenicity and teratogenicity. Despite its toxicity, the drug seems to have some effectiveness in the treatment of Hodgkin's disease.

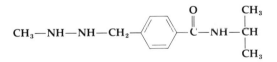

Procarbazine

Imidazole carboxamide, although strictly investigational and of unknown mechanism of action, shows some activity in the treatment of malignant melanoma.

CHOICE OF DRUGS IN CANCER CHEMOTHERAPY

In addition to the use of surgery and radiation, various drugs may be effective in the treatment of malignancies. In fact, chemotherapy is considered the primary method of treatment in the following conditions: choriocarcinoma of the female, Wilms' tumor, acute and chronic leukemias, multiple myeloma, and polycythemia vera.

As a general rule, the drugs of choice for various malignancies change rapidly in the light of statistics accumulated by cancer chemotherapy study groups. This is particularly true for possible synergistic combinations.

Chronic myelocytic leukemia responds to a number of drugs. In order of preference they are busulfan, chlorambucil, and mecaptopurine. It is believed that the drugs are as effective as irradiation and can be substituted for each other as resistance develops.

Chronic lymphocytic leukemia may be treated with irradiation or drugs when the disease becomes progressive. Chlorambucil is preferred by many experts. In resistant cases, corticosteroids may be useful, and among these prednisone in large doses is favored by many.

Table 55-2. Dosage and toxicity of some antimetabolites, antibiotics, hormones, and *Vinca* alkaloids*

Drug	Route of administration	Usual dose	Toxic effects
Antimetabolites			
Methotrexate	Oral and intravenous	2.5 mg. daily for leukemia 10-30 mg. daily for chorio-carcinoma	Stomatitis, enteritis, bone marrow depression, alopecia skin rash; leucovorin is a useful antidote if given within a few hours after methotrexate
Fluorouracil	Intravenous	15 mg./kg. daily for 4 days	Stomatitis, enteritis, leukopenia, hemorrhages
Mercaptopurine	Oral	2.5 mg./kg. daily	Stomatitis, enteritis, jaundice bone marrow depression
Antibiotic			
Actinomycin D	Intravenous	75 μg/kg. total dose in 5 days	Vomiting, stomatitis, enteritis, leukopenia, alopecia
Hormones			
Diethylstilbestrol	Oral	1-5 mg. three times/day	Nausea, vomiting, feminization, hypercalcemia
Fluoxymesterone	Oral	10 mg. three times/day	Masculinization, hirsutism, fluid retention, hypercalcemia
Prednisone	Oral	1 mg./kg. daily	Cushing-type effects
Vinca alkaloids			
Vinblastine	Intravenous	0.10-0.15 mg./kg. weekly	Nausea, vomiting, stomatitis, leukopenia; alopecia
Vincristine	Intravenous	0.02-0.05 mg./kg. weekly	Nausea, vomiting, neurotoxic effects, leukopenia; alopecia

* Based on data from several sources.

Acute leukemias of children respond well to antimetabolites such as methotrexate. The acute lymphoblastic leukemias are also responsive to corticosteroids and vincristine. Other drugs are being used also, but nitrogen mustards are ineffective. In acute myeloblastic and monocytic leukemias, mercaptopurine has been found useful; cytarabine has been effective in causing remissions in acute granulocytic leukemias of adults.

Hodgkin's disease and *lymphosarcoma* are often treated with chlorambucil, TEM, mechlorethamine hydrochloride, methotrexate, vinblastine, and corticosteroids. Occasional favorable response is obtained but no definite prolongation of life.

Multiple myeloma responds to the alkylating agents such as cyclophosphamide or melphalan. Prednisone is useful also, as is vincristine.

Choriocarcinoma is most effectively treated with methotrexate or in resistant cases with actinomycin D. Vinblastine may be useful when the two preferred agents become ineffective.

Regional cancer chemotherapy by means of intra-arterial nitrogen mustards or methotrexate with folinic acid is being used with some favorable results in selected patients.

Malignant effusions are often treated with mechlorethamine instillations, although quinacrine solutions may also be effective.

References

1 Ansfield, F. J., Schroeder, J. M., and Curreri, A. R.: Five years' clinical experience with 5-fluorouracil, J.A.M.A. 181:295, 1962.

2 Burchenal, J. H.: The treatment of leukemia, Bull. N. Y. Acad. Med. 30:429, 1954.

3 Cortes, E. P., Holland, J. F., Wang, J. J., and Sinks, L. F.. Doxorubicin in disseminated osteosarcoma, J. A. M. A. 221:1132, 1972.

4 Farber, S., Toch, R., Sears, E. M., and Pinkel, D.: Advances in chemotherapy of cancer in man, Advances Cancer Res. 4:1, 1956.

5 Goodman, L. S., Wintrobe, M. M., Dameshek, W., Goodman, M. J., Gilman, A., and McLennan, M. T.: Nitrogen mustard therapy, J.A.M.A. 132:126, 1946.

6 Hersh, E. M., Whitecar, J. P., McCredie, K. B., Bodey, G. P., and Freireich, E. J.: Chemotherapy, immunocompetence, immunosuppression and prognosis in acute leukemia, New Eng. J. Med. 285:1211, 1971.

7 Karnofsky, D. A., and Burchenal, J. H.: Present status of clinical cancer chemotherapy, Amer. J. Med. 8:767, 1950.

8 Kidd, J. G.: Regression of transplanted lymphomas induced *in vivo* by means of normal guinea pig serum. I. Course of transplanted cancers of various kinds in mice and rats given guinea pig serum, horse serum or rabbit serum, J. Exp. Med. 98:565, 1953.

9 Philips, F. S.: Recent contributions to the pharmacology of bis(2-haloethyl) amines and sulfides, J. Pharmacol. Exp. Ther. 99:281, 1950.

10 Rundles, R. W.: Triethylene melamine (TEM) therapy in malignant diseases, GP 9:75, 1954.

11 Selawry, O. S., and Hananian, J.: Vincristine treatment of cancer in children, J.A.M.A. 183:741, 1963.

12 Shnider, B. I., and Gold, C. L.: Recent developments in cancer chemotherapy, Med. Ann. D. C. 28:637, 1959.

Recent reviews

13 Busch, H., and Lane, M.: Chemotherapy, Chicago, 1967, Year Book Medical Publishers, Inc.

14 DeVita, V. T., and Rall, D. P.: Pharmacologic aspects of the chemotherapy of solid tumors, Pharmacol. Physicians 2(9):1, 1968.

14a DeVita, V. T., and Schein, P. S.: The use of drugs in combination for the treatment of cancer, New Eng. J. Med. 288:998, 1973.

15 Farber, S.: Chemotherapy in the treatment of leukemia and Wilms' tumor, J.A.M.A. 198:826, 1966.

16 Folkman, J.: Tumor angiogenesis: therapeutic implications, New Eng. J. Med. 285:1182, 1971.

17 Frei, E., and Loo, T. L.: Pharmacologic basis for the chemotherapy of leukemia, Pharmacol. Physicians 1(5):1, 1967.

18 Heidelberger, C.: Cancer chemotherapy with purine and pyrimidine analogues, Ann. Rev. Pharmacol. 7:101, 1967.

19 Hiatt, H. H.: Cancer chemotherapy—present status and prospects, New Eng. J. Med. 276: 157, 1967.

20 Hitchings, G. H.: A quarter century of chemo-therapy, J.A.M.A. **209**:1339, 1969.

21 Hitchings, G. H., and Elion, G. B.: Chemical suppression of the immune response, Pharmacol. Rev. **15**:365, 1963.

22 Honeycutt, W. M., Jansen, T., and Dillaha, C. J.: Topical antimetabolites and cytostatic agents, Cutis **6**:63, 1970.

23 Huggins, C.: The hormone-dependent cancers, J.A.M.A. **186**:481, 1963.

23a Krakoff, I. H.: Cancer chemotherapeutic agents, CA **23**:208, 1973.

24 Miller, E. C., and Miller, J. A.: Mechanisms of chemical carcinogenesis: nature of proximate carcinogens and interactions with macromole-cules, Pharmacol. Rev. **18**:805, 1966.

25 Moore, F. D.: New problems for surgery, Science **144**:388, 1964.

26 Oliverio, V. T., and Zubrod, C. G.: Clinical pharmacology of the effective antitumor drugs, Ann. Rev. Pharmacol. **5**:335, 1965.

27 Penman, S.: Ribonucleic acid metabolism in mammalian cells, New Eng. J. Med. **276**:502, 1967.

28 Pitot, H. C.: Some biochemical aspects of malignancy, Ann. Rev. Biochem. **35**:335, 1966.

29 Santos, G. W.: The pharmacology of immuno-suppressive drugs, Pharmacol. Physicians **2**(8): 1, 1968.

SECTION TEN

PRINCIPLES OF IMMUNOPHARMACOLOGY

56 Principles of immunopharmacology

With the current interest in organ transplantation, the term immunopharmacology brings to mind primarily the study of immunosuppressive drugs. This view of the subject is much too restricted, however. As defined in this discussion, immunopharmacology encompasses not only the study of all drug effects on the immune process but also the formation and release of the chemical mediators involved in the genesis of immune injury.

It has been pointed out[17] that the control of disease by immunologic means has two objectives, the production of *desired immunity* and the elimination of *undesired immune reactions*. The first of these objectives is achieved by *immunization procedures* rather than drugs. For this reason, discussions of immunopharmacology are more concerned with the chemical basis of *undesired* immune reactions and their possible elimination by means of drugs.

IMMUNOSUPPRESSIVE AGENTS

Several groups of drugs have been used clinically for the purpose of suppressing the immune response. The most important are:

1. Corticosteroids
2. Cytotoxic drugs
   a. Antimetabolites: mercaptopurine and azathioprine (Imuran)
   b. Alkylating agents: cyclophosphamide (Cytoxan) and nitrogen mustard
   c. Folic acid antagonists: methotrexate

In addition to these drugs, radiation and antilymphocytic serum (ALS) are also potent immunosuppressive agents.

Mode of action

There is general agreement on certain features of the mode of action of the immunosuppressive drugs,[23] which can be summarized as follows:

1. The cytotoxic drugs tend to destroy replicating cells. They have been classified as *cell cycle drugs* and *noncycle drugs*. The cell cycle drugs destroy *only* rapidly multiplying cells, whereas the noncycle drugs are injurious to nonreplicating cells as well. The antimetabolites and folic acid antagonists act only on dividing cells; the alkylating agents, being noncycle drugs, cause depletion in the total number of small lymphocytes.

2. Immunosuppressive agents inhibit the primary immune response more readily than an established immune state or an anamnestic response. Their main effect on antibody synthesis is exerted during the time when the antigen converts its clone of lymphocytes to antibody-producing cells.

657

3. Various components of the immune response are not equally affected by all suppressive drugs. Delayed hypersensitivity and IgG synthesis can be inhibited selectively. For example, mercaptopurine and antilymphocyte serum can inhibit the development of delayed hypersensitivity without blocking IgG synthesis.[1] These selective effects also depend on the dose of the drug. Mercaptopurine in small doses may block delayed hypersensitivity, in larger doses it prevents the formation of IgG antibodies. Even larger doses are required for blocking the formation of IgM antibodies. These facts suggest varying susceptibility of different cell lines involved in the immune process. Immunosuppressive drugs are generally ineffective against differentiated cells that produce antibodies or carry immunologic memory.

4. The goal of immunosuppressive therapy is the development of drug-induced immune tolerance to specific antigens, with conservation of other immunologic capabilities.

5. Immunosuppressive drugs have many adverse effects. These are not unexpected because immune processes are important defenses against infections and may play a role in protecting the individual against neoplastic cells as well.

CELLULAR ASPECTS OF THE IMMUNE RESPONSE

To understand some of the concepts of immunopharmacology, it is necessary to review briefly the current views on cellular events in the immune response.

As shown in Fig. 56-1, the first step in the immune response is the ingestion and processing of the antigen by a macrophage. Some sort of interaction between the antigen and the macrophage is necessary for lymphocytes to respond to the antigen, which may be on the surface of the macrophage. The small lymphocytes, on exposure to the surface antigen, undergo several cell divisions. Some of them become plasma cells and form humoral antibodies, and others become involved in cellular immunity, delayed hypersensitivity, and immunologic memory.

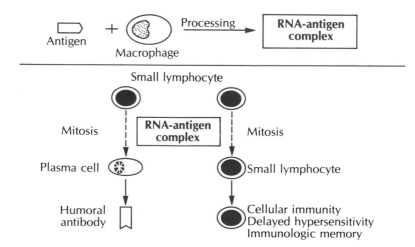

Fig. 56-1. Schema of development of humoral and cellular immunity.

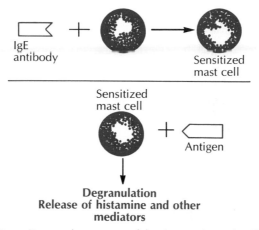

Fig. 56-2. Schema of mediator release caused by interaction of cell-bound IgE antibody and antigen.

EFFECTOR MECHANISMS AND MEDIATORS IN IMMUNE INJURY

Several types of immune injury are recognized, each having characteristic effector mechanisms. Some of the latter are (1) anaphylaxis, (2) cytolysis, (3) immune-complex reactions, and (4) delayed hypersensitivity.

Anaphylactic mechanisms

The antibody in anaphylactic reactions is largely of the IgE type, which attaches itself to cells such as mast cells and leukocytes. When exposed to the antigen, the sensitized mast cells release vasoactive mediators, among which histamine appears the most important. The slow-reacting substance (SRS), an acidic lipid, may not originate from mast cells. In the rat[13] it is released by polymorphonuclear leukocytes. Serotonin is probably not present in human mast cells.

The release of histamine from human basophils or mast cells does not require complement when these cells are sensitized by IgE antibodies. On the other hand, if antibodies are prepared against mast cells, they will attack these cells and cause histamine release by a cytolytic mechanism that requires complement.

Cytolytic mechanisms

Cytolytic mechanisms are involved in the pathogenesis of various types of hemolytic anemia, thrombocytopenia, and leukopenia. The antigen may be a constituent of the cell, such as the Rh factor, or a drug attached to the cell. The antibodies are of the IgE variety except for the cold hemagglutinins (IgM). Complement is not required for cytolysis except when cold agglutinins are involved.

Immune-complex mechanisms

Immune-complex mechanisms are most clearly seen in acute and chronic glomerulonephritis and in serum sickness. Soluble antigen-antibody complexes may be deposited in the glomerular basement membranes where they activate the complement system. Leukotactic factors are generated, which attract polymorphonuclear leukocytes. The release of lytic enzymes from leukocytic lysosomes leads to digestion of the basement membrane.[2] There are variations on this theme. The antibodies may be directed against the basement membrane. In other instances the continued deposit formation leads to membranous glomerulonephritis.

The antibodies involved in immune-complex disease are of the IgG and IgM type, and complement plays an important role in the immunologic injury.

Delayed hypersensitivity mechanisms

The clinical condition that is a prime example of delayed hypersensitivity is *contact dermatitis*. Similar mechanisms are involved also in the rejection of grafts and in the tuberculin reaction.

No humoral antibodies are involved in this type of reaction. Instead, sensitized small lymphocytes are responsible for recognizing the antigen. In addition, large numbers of nonsensitized mononuclear cells that accumulate at the site over a period of 24 to 48 hours act as the "inflammatory cells." The slow accumulation of these cells explains the delayed nature of the reaction. The mechanism of their accumulation may be related to the observation that sensitized lymphocytes exposed to the antigen *in vitro* release a factor (migration-inhibition factor) that causes macrophages to stick to capillary tubes, thus preventing their migration. There are other mediators of delayed hypersensitivity, such as lymphotoxin.[7] The role of the so-called lymph node–permeability factor is questionable and nonspecific.

DRUG EFFECTS ON THE VARIOUS TYPES OF IMMUNE INJURY

Anaphylactic mechanisms are not susceptible to cytotoxic drugs for a number of reasons. These reactions depend on preformed antibodies, and the reactions are of the immediate type. Although it is possible that long-continued administration of cytotoxic drugs would have some effect, the toxicity of these agents precludes their prolonged administration.

The therapeutic approaches to anaphylactic injury are aimed at (1) the development of blocking antibodies by hyposensitization, (2) inhibition of the release of vasoactive mediators, and (3) prevention of the effect of the mediators such as histamine.

The widely employed hyposensitization procedures are believed to increase the formation of blocking antibodies (IgG) that may bind the allergen. It is possible that other mechanisms are involved also. In the rapid desensitization to an antigen such as a serum in an individual known to be hypersensitive to it, there must clearly be other mechanisms involved than the production of blocking antibodies.

Disodium cromoglycate (Intal) is a chroman derivative that is claimed to inhibit the release of vasoactive mediators caused by interaction of antigen with reaginic antibodies.[13] When administered by inhalation, it exerts some therapeutic effect in asthma, which is demonstrable statistically in controlled series. That it is not a powerful therapeutic agent is indicated by some conflict of opinion about its efficacy.

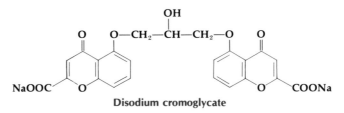

Disodium cromoglycate

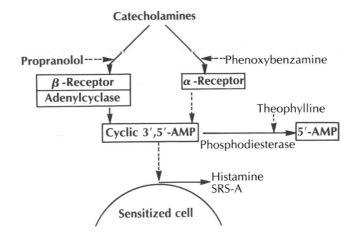

Fig. 56-3. Inhibitory effect of cyclic 3',5'-AMP on mediator release and the influence of some drugs. Broken arrow indicates an inhibitory effect.

Diethylcarbamazine (Hetrazan) also appears to inhibit the release of slow-reacting substance.[13] Both these drugs are extremely weak therapeutic agents, but their mode of action is of great interest because they may point the way to new approaches to allergy and anaphylaxis.

Of great interest are observations indicating that histamine release from human leukocytes and animal mast cells is inhibited by drugs that are expected to raise intracellular cyclic AMP levels. Isoproterenol and theophylline, widely used in the treatment of asthma, have an inhibitory activity on histamine release by allergens from human leukocytes.[6] Although the relative importance of their action on release processes in relation to their bronchodilator action is impossible to state under clinical conditions, these observations have stimulated much research on the role of the beta adrenergic system in the allergic diathesis.[18]

There is not much known about drug effects on cytolysis. On the other hand, drugs may act at several sites in immune-complex disease. Immunosuppressive drugs may reduce the antibody levels and lower the number of granulocytes. It is of great interest that agranulocytic animals do not develop glomerulonephritis despite the presence of complexes in the circulation. Corticosteroids are employed in the treatment of glomerulonephritis. Their action is attributed to stabilization of granulocytic lysosomes, which are believed to play an important role in damaging the basement membrane of the glomeruli. Theoretical approaches to immune-complex disease include also the use of decomplementing agents. A glycoprotein extracted from cobra venom depletes the third component of complement,[11] a finding of great experimental interest.

Delayed hypersensitivity is susceptible to several drugs. The immunosuppressive drugs such as the antimetabolites have important effects on the nonsensitized inflammatory cells. This is understandable, since the inflammatory cells are short-lived and have very active nucleic acid metabolism.[17]

IMMUNOSUPPRESSIVE AND ANTI-INFLAMMATORY DRUG ACTIONS

There is commonly an overlap in the anti-inflammatory and immunosuppressive effects of various drugs. For example, the corticosteroids have both actions. Mercaptopurine treatment reduces the number of mononuclear cells at inflammatory sites[15] in animal experiments.

The simplest way to explain the overlap is to consider that the immune injury leads to inflammation as a consequence of the activity of "inflammatory" cells. Drugs that reduce the number of these cells or inhibit their activities may exert both anti-inflammatory and apparent immunosuppressive effects. The cytotoxic drugs inhibit the multiplication of cells, whereas the milder anti-inflammatory drugs may exert more subtle effects on the inflammatory cells or may block the actions of their products. *Theoretically,* the anti-inflammatory drugs may block the effects of leukotactic factors on inflammatory cells, or they may inhibit the elaboration of mediators by these cells. They may also block the action of the mediators. No simple theory such as that of lysosomal stabilization[21] is sufficient to account for the vast differences in the spectrum of activity of the various types of anti-inflammatory drugs (p. 482).

CLINICAL APPLICATIONS

From the foregoing discussion it should be clear that some types of immune injury may be ameliorated by drug therapy. Some of the examples will be discussed briefly.

Rh hemolytic disease of the newborn is prevented very successfully by Rh_0 (D) immune globulin (RhoGAM). It is used for the passive immunization of the mother to prevent the formation of antibodies. It is injected within 72 hours after birth of an Rh_0-positive (D-positive or D^u-positive) baby to a mother who is negative with respect to these factors.

Acute glomerulonephritis is often treated with corticosteroids (prednisone) and occasionally with other immunosuppressive agents. The same is true for idiopathic thrombocytopenic purpura and autoimmune hemolytic anemia.

Renal transplantation has been greatly aided by the availability of azathioprine (Imuran), prednisone, and antilymphocytic serum (ALS). These drugs are used also in the transplantation of other organs.

The usefulness of drugs in the management of allergic and rheumatic diseases has been commented on in Chapters 16 and 26.

References

1 Borel, Y., and Schwartz, R. S.: Inhibition of immediate and delayed hypersensitivity by 6-mercaptopurine, J. Immun. **92**:754, 1965.

2 Dixon, F. J.: The pathogenesis of glomerulonephritis, Amer. J. Med. **44**:493, 1968.

3 Gowans, J. L., and McGregor, D. D.: Immunological activities of lymphocytes, Progr. Allerg. **9**:1, 1965.

4 Ishizaka, K.: The identification and significance of gamma E, Hosp. Practice **4**:70, 1969.

5 Johnson, A. R., and Moran, N. C.: Inhibition of the release of histamine from rat mast cells: the effect of cold and adrenergic drugs on release of histamine by compound 48/80 and antigen, J. Pharmacol. Exp. Ther. **175**:632, 1970.

6 Lichtenstein, L. M.: Mechanism of allergic histamine release from human leukocytes. In Austen,

K. F., and Becker, E. L., editors: Biochemistry of the acute allergic reactions, Philadelphia, 1967, F. A. Davis Co.

7 Mackaness, G. B., and Blanden, R. V.: Cellular immunity, Progr. Allerg. **11**:89, 1967.

8 Makinodan, T., Santos, G. W., and Quinn, R. P.: Immunosuppressive drugs, Pharmacol. Rev. **22**:189, 1971.

9 Medawar, P.: Antilymphocyte serum: its properties and potentials, Hosp. Practice **4**:26, 1969.

10 Mota, I.: The mechanism of anaphylaxis. I. Production and biological properties of "mast cell sensitizing" antibody, Immunology **7**:681, 1964.

11 Muller-Eberhard, H. J.: Chemistry and reaction mechanisms of complement, Advances Immun. **8**:1, 1968.

12 Novack, S. N., and Pearson, C. M.: Cyclophos-

phamide therapy in Wegener's granulomatosis, New Eng. J. Med. **284**:938, 1971.

13 Orange, R. P., and Austen, K. F.: Pharmacologic dissociation of immunologic release of histamine and slow-reacting substance of anaphylaxis in rats, Proc. Soc. Exp. Biol. Med. **129**:836, 1968.

14 Orange, R. P., Valentine, M. D., and Austen, K. F.: Antigen-induced release of slow-reacting substance of anaphylaxis in rats prepared with homologous antibody, J. Exp. Med. **127**:767, 1968.

15 Page, A. R., Condie, R. M., and Good, R. A.: Effect of 6-mercaptopurine on inflammation, Amer. J. Path. **40**:519, 1962.

16 Piper, P. J., and Vane, J. R.: Release of additional factors in anaphylaxis and its antagonism by antiinflammatory drugs, Nature **223**:29, 1969.

17 Schwartz, R. S.: Therapeutic strategy in clinical immunology, New Eng. J. Med. **280**:367, 1969.

18 Szentivanyi, A.: The beta adrenergic theory of the atopic abnormality in bronchial asthma, J. Allerg. **42**:203, 1968.

19 Uhr, J. W., and Moller, G.: Regulatory effects of antibody on antibody formation, Advances Immun. **8**:81, 1968.

20 Ward, P. A., and Zwaifler, M. J.: Complement-derived leukotactic factors in inflammatory synovial fluids of humans, J. Clin. Invest. **50**:606, 1971.

21 Weissmann, G.: Structure and function of lysosomes, Rheumatology **1**:1, 1967.

22 Weissmann, G.: Lysosomal mechanisms of tissue injury in arthritis, New Eng. J. Med. **286**:141, 1972.

23 Winkelstein, A.: Principles of immunosuppressive therapy, Bull. Rheum. Dis. **21**:627, 1971.

SECTION ELEVEN

POISONS AND ANTIDOTES

57

Poisons and antidotes

The incidence of poisoning has been increasing as a result of the introduction of a variety of new drugs and various chemicals for industrial and home use. A poison is generally defined as a compound that in relatively small quantities and by a chemical action can cause death or disability. According to this definition, there is essentially no difference between a drug and a poison. In large enough doses any drug can cause death or disability.

Toxicology is the science of poisons and poisonings. It may be considered a branch of pharmacology, since the latter discipline also deals with the adverse effects of drugs. A practical reason for the existence of a separate discipline has to do with the fact that many highly specialized procedures are used for laboratory diagnosis of poisonings. These require special laboratories staffed by properly trained toxicologists.

ORDER OF FREQUENCY OF POISONOUS AGENTS

According to recent experience, drug intoxication in the adult usually involves one of five common drugs[15]: barbiturates, salicylates, glutethimide, meprobamate, or phenothiazines. Three other drugs are important causes of self-induced poisoning: scopolamine, bromides, and ethylene glycol.

In addition, poisoning caused by heavy metals continues to be a serious problem, particularly in children. Metals and also thousands of synthetic organic chemicals are receiving increased attention as environmental contaminants. They are not only present in air, water, and soil but often become concentrated in the food chain.

DIAGNOSIS OF POISONING

The diagnosis of poisoning is often difficult. It is based on the history, physical examination or pathologic changes, and laboratory procedures. The investigation should include personal, occupational, and family history. Physical examination and pathologic changes may be quite characteristic for certain types of poisoning. In many instances, however, laboratory procedures are essential in order to make a definitive diagnosis.

An increasingly important problem is that the physician may know the trade name of a preparation that caused the poisoning without knowing the chemical nature of the compounds contained in such a preparation. The development of poison control centers, where extensive files are maintained on the composition of various chemical and pharmaceutic preparations, may be an important step in helping the physician in poisoning cases.

667

PRINCIPLES OF TREATMENT IN POISONING CASES

In general, treatment of poisoning is based on removal of the poison, administration of antidotes, and symptomatic management.

Removal of orally administered poisons may be of great importance if the patient is seen within a few hours after swallowing the noxious agent.

Several procedures are available for emptying the stomach. Gastric lavage is widely used, but its effectiveness is not as great as generally believed. Considerable amounts of a poison may remain in the stomach despite gastric lavage. The use of emetic drugs is of considerable value in poisoning cases.

Emetics. The two drugs that are recommended for the induction of vomiting in poisoning cases are apomorphine and syrup of ipecac. Cupric sulfate is effective also, but its use may be hazardous.

Apomorphine hydrochloride is injected by the subcutaneous route in a dose of 0.1 mg./kg. It induces vomiting within a few minutes by an action on the chemoreceptor trigger zone in the medulla. The emetic effect of the drug is prevented by the pheno-thiazine antiemetics. Apomorphine may cause respiratory depression, which may be antagonized by the narcotic antagonists. Apomorphine hydrochloride NF is available in tablets containing 6 mg. to be prepared for hypodermic use.

Contraindications to the use of apomorphine include shock, coma, advanced age, and ingestion of corrosive substances and probably petroleum distillates.

Ipecac syrup is administered orally in a dosage of 20 ml. for adults and 15 ml. in children over 1 year of age. The emetic effectiveness increases if ingestion of the drug is followed by 200 ml. of water. Ipecac acts locally and also on the chemoreceptor trigger zone. It usually induces vomiting within 20 to 30 minutes. Pediatricians recommend having syrup of ipecac available in the home, since the drug may be very useful in poisonings in children. Ipecac Syrup is a USP preparation. Just as other emetics, syrup of ipecac is contraindicated in comatose patients and after the ingestion of corrosive poisons or petroleum distillates. Activated charcoal adsorbs and inactivates ipecac, and the two should not be administered simultaneously.

ANTIDOTES

Antidotes are used for prevention of absorption of the poison and for inactivating it or opposing its action following absorption. Antidotes are usually classified as chemical or physiologic. The former actually combine with the poisons, whereas the latter oppose its actions.

Until recently, chemical antidotes could serve only for inactivation of the poison in the stomach. Important developments have taken place in recent years in the field of systemically active chemical antidotes. The most important examples are dimercaprol, calcium disodium edetate, and penicillamine. Protective agents against radiation may also be looked upon as antidotes against free radicals produced by radiation. An example of such a drug is 2-aminoethylisothiuronium (AET).

For inactivation of poisons in the gastric contents, one of the most widely used compounds is tannic acid, which can precipitate certain metals and alkaloids. Strong tea will precipitate strychnine, cinchona alkaloids, apomorphine, and also, to a slight extent, cocaine. Salts of zinc, cobalt, copper, mercury, lead, and nickel are also precipitated by strong tea.

Milk and egg white are useful in treatment of poisoning due to mercuric chloride and phenols. Administration of these antidotes should be followed by gastric lavage in order to prevent slow absorption of the bound poison.

Adsorbents such as activated charcoal may also be useful. Following administration of adsorbents, a saline cathartic may be advantageous. Magnesium sulfate or sodium sulfate may be antidotal in poisoning due to barium or lead.

The development of the chemical antidotes dimercaprol and calcium disodium edetate, which are effective against metal poisons even after they are absorbed, represents a brilliant feat of pharmacologic research.

DIMERCAPROL

Dimercaprol (BAL) was developed during World War II in Great Britain.[12] It was the outgrowth of studies directed at finding effective antidotes against the arsenic-containing vesicant lewisite. It was known previously that arsenicals combine with sulfhydryl groups, and when the effect of arsenicals on the sulfhydryl content of keratin was investigated, it was found that each atom of the metal combined with two of these thiol groups. This fact suggested that a dithiol with adjacent sulfhydryl groups might be efficient as an antidote. A number of such compounds were synthesized, and dimercaptopropanol, known at present as dimercaprol, was found to be most effective.

$$CH_2\!-\!SH$$
$$CH\!-\!SH$$
$$CH_2\!-\!OH$$

Dimercaprol

The greater antidotal action of dithiols, when compared with cysteine and other monothiols, is related to the fact that the former produce a ring structure of great stability in combination with the metal.

Dimercaprol is effective in the treatment of poisoning by compounds of mercury, arsenic, and gold. Its usefulness is not certain in antimony and bismuth poisoning. Dimercaprol should not be used in the treatment of poisoning caused by cadmium, iron, or selenium. In the case of cadmium, it has been shown that dimercaprol complexes are more toxic than the metal by itself. The drug is not recommended for the treatment of lead poisoning because calcium disodium edetate is much more effective. It may have some usefulness, however, in the management of lead encephalopathy.

Therapeutic objectives in use. There are two major therapeutic objectives in the use of dimercaprol. First, the antidote can protect essential enzymes in the tissues from circulating metallic poisons by forming stable combinations with the poisonous agent. A second objective is to promote the excretion of the metal in the form of its dimercaprol complexes and thereby decrease the quantity of the poison in the body. Depending on the interval between the poisoning and the institution of treatment, one or the other of these objectives may be more important.

Metabolism. Dimercaprol is rapidly metabolized in the body. When a dose of as much as 3 mg./kg. is administered every 4 hours, there is no cumulative toxicity. Liver damage increases the toxicity of dimercaprol. The drug is contraindicated in severe renal insufficiency also, although metabolic inactivation is more important than renal excretion in its disposition.

669

Toxicity and hypersensitivity. Dimercaprol is a potentially dangerous drug. Even doses of less than 100 mg./kg. can cause swift death in animals. It is believed that in these high concentrations the drug inhibits metal-containing enzymes that are essential in cellular respiration.

Adverse effects of dimercaprol include pain at the site of injection, weakness, nausea, salivation, elevation of blood pressure, coma, and convulsions. Large doses may cause vascular collapse as a consequence of capillary damage. Alkalinization of the urine is claimed to protect against dissociation of the dimercaprol-metal complex and nephrotoxicity.

Preparations. Dimercaprol (BAL) is available in peanut oil for injection, 100 mg./ml. Dosage varies from 3 to 5 mg./kg. intramuscularly for the initial injection. Administration is repeated one to four times daily, depending on the nature and severity of the poisoning.

CALCIUM DISODIUM EDETATE AND DISODIUM EDETATE

Ethylenediamine tetraacetic acid and its salt disodium edetate are powerful chelating agents that form a highly stable complex with calcium. Despite the high stability of the chelate, calcium is displaced from it by lead, zinc, chromium, copper, cadmium, manganese, and nickel. Calcium disodium edetate is useful primarily in the treatment of lead poisoning.

Disodium edetate (Endrate) is quite dangerous when injected intravenously, since it chelates calcium and may lead to hypocalcemia that may be fatal. It has been used for lowering serum calcium concentrations in various clinical conditions, but this should be done only by experts.

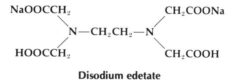

Disodium edetate

Calcium disodium edetate is administered by intravenous drip for two or three days in the treatment of lead poisoning. It promotes the renal excretion of the lead chelate, which is demonstrable within a few hours and becomes maximal in a day or two. Increased lead excretion may have diagnostic importance in lead encephalopathy when the diagnosis is uncertain. For diagnostic purposes the drug may be injected by the intramuscular route. Oral administration of calcium disodium edetate for the treatment of lead poisoning is not effective and may even be hazardous.

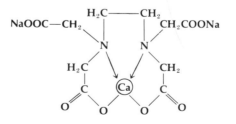

Calcium disodium edetate

Metabolism. In contrast to dimercaprol, calcium disodium edetate is not metabolized in the body and is excreted as a soluble metal complex in the urine.

670

Adverse effects. Adverse effects of calcium disodium edetate include renal damage, hypersensitivity reactions, and transient bone marrow depression.

Preparations. Calcium disodium edetate (Calcium Disodium Versenate) is avail able as a solution, 200 mg./ml. in 5 ml. containers, to be diluted for intravenous infusion. Disodium edetate (Endrate) is prepared as a solution for injection, 150 mg./ml. in 20 ml. containers.

PENICILLAMINE

Penicillamine (Cuprimine) and its acetyl derivatives can chelate copper and other metals. It is used at the present time for removal of copper in hepatolenticular degeneration (Wilson's disease). Penicillamine chelates not only copper but other metals such as mercury, lead, and iron. Since other antidotes are more effective, the drug is recommended only for the removal of copper.

For an action unrelated to metal chelation, penicillamine has some usefulness in cystinuria because it forms soluble complexes with cystine and facilitates its excretion in a soluble form.

Adverse effects of penicillamine are hypersensitivity reactions, rashes, arthralgia, and the nephrotic syndrome.

Penicillamine (Cuprimine) is available in capsules containing 250 mg. Dosage for adults is 250 mg. four times daily, with gradual increase but not to exceed a daily dose of 4 to 5 Gm.

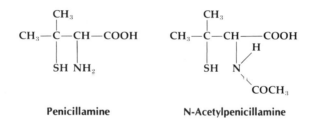

Penicillamine   N-Acetylpenicillamine

DEFEROXAMINE MESYLATE

Deferoxamine mesylate (Desferal) is a chelating agent used in the treatment of iron poisoning and for the removal of iron from the body (p. 534). The drug may be injected intramuscularly or by intravenous infusion. It has great affinity for iron in the ferric form. The drug is toxic and should not be used unless the severity of the poisoning justifies it. Deferoxamine mesylate (Desferal) is available as a powder for injection, 500 mg.

ESSENTIAL FEATURES OF CERTAIN POISONINGS

The toxic effects of the five drugs most commonly causing drug intoxication in the adult (p. 672) are summarized in Table 57-1. The essential features of some other poisonings are discussed in this section.

SCOPOLAMINE AND ATROPINE INTOXICATION

Scopolamine intoxication is not uncommon because the drug is contained in some proprietary hypnotic preparations (Sominex). The symptoms induced by scopolamine

Table 57-1. Essential features of common poisons*

Drug	Oral fatal dose (estimated)	Lethal blood levels (estimated)	Effects	Therapy
Barbiturates				
Short-acting	3 Gm.	3.5 mg.%	Respiratory depres-	Respiratory assist-
Long-acting	5 Gm.	8.0 mg.%	sion, hypotension, renal shutdown, hypothermia, pneumonia	ance, diuresis, dialysis
Glutethimide	10 Gm.	3.0 mg.%	Apnea, mydriasis, hypotension, flaccid paralysis	Gastric lavage, respiratory assistance, diuresis, dialysis
Salicylates	10-20 Gm.	50 mg.%	Hyperventilation, respiratory alkalosis, metabolic acidosis (later), hypoprothrombinemia	Alkaline diuresis, vitamin K, dialysis
Phenothiazines	50 mg./kg. of chlorpromazine or equivalent	Unknown	Miosis, irritability	Supportive control of convulsions
Meprobamate	12 Gm.	Unknown	Hypotension, respiratory depression, coma	Respiratory assistance, dialysis

*Based on data from Castell, D. O., and Morrison, C. C.: Resident Physician **13**:66, 1967.

and atropine have been discussed (p. 125). They include delirium, dilated pupils, tachycardia, dry mouth and skin, and hyperirritability. Injection of 10 to 30 mg. of methacholine has no effect on salivation, sweating, or activity of the intestinal tract. Treatment consists of sponging for high temperature and sedation for convulsions.

BROMIDE INTOXICATION

The toxic dose is about 30 Gm. or a blood level of 200 mg.%. The drug is cumulative. Delirium, mental confusion, respiratory depression, and hypotension should suggest the possibility of bromide intoxication. Treatment is based on the administration of solutions containing sodium chloride.

ETHYLENE GLYCOL INTOXICATION

Ethylene glycol is contained in antifreeze preparations. Its lethal dose is about 100 ml. Ethylene glycol is metabolized to oxalate. Acidosis occurs and methemoglobinemia may be present. The symptoms vary according to the stage of intoxication. In the first stage, hyperactivity of the central nervous system followed by coma is characteristic. In the second stage, cardiac and pulmonary signs with tachypnea, cyanosis, and possibility of pulmonary edema predominate. The third stage is characterized by renal failure with the deposition of calcium oxalate crystals in the renal tubules. Diagnosis is facilitated when such crystals are found in the urine. Treatment is based initially on gastric lavage and the administration of sodium lactate or bicarbonate for acidosis and methylene blue for methemoglobinemia.[11] Dialysis may be quite useful for removal of the poison and treatment of renal failure. Ethyl alcohol is claimed to compete with liver enzymes that metabolize ethylene glycol, but its use is still experimental.[11]

CARBON MONOXIDE POISONING

Carbon monoxide, a colorless and odorless gas, has a great affinity for hemoglobin. The resulting carboxyhemoglobin is unavailable for oxygen transport. The affinity of carbon monoxide for hemoglobin may be 200 to 300 times as great as that of oxygen. As a consequence, inhalation of even low concentrations of the gas can produce markedly elevated levels of carboxyhemoglobin. Serious toxic effects result when 40% of hemoglobin has been changed to carboxyhemoglobin.

The symptoms of carbon monoxide poisoning consist of impairment of vision, headache, tachycardia, hyperpnea, and eventually coma and death when about 60% of the hemoglobin is in the form of carboxyhemoglobin. The skin shows the characteristic cherry-red cyanosis due to the red color of carboxyhemoglobin.

Treatment consists of transferring the patient to fresh air, giving artificial respiration, and administering 100% oxygen.

CYANIDE POISONING

The cyanide ion has a great affinity for respiratory enzymes. Its rapid lethal action is probably due to inactivation of the enzyme cytochrome oxidase, which is very susceptible to this poison.

The lethal effect of hydrocyanic acid is extremely rapid, and the opportunities for treatment hardly exist. When potassium or sodium cyanide are ingested, the lethal dose appears to be 50 to 100 mg., and the rapidity of the lethal effect is dependent on the dose swallowed and the speed of gastrointestinal absorption, which is in turn influenced by the nature of the gastric contents.

In acute cyanide poisoning, death occurs suddenly, usually with terminal convulsions. In less severe cases gastrointestinal disturbances may be present, with or without convulsions. There is no agreement on the existence of chronic cyanide poisoning. Workers exposed to cyanide in industry may complain of a variety of gastrointestinal and neurologic disturbances. Dermatitis also occurs.

Cyanide poisoning can be treated very effectively if there is opportunity for almost immediate therapy after the poison has been swallowed. In addition to gastric lavage for removal of unabsorbed cyanide, therapy is aimed at binding and inactivating the poison.

It has been shown that methemoglobin has great affinity for cyanide, forming cyanmethemoglobin.[3] Methemoglobin can be produced by inhalation of amyl nitrite and intravenous injection of about 300 mg. of sodium nitrite in a 3% solution. If this is followed by intravenous injection of sodium thiosulfate, 12.5 to 25 Gm. in a 25% solution, it is possible to protect the individual against several lethal doses of cyanide. This combined treatment could protect dogs against as many as twenty lethal doses of sodium cyanide.

Other measures such as artificial respiration and vasoconstrictors are also important, and the antidotes may have to be given repeatedly if symptoms recur.

HEAVY METAL POISONING

Many of the metals in common economic usage have adverse effects on the environment and health. Most troublesome of these are the "heavy metals" such as lead and mercury. These metals in their elemental form are generally not absorbed from the gastrointestinal tract. Their salts, however, may be rapidly absorbed and cause poisoning. They may enter the body also through the skin and by inhalation.

The heavy metals, in general, have an affinity for sulfhydryl groups, which are essential in many enzyme systems. Although the symptoms of metal intoxication depend on the particular metal, as a generalization it may be stated that the kidneys, gastrointestinal tract, and brain are commonly affected.

The insidiousness of metal poisoning is well exemplified by the current concern with the environmental effects of mercury. This metal was considered quite inert in its elemental form until recently. It was generally believed that if mercury were discharged into water it would settle and remain quite harmless at the bottom. In 1960 it was reported that 111 people died or suffered neurologic damage in Minamata, Japan, as a consequence of eating shellfish contaminated by mercury discharged into the bay by a plastics manufacturer. Swedish studies have shown that metallic mercury can be changed by bacteria into methyl mercury that can enter the food cycle and become concentrated a thousandfold in fish. In 1970 high levels of mercury were discovered in fish in the United States. This creates considerable concern because the organic mercurials may accumulate in the vital organs of man.

Arsenicals containing trivalent arsenic were widely used in the treatment of syphilis in the recent past. Neoarsphenamine and oxophenarsine (Mapharsen) were most important. Toxic effects from administration of trivalent arsenicals consist of nitritoid reactions, liver damage, neuritis, and bone marrow depression. The antidote is dimercaprol.

Pentavalent arsenicals such as tryparsamide were also used in some types of syphilis. Carbarsone is still used by mouth in the treatment of amebiasis. On a weight basis, the pentavalent compounds are much less toxic than the trivalent arsenicals. They are only moderately well absorbed from the intestine and are slowly changed in the body to trivalent arsenicals. Dimercaprol is the best antidote for poisoning caused by any arsenical.

Bismuth compounds have also been used in the treatment of syphilis. Bismuth subsalicylate in oil given by intramuscular injection was popular but is now obsolete. Bismuth subcarbonate is sometimes used by mouth in doses of 1 to 3 Gm. in the treatment of diarrhea. It is not absorbed significantly from the intestine. Bismuth subnitrate was also employed for this purpose but was abandoned because nitrite poisoning with methemoglobinemia could occur as a consequence of bacterial action on bismuth subnitrate. Bismuth poisoning is characterized by stomatitis and by renal and hepatic damage. Dimercaprol is of questionable value as an antidote.

Mercurials are now obsolete for the treatment of syphilis. They are still used as diuretics and as disinfectants and antiseptics. Mercurial poisoning is characterized by stomatitis, kidney damage to the point of anuria, and damage to the intestinal mucosa. The antidote is dimercaprol. The environmental role of mercury is of great current concern.

Antimonials such as antimony potassium tartrate (tartar emetic) and stibophen (Fuadin) are still used in the treatment of schistosomiasis and some other tropical diseases. The toxicity of antimony is similar to that of arsenic. Dimercaprol is of questionable antidotal value in cases of poisoning caused by these metals.

Thallium is employed as a rodenticide and ant poison. Ingestion leads to serious poisoning, of which loss of hair is a characteristic feature. The usual metal-binding antidotes are ineffective in thallium poisoning.

Lead poisoning

Lead poisoning is usually a chronic occupational disease. Acute poisoning, characterized by encephalopathy, is a rare disorder and may occur in children and also in young adults who are exposed to a large dose of lead compounds. Dimercaprol in combination with calcium disodium edetate may be useful as an antidote.

The most common symptoms and signs in lead poisoning are abdominal pain (lead colic), weakness, gingival lead line, pyorrhea, and muscle weakness of the extensors of the wrists. In addition, anemia, porphyrinuria, and stippling of erythrocytes can be demonstrated, and vague cerebral disturbances occur.

The smooth muscle contraction in lead colic is generally attributed to an effect of lead on this tissue. Some studies indicate that lead has a profound influence on porphyrin metabolism, and it is of interest that in porphyria abdominal pain is common. Coproporphyrin III has been found in large quantities in the urine of patients with lead poisoning.[9]

The most important drug in treatment of lead poisoning is calcium disodium edetate. Prior to the introduction of this drug, treatment of lead poisoning was dominated by certain concepts of induced deposition of lead in bones and mobilization of lead from these storage sites (so-called *deleading*).

MISCELLANEOUS POISONS
Chlorinated hydrocarbon insecticides

A variety of chlorinated hydrocarbons are used as insecticides. Some of these are chlorophenothane (DDT), chlordane, hexachlorocyclohexane (lindane), dieldrin, and others. These insecticides may be absorbed when ingested. Being lipid soluble, they can penetrate through the skin. They are stored in body fat. Large doses of these compounds produce convulsions and death. Smaller amounts may cause tremors and hyperirritability.

Although the acute toxicity of the chlorinated insecticides is not very great (their lethal dose being of the order of 50 to 300 mg./kg. in animals), there is some concern over the cumulation of these compounds in body fat and their possible adverse chronic effects on health and/or environment. The cumulation of these compounds in body fat is not unlimited, since their slow degradation eventually will keep up with their entry into the body. As a consequence, the concentration in human fat has become stabilized at levels of about 10 parts per million of DDT and metabolites. The effect of these insecticides on the environment, however, may be considerable, affecting not only insects but also birds that feed on the insects.

Organophosphorus compounds

The organophosphorus compounds are used as insecticides. Their ability to inhibit cholinesterase and the antidotal action of atropine pralidoxime were discussed in Chapter 7.

Organic solvents

The complex aliphatic hydrocarbons contained in kerosene, gasoline, and industrial solvents may cause anesthesia and respiratory depression when inhaled in high concentrations. They may also cause acute pneumonitis when swallowed.

The halogenated aliphatic hydrocarbons can also act as anesthetics and may cause death as a consequence of respiratory depression and cardiovascular collapse. In addition, most halogenated hydrocarbons can damage the liver and the kidneys. Carbon tetrachloride is an important cause of hepatic damage. Evidence is increasing that this is a direct action on the liver cells.

It is of great interest that mammalian tissues can reduce carbon tetrachloride to chloroform to some extent.[2] Also, chloroform is reduced to methylene chloride, at least in vitro. There may be a connection between the hepatotoxicity of the alkyl halides and their metabolic handling.

Nicotine

Nicotine is used as an insecticide. Its poisonous properties are characterized by nausea, vomiting, and initial rise of blood pressure caused by ganglionic stimulation and norepinephrine release, followed by ganglionic paralysis with fall of blood pressure. Death results from respiratory paralysis. Thromboangiitis and tobacco amblyopia have been attributed to chronic nicotine poisoning.

Treatment of nicotine poisoning is supportive, with emphasis on artificial respiration. There is no specific antidote for nicotine.

References

1 Adams, D. A., Goldman, R., Maxwell, M. H., and Latta, H.: Nephrotic syndrome associated with penicillamine therapy of Wilson's disease, Amer. J. Med. **36**:330, 1964.

2 Butler, T. C.: Reduction of carbon tetrachloride in vivo and reduction of carbon tetrachloride and chloroform in vitro by tissues and tissue constituents, J. Pharmacol. Exp. Ther. **134**:311, 1961.

3 Chen, K. K., and Rose, C. L.: Nitrite and thiosulfate therapy in cyanide poisoning, J.A.M.A. **149**:113, 1952.

4 Foreman, H., Finnigan, C., and Lushbaugh, C. C.: Nephrotoxic hazard from uncontrolled edathamil calcium-disodium therapy, J.A.M.A. **160**:1042, 1956.

5 Kehoe, R. A.: Misuse of edathamil calcium-disodium for prophylaxis of lead poisoning, J.A.M.A. **157**:341, 1955.

6 Mandelbaum, J. M., and Simon, N. M.: Severe methyprylon intoxication treated by hemodialysis, J.A.M.A. **216**:139, 1971.

7 Milthers, E.: Poisoning in childhood, Danish Med. Bull. **10**:132, 1963.

8 Murphy, J. V.: Intoxication following the ingestion of elemental zinc, J.A.M.A. **212**:2119, 1970.

9 Parkinson, E. S., and Cholak, J.: Problems in the analysis of urinary coproporphyrin III, Industr. Hyg. Quart. **13**:158, 1952.

10 Penneys, N. S., Israel, R. M., and Indgin, S. M.: Contact dermatitis due to 1-chloroacetophenone and chemical mace, New Eng. J. Med. **281**:413, 1969.

11 Peterson, D. I., Peterson, J. E., Hardinge, M. G., and Wacker, W. E. C.: Experimental treatment of ethylene glycol poisoning, J.A.M.A. **186**:955 1963.

12 Stocken, L. A., and Thompson, R. H. S.: Reactions of British anti-lewisite with arsenic and other metals in living systems, Physiol. Rev. **29**:168, 1949.

13 Von Oettingen, W. F.: Poisoning: a guide to clinical diagnosis and treatment, Philadelphia, 1958, W. B. Saunders Co.

Recent reviews

14 Arena, J. M.: Treatment of some common household poisonings, Pharmacol. Physicians **3**(9):1, 1969.

15 Castell, D. O., and Morrison, C. C.: Common adult poisons, Resident Physician **13**:66, 1967.

16 Clemmesen, C.: Treatment of narcotic intoxication. Results and principles of the "Scandinavian" method, especially concerning stimulation, Danish Med. Bull. **10**:132, 1963.

17 Dimijian, G. G., and Radelat, F. A.: Evaluation and treatment of the suspected drug user in the emergency room, Arch. Intern Med. 125:162, 1970.

18 Done, A. K.: Clinical pharmacology of systemic antidotes, Clin. Pharmacol. Ther. 2:750, 1961.

19 Done, A. K.: Pharmacologic principles in the treatment of poisoning, Pharmacol. Physicians 3(7):1, 1969.

20 Gosselin, R. E., and Smith, R. P.: Trends in the therapy of acute poisonings, Clin. Pharmacol. Ther. 7:279, 1966.

21 Hollister, L. E.: Overdoses of psychotherapeutic drugs, Clin. Pharmacol. Ther. 7:142, 1966.

22 Lamanna, C., and Carr, J. C.: The botulinal, tetanal, and enterostaphylococcal toxins: A review, Clin. Pharmacol. Ther. 8:286, 1967.

23 Maher, J. F.: Nephrotoxicity of drugs and chemicals, Pharmacol. Physicians 4:1, 1970.

24 Medved, L. I., and Kagan, J. S.: Toxicology, Ann. Rev. Pharmacol. 6:293, 1966.

25 Modell, W.: Drug-induced diseases, Ann. Rev. Pharmacol. 5:285, 1965.

26 Pathak, M. A., and Fitzpatrick, T. B.: Photosensitivity caused by drugs, Rational Drug Ther. 6:1, June, 1972.

27 Russell, F. E.: Pharmacology of animal venoms, Clin. Pharmacol. Ther. 8:849, 1967.

28 Schreiner, G. E.: Dialysis of poisons and drugs —annual review, Trans. Amer. Soc. Artif. Organs 16:544, 1970.

29 Sherlock, S.: Hepatic reactions to therapeutic agents, Ann. Rev. Pharmacol. 5:429, 1965.

30 Zavon, M. R., Hine, C. H., and Parker, K. D.: Chlorinated hydrocarbon insecticides in human body fat in the United States, J.A.M.A. 193:181, 1965.

31 Zbinden, G.: Experimental and clinical aspects of drug toxicity, Advances Pharmacol. 2:1, 1963.

SECTION TWELVE

DRUG INTERACTIONS

58 Drug interactions

Discussions on drug interactions often begin with frightening statistics on the large number of drugs taken by most patients and the dire consequences that may result from drug interactions. What is usually not mentioned is the justification for using several drugs concomitantly in many patients, the beneficial nature of many drug interactions, and the uncritical manner in which many supposedly adverse drug interactions are reported in the literature.

The uninitiated could get the impression when examining large and complex tables of drug interactions that the problem is not only vast but is almost beyond the ability of the physician to handle. What is often not recognized is that the majority of interactions listed in such tables are trivial and create no problems to the physician, who adjusts dosages to the patient's needs and is alert to any adverse effects.

The clinically significant drug interactions can be minimized by avoiding combinations of drugs known to be incompatible according to the current pharmacologic literature and tables of drug interactions such as the one presented in this chapter. It should be possible to develop systems in hospital pharmacies that would prevent the dispensing of incompatible drugs. Ultimately, however, it is the physician's familiarity with the current clinical literature and his understanding of the mechanisms underlying drug interactions that are more likely to prevent their occurrence.

Adverse drug reactions based on drug interactions are not always iatrogenic. Self-medication with over-the-counter drugs may be a contributing factor. In addition, environmental contaminants such as the chlorinated insecticides (DDT) may stimulate drug metabolism by hepatic microsomal enzymes and could conceivably contribute to unusual reactions to drugs.

MECHANISMS UNDERLYING ADVERSE EFFECTS OF DRUG INTERACTIONS

A drug may influence the effect of another drug by several different mechanisms. The influences may be exerted on (1) intestinal absorption, (2) competition for plasma protein binding, (3) metabolism or biotransformation, (4) adrenergic neuronal uptake, (5) action at the receptor site, (6) renal excretion, and (7) alteration of electrolyte balance.

Intestinal absorption. Antacids that contain calcium, magnesium, or aluminum interfere with the absorption of tetracycline, which forms a chelate with the metals. Aluminum-containing antacids interfere with the absorption of phosphate. Carbonates and phytates (cereals) prevent the absorption of iron. Cholestyramine may interfere with the absorption of phenylbutazone, warfarin,[82] and thyroxine.

Antacids may influence drug absorption also by changing the lipid-soluble non-ionized moiety of weak acids and bases in the gastrointestinal tract. It should be recalled (p. 18) that the lipid-soluble, nonionized fraction is much better absorbed. Because of this, antacids would be expected to diminish the absorption of weak acids such as phenylbutazone, nitrofurantoin, sulfonamides, and some barbiturates and oral anticoagulants.

Other gastrointestinal drug interactions may be of clinical significance. Antibiotics that alter the bacterial flora in the intestine may decrease the formation of vitamin K and thus increase the anticoagulant action of the coumarins. Folate deficiency may result from the use of drugs which inhibit the intestinal conjugase that breaks down the polyglutamate portion of the naturally occurring folic acid. By this mechanism, megaloblastic anemia may result in some patients after the use of diphenylhydantoin or triamterene. Mineral oil may interfere with the absorption of vitamin D.

Direct chemical interactions may occur not only in the gastrointestinal tract but also when drugs are mixed for intravenous infusions. Unstable drugs such as methicillin or levarterenol should not be mixed with other drugs without consideration of possible direct drug interactions. Carbenicillin inactivates gentamicin when mixed for intravenous infusion.

Competition for plasma protein binding. Many drugs are bound to plasma proteins to varying degrees, and the bound fraction fails to exert pharmacologic effects. For example, two antibiotics having the same potency in a protein-free culture medium will have vastly different clinical effectiveness if their affinities for plasma proteins differ greatly.[3,37]

Certain drugs compete for the same binding sites on plasma proteins. As a consequence, one drug may displace another, thus increasing the latter's free fraction and pharmacologic effectiveness. Tolbutamide can be displaced from its plasma binding by bishydroxycoumarin, resulting in severe hypoglycemia.[36,58,61] Chloral hydrate increases the anticoagulant action of warfarin because its metabolite, trichloroacetic acid, competes with the anticoagulant for plasma protein binding.[56]

Metabolism or biotransformation. The inhibition of the metabolism of one drug by another is a well-established mechanism of enhanced drug effect.[70] By their enzyme-inhibiting action, the anticholinesterases enhance the actions by acetylcholine, succinylcholine, and some other choline esters. Allopurinol inhibits xanthine oxidase and thus increases the plasma levels of mercaptopurine and azathioprine. The MAO inhibitors have caused severe reactions by preventing the destruction of tyramine in the body.[75,82,85]

Many drugs can accelerate their metabolism and also that of other drugs by induction of hepatic microsomal enzymes (p. 28). Phenobarbital accelerates the metabolism of coumarin anticoagulants, diphenylhydantoin, griseofulvin, cortisol, estrogens, androgens, and progesterone. In addition to the barbiturates, gluthetimide, diphenylhydantoin, and the chlorinated hydrocarbon insecticides such as DDT are enhancers of drug metabolism (p. 675).

Enzyme induction by phenobarbital and other drugs not only leads to a decreased effectiveness of drugs. It may also result in catastrophes when the inducer is discontinued without changing the dose of the second drug. For example, if phenobarbital is suddenly discontinued without lowering the dosage of a coumarin anticoagulant, severe hemorrhagic episodes may develop (Fig. 4-3).

Adrenergic neuronal uptake. Amphetamine and guanethidine are transported by the same mechanism across the adrenergic neuronal membrane. Because of this, amphetamine may prevent the antihypertensive action of guanethidine. The tricyclic antidepressants have a "cocainelike" blocking effect on the amine uptake mechanism and may nullify the antihypertensive effect of guanethidine by preventing its uptake into the adrenergic neuron.[26, 40, 44, 82]

Action at the receptor site. The numerous examples of additive effects or various antagonisms resulting from action at the receptor site do not represent great problems if the drugs are administered by persons well versed in pharmacology (p. 11).

Renal excretion. There are several interesting examples of drug interactions resulting from an influence on renal tubular reabsorption. The best example, of course, is the inhibition of penicillin excretion by probenecid. Interference in the uricosuric action of probenecid by small doses of salicylates and the promotion of phenobarbital clearance after sodium bicarbonate administration are other examples of one drug's influencing the renal excretion of another.

Acidification of the urine after the oral administration of ammonium chloride or alkalinization following sodium bicarbonate may have a demonstrable effect on the renal clearance of several drugs, but the quantitative importance of such knowledge in therapeutics is not great except in phenobarbital poisoning.

Alteration of electrolyte balance. A drug may alter the concentration of many different constituents of the body, thus influencing the action of another drug. Some of the best examples originate from the area of fluid and electrolyte balance. Hypokalemia caused by the thiazide diuretics promotes arrhythmias when digitalis compounds are employed. Ammonium chloride administration reestablishes the effectiveness of mercurial diuretics when blunted by metabolic alkalosis.

The sudden release of catecholamines by reserpine may precipitate arrhythmias in a patient who has been on digitalis therapy. A patient treated with MAO inhibitors is vulnerable to drugs such as amphetamine that cause release of catecholamines from nerve endings because the concentration of the catecholamines at these stores is elevated and more is available for release.

INTERACTIONS IN VARIOUS DRUG CATEGORIES

Most drug interactions present themselves in therapeutics as either an enhanced or diminished drug effect. The enhanced drug effects may manifest themselves as idiosyncratic responses that may occasionally have catastrophic consequences (Table 58-1).

Diminished responses resulting from drug interactions are generally not very dra-

Table 58-1. Clinically observed adverse effects based on drug interactions

Major symptoms	Drugs involved
Hypertensive crisis	MAO inhibitors + tyramine (cheese)
	MAO inhibitors + methamphetamine
Hemorrhagic episodes	Warfarin + phenylbutazone
	Warfarin + phenyramidol
Respiratory paralysis	Neomycin + succinylcholine
	Neomycin + ether
Hypoglycemic reaction	Tolbutamide + phenylbutazone
	Tolbutamide + sulfisoxazole
Cardiac arrhythmias	Digitalis + chlorothiazide
	Digitalis + reserpine

matic. It can happen, however, that manipulations of dosage necessitated by drug interactions may have serious consequences when one of the drugs is discontinued without simultaneous adjustment of the dosage of the other drug. For example, chloral hydrate stimulates the metabolism of several coumarin anticoagulants.[14] If the dosage of the coumarin is increased over a period of several days and then chloral hydrate is suddenly discontinued, the anticoagulant effect may become excessive and bleeding will follow. But the interactions of chloral hydrate with the oral anticoagulants may be more complex than previously thought. The metabolic product of chloral hydrate, trichloroacetic acid, interferes with the binding of warfarin to plasma proteins. Increased anticoagulation may result,[56,78] which is the opposite of the interaction resulting from increased metabolism of bishydroxycoumarin just described.

The clinically significant drug interactions are listed in Table 58-2 along with their probable mechanisms. The table is only a quick survey, and for details the original references should be consulted.

Table 58-2. Clinically significant drug interactions

First drug	Second drug(s)	Possible result	Mechanism*
Analgesics			
Aspirin	Anticoagulant	Enhanced anticoagulation	2
	Sulfonylureas	Enhanced hypoglycemia	2
	p-Aminosalicylate	PAS toxicity	2
	Probenecid	Decreased uricosuria	6
Phenylbutazone	Anticoagulant	Enhanced anticoagulation	2
	Sulfonylurea	Enhanced hypoglycemia	2, 3
	Estrogen, androgen	Decreased hormonal effects	3
Phenyramidol	Anticoagulant	Enhanced anticoagulation	3
Morphine	Phenothiazine	Enhanced analgesia	5
Meperidine	Atropine	Enhanced atropine effect	5
Propoxyphene	Amphetamine	Enhanced amphetamine effect	5
Anticoagulants			
Coumarin drugs	Aspirin, acetaminophen, clofibrate, phenylbutazone, indomethacin, methyldopa, methylphenidate, quinidine	Enhanced anticoagulation	2
	Barbiturates, glutethimide, griseofulvin, meprobamate	Decreased anticoagulant effect	3
	Chloral hydrate	Increased or decreased anticoagulant effect	2, 3
	Vitamin K	Decreased anticoagulant effect	5
Heparin	Polymyxin	Incompatibility in IV solution	8
Antimicrobials			
Aminoglycosides	d-Tubocurarine	Enhanced tubocurarine effect	5

*Mechanisms: 1 = interference with gastrointestinal absorption; 2 = plasma protein binding competition; 3 = metabolism or biotransformation; 3a = enzyme induction; 4 = adrenergic neuronal uptake; 4a = depletion of catecholamines at adrenergic neuron; 5 = action at receptor site or related to end-organ response; 6 = renal excretion; 7 = alteration of electrolyte balance; 8 = direct combination; 9 = inhibition of protein synthesis.

Table 58-2. Clinically significant drug interactions — cont'd

First drug	Second drug(s)	Possible result	Mecha-nism*
Cephalothin	Barbiturates, erythromycin, tetracycline	Incompatibility in IV solution	8
Chloramphenicol	Barbiturates, diphenyl-hydantoin,	Enhanced sedation	3
	Anticoagulants	Enhanced anticoagulation	3
	Penicillin	Antibiotic antagonism (some infections)	5
	Diphtheria or tetanus toxoid	Decreased immune response	9
Furazolidine	Amphetamine, methyldopa, sympatho-mimetics, tyramine	Hypertension, excitement	3
Griseofulvin	Phenobarbital	Decreased phenobarbital effect	3
Penicillin G	Sulfonamides, tetracycline	Antibiotic antagonism (some infections)	5
Polymyxin B	d-Tubocurarine, succinylcholine	Muscle paralysis	5
Sulfonamides	Aspirin, phenylbutazone	Sulfonamide toxicity	2
	Anticoagulants	Enhanced anticoagulation	2
	Sulfonylureas	Enhanced hypoglycemia	2
Tetracycline	Antacids	Decreased absorption	1
Antihistamines			
Antihistaminic drugs	Alcohol, reserpine, phenothiazines	Enhanced sedation	5
	Atropine	Enhanced atropine effects	5
Anticonvulsants			
Diphenylhydantoin	Bishydroxycoumarin, chloramphenicol, methylphenidate, phenyramidol	Enhanced diphenylhydantoin effect	3
	Phenobarbital	Decreased diphenyl-hydantoin effect	3
Antidepressants			
MAO inhibitors	Tyramine, amphetamine, levodopa, methyldopa, sympathomimetics	Hypertension, excitement	3
Tricyclic drugs	Guanethidine	Decreased guanethidine effect	4
	MAO inhibitor	Enhanced MAO inhibitor toxicity	5
	Phenothiazines, antianxiety drugs	Additive effect	5
Antihypertensives			
Guanethidine	Sympathomimetics, amphetamine	Hypertensive crisis	4
	Levarterenol	Enhanced levarterenol effect	4
	Tricyclic antidepressants	Decreased guanethidine effect	4

Continued.

Table 58-2. Clinically significant drug interactions — cont'd

First drug	Second drug(s)	Possible result	Mecha-nism*
Methyldopa	Sympathomimetics	Decreased methyldopa effect	5
Pargyline (same as MAO inhibitors)	MAO inhibitors	Decreased methyldopa effect	3
Reserpine	Sympathomimetics, tricyclic drugs	Decreased reserpine effect	5
	Indirect sympathomimetics, metaraminol	Decreased metaraminol effect	4a
	Anesthetic	Hypotension	4a
	Levarterenol	Enhanced levarterenol effect	5
Antineoplastic agents			
Mercaptopurine	Allopurinol	Enhanced mercaptopurine effect	3
Methotrexate	Aspirin, sulfonamides	Enhanced methotrexate toxicity	2
Digitalis			
Digitalis preparations	Thiazides, calcium	Digitalis toxicity	7
	Reserpine	Arrhythmias	5
	Phenobarbital	Decreased digitalis effect	3a
Diuretics			
Thiazides	Digitalis	Digitalis toxicity	7
	Antihypertensive drugs	Enhanced antihypertensive effect	5
	Sulfonylureas	Antagonism of hypoglycemia	5
	Curare drugs	Enhanced curare effects	7
Mercurials	Ammonium chloride	Enhanced diuresis	7
	Alkalinizing agents	Decreased diuresis	7
Ethacrynic acid	Aminoglycosides	Ototoxicity	5
Antianxiety and antipsychotic drugs			
Benzodiazepines	Alcohol, hypnotics, phenothiazines, tricyclic antidepressants	Enhanced sedation	5
Phenothiazines	Alcohol, hypnotics, narcotics, antihistamines, tricyclic antidepressants	Enhanced sedation	5
	Antihypertensives	Enhanced antihypertensive effect	5
	Convulsants	Lowered convulsive threshold	5
Hormones			
Insulin	Oral hypoglycemics, propranolol, MAO inhibitors	Enhanced hypoglycemic effect	5
Corticosteroids	Barbiturates, diphenyl-hydantoin, antihista-mines	Decreased corticosteroid effect	3a
Estrogens, progestogens	Androgens	Antagonism of androgen anticancer effect	5
	Clofibrate	Decreased hypocholestero-lemic effect	3

Table 58-2. Clinically significant drug interactions—cont'd

First drug	Second drug(s)	Possible result	Mecha-nism*
Hypnotics			
Phenobarbital	Anticoagulants, diphenyl-hydantoin, griseofulvin, hypnotics, cortico-steroids	Decreased drug effects	3a
	Alcohol, phenothiazines, antianxiety drugs	Enhanced sedation	5
Chloral hydrate	Alcohol	Enhanced sedation	5
	Anticoagulant	Increased or decreased anticoagulant effect	2, 3
Uricoscuric agents			
Probenecid	Aspirin, ethacrynic acid	Decreased uricosuria	5
	Penicillin	Enhanced penicillin levels	5

SIGNIFICANCE OF ADVERSE DRUG REACTIONS

Some drug interactions such as those in Table 58-1 may be life-threatening, whereas others are unimportant and require only a simple adjustment in the dosage. An important determinant of the seriousness of an interaction is the therapeutic margin of the drugs involved. With anticoagulants, oral hypoglycemic drugs, digitalis, and antiarrhythmic drugs the margin of safety is not great, and relatively small changes in plasma concentration resulting from drug interactions could have catastrophic effects. On the other hand, drugs with great margins of safety do not cause serious problems as a consequence of drug interactions. This principle should be kept in mind when examining large tables of drug interactions.

References

1 Aggeler, P. M., O'Reilly, R. A., Leong, L., and Kowitz, P. E.: Potentiation of anticoagulant effect of warfarin by phenylbutazone, New Eng. J. Med. **276**:496, 1967.

2 Antilitz, A. M., Tolentino, M., and Kosai, M. F.: Effect of butabarbital on orally administered anticoagulants, Curr. Ther. Res. **10**:70, 1968.

3 Anton, A. H.: The relation between the binding of sulfonamides to albumin and their antibacterial efficacy, J. Pharmacol. Exp. Ther. **129**:282, 1960.

4 Asatoor, A. M., Levi, A. J., and Milne, M. D.: Tranylcypromine and cheese, Lancet **2**:733, 1963.

5 Blackwell, B.: Hypertensive crisis due to monoamine-oxidase inhibitors, Lancet **2**:849, 1963.

6 Blackwell, B., Marley, E., and Ryle, A.: Hypertensive crisis associated with monoamine-oxidase inhibitors, Lancet **1**:722, 1964.

7 Brachfeld, J., Wirtshafter, A., and Wolfe, S.: Imipramine-tranylcypromine incompatibility; near-fatal toxic reaction, J.A.M.A. **186**:1172, 1963.

8 Busfield, D., Child, K. J., Atkinson, R. M., and Tomich, E. G.: An effect of phenobarbitone on blood-levels of griseofulvin in man, Lancet **2**:1042, 1963.

9 Carter, S. A.: Potentiation of the effect of orally administered anticoagulants by phenyramidol hydrochloride, New Eng. J. Med. **273**:423, 1965.

10 Catalano, P. M., and Cullen, S. I.: Warfarin antagonism by griseofulvin, Clin. Res. **14**:266, 1966.

11 Chen, W., Vrindten, P. A., Dayton, P. G., and Burns, J. J.: Accelerated aminopyrine metabolism in human subjects pretreated with phenylbutazone, Life Sci. **1**:35, 1962.

12 Christensen, L. K., Hansen, J. M., and Kristensen, M.: Sulphaphenazole-induced hypogly-

caemic attacks in tolbutamide-treated diabetics, Lancet 2:1298, 1963.

13 Cucinell, S. A., Conney, A. H., Sansur, M., and Burns, J. J.: Drug interactions in man. I. Lowering effect of phenobarbital on plasma levels of bishydroxycoumarin (Dicumarol) and diphenylhydantoin (Dilantin), Clin. Pharmacol. Ther. 6:420, 1965.

14 Cucinell, S. A., Odessky, L., Weiss, M., and Dayton, P. G.: The effect of chloral hydrate on bishydroxycoumarin metabolism, J.A.M.A. 197: 366, 1966.

15 Cullen, S. I., and Catalano, P. M.: Griseofulvin-warfarin antagonism, J.A.M.A. 199:582, 1967.

16 Dayton, P. G., Tarcan, Y., Chenkin, T., and Weiner, M.: The influence of barbiturates on coumarin plasma levels and prothrombin response, J. Clin. Invest. 40:1797, 1961.

17 Domino, E. F., Sullivan, T. S., and Luby, E. D.: Barbiturate intoxication in a patient treated with a MAO inhibitor, Amer. J. Psychiat. 118:941, 1962.

18 Eisen, M. J.: Combined effect of sodium warfarin and phenylbutazone, J.A.M.A. 189:64, 1964.

19 Elis, J., Laurence, D. R., Mattie, H., and Prichard, B. N. C.: Modification by monoamine oxidase inhibitors of the effect of some sympathomimetics on blood pressure, Brit. Med. J. 2:75, 1967.

20 Field, J. B., Ohta, M., Boyle, C., and Remer, A.: Potentiation of acetohexamide hypoglycemia by phenylbutazone, New Eng. J. Med. 277:889, 1967.

21 Fox, S. L.: Potentiation of anticoagulants caused by pyrazole compounds, J.A.M.A. 188:320, 1964.

22 Garrettson, L. K., Perel, J. M., and Dayton, P. G.: Methylphenidate interaction with both anticonvulsants and ethyl biscoumacetate, J.A.M.A. 207:2053, 1969.

23 Gessner, P. K.: Antagonism of the tranylcypromine-meperidine interaction by chlorpromazine in mice, Europ. J. Pharmacol. 22:187, 1973.

24 Goldberg, L. I.: Monamine oxidase inhibitors, J.A.M.A. 190:456, 1964.

25 Goss, J. E., and Dickhaus, D. W.: Increased bishydroxycoumarin requirements in patients receiving phenobarbital, New Eng. J. Med. 273:1094, 1965.

26 Gulati, O. D., Dave, B. T., Gokhale, S. D., and Shah, K. M.: Antagonism of adrenergic neuron blockade in hypertensive subjects, Clin. Pharmacol. Ther. 7:510, 1966.

27 Hansen, J. M., Kristensen, M., Skovsted, L., and Christensen, L. K.: Dicoumarol-induced diphenylhydantoin intoxication, Lancet 2:265, 1966.

28 Hodge, J. V., Nye, E. R., and Emerson, G. W.: Monoamine-oxidase inhibitors, broad beans, and hypertension, Lancet 1:1108, 1964.

29 Horwitz, D., Goldberg, L. I., and Sjoerdsma, A.: Increased blood pressure responses to dopamine and norepinephrine produced by monoamine oxidase inhibitors in man, J. Lab. Clin. Med. 56:747, 1960.

30 Horwitz, D., Lovenberg, W., Engelman, K., and Sjoerdsma, A.: Monoamine oxidase inhibitors, tyramine, and cheese, J.A.M.A. 188:1108, 1964.

31 Hunninghake, D. B., and Azarnoff, D. L.: Drug interactions with warfarin, Arch. Intern. Med. 121:349, 1968.

32 Jawetz, E.: The use of combinations of antimicrobial drugs, Ann. Rev. Pharmacol. 8:151, 1968.

33 Kane, F. J., and Taylor, T. W.: A toxic reaction to combined Elavil-Librium therapy, Amer. J. Psychiat. 119:1179, 1963.

34 Kinoshita, F. K., Frawley, J. P., and DuBois, K. P.: Quantitative measurement of induction of hepatic microsomal enzymes by various dietary levels of DDT and toxaphene in rats, Toxic. Appl. Pharmacol. 9:505, 1966.

35 Koch-Weser, J.: Quinidine-induced hypoprothrombinemic hemorrhage in patients on chronic warfarin therapy, Ann. Intern. Med. 68:511, 1968.

36 Kristensen, M., and Hansen, J. M.: Potentiation of the tolbutamide effect by dicumarol, Diabetes 16:211, 1967.

37 Kunin, C. M.: Clinical pharmacology of the new penicillins. II. Effect of drugs which interfere with binding to serum proteins, Clin. Pharmacol. Ther. 7:180, 1966.

38 Landauer, A. A., Milner, G., and Patman, J.: Alcohol and amitriptyline effects on skills related to driving behavior, Science 163:1467, 1969.

39 Lees, F., and Burke, C. W.: Tranylcypromine, Lancet 1:13, 1963.

40 Leishman, A. W. D., Mathews, H. C., and Smith, A. J.: Antagonism of guanethidine by imipramine, Lancet 1:112, 1963.

41 MacDonald, M. G., and Robinson, D. S.: Clinical observations of possible barbiturate interference with anticoagulation, J.A.M.A. 204:97, 1968.

42 MacDonald, M. G., Robinson, D. S., Sylvester, D., and Jaffe, J. J.: The effects of phenobarbital, chloral betaine, and glutethimide administration on warfarin plasma levels and hypoprothrombinemic responses in man, Clin. Pharmacol. Ther. 10:80, 1969.

43 Mason, A.: Fatal reaction associated with tra-

nylcypromine and methylamphetamine, Lancet 1:1073, 1962.

44 Mitchell, J. R., Arias, L., and Oates, J. A.: Antagonism of the antihypertensive action of guanethidine sulfate by desipramine hydrochloride, J.A.M.A. 202:973, 1967.

45 Nour-Eldin, F., and Lewis, F. J. W.: Tolerance to phenindione of patients with different thromboembolic disorders, Acta Haemat. 32:338, 1964.

46 Oakley, D. P., and Lautch, H.: Haloperidol and anticoagulant treatment, Lancet 2:1231, 1963.

47 Odell, G. B.: Studies in kernicterus. I. The protein binding of bilirubin, J. Clin. Invest. 38: 823, 1959.

48 Olesen, O. V.: The influence of disulfiram and calcium carbimide on the serum diphenylhydantoin, Arch. Neurol. 16:642, 1967.

49 Oliver, M. F., Roberts, S. D., Hayes, D., Pantridge, J. F., Suzman, M. M., and Bersohn, I.: Effect of atromid and ethyl chlorophenoxyisobutyrate on anticoagulant requirements, Lancet 1:143, 1963.

50 Owens, J. C., Neely, W. B., and Owen, W. R.: Effect of sodium dextrothyroxine in patients receiving anticoagulants, New Eng. J. Med. 266:76, 1962.

51 Penlington, G. N.: Droperidol and monoamine-oxidase inhibitors, Brit. Med. J. 1:483, 1966.

52 Pettinger, W. A., Soyangco, F. G., and Oates, J. A.: Inhibition of monoamine oxidase in man by furazolidone, Clin. Pharmacol. Ther. 9:442, 1968.

53 Pyörälä, K., and Kekki, M.: Decreased anticoagulant tolerance during methandrostenolone therapy, Scand. J. Clin. Lab. Invest. 15:367, 1963.

54 Robinson, D. S., and MacDonald, M. G.: The effect of phenobarbital administration on the control of coagulation achieved during warfarin therapy in man, J. Pharmacol. Exp. Ther. 153:250, 1966.

55 Schrogie, J. J., and Solomon, H. M.: The anticoagulant response to bishydroxycoumarin. II. The effect of D-thyroxine, clofibrate, and norethandrolone, Clin. Pharmacol. Ther. 8:70, 1967.

56 Sellers, E. M., and Koch-Weser, J.: Potentiation of warfarin-induced hypoprothrombinemia by chloral hydrate, New Eng. J. Med. 283:828, 1970.

57 Shapiro, S., Redish, M. H., and Campbell, H. A.: The prothrombinopenic effect of salicylate in man, Proc. Soc. Exp. Biol. Med. 53:251, 1943.

58 Silverman, W. A., Anderson, D. H., Blanc, W. A., and Crozier, D. N.: A difference in mortality rate and incidence of kernicterus among premature infants allotted to two prophylactic antibacterial regimens, Pediatrics 18:614, 1956.

59 Solomon, H. M., and Schrogie, J. J.: The effect of phenyramidol on the metabolism of bishydroxycoumarin, J. Pharmacol. Exp. Ther. 154: 660, 1966.

60 Solomon, H. M., and Schrogie, J. J.: Change in receptor site affinity: a proposed explanation for the potentiating effect of D-thyroxine on the anticoagulant response to warfarin, Clin. Pharmacol. Ther. 8:797, 1967.

61 Solomon, H. M., and Schrogie, J. J.: The effect of various drugs on the binding of warfarin-^{14}C to human albumin, Biochem. Pharmacol. 16: 1219, 1967.

62 Stowers, J. M., Constable, L. W., and Hunter, R. B.: A clinical and pharmacological comparison of chlorpropamide and other sulfonylureas, Ann. N. Y. Acad. Sci. 74:689, 1959.

63 Vesell, E. S., and Page, J. G.: Genetic control of the induction of an hepatic microsomal drug metabolizing enzyme in man, J. Clin. Invest. 48:2202, 1969.

64 Vigran, I. M.: Dangerous potentiation of meperidine hydrochloride by pargyline hydrochloride, J.A.M.A. 187:953, 1964.

65 Vital Brazil, O., and Corrado, A. P.: The curariform action of streptomycin, J. Pharmacol. Exp. Ther. 120:452, 1957.

Recent reviews

66 Azarnoff, D. L., and Hurwitz, A.: Drug interactions, Pharmacol. Physicians 4(2):1, 1970.

67 Bressler, R.: Combined drug therapy, Amer. J. Med. Sci. 255:89, 1968.

68 Brodie, B. B.: Displacement of one drug by another from carrier or receptor sites, Proc. Roy. Soc. Med. 58:946, 1965.

69 Brodie, B. B.: Physicochemical and biochemical aspects of pharmacology, J.A.M.A. 202: 600, 1967.

70 Burns, J. J., and Conney, A. H.: Enzyme stimulation and inhibition in the metabolism of drugs, Proc. Roy. Soc. Med. 58:955, 1965.

71 Conney, A. H.: Pharmacological implications of microsomal enzyme induction, Pharmacol. Rev. 19:317, 1967.

72 Drug interactions that can affect your patients, Patient Care 4:91, Oct. 31, 1970.

73 Ellenhorn, M. J., and Sternad, F. A.: Problems of drug interactions, J. Amer. Pharm. Ass. 6:62, 1966.

74 Fowler, T. J.: Some incompatibilities of intravenous admixtures, Amer. J. Hosp. Pharm. 24: 450, 1967.

75 Gillette, J. R.: Biochemistry of drug oxidation and reduction by enzymes in hepatic endoplasmic reticulum, Advances Pharmacol. 4:219, 1966.

76 Hansten, P. D.: Drug interactions, Philadelphia, 1973, Lea & Febiger.

77 Hussar, D. A.: Therapeutic incompatibilities: drug interactions, Amer. J. Pharm. **139**:215, 1967.

78 Koch-Weser, J., and Sellers, E. M.: Drug interactions with coumarin anticoagulants, New Eng. J. Med. **285**:487, 547, 1971.

79 Krakoff, I. H.: Clinical pharmacology of drugs which influence uric acid production and excretion, Clin. Pharmacol. Ther. **8**:124, 1967.

80 Mannering, G. J.: Significance of stimulation and inhibition of drug metabolism in pharmacological testing. In Burger, A., editor: Selected pharmacological testing methods, New York, 1968, Marcel Dekker, Inc.

81 Melmon, K. L.: Preventable drug reactions — causes and cures, New Eng. J. Med. **284**:1361, 1971.

82 Morelli, H. F., and Melmon, K. L.: The clinician's approach to drug interactions, Calif. Med. **109**:380, 1968.

83 Remmer, H., Estabrook, R. W., Schenkman, J., and Greim, H.: Reaction of drugs with microsomal liver hydroxylase: its influence on drug action, Naunyn Schmiedeberg Arch. Pharm. Pharm. Exp. Path. **259**:98, 1968.

84 Sellers, E. M., and Koch-Weser, J.: Kinetics and clinical importance of displacement of warfarin from albumin by acidic drugs, Ann. N. Y. Acad. Sci. **179**:213, 1971.

85 Sjöqvist, F.: Psychotropic drugs. II. Interaction between monoamine oxidase (MAO) inhibitors and other substances, Proc. Roy. Soc. Med. **58**:967, 1965.

SECTION THIRTEEN

PRESCRIPTION WRITING AND DRUG COMPENDIA

59

Prescription writing and drug compendia

PRESCRIPTION WRITING

A prescription is a written order given by a physician to a pharmacist. In addition to the name of the patient and that of the physician, the prescription should contain the name or names of the drugs ordered and their quantities, instructions to the pharmacist, and directions to the patient.

The art of prescription writing has been declining in modern medicine as a result of several developments. Most of the preparations are compounded today by pharmaceutical companies, and the pharmacist's role in most cases consists only of dispensing. Also, the practice of writing long, complicated prescriptions containing many active ingredients, adjuvants, correctives, and various vehicles has been abandoned in favor of using single pure compounds. Even when combinations of several active ingredients are desirable, the pharmaceutical companies often have available several forms of suitable combinations. It may be said that this practice deprives the physician of the opportunity to adjust the various components of a mixture to the individual requirements of the patient. The custom of prescribing trademarked mixtures also has other disadvantages. The physician may be so accustomed to prescribing a mixture of drugs by a trade name that he may not be quite certain about the individual components of it, some of which may be unnecessary or undesirable in a given case.

Drugs may be prescribed by their official names, which are *United States Pharmacopeia* (USP) or *National Formulary* (NF); by their nonofficial generic names, which are *New Drugs* (ND), formerly *New and Nonofficial Drugs* (NND), or *United States Adopted Name* (USAN); or by a manufacturer's trade name. The designation USAN has been recently coined for generic or nonproprietary names adopted by the American Medical Association–United States Pharmacopeia Nomenclature Committee in cooperation with the respective manufacturers. Adoption of USAN names does not imply endorsement of the product by the American Medical Association Council on Drugs or by the United States Pharmacopeia.

There is considerable advantage to prescribing drugs by their official or generic names. This often allows the pharmacist to dispense a more economical product than a trademarked preparation of one company. It would also eliminate the expense of each pharmacy's maintaining a multiplicity of very similar preparations, a saving that could ultimately benefit the patient.

On the other hand, the physician may have reasons for prescribing one manufacturer's product. This is often the only way in which he can be certain that the preparation given to the patient will be exactly what he intends to use, not only in its active ingredients but even to the point of its appearance and taste. A child who is accustomed to the flavor of a certain vitamin mixture may refuse to swallow a similar product if its taste is different. Also, there are some childlike adults who pay much attention to the physical properties and taste of products to which they are accustomed.

693

Although it is not generally appreciated by physicians, absorption of a drug from the gastrointestinal tract may vary greatly, depending on the manufacturing process used in the preparation of a tablet or capsule. For example, chloramphenicol capsules made by various manufacturers may produce quite different blood levels. The whole problem of generic equivalence needs to be reexamined.

On the whole, the use of generic names is more common in teaching hospitals than in general practice. There is much discussion at present concerning the relative advantages of prescribing by generic names rather than by trade names. The outcome of this debate should be of great interest in medical economics.

PARTS OF PRESCRIPTION

Traditionally a prescription is written in a certain order and consists of four basic parts:

1. *Superscription*—This is simply ℞, the abbreviation for *recipe*, the imperative of *recipere*, meaning "*take thou.*"

2. *Inscription*—This represents the ingredients and their amounts. If a prescription contains several ingredients in a mixture, it is customary to write them in the following order: (1) basis or principal ingredient, (2) adjuvant, which may contribute to the action of the basis, and (3) corrective, which may eliminate some undesirable property of the active drug or the vehicle, which is the substance used for dilution.

3. *Subscription*—This contains directions for dispensing. Often it consists only of *M.*, the abbreviation for *misce*, meaning "*mix.*"

4. *Signature*—This is often abbreviated as *Sig.* and contains the directions to the patient, such as "Take one teaspoonful three times a day before meals." The signature should indicate whether the medicine is intended for external application and whether it has some special poisonous properties. Whenever possible, instructions of a general nature, such as "take as directed," should be avoided since the patient may misunderstand verbal directions given by the physician.

In addition to the basic parts of a prescription, it should have the patient's name and the physician's signature, followed by the abbreviation M.D.

MODERN TRENDS IN PRESCRIPTION WRITING

The parts of the prescription described in the previous paragraphs represent a tradition that is undergoing considerable change. Latin, even in the form of abbreviations, is not really necessary. Its main purpose in the past was to conceal from the patient the nature (and often worthlessness) of a drug. At the present time, prescriptions are written in English. Even such abbreviations as *M.* or *Sig.* may be avoided. It is also advisable to avoid as much as possible the use of the decimal point and state the number of milligrams in a dose instead of using the decimal fraction of a gram.

There are other interesting trends in prescription writing.[2] Much confusion results from the fact that the name of a drug is not spelled out on the label, and therefore the patient knows only that he is taking some sort of pills having certain physical characteristics. The busy physician wastes much time trying to identify medications given to his patients by other physicians. It may not be an exaggeration to say that drug treatment in some instances may be truly double-blind.

To avoid this unsatisfactory development, some physicians ask the pharmacist to name the drug on the label, indicating their wish by checking an appropriate box on the prescription form. They also indicate in another box the number of allowable refills.

OFFICIAL AND NONOFFICIAL PRESCRIPTIONS

A prescription for a preparation listed in the *United States Pharmacopeia* or the *National Formulary* is called an official prescription. If the physician chooses to prescribe such an official mixture, he avoids the necessity of specifying the individual ingredients. He simply writes the name of the preparation, followed by USP or NF, and adds the signature, or label.

In a nonofficial prescription the physician must spell out not only each ingredient but also the quantity of each. This can be done either by indicating the ingredients of a single dose with instructions on the number of such doses to be dispensed or by describing the total quantities of the various ingredients. In the latter instance the instructions to the pharmacist should state that the total amount is to be divided into so many capsules, or in the case of liquid medicines, that they are simply to be mixed, the dose being indicated on the label.

PRESCRIPTIONS AND THE FEDERAL CONTROLLED SUBSTANCES ACT

Until recently, prescriptions for narcotic drugs were regulated by the Harrison Anti-Narcotic Act and the drug abuse control amendments of 1965. These regulations have been replaced by the Federal Controlled Substances Act of 1970 and the regulations issued by the Director of the Federal Bureau of Narcotics and Dangerous Drugs. The new regulations became effective May 1, 1971. The drugs controlled by the Act are placed in five categories, or schedules:

Schedule I. Hallucinogenic substances and some opiates for which there is no current accepted medical use

Schedule II. Drugs of high abuse potential, such as most narcotics of the former Class A group, amphetamines, some closely related compounds, and some barbiturates

Schedule III. Depressants such as barbiturates, nalorphine, straight paregoric, certain amphetamine combination drugs, and narcotics of the former Class B group

Schedule IV. Chloral hydrate, meprobamate, paraldehyde, and some long-acting barbiturates (Generally, the abuse potential for drugs in this schedule is lower than for the representatives of the previous schedules.)

Schedule V. Paregoric combination preparations and other drugs and other compounds for which the abuse potential is lower than for members of schedule IV

All prescriptions for controlled drugs (schedules II to V) must contain the full name and address of the patient, full name, address, and BNDD (Bureau of Narcotics and Dangerous Drugs) number of the prescribing doctor, signature of the prescribing doctor, and date. Prescriptions for schedule II drugs are not refillable. Schedules III and IV drugs may be refilled up to five times within 6 months of initial issuance if so authorized by the prescribing physician. Prescriptions for schedule V drugs may be refilled as authorized by the prescribing physician.

TYPICAL PRESCRIPTIONS

Two examples of prescriptions are shown on p. 696.

DRUG COMPENDIA

Authoritative information on drugs can be found in the *United States Pharmacopeia* and the *National Formulary* as well as in many textbooks of pharmacology. The *United*

John Doe, M.D.
555 Medical Arts Building
City

Telephone: EM 1-4282

Name   David Smith   Date   May 9, 1970

Address   201 Hall Street   Age   37

℞

Tetracycline USP, 250 mg.
Dispense twenty capsules
Label: Take one capsule four times a day

Reg. No. _____   John Doe, M.D.

John Doe, M.D.
555 Medical Arts Building
City

Telephone: EM 1-4282

Name   David Smith   Date   May 9, 1970

Address   201 Hall Street   Age   37

℞   Gm. or ml.

Ammonium chloride   12
Terpin Hydrate Elixir,
   to make   120
M.
Label: Take one teaspoonful in
       half glass of water for cough
       every 4 hours if necessary

Reg. No. _____   John Doe, M.D.

States Pharmacopeia and the National Formulary are referred to as official publications. The official position of these compendia is based on the Federal Food, Drug and Cosmetic Act of 1938, which states that any drug described in these compendia must conform to the specifications laid down in these publications.

The United States Pharmacopeia was first published in 1820. It and the National Formulary became official in 1906, when they were so designated by the first Food and Drug Act. The United States Pharmacopeia is revised by physicians, pharmacists, and medical scientists who are elected by delegates to the United States Pharmacopeial Convention. The delegates originate from schools of medicine and pharmacy, from medical and pharmaceutical societies, and from some departments of the government.

In order for a drug to be included in the *United States Pharmacopeia* there must be good evidence for its therapeutic usefulness or its pharmaceutic necessity. When a physician prescribes a drug listed in the *United States Pharmacopeia*, he may be certain that he is using a compound of recognized therapeutic benefit and of high standards of purity.

The *National Formulary* is published by the American Pharmaceutical Association. The criteria for inclusion of a drug are based not exclusively on therapeutic value but on extent of use.

AMA Drug Evaluations 1973 is a valuable source of information on most drugs that are available in the United States. It is particularly useful in checking on currently accepted therapeutic practices and available preparations.

If a physician could limit his use of drugs to those that are listed in the *United States Pharmacopeia* or those that have been recommended by *AMA Drug Evaluations 1973*, he would be protected against unfounded claims or the power of advertising. When a new drug represents a great therapeutic advance, the physician may be unable to wait for such authoritative reviews. He must often rely on the written or verbal statements of recognized experts in the field. In any case, he should not depend solely on the advertising literature or drug circulars and package inserts.

References

1 Cutting, W.: A note on names, Clin. Pharmacol. Ther. 5:569, 1963.

2 Friend, D. G.: Principles and practices of prescription writing, Clin. Pharmacol. Ther. 6:411, 1965.

APPENDIX

DRUG BLOOD LEVELS*

The concentration of drugs in the blood is of interest in clinical medicine and in medicolegal situations. The tabular presentation of drug blood levels presented in Table A is intended as a source of information and as a guide to the available literature. It should be recognized that the figures given are often based on a few cases and are subject to change as more information accumulates. Furthermore, the significance of blood levels depends on numerous factors, and the table should be consulted with full recognition of the role of modifying influences.

Importance of drug serum concentrations

The determination of drug serum concentrations is not important when the pharmacologic effects of the drug can be easily monitored. For example, in the use of coumarin anticoagulants or antihypertensive drugs, the effects of the drugs provide a good indication for adequacy of serum levels and dosage. On the other hand, there are drugs that are used prophylactically, such as diphenylhydantoin, quinidine, and others, which provide therapeutic problems in the absence of knowledge of their serum concentrations. The determination of diphenylhydantoin in the serum is useful also for revealing noncompliance with the physician's instructions.

The relationship between serum concentration and its pharmacologic effect is complicated by numerous factors such as (1) tolerance, (2) drug interactions, (3) the underlying disease, (4) protein binding, and (5) active metabolites.

The role of tolerance, drug interactions, and underlying disease in modifying the relationship between serum concentration and drug effect is easily understood. The importance of protein binding and the role of active metabolites are not always appreciated.

The role of protein binding is illustrated by the following problem.

Problem A: The therapeutic concentration of diphenylhydantoin is 20 mg./L. It is about 95% bound to serum albumin. In the case of uremia, hypoalbuminemia, or the presence of other drugs that displace diphenylhydantoin from its binding site, the bound fraction could go down to 90%. What will be the effect on the free drug fraction and the potential toxicity of diphenylhydantoin? If the total diphenylhydantoin concentration in the serum is reported to be 20 mg./L, the free fraction will be 2 mg., which is twice as much as it would be with normal albumin binding and could be toxic.[18]

The complicating effect of active metabolites is demonstrated in the case of propranolol. This drug is metabolized to 4-hydroxy-propranolol, which is an active beta blocker. If one knows the serum concentration of propranolol, he may still not be able

---

*Much of this information has been compiled and kindly provided by Dr. Charles L. Winek, Chief Toxicologist, County of Allegheny, and Professor of Toxicology, Duquesne University.

to state the intensity of beta blockade. Other complicating factors may result from the application of radioimmunoassays. In a few instances the biologic activity — usually of an endogenous compound — and the concentration as measured by radioimmunoassay do not correlate well.

Definition of blood levels

Therapeutic blood level the concentration of drug present in the blood, serum, or plasma after therapeutically effective dosage in man. The values in the table are generally those reported with oral administration of the drug.

Toxic blood level the concentration of drug in the blood, its serum or plasma associated with serious toxic symptoms in man.

Lethal blood level the concentration of drug in blood, serum, or plasma that has been reported to cause death or is so far above reported therapeutic or toxic concentrations that it might cause death in man.

• • •

Table A gives the therapeutic, toxic, and lethal blood levels of a large number of drugs. In addition, Table B presents serum concentrations of some cardiac drugs.

Table A. Drug blood levels*

Drug	Therapeutic	Toxic	Lethal
Acetaminophen (Tylenol)	1-2 mg.% [10, 23]	—	—
Acetohexamide (Dymelor)	2.1-5.6 mg.% [21]	—	—
Amitriptyline (Elavil)	—	40 μg%	1.0-2.0 mg.% [16]
Aminophylline	2-10 mg.% [14]	—	—
Amphetamine		—	0.2 mg.% [3]
Barbiturates			
Short-acting	0.1 mg.%	0.7 mg.%	1 mg.%
Intermediate-acting	0.1-0.5 mg.%	1-3 mg.%	3 mg.%
Phenobarbital	Ca. 1.0 mg.%	4-6 mg.%	8-15 mg.%
Barbital	Ca. 1.0 mg.%	6-8 mg.%	10 mg.%
Bromide	5.0 mg.%	50 mg.%	200 mg.%
Carbon monoxide	—	15-35%	50%
Chloral hydrate	1.0 mg.%	10 mg.%	25 mg.%
Chlordiazepoxide (Librium)	0.1-0.2 mg.% [19]	0.55 mg.%	2 mg.%
Chlorpheniramine	—	2-3 mg.%	—
Chlorpromazine (Thorazine)	0.05 mg.%	0.1-0.2 mg.%	0.3-1.2 mg.% [8, 12]
Chlorpropamide (Diabinese)	3.0-14.0 mg.% [21]	—	—
Desipramine (Norpramin)	0.059-0.14 mg.% [25]	—	0.3 mg % [24]
Dextropropoxyphene (Darvon)†	2.5-20.0 μg%	—	5.7 mg.% [4]
Diazepam (Valium)	0.05-0.25 mg.% [19]	0.5-2.0 mg %	2.0 mg.%
Diphenylhydantoin (Dilantin)	0.6-1.7 mg.%	2-5 mg.%	10 mg.%
Ethanol	—	0.15%	0.35%
Ethchlorvynol (Placidyl)	Ca. 0.5 mg.%	2 mg.%	15 mg.%
Ethyl ether	90-100 mg.% [17]	—	140-180 mg.% [17]
Glutethimide (Doriden)	0.02 mg.%	1-8 mg.%	3-10 mg.%
Imipramine (Tofranil)	0.2-0.6 mg.%	—	—

*Modified from Winek, C. L.: Clin. Toxicol. 3:541, 1970.
†Liver levels are about 20 times higher than blood levels.
— = Not established.

Continued.

Table A. Drug blood levels — cont'd

Drug	Therapeutic	Toxic	Lethal
Iron	50 mg.% (RBC)	0.6 mg.% (serum)	—
Meperidine (Demerol)	60-65 μg%[9]	0.5 mg.%	Ca. 3 mg.%
Meprobamate	1 mg.%	10 mg.%	20 mg.%
Methamphetamine	—	—	4 mg.%[16]
Methapyrilene	—	3-5 mg.%	—
Methaqualone	0.5 mg.%	1-3 mg.%	3 mg.%
Methyprylone (Noludar)	1.0 mg.%[19]	3-6 mg.%	10 mg.%
Morphine	—	—	0.005 mg.%[4] (free morphine)
Nicotine	—	1 mg.%[4]	0.5-5.2 mg.%[3]
Nitrofurantoin (Furadantin)	0.18 mg.%[15]	—	—
Oxazepam (Serax)	0.1-0.2 mg.%[11]	—	—
Paraldehyde	Ca. 5.0 mg.%	20-40 mg.%	50 mg.%
Pentazocine (Talwin)	0.014-0.016 mg.%[2]	—	—
Phenylbutazone (Butazolidin)	Ca. 10 mg.%[6]	—	—
Probenecid (Benemid)	10-20 mg.%[7]	—	—
Quinidine	0.3-0.6 mg.%	—	—
Quinine	—	—	1.2 mg.%[4]
Salicylate (acetylsalicylic acid)	2-10 mg.%	15-30 mg.%	50 mg.%
Sulfadimethoxine (Madribon)	8-10 mg.%[19]	—	—
Sulfisoxazole (Gantrisin)	9-10 mg.%[19]	—	—
Thioridazine (Mellaril)	—	0.1 mg.%[6]	—
Tolbutamide (Orinase)	5.3-9.6 mg.%[21]	—	—
Trimethobenzamide (Tigan)	0.1-0.2 mg.%[19]	—	—

Table B. Serum concentrations of some cardiac drugs*

Drug	Therapeutic range mg./L.	Toxic range mg./L.
Digoxin	1-2†	Variable†
Digitoxin	20†	Variable†
Quinidine	4	8
Diphenylhydantoin	10-20	25
Procainamide	6	10
Lidocaine	2	6

*Based on data from Koch-Weser, J., and Klein, S. W.: J.A.M.A. **215**:1454, 1971; Beller, G. A., Smith, T. W., Abelmann, W. H., Haber, E., and Hood, W. B.: New Eng. J. Med. **284**:989, 1971; and Shand, D. G., Nuckolls, E. M., and Oates, J. A.: Clin. Pharmacol. Ther. **11**:112, 1970.

†The therapeutic and toxic effects of digoxin and digitoxin are greatly influenced by the level of serum potassium, hypercalcemia, hypomagnesemia, catecholamines, and acid-base disturbances.

References

1 Beller, G. A., Smith, T. W., Abelmann, W. H., Haber, E., and Hood, W. B.: Digitalis intoxication: a prospective clinical study with serum level correlations, New Eng. J. Med. **284**:989, 1971.

2 Berkowitz, B. A., Asling, J. H., Shnider, S. M., and Way, E. L.: Relationship of pentazocine plasma levels to pharmacological activity in man, Clin. Pharmacol. Ther. **10**:320, 1969.

3 Clarke, E. G. C.: Isolation and identification of drugs in pharmaceuticals, body fluids, and postmortem material, London, 1969, The Pharmaceutical Press.

4 Collom, W. D.: Personal communication, 1969.

5 Cravey, R. H., and Baselt, R. C.: Methamphetamine poisoning, J. Forensic Sci. Soc. 8:110, 1968.

6 Curry, A.: Poison detection in human organs, ed. 2, Springfield, Ill., 1969, Charles C Thomas, Publisher.

7 Dayton, P. G., Yu, T. F., Chen, W., Berger, L., West, L. A., and Gutman, A. B.: The physiological disposition of probenecid, including renal clearance, in man, studied by an improved method for its estimation in biological material, J. Pharmacol. Exp. Ther. 140:278, 1963.

8 Fatteh, A. J.: Therapeutic serum concentrations of meperidine (Demerol), Forensic Med. 11:120, 1964.

9 Fochtman, F. W., and Winek, C. L.: J. Forensic Sci. 14:213, 1969.

10 Gwilt, J. R., Robertson, A., and McChesney, E. W.: Determination of blood and other tissue concentrations of paracetamol in dog and man, J. Pharm. Pharmacol. 15:440, 1963.

11 Hausner, E. P., Shafer, C. L., Corson, M., Johnson, O., Trujillo, T., and Langham, W.: Clinical evaluation of dicumarinyl derivatives with metabolic study of radioactively labeled anticoagulants in animals, Circulation 3:171, 1951.

12 Hollister, L. E., and Kosek, J. C.: Sudden death during treatment with phenothiazine derivatives, J. A. M. A. 192:1035, 1965.

13 Koch-Weser, J., and Klein, S. W.: Procainamide dosage schedules, plasma concentrations and clinical effects, J. A. M. A. 215:1454, 1971.

14 Lillehei, J. P.: Aminophylline: oral vs. rectal administration, J. A. M. A. 205:530, 1968.

15 Loughridge, L. W.: Peripheral neuropathy due to nitrofurantoin, Lancet 2:1133, 1962.

16 McBay, A.: Personal communication, 1967.

17 Ohio Chemical: Historical and clinical data on the inhalation anesthetic agents, Madison, Wis., 1966.

18 Reidenberg, M. M.: Protein binding of diphenylhydantoin and desmethylimipramine in plasma from patients with poor renal function, New Eng. J. Med. 285:264, 1971.

19 Roche Laboratories: Product reference manual, Nutley, New Jersey.

20 Shand, D. G., Nuckolls, E. M., and Oates, J. A.: Propranolol plasma levels in adults, Clin. Pharmacol. Ther. 11:112, 1970.

21 Sheldon, J., Anderson, J., and Stoner, L.: Serum concentration and urinary excretion of oral sulfonylurea compounds: relation to diabetic control, Diabetes 14:362, 1965.

22 Thomson, P. D., Rowland, M., and Melmon, K. L.: Influence of heart failure, liver disease, and renal failure on the disposition of lidocaine in man, Amer. Heart J. 82:417, 1971.

23 Weikel, J. H.: J. Amer. Pharm. Ass. 47:477, 1958.

24 Wilson, W. J.: 1966 (through ref. 16).

25 Yates, C. M., Todrick, A., and Tait, A. C.: Aspects of the clinical chemistry of desmethylimiprimine in man, J. Pharm. Pharmacol. 15:432, 1963.

Recent review

26 Koch-Weser, J.: Serum drug concentrations as therapeutic guides, New Eng. J. Med. 287:227, 1972.

COMPARISON OF SELECTED EFFECTS OF COMMONLY ABUSED DRUGS

Some selected effects of commonly abused drugs are summarized in Table C. This table is intended for quick reference only. Greater detail on the subject is available in Chapter 25 dealing with contemporary drug abuse.

Table C. Comparison of selected effects of commonly abused drugs*

Drug category	Physical dependence	Characteristics of intoxication
Opiates (see p. 284 for classification)	Marked	Analgesia with or without depressed sensorium; pinpoint pupils (tolerance does not develop to this action); patient may be alert and appear normal; respiratory depression with overdose
Barbiturates	Marked	Patient may appear normal with his usual dose, but narrow margin between dose needed to prevent withdrawal symptoms and toxic dose is often exceeded and patient appears "drunk," with drowsiness, ataxia, slurred speech, and nystagmus on lateral gaze; pupil size and reaction normal; respiratory depression with overdose
Nonbarbiturate sedatives Glutethimide (Doriden)	Marked	Pupils dilated and reactive to light; coma and respiratory depression prolonged; sudden apnea and laryngeal spasm common
Antianxiety agents† ("minor tranquilizers")	Marked	Progressive depression of sensorium as with barbiturates; pupil size and reaction normal; respiratory depression with overdose
Ethanol	Marked	Depressed sensorium, acute or chronic brain syndrome, odor on breath, pupil size and reaction normal
Amphetamines	Mild to absent	Agitation, with paranoid thought disturbance in high doses; acute organic brain syndrome after prolonged use; pupils dilated and reactive; tachycardia, elevated blood pressure, with possibility of hypertensive crisis and CVA; possibility of convulsive seizures

*Modified from Dimijian, G. G.: Drug Ther. **1:**7, 1971.
†Meprobamate (Equanil), chlordiazepoxide (Librium), diazepam (Valium), ethchlorvynol (Placidyl), and ethinamate (Valmid).

Characteristics of withdrawal	"Flashback" symptoms	Masking of symptoms of illness or injury during intoxication
Rhinorrhea, lacrimation, and dilated, reactive pupils, followed by gastrointestinal disturbances, low back pain, and waves of gooseflesh; convulsions not a feature unless heroin samples were adulterated with barbiturates	Not reported	An important feature of opiate intoxication, due to analgesic action, with or without depressed sensorium
Agitation, tremulousness, insomnia, gastrointestinal disturbances, hyperpyrexia, blepharoclonus (clonic blink reflex), acute brain syndrome, major convulsive seizures	Not reported	Only in presence of depressed sensorium or after onset of acute brain syndrome
Similar to barbiturate withdrawal syndrome, with agitation, gastrointestinal disturbances, hyperpyrexia, and major convulsive seizures	Not reported	Same as in barbiturate intoxication
Similar to barbiturate withdrawal syndrome, with danger of major convulsive seizures	Not reported	Same as in barbiturate intoxication
Similar to barbiturate withdrawal syndrome, but with less likelihood of convulsive seizures	Not reported	Same as in barbiturate intoxication
Lethargy, somnolence, dysphoria, and possibility of suicidal depression; brain syndrome may persist for many weeks	Infrequently reported	Drug-induced euphoria or acute brain syndrome may interfere with awareness of symptoms of illness or may remove incentive to report symptoms of illness

Continued.

Table C. Comparison of selected effects of commonly abused drugs—cont'd

Drug category	Physical dependence	Characteristics of intoxication
Cocaine	Absent	Paranoid thought disturbance in high doses, with dangerous delusions of persecution and omnipotence; tachycardia; respiratory depression with overdose
Marihuana	Absent	Milder preparations: drowsy, euphoric state with frequent inappropriate laughter and disturbance in perception of time or space (occasional acute psychotic reaction reported); stronger preparations such as hashish: frequent hallucinations or psychotic reaction; pupils normal, conjunctivae injected (marihuana preparations frequently adulterated with LSD, tryptamines, or heroin)
Psychotomimetics (LSD, STP, tryptamines, mescaline, morning glory seeds)	Absent	Unpredictable disturbance in ego function, manifest by extreme lability of affect and chaotic disruption of thought, with danger of uncontrolled behavioral disturbance; pupils dilated and reactive to light
Anticholinergic agents	Absent	Nonpsychotropic effects such as tachycardia, decreased salivary secretion, urinary retention, and dilated, nonreactive pupils plus depressed sensorium, confusion, disorientation, hallucinations, and delusional thinking
Inhalants*	Unknown	Depressed sensorium, hallucinations, acute brain syndrome; odor on breath; patient often with glassy-eyed appearance

*The term "inhalant" is used to designate a variety of gases and highly volatile organic liquids, including the sprayed into the nasopharynx (droplet transport required) and substances that must be ignited prior to inhalation

Characteristics of withdrawal	"Flashback" symptoms	Masking of symptoms of illness or injury during intoxication
Similar to amphetamine withdrawal	Not reported	Same as in amphetamine intoxication
No specific withdrawal symptoms	Infrequently reported	Uncommon with milder preparations; stronger preparations may interfere in same manner as psychotomimetic agents
No specific withdrawal symptoms; symptomatology may persist for indefinite period after discontinuation of drug	Commonly reported as late as 1 year after last dose	Affective response or psychotic thought disturbance may remove awareness of, or incentive to report, symptoms of illness
No specific withdrawal symptoms; mydriasis may persist for several days	Not reported	Pain may not be reported as a result of depression of sensorium, acute brain syndrome, or acute psychotic reaction
No specific withdrawal symptoms	Infrequently reported	Same as in anticholinergic intoxication

aromatic glues, paint thinners, gasoline, some anesthetic agents, and amyl nitrite. The term excludes liquids (such as marihuana).

INDEX

A

Index

Index

Durabolin; *see* Nandrolone phenpropionate
Dydrogesterone, characteristics and preparations, 520
Dynapen; *see* Dicloxacillin
Dyphylline as bronchodilator, 451
Dyrenium; *see* Triamterene
Dysleptic drugs, abuse of, 314-318

E

Echothiophate, structural formula, 83
Ecolid; *see* Chlorisondamine
Edathamil calcium disodium in acute iron poisoning, 534
Edecrin; *see* Ethacrynic acid
Edrophonium chloride
  diagnostic uses, 88
  in myasthenia gravis, 82-83
  structural formula, 82
Effector mechanisms and mediators in immune injury, 659-660
Effectors, response of, to chemical mediators, 64-65
Efficacy
  drug, quantitative aspects of, 8, 9
  of general anesthetics, 351
Effusions, malignant, 653
Egg white as poison antidote, 669
5,8,11,14-Eicosatetraenoic acid, structural formula, 216
8,11,14-Eicosatrienoic acid, structural formula, 215
Elavil; *see* Amitriptyline hydrochloride
Electrocardiogram
  effects of digitalis on, 380
  effects of quinidine on, 394, 395
  effects of varying calcium levels on, graph, 503
  effects of varying serum potassium levels on, 433
Electrolyte balance, alterations of, in drug interactions, 683
Electrolytes and water
  metabolism of, effects of cortisol on, 481-482
  renal handling of, effect of mercurial diuretics on, 427
Electron transport of NADPH to cytochrome P_{450}, 28
Electrophysiologic basis of antiarrhythmic action, 391-393
Eledoisin, 214
Elipten; *see* Aminoglutethimide
Elixophyllin; *see* Theophyllin elixir
Elkosin; *see* Sulfisomidine
Elorine; *see* Tricyclamol
Emetic effect of morphine, 287
Emetics in treatment of poisoning, 668
Emetine
  for intestinal amebiasis, 622
  for sheep liver fluke, 630
Emivan; *see* Ethamivan
Emodin
  compounds of, as cathartics, 458-459
  structural formula, 458
End plate potential, 142
  effect of curarine on, graph, 142
Endocrine and metabolic functions, drugs influencing, 463-551

Endrate; *see* Disodium edetate
Entamoeba histolytica, phases in life cycle of, 621
Enterobiasis, drugs of choice for, 627
Enzyme induction of drugs, 33-35
Enzymes
  drug action on, 7-8
  drug-metabolizing, stimulation of, by drugs and foreign compounds, 33-34
  microsomal, in drug metabolism, 28-29
Eosinophils, effect of epinephrine on, 97-98
Ephedrine
  abuse of, 312
  for asthma, 450
  history, effects, and structural formula, 108-109
Epilepsy
  drugs for, 276-282; *see also* Antiepileptic drugs
  general concept, 276
Epinephrine, 91-107; *see also* Catecholamines
  for asthma, 450
  bronchodilator action, 96-97, 105
  cardiac uses, 105
  cardiovascular effects, 94-96
  effect of
    adrenergic blocking agents on, 151
    on blood pressure and heart rate in man, graphs, 95
    on carbohydrate metabolism, 98-99
    dichloroisoproterenol and phentolamine on blood pressure responses to, tracings, 150
    on eosinophils, 97-98
    on glands, 97
    on renal hemodynamics, 96
  function of, 92
  metabolic actions, 98-99
  metabolism of, 100-102
  neural actions, 97
  occurrence and physiologic functions, 91-92
  pharmacologic actions, 93-99
  preparations and dosage, 107
  reversal of, concept of, 149, 150, 151
  reversal of, by phentolamine, chart, 149
  small dose of, in man, cardiovascular effects, 94
  smooth muscle effects, 97
  structural formula, 91
  therapeutic applications, 104-105
  use of, in local anesthesia, 367
  vasoconstrictor uses, 104
β-H^3-Epinephrine, fate of, in man, table, 101
Epinephrine suspension, preparations and dosage, 107
Epsilon-aminocaproic acid in anticoagulant therapy, 420
Equanil; *see* Meprobamate
Ergocalciferol; *see* Vitamin D_2
Ergonavine
  obstetric use, 210
  structural formula, 208
  use, adverse effects, and preparations, 210
Ergot alkaloids, 208-211
  as alpha adrenergic blocking agents, 153
  chemistry, 209
  pharmacologic effects, 209
  pharmacology of, historical aspects, 208

Index

Index

Index

Index

Index

Resistance of bacteria to chemotherapeutic agents, 557-558
Resistopen; *see* Oxacillin
Resorcinol, 617
Respiration
    depression of, in barbiturate poisoning, 253
    effect of morphine on, 286-287
Respiratory system
    drug effects on, 447-454
    effects of
        barbiturates on, 251
        bronchodilators on, 448-451
        expectorants on, 451
        general anesthetics on, 352
        marihuana on, 307, 308
        mucolytic drugs on, 451
        salicylates on, 331
    paralysis of, due to drug interactions, 683
Rheumatic diseases, drugs for, 337
Rheumatic fever, salicylates for, 330
Rheumatoid arthritis, effectiveness of cortisone and corticotropin in, 477-478
Riboflavin, deficiency, occurrence, and structural formula, 544
Rickets, characteristics of, 547
Rifampin in tuberculosis, 609, 613
Rimifon; *see* Isoniazid
Riopan; *see* Magaldrate
Ritalin; *see* Methylphenidate
Robaxin; *see* Methocarbamol
Robinul; *see* Glycopyrrolate
Rolitetracycline, administration, 592
Romilar; *see* Dextromethorphan
Rondomycin; *see* Methacycline

S

Safety and effectiveness of drugs, 41-52
Safety of general anesthetics, 351
Salbutamol as bronchodilator, 449, 450
Salicylamide
    as aspirin substitute, 333
    structural formula, 328
Salicylates, 328-333
    analgesic effect, 329
    antipyretic effect, 329-330
    antirheumatic and anti-inflammatory effects, 330
    and cortisone, comparison of action, 330
    gastrointestinal effects, 331
    inhibition of action of bradykinin, 329
    metabolic effects, 331-332
    metabolism of, 332
    pharmacologic effects, 329
    and platelet aggregation, 331
    poisoning from, 332-333
        essential features of, 672
    preparations, 333
    respiratory effects, 331
    uricosuric action, 330-331
Salicylic acid
    effects of, 328
    as fungistatic agent, 619
    structural formula, 611

Salt excretion, antihypertensive drugs promoting, 178-179
Saluron; *see* Hydroflumethiazide
Salyrgan; *see* Mersalyl
Sanitizer, definition, 616
Sansert; *see* Methysergide maleate
Sarcolysin; *see* Melphalan
Schistosomiasis, drugs for, 629-630, 633-635
Schizonticides
    blood, 638
    primary tissue, 636, 638
Scopolamine; *see also* Atropine and scopolamine
    intoxication due to, 671-672
    in parkinsonism, 124, 125, 131
Scurvy, characteristics, 545
Secretions, effect of histamine on, 191-192
Sedative-hypnotic effects of antihistaminic drugs, 260
Sedative-hypnotics
    alcohols, 255-256
    bromides, 259
    carbamates, 257
    chloral hydrate and related drugs, 257-258
    cyclic ether, 258-259
    miscellaneous, 259-260
    nonbarbiturate, 245-251, 255-260
        classification, 255
    piperidinediones, 256-257
Sedatives
    anticholinergic, 233
    antihistaminic, 232-233
    definition, 245
    nonbarbiturate, abuse of, 310-311, 702-703
Selective action of drugs, 556
Selectivity of drugs, 9
Semicarbazide, convulsant action, 271
Semilente insulin, 471
Sensitization to chemical mediators by drugs, 64-65
Septrin; *see* Co-trimoxazole
Serax; *see* Oxazepam
Serentil; *see* Mesoridazine
Seromycin; *see* Cycloserine
Serotonin, 71-72, 204-207
    antagonists of, 207-211
    biosynthesis of, 71, 205
    in brains of rabbits, effect of iproniazid on, table, 236
    depletion of, reserpine in, 175
    occurrence and distribution, 204
    pharmacologic effects, 205-206
    in psychopharmacology, 72
    psychotomimetic effects of, 206
    roles of, in health and disease, 206-207
    structural formula, 205
Serpasil; *see* Reserpine
Serum, concentrations of drugs in, importance of, 698-699
Serum sickness
    as delayed allergy, 47
    due to penicillin, 581-582
Sex hormones, anterior pituitary gonadotropins and, 510-525